Designing Resistance Training Programs

FOURTH EDITION

Steven J. Fleck, PhD
University of Wisconsin–Parkside

William J. Kraemer, PhD
University of Connecticut

Human Kinetics

Library of Congress Cataloging-in-Publication Data

Fleck, Steven J., 1951- author.
  Designing resistance training programs / Steven J. Fleck, William J. Kraemer. -- Fourth edition.
      p. ; cm.
  Includes bibliographical references and index.
  I. Kraemer, William J., 1953- author. II. Title.
  [DNLM: 1. Resistance Training. 2. Weight Lifting. QT 260.5.W4]
  GV505
  613.7'1--dc23
                                        2013031094
  ISBN-10: 0-7360-8170-4 (print)
  ISBN-13: 978-0-7360-8170-2 (print)

The web addresses cited in this text were current as of August 2013, unless otherwise noted.

Acquisitions Editor: Roger W. Earle; **Developmental Editor:** Christine M. Drews; **Assistant Editors:** Amy Akin, Amanda S. Ewing, Anne E. Mrozek and Melissa J. Zavala; **Copyeditor:** Patsy Fortney; **Proofreader:** Red Inc.; **Indexer:** Susan Danzi Hernandez; **Permissions Manager:** Dalene Reeder; **Graphic Designer:** Nancy Rasmus; **Graphic Artist:** Dawn Sills; **Cover Designer:** Keith Blomberg; **Photograph (cover):** Neil Bernstein; **Photographs (interior):** © Human Kinetics, unless otherwise noted; **Photo Asset Manager:** Laura Fitch; **Photo Production Manager:** Jason Allen; **Art Manager:** Kelly Hendren; **Associate Art Manager:** Alan L. Wilborn; **Illustrations:** © Human Kinetics, unless otherwise noted; **Printer:** Courier Companies, Inc.

Printed in the United States of America   10 9 8 7 6 5 4 3 2 1

The paper in this book was manufactured using responsible forestry methods.

Human Kinetics
Website: www.HumanKinetics.com

United States: Human Kinetics
P.O. Box 5076
Champaign, IL 61825-5076
800-747-4457
e-mail: humank@hkusa.com

Canada: Human Kinetics
475 Devonshire Road Unit 100
Windsor, ON N8Y 2L5
800-465-7301 (in Canada only)
e-mail: info@hkcanada.com

Europe: Human Kinetics
107 Bradford Road
Stanningley
Leeds LS28 6AT, United Kingdom
+44 (0) 113 255 5665
e-mail: hk@hkeurope.com

Australia: Human Kinetics
57A Price Avenue
Lower Mitcham, South Australia 5062
08 8372 0999
e-mail: info@hkaustralia.com

New Zealand: Human Kinetics
P.O. Box 80
Torrens Park, South Australia 5062
0800 222 062
e-mail: info@hknewzealand.com

E4758

Steve Fleck: To my brother, Glenn; nephew, Brian; and niece, Jessica, all of whom left us too soon. Their passing has taught me the importance of enjoying each day and that making a contribution in life needs to be done every day.

William Kraemer: To my wife, Joan, and to my children, Daniel Louis, Anna Mae, and Maria Rae—your love is the foundation of my life.

CONTENTS

PREFACE

We welcome you to our fourth edition of *Designing Resistance Training Programs*, which over the years has been a solid resource in the field of exercise and sport science. This textbook has been used by a wide variety of readers seriously interested in resistance training, including undergraduate students in resistance training theory courses, strength coaches, and personal trainers, in addition to sport scientists wanting to further their understanding of the scientific basis of resistance training. Because the concept of individualization is so important in designing a resistance training program, this text has also been highly individualized for many needs and settings. Ultimately, it provides the tools for understanding and designing resistance training programs for almost any situation or need. It also offers a comprehensive background in resistance training program design from both scientific and practical perspectives. We hope you will gain an understanding of the dynamic nature of the program design process and will pick up on the many subtleties involved in bringing the science of resistance training into practice.

What Is New in the Fourth Edition?

All chapters of this fourth edition have been updated given that research in the field of resistance training has moved forward quickly as exercise and sport scientists from all parts of the world have advanced knowledge in this field. This new edition combines the knowledge from the past with the dramatic amount of new information that has come to light over the past several years. Thus, readers of our previous editions will find important updates to fill in the blanks of the past and further their understanding of the growing field of resistance training and program design.

In the early 1980s we were both struck with the importance of understanding how to design a resistance training program. We sought to develop a scientifically based theoretical paradigm to help people understand how to design training programs. This resulted in identifying the acute program variables to address when developing a training session and the need to manipulate these variables over time so that the desired chronic training adaptations occur. This paradigm provided the theoretical framework for both practical applications and the scientific study of resistance training. Our own work with athletes and in the laboratory has benefited from this more quantitative approach to resistance training, and we have been overwhelmed through the years at its acceptance and use by a multitude of practitioners and scientists.

This edition explores both the acute program variables and their chronic manipulation using the most recent information available. Because we both understand that the process of program design is related to the art of using science, previous editions attempted to use the science of resistance training to understand and further develop resistance training program design. This fourth edition continues in this vein and adds recent information. Over the years students, instructors, strength coaches, personal trainers, and even those just interested in what they are doing in the weight room have found this book to be a valuable reference as well as a good read. We believe this edition will not disappoint.

We have added two types of sidebars:

- Practical Question boxes look at questions resistance training professionals and coaches are likely to ask and apply the latest research to answer those questions.
- Research boxes explain research findings and apply those findings to resistance training and program design.

Since our last edition, the number of scientific studies concerning some aspect of resistance training has grown almost exponentially. Thus,

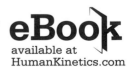
eBook
available at
HumanKinetics.com

this textbook can no longer be a comprehensive source for such a dramatic amount of new data. Rather, we have used this large database to continue to mature and develop the concepts we put forth in our previous editions. The field is clearly moving forward at what might be called warp speed, with the interest in resistance training as great as ever and growing worldwide. This textbook will give you information and tools to help you evaluate resistance training programs and better understand the context and efficacy of the information you receive from the Internet, magazines, television, radio, videos, and infomercials concerning resistance training. More than ever we need a paradigm for understanding the information now available in this growing field.

Organization

We have added information and reorganized all of the chapters of this book. Chapter 1 concerns the basic principles of resistance training and exercise prescription. This chapter lays the foundation for all subsequent chapters. For example, one of the hallmarks of resistance training is the concept of training specificity, which affects everything from the cellular-level events in the muscle to the performance of athletic skills. Chapter 2 provides a detailed examination of the types of strength training from isometrics to eccentrics and makes unique comparisons among types of resistance training to help you understand how muscle action type influences adaptations and performance changes.

It is vital that you have an understanding of basic physiology and the adaptations to resistance training to be able to use new information in the future and put into context expected training outcomes from resistance training. You need to understand what causes strength gains in the first weeks of training and after months or years of training, as well as what you can expect in terms of muscle hypertrophy in the first six weeks of a program. A fundamental understanding of basic physiology will help you distinguish fact from fiction when assessing the physical changes that occur with resistance training. Chapter 3 provides this comprehensive and important view of resistance training from a physiological perspective. This chapter is one of the few in the literature to present such a perspective and offers a new look at some basic concepts in physiological science.

This chapter also provides students studying kinesiology, exercise and sport sciences, and physical education a chance to integrate what they have learned from their courses in anatomy, physiology, and exercise physiology into an understanding of the acute response to and chronic adaptations that result from resistance training.

Because resistance training is only one component of a total conditioning program, we believe it is very important to show you how resistance training programs interact with other conditioning components such as aerobic training, interval training, and flexibility training. Chapter 4 offers an overview of important conditioning components and explains how they interact with, and whether they are compatible with, resistance training.

Chapter 5 presents the design of a single workout session. Proper design of each session is important because individual sessions are the building blocks of long-term training programs. This chapter addresses the acute program variables in detail as we continue using a specific paradigm to help you understand what you are asking someone to do in the weight room and why. The discussion starts with a needs analysis to help you develop a sound rationale for using the acute program variables and set reasonable training goals.

Chapter 6 presents an overview from a scientific perspective of some of the many popular resistance training systems so you can understand them in terms of the acute program variables presented in chapter 5. In chapter 6 you get to apply what you learned about program variables in chapter 5 to a variety of training systems. The skill of evaluating programs based on an analysis of the acute variable used will help you assess the value of the many new programs and systems to which you are exposed each year. This process allows you to predict the potential physiological stress of, and extrapolate realistic training adaptations for, programs that may not have been studied scientifically.

Chapter 7 explores advanced training strategies and explains how to manipulate training variables as the trainee progresses in a long-term resistance training program. Principles such as periodization are important to this process. Work from laboratories around the world, including our own, has shown that without variation in training, adaptations and gains can plateau well before the person's potential has been reached. We also cover the popular topic of plyometrics and power-type training, which are important components of many training strategies used today.

Rest is crucial at some points in any resistance training program. It can, however, result in detraining or loss of training adaptations and performance gains, especially when training is stopped or significantly reduced. How does this affect the average person, fitness enthusiast, or athlete? What about training in-season? How long can one go without working out or with reduced training before losing fitness gains? These are some of the questions addressed in chapter 8 to help you plan rest into long-term training without experiencing a significant loss of fitness or performance gains.

In the final three chapters we take a careful look at resistance training exercise prescription in several populations. Chapter 9 addresses women and resistance training. Although women undertaking resistance training are similar to men in many respects, some sex differences do exist. The exercise prescription process must take these factors into account to bring about optimal gains. This theme continues in chapter 10, which addresses resistance training in children and adolescents. The benefits of resistance training are clearly established for children of all ages, but this unique population requires careful consideration to create programs that are safe and effective. Given the epidemic of obesity and inactivity in children today, resistance training is a fun way to attract more children to an active lifestyle. This chapter helps create the proper mind-set for working with young children and adolescents to ensure that they are not viewed as little adults, which can result in ineffective or unsafe programs.

We end the book by addressing those at the other end of the age continuum, older adults. This area of study is important because people are living longer and it is clear that even the very old can safely perform and receive benefits from resistance training, in terms of both health and performance. This population requires particular program design considerations to achieve optimal health and performance gains. For example, joint compression and pain are problems that must be addressed with this group to ensure the successful use of and adherence to resistance training programs.

Designing Resistance Training Programs is a literature-based book that can be a cornerstone in your understanding of this topic. We understand that the ideas, philosophies, and approaches to resistance training change by the day; ultimately, science-based knowledge creates the stability needed for designing effective resistance training programs for any population from children to elite athletes. We have provided extensive literature citations and selected readings to give you a context of what is being explored and a historical feel for the field. This book will be an important component in your preparation for designing resistance training programs. We wish you good reading and good training!

Instructor Resources

Designing Resistance Training Programs, Fourth Edition, comes with a full array of instructor ancillaries, including an instructor guide, presentation package, image bank, and test package.

- The instructor guide includes a sample course syllabus, sample lecture outlines, suggestions for class projects and student assignments, and ideas for presenting important key concepts.

- The presentation package features hundreds of full-color PowerPoint slides that highlight the most important concepts and selected text, figures, and tables from the book.

- The image bank includes almost all of the figures, content photos, and tables from the text, sorted by chapter. Images can be used to develop a customized presentation based on specific course requirements. A blank PowerPoint template is provided so instructors can quickly insert images from the image bank to create their own presentations.

- The test package includes a bank of 110 questions. The test package is available for download in three different formats: Rich Text Format (.rtf) for use with word processing software such as Microsoft Word, Respondus, and LMS format.

All of the ancillaries are accessible at www.HumanKinetics.com/DesigningResistanceTrainingPrograms.

ACKNOWLEDGMENTS

I would like to acknowledge the many friends, colleagues, coaches, and athletes who have shared their knowledge and experiences with me concerning resistance training. Their collective knowledge and experience helped shape the belief that designing resistance training programs requires a mix of science and experience. I would also like to acknowledge my wife, Maelu; mother, Elda; father, Marv; and my brothers and sisters, who have always seemed to understand the space I needed to pursue my professional career.

Steve Fleck

The study of resistance training has been a career-long passion for me. I have been blessed to have had both secondary and college coaching experiences that helped to shape the context for the implementation of science into resistance training program designs. I have been fortunate to have been a coach and then a scientist to see the transformation of the field in bridging the gap between the laboratory and the field practices. In reality, to individually acknowledge everyone in my career who has had a very important influence that has shaped me as a person, former coach, and then as a scientist would be too unwieldy to give proper credit and fair acknowledgement. So, to my friends and scientific collaborators, your support, help, and insights have made it possible to succeed in this field. To the multitude of graduate students at three universities and especially to my current and former doctoral students, the Kraemer Laboratory family, you have given me extraordinary satisfaction and pride. Finally, to my friend, Steve Fleck, my former college football teammate, it has been a great ride with this book and our work together and having had the opportunity to see the acceptance of resistance training realized in our field and in the world today. To our readers, enjoy this book, and God bless you all.

William J. Kraemer

Basic Principles of Resistance Training and Exercise Prescription

---

After studying this chapter, you should be able to

1. define basic terms commonly used in the design of resistance training programs,
2. demonstrate the three types of muscle actions,
3. explain the use of voluntary muscle actions and their role in bringing about optimal gains in strength or muscle hypertrophy,
4. discuss principles of program design, including intensity, training volume, rest periods, specificity, periodization, and progressive overload, and
5. discuss the importance of safety, including proper spotting, breathing, technique, range of motion, and equipment.

Resistance training, also known as strength or weight training, has become one of the most popular forms of exercise for enhancing physical fitness as well as for conditioning athletes. The terms *strength training, weight training,* and *resistance training* have all been used to describe a type of exercise that requires the body's musculature to move (or attempt to move) against an opposing force, usually presented by some type of equipment. The terms *resistance training* and *strength training* encompass a wide range of training modalities, including body weight exercises, the use of elastic bands, plyometrics, and hill running. The term *weight training* typically refers only to resistance training using free weights or some type of weight training machine.

The increasing number of health club, high school, and college resistance training facilities attests to the popularity of this form of physical conditioning. Those who participate in resistance training programs expect them to produce certain health and fitness benefits, such as increased strength, increased fat-free mass, decreased body fat, and improved physical performance in either a sporting activity or daily life activities. Other health benefits, such as changes in resting blood pressure, blood lipid profile, and insulin sensitivity, can also occur. A well-designed and consistently performed resistance training program can produce all of these benefits while emphasizing one or several of them.

The fitness enthusiast, recreational weight trainer, and athlete all expect gains in strength or muscle size (muscle hypertrophy) from a resistance training program. Many types of resistance training modalities (e.g., isokinetic, variable resistance, isometric, plyometric) can be used to accomplish these goals. In addition, a variety of training systems or programs (i.e., combinations of sets, repetitions, and resistances) can produce significant increases in strength or muscle hypertrophy as long as an effective training stimulus is presented to the neuromuscular system. The effectiveness of a specific type of resistance training system or program depends on its efficacy and proper use in the total exercise prescription or program. Fitness gains will continue as long as the training stimulus remains effective, which requires increasing the difficulty (i.e., progressive overload) in some manner and using periodized programs.

Most athletes and fitness enthusiasts expect the gains in strength and power produced by a resistance training program to result in improved sport or daily life activity performance. Resistance training can improve motor performance (e.g., the ability to sprint, throw an object, or climb stairs), which can lead to better performance in various games, sports, and daily life activities. The amount of carryover from a resistance training program to a specific physical task depends on the specificity of the program. For example, multijoint exercises, such as clean pulls from the knees, have greater carryover to vertical jump ability than isolated single-joint exercises, such as knee extensions and leg curls. Both multijoint and single-joint exercises increase the strength of the quadriceps and hamstring muscle groups. However, the greater similarity of biomechanical movement and muscle fiber recruitment patterns between a multijoint exercise and most sporting or daily life activities results in greater specificity and carryover. In general, multijoint exercises have a greater specificity and carryover to motor performance tasks than single-joint exercises do.

Body composition change is also a goal of many fitness enthusiasts and athletes engaged in resistance training programs. Normally, the changes desired are a decrease in the amount of body fat and an increase in fat-free mass. However, some people also desire a gain or loss in total body weight. Body composition changes are associated with not only increases in physical performance, but also health benefits. Fitness enthusiasts, and to a lesser extent athletes, may also be interested in the health benefits of weight training, such as adaptations that reduce the risk for disease. For example, decreased resting blood pressure is associated with a decreased risk for cardiovascular disease. The success of any program in bringing about a specific adaptation depends on the effectiveness of the training stimulus produced by that program. All of the preceding changes can be achieved by a properly designed and performed resistance training program.

Resistance training can produce the changes in body composition, strength, power, muscle hypertrophy, and motor performance that many people desire, as well as other health benefits. To achieve optimal changes in these areas, people must adhere to some basic principles that apply regardless of the resistance modality or the type of system or program.

Different people desire different changes from a resistance training program. Bodybuilders mostly desire increased fat-free mass and decreased percent body fat. Other athletes may desire improved power or motor performance, and fitness enthusiasts often desire the aforementioned changes as well as health benefits such as decreased blood pressure and positive changes to the blood lipid profile.

Basic Definitions

Before discussing the principles of resistance training, we will define some basic terms commonly used in describing resistance training programs and principles. Having multiple meanings for the same term leads to misunderstanding. This is why terminology is so important when communicating with others interested in strength and conditioning.

- When a weight is being lifted, the major muscles involved are shortening, or performing a **concentric muscle action** (see figure 1.1a). During a concentric muscle action, force is developed and shortening of the muscle occurs; therefore, the word *contraction* is also appropriate for this type of muscle action.

- When a weight is being lowered in a controlled manner, the major muscles involved are developing force and lengthening in a controlled manner; this is termed an **eccentric muscle action** (see figure 1.1b). Muscles can only shorten or lengthen in a controlled manner; they cannot push against the bones to which they are attached. In most exercises, gravity pulls the weight back to the starting position. To control the weight as it returns to the starting position, the muscles must lengthen in a controlled manner; otherwise, the weight will fall abruptly.

- When a muscle is activated and develops force, but no visible movement at the joint occurs, an **isometric muscle action** takes place (see figure 1.1c). This can occur when a weight is held sta-

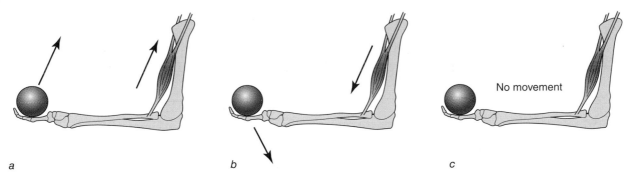

FIGURE 1.1 Major types of muscle actions. *(a)* During a concentric muscle action, the muscle shortens. *(b)* During an eccentric muscle action, the muscle lengthens in a controlled manner. *(c)* During an isometric muscle action, no movement of the joint occurs, and no shortening or lengthening of the total muscle takes place.

tionary or when a weight is too heavy to lift any farther. Maximal isometric action force is greater than maximal concentric force at any velocity of movement, but less than maximal eccentric force at any movement velocity.

- A **repetition** is one complete motion of an exercise. It normally consists of two phases: the concentric muscle action, or lifting of the resistance, and the eccentric muscle action, or lowering of the resistance. However, in some exercises a complete repetition may involve several movements and thus several muscle actions. For example, a complete repetition of the power clean requires concentric muscle actions to accelerate the weight so it can be caught at a shoulder-height position, eccentric muscle actions as the knees and hips flex to drop underneath the weight, and then concentric actions to assume a full standing position.

- A **set** is a group of repetitions performed continuously without stopping or resting. Although a set can consist of any number of repetitions, sets typically range from 1 to 15 repetitions.

- A **repetition maximum,** or **RM,** is the maximal number of repetitions per set that can be performed in succession with proper lifting technique using a given resistance. Thus, a set at a certain RM implies that the set is performed to momentary voluntary fatigue usually in the concentric phase of a repetition. The heaviest resistance that can be used for one complete repetition of an exercise is called 1RM. A lighter resistance that allows completion of 10, but not 11, repetitions with proper exercise technique is called 10RM.

- A **repetition training zone** is a range of typically three repetitions (e.g., 3-5, 8-10). When performing the repetitions in a repetition training zone, the resistance used can allow the person to perform the desired number of repetitions with relative ease or can result in momentary voluntary failure. If the resistance used results in momentary voluntary failure, the repetition training zone is termed an **RM training zone.** However, using an RM training zone does not necessarily result in a set to failure. For example, using an 8- to 10RM training zone for 8 repetitions is not training to failure; performing 10 repetitions may bring the person close to failure.

- **Power** is the rate of performing work (see box 1.1). During a repetition, power is defined as the weight lifted multiplied by the vertical distance the weight is lifted divided by the time to complete the repetition. Power can be increased by lifting the same weight the same vertical distance in a shorter period of time. Power can also be increased by lifting a heavier resistance the same vertical distance in the same period of time as a lighter resistance. Normally, factors such as arm and leg length limit the ability to increase power by moving a weight a greater distance. Thus, the only ways to increase power are to increase movement speed or lift a heavier resistance with the same or greater movement speed than one would use with a lighter resistance.

- **Maximal strength** is the maximal amount of force a muscle or muscle group can generate in a specified movement pattern at a specified velocity (Knuttgen and Kraemer 1987). In an exercise such as the bench press, 1RM is a measure of strength at a relatively slow speed. The classic strength–velocity curve indicates that as the concentric velocity increases, maximal strength decreases (see chapter 3). On the other hand, as eccentric

? BOX 1.1 PRACTICAL QUESTION

What Is the Difference Between Work and Power?

Work is defined as force multiplied by the distance a weight or resistance is moved. Power is the rate of doing work, or work divided by time. Work can be increased by increasing the distance a weight is moved or increasing the weight or resistance being moved. Power can be increased the same way work is increased, or by decreasing the time in which a certain amount of work is performed. If the time to perform a certain amount of work is decreased by half, power doubles. Work and power can be calculated for a resistance training exercise and are normally calculated for the concentric phase of a repetition. If 100 kg (220 lb) is lifted 0.9 m vertically in two seconds during a bench press, the work performed is 90 kg $\cdot$ m^{-1} (100 kg $\times$ 0.9 m) or 882.9 joules (1 kg $\cdot$ m^{-1} = 9.81 joules). The average power during the concentric phase is 45 kg $\cdot$ m$^{-1}\cdot$ sec^{-1} (100 kg $\times$ 0.9 m / 2 sec) or 441.5 watts (1 watt = 1 joule $\cdot$ s^{-1}). During weight training exercises high-speed video recording or some other means is needed for accurately determining the time and distance a weight is moved to accurately determine work and power. In some exercises, such as the bench press as in this example, ignoring the mass of the body parts moved results in little error in calculating work and power. But in other exercises, such as a squat, in which the mass of the body parts moved is high, not including the mass of the body parts moved does result in a significant amount of error when calculating work and power.

velocity increases, maximal strength increases and then plateaus.

Maximal Voluntary Muscle Actions

Maximal voluntary muscle actions, or performing sets to failure, appears to be an effective way to increase muscular strength (see the discussion of dynamic constant external resistance training in chapter 2). This does not mean that the maximal resistance possible for one complete repetition (1RM) must be lifted. Performing **maximal voluntary muscle actions** means that the muscle generates as much force as its present fatigue level will allow. The force a partially fatigued muscle can generate during a maximal voluntary muscle action is not as great as that of a nonfatigued muscle. The last repetition in a set to momentary concentric failure is thus a maximal voluntary muscle action, even though the force produced is not the absolute maximum because the muscle is partially fatigued.

Many resistance training systems use momentary concentric failure, or RM resistance, to ensure the performance of maximal voluntary muscle actions. This does result in increases in strength, power, or local muscular endurance (see chapter 2). As a result of daily variation in strength due to a variety of factors (e.g., fatigue from other types of training, a poor night's sleep), many programs use repetition training zones or RM training zones to prescribe training resistances for a set.

A training zone encompasses a small number of repetitions, such as a 4-6 zone or an 8-10 zone, and does not necessarily result in momentary concentric failure. An RM training zone also encompasses a small range of repetitions, but does result in momentary concentric failure. One rationale to use training zones instead of RM training zones is that always carrying sets to failure may result in less than optimal increases in power (see chapter 6). Training zones and RM training zones allow for day-to-day variations in strength, whereas prescribing a true repetition maximum, such as 6RM, requires that the lifter perform exactly six repetitions. The lifter can be instructed to perform a minimum of six repetitions or more if possible, or as close to six repetitions as possible. Prescribing the number of repetitions per set in this manner results in prescribing an RM training zone or sets to momentary voluntary fatigue.

Maximal increases in strength can occur without maximal voluntary muscle actions or sets carried to failure in all training sessions or even no training sessions. This is true for seniors (Hunter et al. 2001) as well as healthy adults (Izquierdo et al. 2006). In seniors equivalent strength and fat-free mass gains occur when performing maximal voluntary muscle actions during all three training sessions per week and during only one of three training sessions per week. In healthy adults, not performing sets to failure resulted in equivalent maximal strength gains as well as greater power gains after a peaking training phase compared to carrying sets to failure (see chapter 6). Thus, performing sets to voluntary fatigue is not a prerequisite for strength gains. However, how far from failure (the number of repetitions prior to being unable to continue) a set can be terminated and still result in optimal maximal strength gains is not known. So generally, it is recommended that sets be carried at least close to failure at some point in a training program.

In some exercises, performance of maximal voluntary muscle actions does not necessarily mean that the last repetition in a set is not completed. For example, when some muscle fibers become fatigued during power cleans, the velocity of the bar decreases and the weight is not pulled as high as it could be during the first repetition of a set even though the trainee is exerting maximal effort. Because the trainee developed maximal force in a partially fatigued state, by definition this is a maximal voluntary muscle action.

Some resistance training machines have been specifically designed to force the muscle to perform maximal voluntary muscle actions either through a greater range of motion or for more repetitions in a set. Developments in equipment such as variable resistance, variable variable resistance, and isokinetic equipment (see chapter 2) attest to a belief in the necessity for close to maximal voluntary muscle actions in training. All competitive Olympic weightlifters, powerlifters, and bodybuilders use maximal voluntary muscle actions at some point in their training programs. They recognize the need for such actions at some point in the training process to bring about optimal gains in strength or muscle hypertrophy. However, strength gains and hypertrophy can clearly occur without carrying sets to absolute failure.

Intensity

The **intensity** of a resistance training exercise is estimated as a percentage of the 1RM or any RM resistance for the exercise. The minimal intensity that can be used to perform a set to momentary voluntary fatigue in young, healthy people to result in increased strength is 60 to 65% of 1RM (McDonagh and Davies 1984; Rhea et al. 2003). However, progression with resistances in the 50 to 60% of 1RM range may be effective and may result in greater 1RM increases than the use of heavier resistances in some populations (e.g., in children and senior women; see chapters 10 and 11). Additionally, approximately 80% of 1RM results in optimal maximal strength gains in weight-trained people (Rhea et al. 2003). Performing a large number of repetitions with a very light resistance will result in no or minimal strength gain. However, the maximal number of repetitions per set of an exercise that will result in increased strength varies from exercise to exercise and from muscle group to muscle group. For example, the maximal number of repetitions possible at 60% of 1RM by trained men in the leg press is 45.5 and for the arm curl is 21.3 (see table 1.1).

In addition, training level may also affect the number of repetitions performed in a weight machine exercise; trained men and women typically perform more repetitions at a given percentage of 1RM than untrained men and women do (Hoeger et al. 1990). *Trained* was defined very heterogeneously as having two months to four years of training experience. Thus, it appears that when using a percentage of 1RM resistance, the

TABLE 1.1 Number of Repetitions to Concentric Failure at Various Percentages of an Exercise

Hoeger et al. 1990	Leg press 60% of 1RM	Leg press 80% of 1RM	Bench press 60% of 1RM	Bench press 80% of 1RM	Arm curl 60% of 1RM	Arm curl 80% of 1RM
Untrained	33.9	15.2	19.7	9.8	15.3	7.6
Trained	45.5	19.4	22.6	12.2	21.3	11.4
Shimano et al. 2006	**Squat 60% of 1RM**	**Squat 80% of 1RM**	**Bench press 60% of 1RM**	**Bench press 80% of 1RM**	**Arm curl 60% of 1RM**	**Arm curl 80% of 1RM**
Untrained	35.9	11.8	21.6	9.1	17.2	8.9
Trained	29.9	12.3	21.7	9.2	19.0	9.1

The average number of repetitions possible at percentages of 1RM in machine exercises and free weight barbell exercises.

number of repetitions possible is higher with larger muscle groups and in trained people when using weight machines. However, not all studies confirm that the number of repetitions possible at a percentage of 1RM increases with training; the percentage of 1RM used for a 10RM in machine exercises was generally unchanged in previously untrained women after 14 weeks of training (Fleck, Mattie, and Martensen 2006).

When trained men perform barbell free weight exercises, more repetitions per set are also possible with large-muscle-group exercises (squat and bench press) than with small-muscle-group exercises (arm curl). However, cross-sectional data indicate that trained men may perform fewer repetitions at given percentages than untrained men in the squat but not in other exercises (table 1.1). Also, 12 weeks of weight training of American football players did not increase the number of repetitions possible at 60, 70, 80 and 90% of 1RM in the bench press (Brechue and Mayhew 2009), but did increase the number of repetitions possible at 70% of 1RM in the squat (Brechue and Mathew 2012). On average, similar free weight and machine exercises, such as barbell and machine arm curls, produce similar results in the number of repetitions possible at a specific percentage of 1RM except for the squat, in which typically fewer repetitions than the leg press were performed by trained and untrained men, probable due to less low back use in the leg press.

Thus, RMs or RM training zones vary from exercise to exercise, between men and women, between similar machine and free weight exercises and possibly with training status. It is also important to note that a great deal of individual variation exists in the number of repetitions possible at a percentage of 1RM in all exercises (as shown by the large standard deviations in the aforementioned studies). These factors need to be considered when the percentage of 1RM or RM training zones are used to prescribe training intensity and volume.

Lower intensities, with resistance moved at a fast velocity, are used when training for power (see chapter 7). This is in large part because, in many exercises, lower intensities (light resistance) allow faster velocities of movement and result in higher power output than other combinations of intensity and velocity of movement. This is true for both multijoint and single-joint exercises (Komi 1979), but typically, multijoint exercises are used when training for power.

Unlike the intensity of endurance exercise, the intensity of resistance training is not estimated by heart rate during the exercise. Heart rate during resistance exercise does not consistently vary with the exercise intensity (see figure 1.2). Heart rate attained during sets to momentary voluntary fatigue at 50 to 80% of 1RM can be higher than heart rate attained during sets with 1RM or sets performed to momentary voluntary fatigue at higher percentages of 1RM (Fleck and Dean 1987). Heart rate during training is different with various types of weight training programs (Deminice et al. 2011). Maximal heart rate attained during a training session using three sets of 10RM and 90-second rest periods between sets and exercises, and performing all the arm exercises followed by all the leg exercises, results in a mean heart rate of 117 beats per minute (60% of maximal heart rate). Performing the same exercises for the same number of sets with the same resistance with an alternating arm–leg exercise order with little rest between exercises results in a mean heart rate of 126 beats per minute (65% of maximal heart rate). In both training sessions the same intensity, number of sets, and repetitions were performed. The difference in heart rate was due to the use of exercise order and rest period lengths and not to differences in training intensity or volume, which is the next concept discussed. Recovering between sets and exercises to a specific heart rate, however,

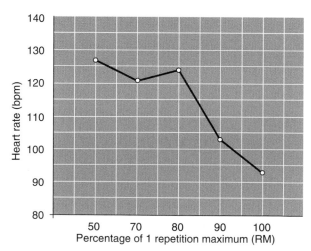

FIGURE 1.2 Maximal heart rate of a moderately trained group of males during knee extension sets to momentary voluntary fatigue at various percentages of 1RM. The heart rate does not reflect the intensity (% of 1RM) of the exercise.

Based on Fleck and Dean 1987.

has been used to determine the rest period length between sets and exercises (Piirainen et al. 2011).

Training Volume

Training volume is a measure of the total amount of work (in joules) performed in a training session, a week of training, a month of training, or some other period of time. Training frequency (number of training sessions per week, month, or year), training session duration, number of sets, number of repetitions per set, and number of exercises performed per training session all have a direct impact on training volume. The simplest method to estimate volume is to add the number of repetitions performed in a specific time period, such as a week or a month of training. Volume can also be estimated by the total amount of weight lifted. For example, if 100 lb (45 kg) are used to perform 10 repetitions, the volume of training is 1,000 lb (450 kg) (10 repetitions multiplied by 100 lb, or 45 kg).

Training volume is more precisely determined by calculating the work performed. Total work in a repetition is the resistance multiplied by the vertical distance the weight is lifted. Thus, if 100 lb (45 kg or 445 N) is lifted vertically 3 ft (0.9 m) in a repetition, the volume or total work is 100 lb multiplied by 3 ft or 300 ft · lb (445 N × 0.9 m = 400 J). Training volume for a set of 10 repetitions in this example is 300 ft · lb (400 J) per repetition

multiplied by 10 repetitions, which equals 3,000 ft · lb (4,000 J). The calculation of training volume is useful in determining the total training stress.

A relationship exists between higher training volumes and training outcomes, such as muscle hypertrophy, decreased body fat, increased fat-free mass, and even motor performance. Larger training volumes may also result in a slower loss of strength gains after cessation of training (Hather, Tesch et al. 1992). Thus, training volume is a consideration when designing a resistance training program (see box 1.2).

Rest Periods

Rest periods between sets of an exercise, between exercises, and between training sessions allow recovery and are important for the success of any program. The rest periods allowed between sets and between exercises during a training session are in large part determined by the goals of the training program. Rest period length affects recovery and blood lactate, a measure of acidity, as well as the hormonal responses to a training session (see chapter 3). The rest periods between sets and exercises, the resistance used, and the number of repetitions performed per set all affect the design and goals of the program (see chapter 5). In general, if the goal is to emphasize the ability to exhibit maximal strength, relatively long rest periods (several minutes), heavy resistances, and

 BOX 1.2 **RESEARCH**

Training Volume Affects Strength Gains

Strength gains are affected by total training volume. Several meta-analyses have concluded that training programs that use multiple sets of an exercise result in greater increases in strength than single-set programs do (Peterson et al. 2004; Rhea et al. 2003; Wolfe, LeMura, and Cole 2004). But increasing the number of sets performed is only one way of increasing training volume. Training volume is also affected by other training variables, such as training frequency. Performing nine exercises during six weeks of training for either three days per week with two sets of 10 repetitions (10RM) or two days per week with three sets of 10 repetitions (10RM) results in the same total training volume (six sets of 10 repetitions of each exercise per week). The only difference between the programs is training frequency. No significant difference in 1RM bench press or back squat was shown between training programs. The authors concluded that total training volume is more important than other training variables, such as training frequency and number of sets, to bring about maximal strength gains (Candow and Burke 2007).

Candow, D.G., and Burke, D.G. 2007. Effect of short-term equal-volume resistance training with different workout frequency on muscle mass and strength in untrained men and women. *Journal of Strength and Conditioning Research* 21: 204-207.

one to six repetitions per set are suggested. When the goal is to emphasize the ability to perform high-intensity exercise for short periods of time, rest periods between sets should be less than one minute. Repetitions and resistance can range from 10 to 25 repetitions per set, depending on the type of high-intensity ability the person wishes to enhance. If enhancement of long-term endurance (aerobic power) is the goal, then circuit-type resistance training with short rest periods (less than 30 seconds), relatively light resistances, and 10 to 15 repetitions per set is one training prescription.

Shorter rest period lengths do result in an overall shorter training session. If the same session is performed with one-minute rest periods rather than two-minute rest periods between sets and exercises, the session is completed in about half the time. This may be important for trainees with limited time in which to train. However, other training variables, such as the number of repetitions per set, may be affected (see box 1.3). Trainees must also make sure that exercise technique is not compromised by short rest periods; greater fatigue levels can result in improper technique, which may increase the potential for injury.

Many fitness enthusiasts and some athletes allow one day of recovery between resistance training sessions for a particular muscle group. This

BOX 1.3 RESEARCH

Shorter Rest Periods Significantly Affect Training Volume

Short rest periods between sets and exercises offer the advantage of completing a training session in less time. Fatigue as the training session progresses decreases training volume as indicated by a decrease in number of repetitions possible with a specific intensity. Figure 1.3 presents the number of repetitions possible at 8RM as a training session progresses. Three-minute rest periods allow significantly more repetitions per set than one-minute rest periods. The number of repetitions possible in a set decreases substantially in successive sets of an exercise and particularly when two exercises involving the same muscle groups are performed in succession. Rest periods as well as exercise order affect training volume by affecting the number of repetitions performed per set.

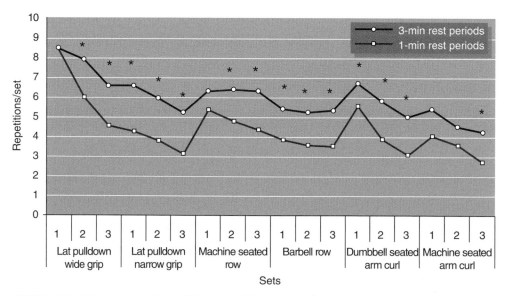

FIGURE 1.3 The number of repetitions possible in a training session with one- and three-minute rest periods between sets and exercises.

* = significant difference in repetitions with one- and three-minute rest periods in the same set.

Adapted, by permission, from R. Miranda, S.J. Fleck, et al., 2007, "Effect of two different rest period lengths on the number of repetitions performed during resistance training," *Journal of Strength and Conditioning Research* 21:1032-1036.

is a good general rule, although some evidence indicates that other patterns of training sessions and recovery periods are equally or even more beneficial (see the discussion of rest periods between workouts in chapter 5 and the discussion of two training sessions per day in chapter 7). A practical indication of the need for more rest between training sessions is residual muscular soreness. When muscular soreness interferes with performance in the following training session, the rest between training sessions was probably insufficient.

Velocity Specificity

Many coaches and athletes maintain that some resistance training should be performed at the velocity required during the actual sporting event. For many sporting events this means a high velocity of movement. **Velocity specificity** is the concept that resistance training produces its greatest strength and power gains at the velocity at which the training is performed (see chapter 7 for a discussion of movement speed and power development). However, if the training goal is to increase strength at all velocities of movement and only one training velocity is to be used, an intermediate velocity is the best choice. Thus, for someone interested in general strength, an intermediate training velocity is generally recommended. However, training at a fast velocity against light resistance and training at a slower velocity against heavy resistance both demonstrate velocity-specific strength gains. Thus, velocity-specific training to maximize strength and power gains at velocities needed during competition is appropriate for athletes at some point in their total training programs. If strength and power need to be maximized across velocities ranging from slow to very fast, training at several velocities of movement should be performed.

Muscle Action Specificity

If a person trains isometrically and progress is evaluated with a static muscle action, a large increase in strength may be apparent. However, if progress is evaluated using concentric or eccentric muscle actions, little or no increase in strength may be demonstrated. This is termed muscle action specificity or testing specificity. **Muscle action specificity** indicates that gains in strength are in part specific to the type of muscle action used in training (e.g., isometric, variable resistance, isokinetic). **Testing specificity** is a similar term referring to the fact that strength increases are higher when tested using an exercise or muscle action performed during training and less when tested using an exercise or muscle action involving the same muscle groups, but not performed during training. Testing specificity is also apparent when testing and training are performed using the same exercise but different types of equipment, such as training with a machine bench press and testing with a free weight bench press.

The specificity of strength gains is caused by neural adaptations resulting in the ability to recruit the muscles in the most efficient way to perform a particular type of muscle action or exercise (see the discussion of nervous system adaptations in chapter 3). Generally, fitness gains are evaluated with an exercise performed during training, and the training program for a specific sport or activity should include the types of muscle actions encountered in that sport or activity. For example, isometric muscle actions are frequently performed while wrestling, so it is beneficial to incorporate some isometric training into the resistance training program of wrestlers.

Muscle Group Specificity

Muscle group specificity simply means that each muscle group requiring strength gains or other adaptations to the training program must be trained. In other words, the muscle tissue in which adaptations are desired must be activated or recruited by the exercises performed during training (see chapter 3). If an increase in strength is desired in the flexors (biceps group) and extensors (triceps) of the elbow, exercises for both muscle groups need to be included in the training program. Exercises in a training program must be specifically chosen for each muscle group in which a training adaptation such as increased strength, power, endurance, or hypertrophy is desired.

Energy Source Specificity

Energy source specificity refers to the concept that physical training may bring about adaptations of the metabolic systems predominantly used to supply the energy needed by muscles to perform a given physical activity. There are two anaerobic sources and one aerobic source of energy for muscle actions. The anaerobic sources of energy supply the majority of energy for high-power, short-duration events such as sprinting 100 m, whereas the aerobic energy source supplies the majority of energy for longer-duration, lower-power events, such as running 5,000 m. If an increase in the ability of a muscle to perform anaerobic exercise is desired, the bouts of exercise should be of short duration and high intensity. To increase aerobic capability, training bouts should be of longer duration and lower intensity. Resistance training is most commonly used to bring about adaptations of the anaerobic energy sources; however, resistance training can cause increases in aerobic capability as indicated by increases in maximal oxygen consumption (see chapter 3). The number of sets and repetitions, the length of rest periods between sets and exercises, and other training variables need to be appropriate for the energy source in which training adaptations are desired (see chapter 5).

Periodization

Periodization, planned variation in the training volume and intensity, is extremely important for continued optimal gains in strength, as well as other training outcomes (see chapter 7). Additionally, changes in other training variables, such as exercise choice (e.g., performing more power-oriented exercises at some point in the training program) and rest period length between sets and

exercises can also be made on a regular basis in a periodized fashion.

Variations in the position of the feet, hands, and other body parts that do not affect the safety of the lifter affect muscle fiber recruitment patterns and can also be used as training variations. The use of several exercises to vary the conditioning stimulus of a particular muscle group is also a valuable way to change muscle fiber recruitment patterns to produce continued increases in strength and muscle fiber hypertrophy (see the discussion of motor unit activation in chapter 3). Periodization is needed for achieving optimal gains in strength and power as training progresses (American College of Sports Medicine 2009; Rhea and Alderman 2004). Considering the factors that can be manipulated, there are an infinite number of possibilities for periodization of resistance training; however, in terms of research, training volume and intensity are the most commonly manipulated variables (see box 1.4).

Progressive Overload

Progressive overload is the practice of continually increasing the stress placed on the body as force, power, or endurance capabilities increase as a result of training. **Progressive resistance** is a similar term that applies specifically to resistance training; the stress of resistance training is gradually increased as fitness gains are achieved with training. The term was developed by physician Capt. Thomas

 BOX 1.4 PRACTICAL QUESTION

Can the Same Training Volume and Intensity Be Used to Create Two Different Periodization Plans?

Training volume and intensity are the most commonly manipulated training variables in research examining the effects of periodized resistance training. These variables are also commonly changed by strength and conditioning professionals when creating programs for athletes or clients. The same average intensity and volume can be used to create very different programs. If three training zones of 12- to 15RM, 8- to 10RM, and 4- to 6RM are used each for one month of training in succession (linear periodization; see chapter 7) with three training days per week, a total of 12 training sessions are performed with each RM training zone. If the same RM training zones are performed one day per week for three months of training (nonlinear periodization), there are also 12 training sessions performed with each of the three training zones. Although the arrangement of training volume and intensity is quite different in these two programs, the total training volume and intensity are equivalent.

Delorme after World War II when he demonstrated in a series of studies that resistance training was an effective medical treatment for rehabilitating wounded soldiers from war-related injuries. Not knowing what to call this form of resistance training in which he carefully increased the resistance used over time, his wife during a dinner conversation on the topic said, "Why don't you call it progressive resistance training," and so the term was created (oral communication with Dr. Terry Todd, University of Texas at Austin). For example, at the start of a training program the 5RM for arm curls might be 50 lb (23 kg), which is a sufficient stimulus to produce an increase in strength. As the program progresses, five repetitions with 50 lb (23 kg) would not be a sufficient stimulus to produce further gains in strength because the trainee can now easily perform five repetitions with this weight. If the training stimulus is not increased in some way at this point, no further gains in strength will occur.

Several methods are used to progressively overload muscles (American College of Sports Medicine 2009). The most common is to increase the resistance to perform a certain number of repetitions. The use of RMs or RM training zones automatically provides progressive overload because as a muscle's strength increases, the resistance necessary for performing an RM or staying within an RM training zone increases. For example, a 5RM or a 4- to 6RM training zone may increase from 50 lb (23 kg) to 60 lb (27 kg) after several weeks of training. However, as discussed earlier, performing sets to failure is not needed to cause increased strength. As long as the resistance used is gradually increased, progressive overload is occurring.

Other methods to progressively overload the muscle include increasing the total training volume by increasing the number of repetitions, sets, or exercises performed per training session; increasing the repetition speed with submaximal resistances; changing the rest period length between exercises (i.e., shortening the rest period length for local muscular endurance training); and changing the training frequency (e.g., performing multiple training sessions per day for a short period of time). To provide sufficient time for adaptations and to avoid overtraining, progressive overload of any kind should be gradually introduced into the training program; sufficient time is needed for the trainee to become accustomed to the training and make physiological adaptations to it.

Safety Aspects

Successful resistance training programs have one feature in common—safety. Resistance training has some inherent risk, as do all physical activities. The chance of injury can be greatly reduced or completely removed by using correct lifting techniques, spotting, and proper breathing; by maintaining equipment in good working condition; and by wearing appropriate clothing.

The chance of being injured while performing resistance training is very slight. Among college American football players (Zemper 1990) the weight room injury rate was very low (0.35 per 100 players per season). Weight room injuries accounted for only 0.74% of the total reported time-lost injuries during the football season. This injury rate may be reduced to even lower levels through more rigorous attention to proper procedures in the weight room (Zemper 1990), such as proper exercise technique and the use of collars with free weight bars. Injury rates in a supervised health and fitness facility that included resistance training as part of the total training program were also very low (0.048 per 1,000 participant-hours) (Morrey and Hensrud 1999). A review of the U.S. Consumer Product Safety Commission National Electronic Injury Surveillance System indicates that 42% of resistance training injuries occur at home (Lombardi and Troxel 1999), and 29 and 16% of resistance training injuries occur at sport facilities and schools, respectively. Muscle sprains and strains during weight training are common injuries in children as well as adults, but increase in frequency with age from 8-13 years to 23-30 years of age (Meyer et al. 2009). Accidental injury is highest in children and decreases with increasing age.

These results indicate that lack of supervision contributes to injury. Exercise techniques involving the shoulder complex also need special attention because 36% of documented resistance training injuries involve the shoulder complex (Kolber et al. 2010). The injury rate even in competitive male and female powerlifters is low compared to that in other sports. The rate of injury in powerlifters was only 0.3 injuries per lifter per year (1,000 hours of training = 1 injury) (Siewe et al. 2011). The rate of injury in the powerlifters increased with age, and women had more injuries than men. Interestingly, the use of weight belts actually increased the rate of lumbar spine injuries most likely due to an overestimation of the degree of protection to the low back weight belts provide when lifting maximal loads. So, although resistance training is a very safe activity, all proper safety precautions should be taken, and supervision should always be present.

Spotting

Proper spotting is necessary for ensuring the safety of the participants in a resistance training program. **Spotting** refers to the activities of people other than the lifter that help ensure the safety of the lifter. Spotters serve three major functions: to assist the trainee with the completion of a repetition if needed, to critique the trainee's exercise technique, and to summon help if an accident does occur. Briefly, the following factors should be considered when spotting:

- Spotters must be strong enough to assist the trainee if needed.

- During the performance of certain exercises (e.g., back squats), more than one spotter may be necessary to ensure the safety of the lifter.

- Spotters should know proper spotting technique and the proper exercise technique for each lift for which they are spotting.

- Spotters should know how many repetitions the trainee is going to attempt.

- Spotters should be attentive at all times to the lifter and to his or her exercise technique.

- Spotters should summon help if an accident or injury occurs.

Following these simple guidelines will aid in the avoidance of weight room injuries. A detailed description of spotting techniques for all exercises is beyond the scope of this text, but spotting techniques for a wide variety of resistance training exercises have been presented elsewhere (Fleck 1998; Kraemer and Fleck 2005).

Breathing

A **Valsalva maneuver** is holding one's breath while attempting to exhale with a closed glottis. This maneuver is not recommended during resistance training exercises because blood pressure rises substantially (see the discussion of acute cardiovascular responses in chapter 3). Figure 1.4 depicts the intra-arterial blood pressure response to maximal

isometric muscle actions during one-legged knee extensions. The blood pressure response during an isometric muscle action in which breathing was allowed is lower than the response observed during either an isometric action performed simultaneously with a Valsalva maneuver or during a Valsalva maneuver in the absence of an isometric muscle action. This demonstrates that the elevation of blood pressure during resistance training is lower when the person breathes during the muscle action compared to when a Valsalva maneuver is performed during the muscle action. Elevated blood pressure increases the afterload on the heart; this requires the left ventricle to develop more pressure to eject blood, which makes the work of the left ventricle more difficult.

Exhaling during the lifting of the resistance and inhaling during the lowering of the resistance are normally recommended, although little difference in the heart rate and blood pressure response during resistance training is observed between that and inhaling during lifting and exhaling during lowering (Linsenbardt, Thomas, and Madsen 1992). During an exercise using 1RM or during the

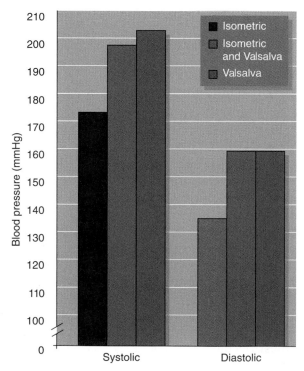

FIGURE 1.4 Systolic and diastolic blood pressure during an isometric action only, simultaneous isometric action and Valsalva maneuver, and Valsalva maneuver only.

$N = 6$.

Unpublished data of authors.

last few repetitions of a set performed to momentary voluntary fatigue, the Valsalva maneuver will occur. However, excessive breath holding should be discouraged.

Proper Exercise Technique

Proper technique for resistance training exercises is partially determined by anatomy and the specific muscle groups being trained. Altering the form of an exercise causes other muscle groups to assist in the movement. This decreases the training stimulus on the muscles normally associated with a particular exercise. Proper technique is altered in several advanced resistance training techniques (e.g., the forced repetition technique), but these techniques are not recommended for beginning resistance trainees (see chapter 6).

Proper technique is also necessary for preventing injury, especially in exercises in which improper technique exposes the low back to additional stress (e.g., squat, deadlift) or in which the resistance can be "bounced" off a body part (e.g., free weight bench press). Improper form often occurs when the lifter performs an exercise with resistances that exceeds his or her present strength capabilities for a certain number of repetitions. If exercise technique deteriorates, the set should be terminated. Proper exercise technique for a large variety of exercises has been described elsewhere (Fleck 1998; Kraemer and Fleck 2005).

Full Range of Motion

Full range of motion refers to performing an exercise with the greatest possible range of movement. Exercises are normally performed with the full range of motion allowed by the body's position and the joints involved. Although no definitive studies are available to confirm this, it is assumed that to develop strength throughout the joint's full range of motion, training must be performed throughout that range. Studies demonstrating joint-angle specificity with isometric training indicate that when training is performed only at a specific joint angle, strength gains are realized in a narrow range around that specific joint angle and not throughout the joint's range of motion (see chapter 2). In advanced training programs joint-angle specificity is used to increase strength and power in a range of motion to increase motor performance (e.g., using quarter squats to develop jumping ability). Some advanced training techniques (e.g., partial repetitions) intentionally limit the range of motion (see chapter 6). However, generally, exercises are performed throughout a full range of motion to ensure strength gains throughout that range.

Resistance Training Shoes

A safe shoe for resistance training does not have to be one specifically designed for Olympic-style lifting or powerlifting, but should have good arch support, a nonslip sole, proper fit, and a sole that is not shock absorbing. The first three of these factors are for safety reasons. The last is important for a simple reason: Force produced by the leg muscles to lift the weight should not be wasted in compressing the shoe's sole. Additionally, if the heel area is very compressible, such as in a running shoe, in some exercises, such as back squats, compression of the heel area during the lift may result in a loss of balance. Shoes designed for cross-training offer all of these characteristics and are appropriate for all but the advanced fitness enthusiast, strength or power athlete, Olympic-style lifter, or powerlifter.

Resistance Training Gloves

Gloves for resistance training cover only the palm area. This protects the palms from catching or scraping on free weight and machine handles, but allows a good grip of the bar or handle with the fingers. Gloves help prevent blisters and the ripping of calluses on the hand. However, they are not mandatory for safe resistance training.

Training Belts

Training belts have a wide back portion that supposedly helps support the lumbar area or low back. They do help support the low back, but not because of the wide back area. Instead, the belt gives the abdominal muscles an object to push against. This helps to raise intra-abdominal pressure, which supports the lumbar vertebrae from the anterior side (Harman et al. 1989; Lander, Hundley, and Simonton 1992; Lander, Simonton, and Giacobbe 1990). Increased intra-abdominal pressure prevents flexion of the lumbar vertebrae, which aids in maintaining an upright posture. Strong abdominal musculature helps to maintain intra-abdominal pressure. When intra-abdominal pressure increases, weak abdominal musculature protrude anteriorly. This results in decreased intra-abdominal pressure and so less support for the lumbar vertebrae. A training belt can be used for exercises that place significant stress on the lumbar area, such as squats and deadlifts. However, it is not necessary for the safe performance of these exercises and should not be used to alleviate technique problems caused by weak abdominal or low back musculature.

Many lifters use weight training belts in inappropriate situations (e.g., lifting light weights or performing exercises not related to low back stress; Finnie et al. 2003). As noted earlier, the use of weight training belts has been shown to increase the injury rate to the lower spine possibly as a result of the belief that they protect competitive lifters as they push their ability with maximal or supra-maximal weights in preparation for competition (Siewe et al. 2011). In addition, electromyographic activity of the lumbar extensor musculature is higher when wearing a belt during squats at 60% of 1RM compared to without a belt. This suggests that a belt does not reduce stress on the low back when using relatively light resistance and therefore should not be used with such resistances (Bauer, Fry, and Carter 1999). If exercises placing a great deal of stress on the low back are to be performed, exercises to strengthen the low back and abdominal regions need to be included in the training program.

Wearing a tightly cinched belt during an activity increases blood pressure (Hunter et al. 1989), which can result in increased cardiovascular stress. Thus, a tightly cinched training belt should not be worn during activities such as riding a stationary bike or during exercises in which the lumbar area is not significantly stressed. Belts should normally not be worn when performing exercises that do not require back support or when using light to moderate resistances (i.e., RMs higher than 6RM or low percentages of 1RM).

Equipment Maintenance

Maintaining equipment in proper operating condition is of utmost importance for a safe resistance training program. Pulleys and cables or belts should be checked frequently for wear and replaced as needed. Equipment should be lubricated as indicated by the manufacturer. Cracked or broken free weight plates, dumbbells, or plates in a machine's weight stack should be retired and replaced. Upholstery should be disinfected daily. The sleeves on Olympic bars and other free weight bars should revolve freely to avoid tearing the skin on a lifter's hands. Equipment in a facility that is not in working order needs to be clearly marked as such. An injury resulting from improper equipment maintenance should never happen in a well-run resistance training facility or program.

Summary

Understandable and clear definitions of terminology are important to any field of study. Clear definitions of weight training terms are necessary for accurate communication and an exchange of ideas among fitness enthusiasts and strength and conditioning professionals. Proper safety precautions, such as spotting and proper exercise technique, are a necessity of all properly designed and implemented resistance training programs. An understanding of the basic terminology and safety aspects of weight training is important when examining the topic of the next chapter, the types of strength training.

SELECTED READINGS

Deminice, R., Sicchieri, T., Mialich, M., Milani, F., Ovidio, P., and Jordao, A.A. 2011. Acute session of hypertrophy-resistance traditional interval training and circuit training. *Journal of Strength and Conditioning Research* 25: 798-804.

Fleck, S.J. 1998. *Successful long-term weight training.* Chicago: NTP/Contemporary Publishing Group.

Fleck, S.J. 1999. Periodized strength training: A critical review. *Journal of Strength and Conditioning Research* 13: 82-89.

Kraemer, W.J., and Fleck, S.J. 2005. *Strength training for young athletes* (2nd ed.). Champaign, IL: Human Kinetics.

Meyer, G.D., Quatman, C.E., Khoury, J., Wall, E.J., and Hewitt, T.E. 2009. Youth versus adult "weightlifting" injuries presenting to United States emergency rooms: Accidental versus non-accidental injury mechanisms. *Journal of Strength and Conditioning Research* 23: 2064-2080.

Types of Strength Training

After studying this chapter, you should be able to

1. define isometric, dynamic constant external resistance, variable resistance, variable-variable resistance, isokinetic, and eccentric training,

2. describe what is known from research concerning the optimal training frequency, volume, and intensity to cause strength increases, motor performance increases, hypertrophy increases and body composition changes with the various types of training,

3. describe considerations unique to each type of training,

4. discuss how the various types of training compare in causing strength increases, motor performance increases, hypertrophy increases and body composition changes, and

5. define and discuss specificity of training factors such as joint angle specificity, velocity specificity, and testing specificity.

Most athletes and fitness enthusiasts perform strength training as a portion of their overall training program. The main interest for athletes is not how much weight they can lift, but whether increased strength and power and changes in body composition brought about by weight training result in better performances in their sports. Fitness enthusiasts may be interested in some of the same training adaptations as athletes, but also in health benefits such as decreased blood pressure and changes in body composition, as well as the lean, fit appearance brought about by weight training.

There are several factors to consider when examining a type of strength training. Does this type of training increase motor performance? Vertical jump tests, a 40 yd sprint, and throwing a ball or medicine ball for distance are common motor performance tests. Is strength increased throughout the full range of motion and at all velocities of movement? Most sports and daily life activities require strength and power throughout a large portion of a joint's range of motion. If strength and power are not increased throughout a large portion

of the range of motion, performance may not be enhanced to the extent that it could be. The majority of athletic events require strength and power at a variety of movement speeds, particularly at fast velocities. If strength and power are not increased over a wide variety of movement velocities, once again, improvements in performance may not be optimal.

Other questions to consider when examining types of strength training include the following: To what extent does the type of training cause changes in body composition, such as the percentage of body fat or fat-free body mass? How much of an increase in strength and power can be expected over a specified training period with this type of training? How does it compare with other training types in the preceding factors?

A considerable amount of research concerning types of resistance training exists. The emergence of conclusions from this research, however, is hampered by several factors. The vast majority of studies have been of short-term duration (8 to 12 weeks) with sedentary or moderately trained people. This makes the direct application of their results to long-term training (years) and highly trained fitness enthusiasts or athletes questionable.

As an example, following one year of training, elite Olympic-style weightlifters show an increase in 1RM snatch ability of 1.5% and in 1RM clean and jerk ability of 2%; they also exhibit an increase in fat-free body mass of 1% or less and a decrease in percent body fat up to 1.7% (Häkkinen, Komi et al. 1987; Häkkinen, Pakarinen et al. 1987b). Following two years of training, elite Olympic-style weightlifters show an increase in their lifting total (total = 1RM snatch + 1RM clean and jerk) of 2.7%, an increase in fat-free body mass of 1%, and a decrease in percent body fat of 1.7% (Häkkinen et al. 1988b). These changes are much smaller than those shown by untrained or moderately trained people in strength and body composition (see table 3.3 in chapter 3) over much shorter training periods. This indicates that causing changes in strength and body composition in highly fit people, such as athletes and advanced fitness enthusiasts, is more difficult than in untrained or moderately trained people. The idea that it is more difficult to increase strength in highly trained people is supported by a meta-analysis of research studies (Rhea et al. 2003) and clearly shown in figure 2.1.

Other factors that can affect gains in strength are the training volume (number of muscle actions or sets and repetitions) performed and the training intensity (% 1RM) used in training. These factors vary considerably from study to study and make interpretation of the results difficult. Additionally, training volume (four vs. eight sets per muscle group for untrained people and athletes, respectively) and training intensity (60 vs. 85% of 1RM for untrained people and athletes, respectively) may not be the same in all populations to bring about maximal strength gains (Peterson, Rhea, and Alvar 2004). Another factor making interpretations and comparisons of studies difficult is the fact that strength increases in different muscle groups do not necessarily occur at the same rate or to the same magnitude with identical training programs (Willoughby 1993). Ultimately, the outcome of any comparison of strength training types depends on the efficacy of the programs used in the comparison.

A comparison of the optimal dynamic constant external resistance training program to a very ineffective isokinetic program will favor the former. Conversely, a comparison of the optimal isokinetic program to a very ineffective dynamic constant external resistance training program will favor the isokinetic program. Ideally, any comparison of strength training types would be of long duration and use the optimal programs, which may change over time. Unfortunately, comparisons of this nature do not exist. Enough research has been conducted, however, to reach some tentative conclusions concerning the types of strength training and how to use them in a training program. This chapter addresses the major research studies and their conclusions.

Isometric Training

Isometric training, or static resistance training, refers to a muscular action during which no change in the length of the total muscle takes place. This means that no visible movement at a joint (or joints) takes place. Isometric actions can take place voluntarily against less than 100% of maximal voluntary action, such as voluntarily holding a light dumbbell at a certain point in an exercise's range of motion or voluntarily generating less than maximal force against an immovable object. An isometric action can also be performed at 100% of maximal voluntary muscle action (MVMA) against an immovable object.

Isometric training is most commonly performed against an immovable object such as a wall or

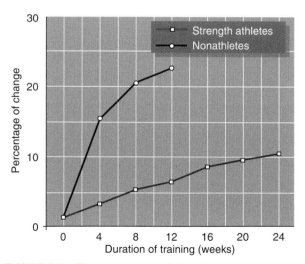

FIGURE 2.1 The percentage of change in maximal squat ability from the pretraining value depends on the pretraining status of the trainees and the duration of training.

Adapted, by permission, from K. Häkkinen, 1985, "Factors influencing trainability of muscular strength during short-term and prolonged training," *National Strength and Conditioning Association Journal* 7: 33.

a weight machine loaded beyond the person's maximal concentric strength. Isometrics can also be performed by having a weak muscle group act against a strong muscle group—for example, activating the left elbow flexors maximally to try to flex the left elbow while simultaneously resisting the movement by pushing down on the left hand with the right hand with just enough force to stop any movement at the left elbow. If the left elbow flexors are weaker than the right elbow extensors, the left elbow flexors would perform an isometric action at a 100% of MVMA. Isometric actions can also be performed after a partial range of motion of a dynamic action in some exercises (see the chapter 6 section Functional Isometrics).

Isometrics came to the attention of the American public in the early 1950s, when Steinhaus (1954) introduced the work of two Germans, Hettinger and Muller (1953). Hettinger and Muller concluded that gains in isometric strength of 5% per week were produced by one daily 66% maximal isometric action performed for six seconds. Gains in strength of this magnitude with such little training time and effort seemed unbelievable. A subsequent review concluded that isometric training leads to static strength gains, and that the gains can be substantial and variable over short duration training periods (Fleck and Schutt 1985; also see table 2.1).

Increases in strength from isometric training may be related to the number of muscle actions performed, the duration of the muscle actions, whether the muscle actions are maximal, and the frequency of training. Because most studies involving isometric training manipulate several of these factors simultaneously, it is difficult to evaluate the importance of any one of them. Enough research has been conducted, however, to suggest

TABLE 2.1 Effects of 100% Maximal Voluntary Contractions on Isometric Strength

Reference	Duration of contraction(s)	Contractions per day	Duration × contractions per day	Number of training days	MVIC increase (%)	MVIC increase % per day	Muscle
Bonde-Peterson 1960	5	1	5	36	0	0	Elbow flexors
Ikai and Fukunaga 1970	10	3	30	100	92	0.9	Elbow flexors
Komi and Karlsson 1978	3-5	5	15-25	48	20	0.4	Quadriceps
Bonde-Peterson 1960	5	10	50	36	15	0.4	Elbow flexors
Maffiuletti and Martin 2001	4	12	48	21	16	0.7	Quadriceps
Alway et al. 1989	10	5-15	50-150	48	44	0.9	Triceps surae
McDonagh, Hayward, and Davies 1983	3	30	90	28	20	0.71	Elbow flexors
Grimby et al. 1973	3	30	90	30	32	1.1	Triceps
Davies and Young 1983	3	42	126	35	30	0.86	Triceps surae
Carolyn and Cafarelli 1992	3-4	30	90-120	24	32	1.3	Quadriceps
Garfinkel and Cafarelli 1992	3-5	30	90-150	24	28	1.2	Quadriceps
Kanehisa et al. 2002	6	12	48	30	60	2.0	Elbow extensors

MVIC = maximal voluntary isometric contraction.

With kind permission from Springer Science+Business Media: *European Journal of Applied Physiology* "Adaptive responses of mammalian skeletal muscle to exercise with high loads," 52: 140, M.J.N. McDonagh and C.T.M. Davies, table 1, copyright 1984; Additional data from Garfinkel and Cafarelli 1992; Carolyn and Cafarelli 1992; Alway et al. 1989; Kanehisa et al. 2002.

recommendations and tentative conclusions concerning isometric training.

Maximal Voluntary Muscle Actions

Increases in isometric strength can be achieved with submaximal isometric muscle actions (Alway, Sale, and McDougall 1990; Davies, Greenwood, and Jones 1988; Davies and Young 1983; Folland et al. 2005; Hettinger and Mueller 1953; Kanehisa et al. 2002; Kubo et al. 2001; Lyle and Rutherford 1998; Macaluso et al. 2000). However, contradictions exist concerning the need for MVMAs because they have been shown to be superior to submaximal voluntary isometric muscle actions in causing strength increases (Rasch and Morehouse 1957; Ward and Fisk 1964), and no difference in strength increases between maximal and submaximal actions have been shown (Kanehisa et al. 2002). There may be adaptational differences depending on how a maximal voluntary isometric action is performed (Maffiuletti and Martin 2001).

Isometric actions can be performed in such a way that maximal force is developed as quickly as possible or that force increases and reaches maximal in a specified time period, such as four seconds. Both types of training result in significant and similar increases in maximal isokinetic and isometric force capabilities. However, electromyographic (EMG) and electrically evoked twitch contractile properties indicate that training in which maximal force is developed in four seconds results in modifications of the nervous system in the periphery (i.e., muscle membrane electrical activity), whereas training by developing maximal force as quickly as possible results in adaptations in contractile muscle properties (i.e., excitation–contraction coupling).

As with other types of resistance training, the effect of the "quality" of the muscle action needs to be further investigated. Generally, MVMAs are used in training healthy people, and submaximal isometric actions are used in rehabilitation programs or remedial strength training programs in which maximal muscular actions are contraindicated.

Number of Muscle Actions and Duration

Hettinger and Muller (1953) proposed that only one 6-second muscle action per day was necessary to produce maximal strength gains. As shown in table 2.1, many combinations in the number and duration of MVMAs result in significant strength gain. The majority of MVMA studies used isometric actions 3 to 10 seconds in duration, with 3 being the least number of muscle actions resulting in a significant strength gain. Similarly, many combinations in the number and duration of submaximal isometric actions can result in increased isometric strength. For example, four sets of six repetitions of two seconds in duration at 50% MVMA (adductor pollicis) and four muscle actions each 30 seconds in duration at 70% MVMA (quadriceps) have resulted in significant increases of isometric strength (Lyle and Rutherford 1998; Schott, McCully, and Rutherford 1995). It is important to note that, generally, these studies used healthy, but non-weight-trained people as subjects.

The duration of the muscle action and the number of training muscle actions per day individually show weaker correlations to strength increases than do duration and number combined (McDonagh and Davies 1984). This means that the total length of the isometric actions performed is directly related to increased strength. It also indicates that optimal gains in strength are the result of either a small number of long-duration muscle actions or a high number of short-duration muscle actions (Kanehisa et al. 2002). As an example, seven daily one-minute muscle actions at 30% of MVMA or 42 three-second MVMAs per training day over a six-week training period both result in about a 30% increase in isometric MVMA (Davies and Young 1983).

However, some information indicates that longer-duration isometric actions may be superior to short-duration actions in causing strength gains (Schott, McCully, and Rutherford 1995). Training the quadriceps at 70% of MVMA with four 30-second actions and four sets of 10 repetitions each three seconds in duration both result in significant isometric strength gains. Even though the total duration of the isometric muscle actions (120 seconds per training session) was identical between the two training programs, the longer-duration isometric actions resulted in a significantly greater increase in isometric strength (median 55 vs. 32% increase). The longer-duration isometric actions resulted in a significant increase in isometric strength after two weeks of training, whereas eight weeks of training was necessary before a significant increase in strength was achieved with the short-duration isometric actions. This indicates that longer-duration submaximal isometric actions may be more appropriate when a quick increase in strength is desired.

During isometric actions, blood flow occlusion does occur and may in part be responsible for increased metabolite concentrations and acidity; this could be a stimulus for greater strength gains from long-duration isometric actions than from short-duration ones (see the section in chapter 6, Vascular Occlusion). The possible role of occlusion as a stimulus for strength gains is shown in studies by Takarada and colleagues. They found that training using 20 to 50% of 1RM while blood flow is occluded results in increased metabolite concentrations, acidity, and serum growth hormone concentrations (Takarada et al. 2000a, 2000b). Training at 30 to 50% of 1RM with blood flow occlusion resulted in a significantly higher blood lactate concentration compared to training at 50 to 80% of 1RM without occlusion, indicating greater concentrations of intramuscular metabolites (Takarada et al. 2000b). Over 16 weeks of training, both programs resulted in significant, but similar, increases in strength. This indicates that blood flow occlusion and the resulting increase in intramuscular metabolites do affect strength increases.

Many studies using isometrics give subjects several seconds to increase the force of the muscle action until they reach the desired percentage of MVMA. This is in part done for safety reasons. Some information, however, indicates that a rapid increase in the isometric force results in significantly greater increases in strength at the training joint angle (Maffiuletti and Martin 2001). During seven weeks of training, some subjects performed isometric actions of the knee extensors by increasing muscle force as rapidly as possible (the action lasted approximately one second), and others increased force to a maximal over four seconds. They experienced an increase in MVMA of 28 and 16%, respectively. Similar and comparable increases in strength were shown at knee angles different from the training angle, and during eccentric and concentric isokinetic testing. Thus, increasing force as quickly as possible during training revealed a significantly greater increase in strength only at the training joint angle.

Collectively, these studies indicate that many combinations of maximal and submaximal isometric muscle action durations and numbers can bring about isometric strength gains. However, in typical training settings with healthy people, per-haps the most efficient use of isometric training time is to perform a minimum of 15 MVMAs or near MVMAs of three to five seconds in duration for three sessions per week as discussed in the next section on training frequency.

Training Frequency

Three training sessions per week using either maximal or submaximal isometric actions result in a significant increase in isometric MVMA (Alway, MacDougall, and Sale 1989; Alway, Sale, and MacDougall 1990; Carolyn and Cafarelli 1992; Davies et al. 1988; Folland et al. 2005; Garfinkel and Cafarelli 1992; Lyle and Rutherford 1998; Macaluso et al. 2000; Maffiuletti and Martin 2001; Schott, McCully, and Rutherford 1995; Weir, Housh, and Weir 1994; Weir et al. 1995). Increases in isometric MVMA over 6 to 16 weeks of training ranged from 8 to 79% in these studies. However, whether three training sessions per week cause maximal increases in strength is not fully substantiated. Hettinger (1961) calculated that alternate-day isometric training is 80% and that once-a-week training is 40% as effective as daily training sessions. Hettinger also concluded that training once every two weeks does not cause increases in strength, although it does serve to maintain strength. Daily training with isometrics is superior to less frequent training (Atha 1981), although the exact percentage of strength superiority is debated and may vary by muscle group and other training variables (e.g., muscle action duration, number of muscle actions). To increase maximal strength, daily isometric training may be optimal; however, two or three training sessions per week will bring about significant increases in maximal strength. Three sessions per week is the routine most frequently used in studies.

Muscle Hypertrophy

Increases in limb circumferences have been used to determine muscle hypertrophy and have been shown to occur as a result of isometric training (Kanehisa and Miyashita 1983a; Kitai and Sale 1989; Meyers 1967; Rarick and Larson 1958). More recently, technologies (computerized tomography, magnetic resonance imaging [MRI]) that more accurately determine muscle cross-sectional area and muscle thickness (ultrasound) have been used to measure changes in muscle hypertrophy due to isometric training.

It is clear that isometric training can result in significant hypertrophy (Wernbom, Augustsson, and Thomee 2007). Quadriceps cross-sectional area (CSA) increases on average 8.9% (range 4.8-14.6%) after 8 to 14 weeks of isometric training (Wernbom, Augustsson, and Thomee 2007). Likewise, significant gains in elbow flexor CSA up to 23% have been shown following isometric training. Increases in CSA are typically accompanied by increases in maximal strength. For example, 12 weeks of training resulted in a significant increase of 8% in knee extensor CSA and a 41% increase in isometric strength (Kubo et al. 2001). As with other training types, strength increases are due to a combination of neural adaptations and hypertrophy as indicated by studies showing significant (Garfinkel and Cafarelli 1992) and nonsignificant (Davies et al. 1988) correlations between increases in strength and CSA.

Whether hypertrophy occurs and the extent to which it occurs may vary from muscle to muscle and by muscle fiber type. Type I and II muscle fiber diameters in the vastus lateralis did not change after isometric training at 100% of MVMA (Lewis et al. 1984). Type I and II fiber areas increased in the soleus approximately 30% after isometric training with either 30 or 100% of MVMA (Alway, MacDougall, and Sale 1989; Alway, Sale, and Mac-Dougall 1990), whereas only the type II fibers of the lateral gastrocnemius increased in area 30 to 40% after an identical isometric training program.

Longer-duration muscle actions may result in greater gains in CSA than shorter-duration muscle actions (Schott, McCully, and Rutherford 1995). Muscle CSA was determined (via computerized tomography) before and after training with four 30-second actions and four sets of 10 repetitions each three seconds in duration. Even though the total duration of the isometric muscle actions (120 seconds per training session) was identical between the two groups, the longer-duration isometric actions resulted in a significant increase in quadriceps CSA (10-11%), whereas the shorter-duration muscular actions resulted in nonsignificant increases (4-7%) in quadriceps CSA. Additionally, maximal MVMAs may result in significantly greater hypertrophy than 60% MVMAs over 10 weeks of training (Kanehisa et al. 2002). This comparison was between 12 muscle actions at 100% MVMA with each action lasting six seconds and four actions at 60% MVMA with each action lasting 30 seconds. So total isometric action duration

per training session was equivalent (120 seconds) between the two training programs. However, when training volume is expressed as the total duration of isometric actions per training session or as the product of training intensity times total duration, no apparent relation between volume and rate of CSA increase was apparent (Wernbom, Augustsson, and Thomee 2007). This indicates that a variety of training intensity and volume can result in significant hypertrophy.

Muscle protein synthesis in the soleus after an isometric action at 40% of MVMA to fatigue (approximately 27 minutes) increases significantly by 49% (Fowles et al. 2000). This finding supports the efficacy of isometric actions inducing muscle hypertrophy. Collectively, this information indicates that muscle hypertrophy of both the type I and type II muscle fibers can occur from isometric training with submaximal and maximal muscle actions of varying durations. Table 2.2 describes guidelines to bring about muscle hypertrophy with various intensities of isometric training.

Joint-Angle Specificity

Gains in strength occur predominantly at or near the joint angle at which isometric training is performed; this is termed **joint-angle specificity**. The majority of research indicates that static strength increases from isometric training are joint-angle specific (Bender and Kaplan 1963; Gardner 1963; Kitai and Sale 1989; Lindh 1979; Meyers 1967; Thepaut-Mathieu, Van Hoecke, and Martin 1988; Weir, Housh, and Weir 1994; Weir et al. 1995; Williams and Stutzman 1959), although lack of joint-angle specificity strength gains have also been shown (Knapik, Mawdsley, and Ramos 1983; Rasch and Pierson 1964; Rasch, Preston, and Logan 1961). Several factors may affect the degree to which joint-angle specificity occurs, including the muscle group(s) trained, the joint angle at which the training is performed, and the intensity and duration of the isometric actions. Joint-angle specificity is normally attributed to neural adaptations, such as increased muscle fiber recruitment at the trained angle and the inhibition of the antagonistic muscles at the trained angle.

Carryover of significant isometric strength increases to other joint angles can vary from 5 to 30 degrees on either side of the joint angle trained depending on the muscle group and joint angle trained (Kitai and Sale 1989; Knapik, Mawdsley, and Ramos 1983; Maffiuletti and Martin 2001;

TABLE 2.2 Guidelines to Increase Hypertrophy With Isometric Training

Training variable	Low intensity	High intensity	Maximal intensity
Intensity	30-50% MVIA	70-80% MVIA	100% MVIA
Repetitions	1	1	10
Sets	2-6 per exercise Progress from 2 to 4-6 sets per muscle group	2-6 per exercise Progress from 2 to 4-6 sets per muscle group	1-3 per exercise Progress from 1 to 3 sets per muscle group
Repetition duration	40-60 sec, and to muscular failure during the final 1-2 sets	15-20 sec, and to muscular failure during the final 1-2 sets	3-5 sec
Rest between repetitions and sets	30-60 sec	30-60 sec	25-30 sec and 60 sec
Training frequency	3-4 sessions per muscle group per week	3-4 sessions per muscle group per week	3 sessions per muscle group per week

MVIA = maximal voluntary isometric action

Adapted from Wernbom, Augustsson, and Thomee 2007.

Thepaut-Mathieu, Van Hoecke, and Martin 1988). Joint-angle specificity (see figure 2.2) may be most marked when the training is performed with the muscle in a shortened position (25-degree angle) and occurs to a smaller extent when the training occurs with the muscle in a lengthened position (120-degree angle) (Gardner 1963; Thepaut-Mathieu, Van Hoecke, and Martin 1988). When training occurs at the midpoint of a joint's range of motion (80-degree angle), joint-angle specificity may occur throughout a greater range of motion (Kitai and Sale 1989; Knapik, Mawdsley, and Ramos 1983; Thepaut-Mathieu, Van Hoeke, and Martin 1988). In addition, twenty 6-second muscle actions result in greater carryover to other joint angles than six 6-second muscle actions do (Meyers 1967). This indicates that the longer the duration of isometric training per training session (i.e., the number of muscle actions multiplied by the duration of each muscle action), the greater the carryover to other joint angles.

Isometric training at one joint angle may not result in dynamic power increases. Isometric training of the knee extensors at one joint angle results in inconsistent and for the most part nonsignificant changes in isokinetic torque across a wide range of movement velocities (Schott, McCully, and Rutherford 1995). However, it has also been reported that isometric training at one joint angle results in significant force increases in dynamic (isokinetic) eccentric and concentric actions (Maffiuletti and Martin 2001) and increases peak power at 40, 60, and 80% of normal weight training 1RM (Ullrich, Kleinoder, and Bruggemann 2010). Thus, isometric

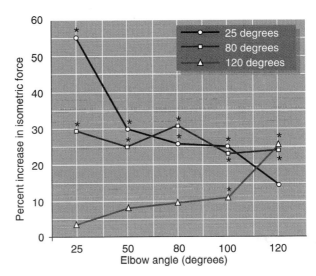

FIGURE 2.2 Percentage gain in the isometric strength of elbow flexors due to isometric training at various elbow angles.

* = significant increase ($p < .05$).

Data from Thépaut-Mathieu et al. 1988.

training at one joint angle may not always result in increased force and power throughout the joint's range of motion. However, isometric training of the elbow flexors and knee extensors at four different joint angles increases static strength at all four joint angles and significantly increases the dynamic power and force (isokinetic) throughout the range of motion at several velocities (45, 150, and 300 degrees per second) (Folland et al. 2005; Kanehisa and Miyashita 1983a). Thus, to ensure an increase in dynamic power and strength throughout a joint's range of motion, a trainee must perform isometric training at several points in a joint's range of motion.

This information on joint-angle specificity offers some practical guidelines for increasing strength and power throughout the entire range of motion. First, the training should be performed at joint-angle increments of approximately 10 to 30 degrees. Second, the total duration of isometric training (the duration of each muscle action multiplied by the number of muscle actions) per session should be long (three- to five-second actions, 15 to 20 actions per session). Third, if isometric actions cannot be performed throughout the entire range of motion, it may be best to perform them with the muscle(s) in a lengthened position rather than a shortened position. It is also possible to use isometric training's joint-angle specificity to increase dynamic strength lifting ability by performing isometric actions at the sticking point of an exercise (see the section Functional Isometrics in chapter 6).

Motor Performance

Maximal isometric strength has shown significant correlations to performance in sports such as basketball (Häkkinen 1987), rowing (Secher 1975), and sprinting (Mero et al. 1981), as well as to countermovement and static jump ability (Häkkinen 1987; Kawamori et al. 2006; Khamoui et al. 2011; Ugarkovic et al. 2002) and dynamic force in a mid-thigh clean pull (Kawamori et al. 2006). However, nonsignificant correlations between maximal isometric strength and dynamic

performance have also been shown. A review (Wilson and Murphy 1996) concluded that the relationship between maximal isometric strength and dynamic performance is questionable, even though some studies demonstrated significant correlations between the rate of force development during an isometric test and dynamic performance. Similarly, isometric tests are not sensitive to training adaptations induced by dynamic activity nor do they consistently discriminate among athletes of differing caliber in the same sport or activity (Wilson and Murphy 1996). The isometric rate of force development (first 50 and 100 ms) in a clean high pull does correlate to peak velocity in a clean high pull, and isometric peak force per kilogram of body mass correlates with vertical jump height and vertical jump peak velocity (Khamoui et al. 2011). All of these correlations, although significant, were moderate ($r = .49-.62$); however, they do indicate that isometric force development in a multijoint movement does correlate to vertical jump and clean pull ability. Thus, although isometric testing may not be the best modality for monitoring changes in dynamic motor performance, if it is used in this manner, an isometric multijoint movement appears to be most appropriate. This information may also indicate that when isometric training is used to increase dynamic motor performance, such as sprinting or vertical jumping, the training should be multijoint in nature. Isometric training and testing is, however, of substantial value if the sport involves a significant amount of isometric action, such as rock climbing (see box 2.1).

BOX 2.1 **RESEARCH**

Rock Climbing and Isometric Strength

Rock climbers use numerous isometric actions—in particular, while gripping a handhold, which involves flexion of the fingers. Maximal isometric force per kilogram of body mass of the fingers is significantly correlated to rock climbing ability (Wall et al. 2004). Additionally, this same measure is significantly greater in climbers of higher ability than in climbers of lesser ability. Climbers perform isometric actions of the fingers when training by gripping handholds (finger board). Isometric actions of the fingers are also recommended to climbers for rehabilitation after an injury to the fingers (Kubiac, Klugman, and Bosco 2006). This is clearly one sport in which isometric actions are very important for successful performance and for rehabilitation after injury.

Kubiak, E.N., Klugman, J.A., and Bosco, J.A. 2006. Hand injuries in rock climbers. *Bulletin of the NYU Hospital for Joint Diseases* 64: 172-177.

Wall, C., Byrnes, W., Starek, J., and Fleck, S.J. 2004. Prediction of performance in female rock climbers. *Journal of Strength and Conditioning Research* 18: 77-83.

Isometric training at one joint angle has been shown to increase motor performance in the novel task of one-legged jumping using only plantar flexion (Burgess et al. 2007); however, it does not consistently increase dynamic motor performance (Clarke 1973; Fleck and Schutt 1985). The lack of any or a consistent increase in motor performance may be due to the inconsistent changes in the rate of force or power, as discussed previously, and the lack of an increase in the limb's maximal velocity of movement with little or no resistance (DeKoning et al. 1982) with isometric training at one joint angle. Other factors that may inhibit isometric strength gains from affecting dynamic motor performance include differences in muscle fiber recruitment patterns between isometric and dynamic actions and mechanical differences, such as little, if any, stretch-shortening cycle during in an isometric action.

Maximal isometric force varies throughout the range of motion of a movement. The correlation between dynamic bench press ability and isometric strength varies drastically with the elbow angle at which the isometric test is performed (Murphy et al. 1995). This has led to the suggestion that isometric testing should be performed at the point within the range of motion at which maximal force is developed. However, the use of such an angle may not demonstrate the highest correlation between isometric strength and dynamic motor performance (Wilson and Murphy 1996). Thus, the exact angle at which isometric strength should be assessed to monitor isometric training to increase motor performance or train to increase motor performance remains unclear.

If isometric actions are used to monitor or increase dynamic motor performance, several suggestions seem warranted. First, as discussed earlier, dynamic power can be increased with isometric training if the isometric actions are performed at several points within the range of motion. Thus, performance of isometric actions at 10- to 20-degree intervals throughout the movement's range of motion may aid in carryover of isometric strength gains to dynamic actions. Second, most dynamic motor performance tasks are multijoint and multi-muscle-group in nature. Thus, multijoint, sport-specific isometric movements, such as a leg press or clean pull movement, should be used to monitor or improve dynamic motor performance tasks. Third, if previous research indicates a point within the range of motion that demonstrates a high significant correlation between isometric strength and a motor performance task, isometric strength should be assessed at this point. If previous research does not indicate such a point, the strongest point within the range of motion can be used as the initial position for isometric strength testing. Fourth, the quick development of maximal force (within one second) at one joint angle has been shown to increase peak power (Ullrich, Kleinoder, and Bruggemann 2010); isometric force in 50 to 100 ms has shown significant correlations to vertical jump ability (Khamoui et al. 2011); and although not significant, a trend for significance ($p = .059$) was shown for an increase in one-legged jumping ability with quick force development of the plantar flexors after isometric training (Burgess et al. 2007). Therefore, the quick development of isometric force may help improve motor performance, but this type of training does carry risks for injury.

Combining Isometric With Other Types of Training

Minimal information is available concerning the effect of combining isometric with other types of training. Combining isometric training of the elbow flexors with power training (resistance moved as fast as possible) at 30 and 60% of maximal force resulted in increased peak power, but the increase was not different from what would result from power training alone (Toji and Kaneko 2004). Combining isometric training of the knee extensors and flexors with weight training in which the concentric repetition phase was performed as fast as possible and the eccentric phase was performed in 0.5 second also resulted in increased peak power at 40, 60, and 80% of 1RM; however, again, the increase in power was not different from what resulted from concentric–eccentric or isometric training alone (Ullrich, Kleinoder, and Bruggemann 2010). Thus, although the information is minimal and used only single-joint movements, no advantage was shown for increasing power by combining isometric with power-type training.

Other Considerations

Long-term isometric training decreases resting blood pressure (Taylor et al. 2003). However, as with all resistance training, a Valsalva maneuver may occur, resulting in an exaggerated blood pressure response during training. Performance of a

Valsalva maneuver should be discouraged because it results in higher blood pressure. As duration, intensity (% MVMA), and muscle mass increase during an isometric action, the blood pressure response increases (Kjaer and Secher 1992; Seals 1993). The increased blood pressure response during high-intensity large-muscle-group isometric exercise can decrease left ventricular function (ejection fraction) (Vitcenda et al. 1990). These factors need to be considered when isometric actions are performed by those with compromised, or potentially compromised, cardiovascular function, such as older trainees.

Because they do not lift or move an actual weight, some trainees may experience motivational problems with isometric training. It is also difficult to evaluate whether the trainees are performing the isometric actions at the desired intensity without feedback on force development. Visual feedback of force development, especially during unfamiliar movements, serves as positive feedback and encourages greater force production during isometric actions (Graves and James 1990). EMG feedback during isometric training is beneficial for increasing strength, but there is wide variability in its effect on strength increases (Lepley, Gribble, and Pietrosimone 2011). Feedback equipment may not be practical in many training situations. However, for isometric actions to be optimal, use of a feedback-monitoring system may be warranted.

Dynamic Constant External Resistance Training

Isotonic is a term traditionally used to describe an action in which the muscle exerts constant tension. Free weight exercises and exercises on various weight training machines that are usually considered isotonic are not isotonic according to this definition. The force exerted by muscles in the performance of such exercises is not constant, but rather varies with the mechanical advantage of the joint(s) involved in the exercise and the acceleration or deceleration of the resistance. Two terms, **dynamic constant external resistance** (DCER) and **isoinertial**, more accurately describe resistance training exercise in which the external resistance does not change in the lifting (concentric) or lowering (eccentric) phase. These terms imply that the weight or resistance being lifted is held constant and not that the force developed by a muscle during the exercise is constant.

On many resistance training machines the weight stack or weight plates have constant values. However, the point at which a cable or strap attaches to a movable handle or foot pad on the machine changes the muscular force needed to move the resistance throughout the exercise's range of motion. If the resistance training machine has circular pulleys (as opposed to noncircular pulleys), even though the muscular force needed to lift the resistance through the range of motion changes, the machine is still termed a DCER or isoinertial machine. With free weights and weight training machines, the external resistance or weight lifted is held constant even though the muscular force varies throughout the exercise movement. Thus, *DCER* and *isoinertial* describe this type of resistance training more accurately than the old term *isotonic*.

Number of Sets and Repetitions

The number of sets and repetitions needed for DCER exercises to result in maximal gains in strength and power, and in body composition changes, has received a great deal of attention from personal trainers, strength coaches, and sport scientists. The search for an optimal number of sets and repetitions assumes several factors: that an optimal number of sets and repetitions actually exists; that once found, it will work for all people and exercises or muscle groups; that it will work equally well in untrained and trained people; and that it will promote maximal increases in strength, power, and local muscular endurance, as well as body composition changes for an indefinite period of time. Acceptance of some of these assumptions would mean, among other things, that periodization of training and different programs for different age groups or training statuses are not necessary. Additionally, the optimal number of sets may be different among muscle groups. Researchers reported no difference in upper-body strength gains between people performing one set and people performing three sets. However, previously untrained men experienced significantly greater strength gains with three sets of exercises of the lower body (Ronnestad et al. 2007); increases in bench press and leg press strength of 3 and 9%, respectively, after performing the same training program for eight weeks (Kerrsick et al. 2009); and increases in bench press and leg press strength of 17 and 79%, respectively, after performing the same daily nonlinear program (Buford et al. 2007).

The vast majority of research studies concerning DCER have used novice, college-age subjects and a relatively short duration of training (8 to 12 weeks, with several lasting 20 to 36 weeks). Pretraining status and the duration of the training affect the results of any weight training program. These factors make interpretation of the studies and drawing conclusions concerning long-term training effects difficult. Common to the vast majority of studies concerning DCER is the use of sets carried to or close to volitional fatigue or the use of an RM resistance at some point in the training program (see chapter 6, Sets to Failure Technique).

Perhaps the earliest studies investigating the effect of varying numbers of sets and repetitions were by Berger in the 1960s; they indicated that optimal increases in 1RM in the bench press and back squat can occur with a variety of numbers of sets and repetitions when sets are carried to failure (Berger 1962b, 1962c, 1963a). The point that various combinations of sets and repetitions can bring about increased strength is well supported by research. Using nonperiodized training numbers of sets ranging from 1 to 6 and numbers of repetitions per set ranging from 1 to 20 have resulted in increased strength (see tables 2.3 and 2.4; Bemben et al. 2000; Calder et al. 1994; Dudley et al. 1991; Graves et al. 1988; Häkkinen 1985; Hass et al. 2000; Humburg et al. 2007; Kraemer et al. 2000; Marx et al. 2001; Schlumberger, Stec, and Schmidtbleicher 2001; Staron et al. 1989, 1994; Willoughby 1992, 1993).

Direct comparisons substantiate the assertion that there is no one optimal combination of nonperiodized sets and repetitions for increasing strength. No significant difference in increases in 1RM were found when training consisted of five sets of three at 3RM, four sets of five at 5RM, or three sets of seven at 7RM (Withers 1970); three sets of two to three, five to six, or nine to ten repetitions at the same respective RM resistance (O'Shea 1966); or one, two, or four sets all at 7 to 12RM (Ostrowski et al. 1997). Various combinations of nonperiodized sets and repetitions per set result in strength increases; however, multiple sets do result in greater strength increases than single sets, and the optimal number of sets varies with training status (see Considerations for All Types of Training later in this chapter).

Training Frequency

Training frequency, the number of sets and repetitions, and the number of exercises per training session determine total training volume. The optimal training frequency, therefore, may depend in part on total training volume per training session. The term *training frequency* is normally used to refer to the number of training sessions per week in which a certain muscle group is trained. This definition is important because it is possible to have daily training sessions and train a particular muscle group or body part from anywhere between not at all to seven sessions per week. Training frequency is defined here as the number of training sessions per week in which a certain muscle group is trained or a particular exercise is performed.

The importance of the definition of *training frequency* is made apparent by comparing an upper- and lower-body split program (see chapter 6) to a total-body weight training routine (Calder et al.

TABLE 2.3 Changes in Bench Press Strength Due to Training

Reference	Sex of subjects	Type of training	Training duration (wk)	Training days/ week	Sets and repetitions	% increase for equipment trained on	Comparative type of equipment	Comparative test % increase
Boyer 1990	F	DCER	12	3	3 wk = 3 × 10RM 3 wk = 3 × 6RM 6 wk = 3 × 8RM	24	VR	23
Brazell-Roberts and Thomas 1989	F	DCER	12	2	3 × 10 (75% of 1RM)	37	—	—
Brazell-Roberts and Thomas 1989	F	DCER	12	3	3 × 10 (75% of 1RM)	38	—	—

>continued

TABLE 2.3 >*continued*

Reference	Sex of subjects	Type of training	Training duration (wk)	Training days/ week	Sets and repetitions	% increase for equipment trained on	Comparative type of equipment	Comparative test % increase
Brown and Wilmore 1974	F	DCER	24	3	8 wk = 1 × 10, 8, 7, 6, 5,4 16 wk = 1 × 10, 6, 5, 4, 3	38	—	—
Calder et al. 1994	F	DCER	20	2	5 × 6- to 10RM	33	—	—
Hostler, Crill et al. 2001	F	DCER	16	2-3	4 wk = 2 × 7RM 4 wk = 3 × 7RM (10 days off) 8 wk = 3 × 7RM	47	—	—
Kraemer et al. 2000	F (college tennis)	DCER	36	3	1 × 8- to 10RM	8	—	—
Kraemer, Häk-kinen et al. 2003	F (college tennis)	DCER	36	2 or 3	3 × 8- to 10RM	17	—	—
Marx et al. 2001	F	DCER	24	3	1 × 8- to 10RM	12	—	—
Kraemer, Maz-zetti et al. 2001e	F	DCER	24	3	Periodized 3 × 3- to 8RM	37	—	—
Kraemer, Maz-zetti et al. 2001e	F	DCER	24	3	Periodized 3 × 8- to12RM	23	—	—
Mayhew and Gross 1974	F	DCER	9	3	2 × 20	26	—	—
Wilmore 1974	F	DCER	10	2	2 × 7-16	29	—	—
Wilmore et al. 1978	F	DCER	10	3	40-55% of 1RM for 30 s	20	—	—
Allen, Byrd, and Smith 1976	M	DCER	12	3	2 × 8, 1 × exhaustion	44	—	—
Ariel 1977	M	DCER	20	5	4 × 3-8	14	—	—
Baker, Wilson, and Carlyon 1994b	M	DCER	12	3	3 × 6	13	—	—
Berger 1962b	M	DCER	12	3	3 × 6	30	—	—
Coleman 1977	M	DCER	10	3	2 × 8- to 10RM	12	—	—
Fahey and Brown 1973	M	DCER	9	3	5 × 5	12	—	—
Gettman et al. 1978	M	DCER	20	3	50% of 1RM, 6 wk = 2 × 10-20 14 wk = 2 × 15	32	IK (12 deg/s)	27
Hoffman et al. 1990	M (college football)	DCER	10	3	4 wk = 4 × 8RM 4 wk = 5 × 6RM 2 wk = 1 × 10, 8, 6, 4, 2RM	2	—	—
Hoffman et al. 1990	M (college football)	DCER	10	4	Same as 3/wk	4	—	—
Hoffman et al. 1990	M (college football)	DCER	10	5	Same as 3/wk	3	—	—
Hoffman et al. 1990	M (college football)	DCER	10	6	Same as 3/wk	4	—	—

Reference	Sex of subjects	Type of training	Training duration (wk)	Training days/ week	Sets and repetitions	% increase for equipment trained on	Comparative type of equipment	Comparative test % increase
Hostler, Crill et al. 2001	M	DCER	16	2 or 3	4 wk = 2 × 7RM 4 wk = 3 × 7RM (10 days off) 8 wk = 3 × 7RM	29	—	—
Rhea et al. 2002	M	DCER	12	3	DNLP 1 × 8- to 10RM 1 × 6- to 8RM 1 × 4- to 6RM each 1 day/wk	20	—	—
Rhea et al. 2002	M	DCER	12	3	DNLP 1 × 8- to 10RM 3 × 6- to 8RM 3 × 4- to 6RM each 3 day/wk	33	—	—
Buford et al. 2007	M and F	DCER	9	3	LP 3 wk = 3 × 8 3 wk = 3 × 6 3 wk = 3 × 4	24	—	—
Buford et al. 2007	M and F	DCER	9	3	DNLP 3 × 8 3 × 6 3 × 4 each 1 day/wk	17	—	—
Kerksick et al. 2009	M	DCER	8	4	4 wk = 3 × 10 4 wk = 3 × 8	3	—	—
Marcinik et al. 1991	M	DCER	12	3	1 × 8- to 12RM	20	—	—
Stone, Nelson et al. 1983	M	DCER	6	3	3 × 6RM	7	—	—
Wilmore 1974	M	DCER	10	2	2 × 7-16	16	—	—
Ariel 1977	M	VR	20	5	4 × 3-8	—	DCER	29
Boyer 1990	F	VR	12	3	3 wk = 3 × 10RM 3 wk = 3 × 6RM 6 wk = 3 × 8RM	47	DCER	15
Coleman 1977	M	VR	10	3	1 × 8- to 12RM	—	DCER[a]	12
Lee et al. 1990	M	VR	10	3	3 × 10RM	20	—	—
Stanforth, Painter, and Wilmore 1992	M and F	VR	12	3	3 × 8- to 12RM	11	IK (1.5 s/con-traction)	17
Fleck, Mattie, and Mar-tensen 2006	F	VVR	14	3	3 × 10RM	28	—	—
Gettman and Ayres 1978	M	IK (60 deg/s)	10	3	3 × 10-15	—	DCER	11
Gettman and Ayres 1978	M	IK (120 deg/s)	10	3	3 × 10-15	—	DCER	9
Gettman et al. 1979	M	IK	8	3	4 wk = 1 × 10 at 60 deg/s 4 wk = 1 × 15 at 90 deg/s	22	DCER	11
Stanforth, Painter, and Wilmore 1992	M and F	IK (1.5 s/ contrac-tion)	12	3	3 × 8- to 12RM	20	VR	11

DCER = dynamic constant external resistance; VR = variable resistance; VVR = variable variable resistance; IK = isokinetic; DNLP = daily nonlinear periodization; LP = linear periodization; RM = repetition maximum; * = values for average training weights.

TABLE 2.4 Changes in Leg Press Strength Due to Training

Reference	Sex of subjects	Type of training	Training duration (wk)	Training days/ week	Sets and repetitions	% increase for equipment trained on	Comparative type of equipment	Comparative test % increase
Brown and Wilmore 1974	F	DCER	24	3	8 wk = 1 × 10, 8, 7, 6, 5, 4 16 wk = 1 × 10, 6, 5, 4, 3	29	—	—
Calder et al. 1994	F	DCER	20	2	5 × 10- to 12RM	21	—	—
Cordova et al. 1995	F	DCER	5	3	1 × 10, 1 × 6, 2 × as many as possible normally up to 11	50	—	—
Kraemer et al. 2000	F (college tennis)	DCER	36	3	1 × 8- to 10RM	8	—	—
Kraemer, Häkkinen et al. 2003	F (college tennis)	DCER	36	2-3	3 × 8- to 10RM	17	—	—
Marx et al. 2001	F	DCER	24	3	1 × 8- to 10RM	11	—	—
Mayhew and Gross 1974	F	DCER	9	3	2 × 10	48[a]	—	—
Staron et al. 1991	F	DCER (vertical leg press)	18 (8 wk, 1 wk off, 10 wk)	2	3 × 6- to 8RM	148	—	—
Wilmore et al. 1978	F	DCER	10	3	40-55% of 1RM for 30 s	27	—	—
Allen, Byrd, and Smith 1976	M	DCER	12	3	2 × 8 1 × exhaustion	71[b]	—	—
Coleman 1977	M	DCER	10	3	2 × 8- to 10RM	17	—	—
Dudley et al. 1991	M	DCER	19	2	4-5 × 6- to 12RM	26	—	—
Gettman et al. 1978	M	DCER	20	3	50% 1RM, 6 wk = 2 × 10-20 14 wk = 2 × 15	—	IK	43
Pipes 1978	M	DCER	10	3	3 × 8	29	VR	8
Sale et al. 1990	M and F	DCER	11 (3 wk off), 11 more, total 22	3	6 × 15- to 20RM (one-legged training)	30	—	—
Tatro, Dudley, and Convertino 1992	M	DCER	19	2	7 wk = 4 × 10- to 12RM 6 wk = 5 × 8- to 10RM 6 wk = 5 × 6- to 8RM	25 (3RM)	—	—
Wilmore et al. 1978	M	DCER	10	3	40-55% of 1RM for 30 s	7	—	—
Rhea et al. 2002	M	DCER	12	3	DNLP 1 × 8- to 10RM 1 × 6- to 8RM 1 × 4- to 6RM each 1 day/wk	26	—	—

Reference	Sex of subjects	Type of training	Training duration (wk)	Training days/ week	Sets and repetitions	% increase for equipment trained on	Comparative type of equipment	Comparative test % increase
Rhea et al. 2002	M	DCER	12	3	DNLP 1 × 8- to 10RM 3 × 6- to 8RM 3 × 4- to 6RM each 3 day/wk	56	—	—
Buford et al. 2007	M and F	DCER	9	3	LP 3 wk = 3 × 8 3 wk = 3 × 6 3 wk = 3 × 4	85	—	—
Buford et al. 2007	M and F	DCER	9	3	DNLP 3 × 8 3 × 6 3 × 4 each 1 day/wk	79	—	—
Kerksick et al. 2009	M	DCER	8	4	4 wk = 3 × 10 4 wk = 3 × 8	9	—	—
Coleman 1977	M	VR	10	3	1 × 10- to 12RM	—	DCER	18
Gettman, Culter, and Strathman 1980	M	VR	20	3	3 × 8	18[c]	IK	17
Lee et al. 1990	M	VR	10	3	3 × 10RM	6	—	—
Pipes 1978	M	VR	10	3	3 × 8	27	DCER	8
Smith and Melton 1981	M	VR	6	4	3 × 10	—	VR[d]	11
Fleck, Mattie, and Martensen 2006	F	VVR	14	3	3 × 10RM	31	—	—
Cordova et al. 1995	F	IK	5	3	2 × 10 at 60, 180, and 240 deg/s	64	—	—
Gettman et al. 1979	M	IK	8	3	4 wk = 1 × 10 at 60 deg/s 4 wk = 1 × 15 at 90 deg/s	38	DCER	18
Gettman, Culter, and Strathman 1980	M	IK	20	3	2 × 12 at 60 deg/s	42	VR	10
Smith and Melton 1981	M	IK	6	4	Sets to 50% exhaustion at 30, 60, and 90 deg/s	—	VR	10
Smith and Melton 1981	M	IK	6	4	Sets to 50% fatigue at 180, 240, and 300 deg/s	—	VR	7

DCER = dynamic constant external resistance; IK = isokinetic; DNLP = daily nonlinear periodization; LP = linear periodization; VR = variable resistance; VVR = variable variable resistance; RM = repetition maximum; a = values for 10RM; b = values for average training weights; c = values for number of weight plates; d = different type of VR equipment.

1994). Trainees in both programs performed the same exercises and numbers of sets and repetitions per exercise. However, those in the total-body program performed all upper- and lower-body exercises in two training sessions per week, whereas those in the split program performed all of the upper-body exercises two days per week and the lower-body exercises on two other days per week resulting in four training sessions per week. Total training volume was not different between the programs, but training frequency was different (unless it is defined as the total number of training sessions performed per week). The two training programs showed no difference in strength gains during the 10 weeks of training. Additionally, the importance of total training volume when examining training frequency is apparent from a comparison of training untrained people two days per week with three sets of each exercise or three days per week with two sets of each exercise for six weeks; no significant difference in 1RM bench press and squat ability or body composition (DEXA) was noted. Training volume was equal (six sets per week of each exercise) in this comparison (Candow and Burke 2007).

The optimal training frequency may be different for different muscle groups. The American College of Sports Medicine recommends a training frequency of two or three sessions per week for major muscle groups (2011). However, comparisons of training frequency for the bench press and squat concluded that three sessions resulted in greater strength increases than one or two sessions (Berger 1962a; Faigenbaum and Pollock 1997). Graves and colleagues (1990) concluded that one session was equally as effective as two or three sessions per week when training for isolated lumbar extension strength. DeMichele and colleagues (1997) found that two sessions per week was equivalent to

three and superior to one when training for torso rotation. These studies indicate that a frequency of three sessions per week is superior to one or two sessions per week when training arm and leg musculature, whereas a frequency of one or two sessions per week results in equivalent gains compared to three sessions per week when training lumbar extension or torso rotation.

In a comparison of varying self-selected training frequencies among collegiate American football players using various body-part training programs over 10 weeks of training (see table 2.5), 1RM bench press ability significantly increased only in the five-sessions-per-week group (Hoffman et al. 1990), and 1RM squat ability significantly increased in the four-, five-, and six-sessions-per-week groups. All training frequencies did result in gains in bench press (2-4%) and squat (5-8%) ability. Examining all of the tests (vertical jump, sum of skinfolds, 2 mi [3.2 km] run, 40 yd sprint, thigh circumference, and chest circumference) pre- and posttraining, the researchers concluded that a frequency of four or five sessions per week results in the greatest overall fitness gains. Note, however, that each muscle group was trained only two or four times per week.

Table 2.6 presents two studies of training frequency. One study (Gillam 1981) compared from one to five training sessions per week. All groups performed a large number of very intense sets (18 sets of 1RM) per training session. Five sessions were shown to be superior in causing increases in 1RM bench press ability compared to the other training frequencies. Additionally, five and three sessions per week showed significantly greater increases than two or one session per week. A study comparing training frequencies of four and three sessions reported significantly greater gains in both sexes with more frequent training sessions (Hunter

TABLE 2.5 **Resistance Training Programs With Three to Six Sessions per Week**

Frequency	Training days	Body parts trained
3	Mon., Wed., Fri.	Total body
4	Mon., Thurs. Tues., Fri.	Chest, shoulders, triceps, neck Legs, back, biceps, forearms
5	Mon., Wed., Fri. Tues., Thurs.	Chest, triceps, legs, neck Back, shoulders, biceps, forearms
6	Mon., Tues., Thurs., Fri. Wed., Sat.	Chest, triceps, legs, shoulders, neck Back, biceps, forearms

Adapted, by permission, from J.R. Hoffman et al., 1990, "The effects of self-selection for frequency of training in a winter conditioning program for football," *Journal of Applied Sport Science Research* 4: 76-82.

1985). Both groups performed all exercises using a 7- to 10RM resistance; the three-sessions-per-week group performing three sets of each exercise per session, and the four-sessions-per-week group performing two sets of each exercise three days per week and three sets one day per week. Thus, total training sets were equivalent between the two groups. Interestingly, the four-sessions-per-week subjects trained two consecutive days twice a week (i.e., Monday and Tuesday, and Thursday and Friday), whereas the three-sessions-per-week subjects trained in the traditional alternate-day method (i.e., Monday, Wednesday, Friday). Results indicate that the necessity of the traditional one day of rest between weight training sessions may not apply to all muscle groups.

Meta-analyses (see box 2.2) of studies in which the majority of subjects trained using DCER concluded that a training frequency of three days per week per muscle group is optimal for untrained people, whereas a frequency of two days per week per muscle group is optimal for recreationally trained nonathletes and trained athletes (Peterson, Rhea, and Alvar 2004, 2005; Rhea et al. 2003). The difference in optimal training frequencies may be due to the higher training volumes used in the studies with trained subjects (Rhea et al. 2003). The results indicate that optimal training frequency may vary with training status and training volume.

Many of the aforementioned studies have design limitations: The majority used beginning resistance exercisers (novice subjects) and examined short training durations (up to 12 weeks), and some studies did not equate the total number of sets and repetitions performed by the various training groups. However, based on the available information, to improve strength, hypertrophy, or local muscular endurance training with DCER, novice trainees should use a total-body program two or three days per week, intermediate trainees

TABLE 2.6 Effect of Training Frequency on 1RM Bench Press

Reference	Sex	Days per week of training and % improvement
Gillam 1981	M	Days 1, 2, 3, 4, 5 % improvement 19, 24, 32⁺, 29, 41*
Hunter 1985	M	Days 3, 4 % improvement 12, 17^
Hunter 1985	F	Days 3, 4 % improvement 20, 33^

* = significantly greater than all other frequencies; + = significantly greater than frequencies 1 and 2; ^ = significantly greater than frequency 3.

BOX 2.2 PRACTICAL QUESTION

What Is a Meta-Analysis?

A meta-analysis is a statistical method to quantitatively analyze the results of a group of studies concerning the same general question (Rhea 2004)—for example, does the number of repetitions per set affect strength and body composition changes, or does training frequency per week affect strength gains? The basic calculation used in a meta-analysis is effect size, which is a measure of the magnitude of change shown between two time points, such as from pre- to posttesting. There are multiple ways to compute the effect size of a study. For example, the effect size for the change in a single group can be calculated as the posttraining mean minus the pretraining mean divided by the pretraining standard deviation. The effect size comparing two groups can be calculated as the posttraining mean of the treatment group minus the posttraining mean of the control group divided by the pretraining standard deviation of the control group. The pretraining standard deviation is used in both calculations because it is unbiased.

Rhea, M.R. 2004. Synthesizing strength and conditioning research: The meta-analysis. *Journal of Strength and Conditioning Research* 18: 921-923.

should use a total-body program three days per week or a split-body routine four days per week, and advanced lifters should train four to six days per week with a variety of split routines to train one to three muscle groups per session (American College of Sports Medicine 2009).

Motor Performance

It has long been known that DCER exercise can increase motor performance. Studies show significant small increases of several percent or less in the following motor performance tests:

- Vertical jump ability (Adams et al. 1992; Campbell 1962; Caruso et al. 2008; Channel and Barfield 2008; Dodd and Alvar 2007; Kraemer et al. 2000; Kraemer, Mazzetti et al. 2001; Kraemer et al. 2003; Marx et al. 2001; Stone, Johnson, and Carter 1979; Stone, O'Bryant, and Garhammer 1981; Taube et al. 2007)

- Standing long jump (Capen 1950; Chu 1950; Dodd and Alvar 2007; Taube et al. 2007)

- Shuttle run (Campbell 1962; Kusintz and Kenney 1958)

- T-agility test (Cressey et al. 2007)

- Short sprint (Capen 1950; Comfort, Haigh, and Matthews 2012; Deane et al. 2005; Dodd and Alvar 2007; Marx et al. 2001; Schultz 1967)

- Baseball throwing velocity (Thompson and Martin 1965)

- Soccer kick and ball velocity (Young and Rath 2011)

- Shot put (Chu 1950; Schultz 1967; Terzis et al. 2008)

Statistically insignificant changes in short sprint time (Chu 1950; Dodd and Alvar 2007; Hoffman et al. 1990; Jullian et al. 2008; Kraemer et al. 2003; Marx et al. 2001) and in vertical jump ability (Hoffman et al. 1990; Marx et al. 2001; Newton, Kraemer, and Häkkinen 1999; Stone, Nelson et al. 1983) and standing long jump ability (Schultz 1967) have also been demonstrated. Perhaps more important from a training perspective, significant increases in softball throwing velocity (Prokopy et al. 2008); team handball throwing velocity, vertical jump ability, and short sprint ability (Marques and Gonzalez-Badillo 2006); tennis serve, forehand, and backhand ball velocity (Kraemer, Ratamess et al. 2000 Kraemer, Häkkinen et al. 2003); and vertical jump ability have been shown when weight training is incorporated into a total training program (sprint, aerobic, agility, plyometrics; see box 2.3). No significant changes were shown when weight training was incorporated into a total training program for athletes (rugby, basketball)

BOX 2.3 RESEARCH

Effects of Resistance Training on Motor Performance

The degree of change in motor performance that occurs in athletes as a result of resistance training is highly variable. Significant changes and nonsignificant changes have been shown in a variety of motor performance tasks when athletes perform weight training in addition to their normal training. How much of a change, if any, depends on a wide variety of factors including the type of weight training program and the specific motor performance task.

In professional team handball players, performance of a 12-week in-season resistance training program increased motor performance and strength (Marques and Gonzalez-Badillo 2006). The program was a multiple-set periodized program performed two or three times per week in addition to sprint, plyometric, and normal skill and technique training. The program resulted in a significant increase in ball-throwing velocity of 6%, in 30 m sprint ability of 3%, and in countermovement jump ability of 13%. Although these changes were significant, they were substantially lower than the significant change in 1RM bench press ability of 27%. This is not unusual given that changes in strength are generally substantially greater than changes in motor performance when resistance training is performed.

Marques, M.C., and Gonzalez-Badillo, J.J. 2006. In-season resistance training and detraining in professional team handball players. *Journal of Strength and Conditioning Research* 20: 563-571.

in short-range (less than 6.25 m) and long-range (more than 6.25 m) basketball shooting ability, vertical jump, and short sprint ability (Gabbett, Johns, and Riemann 2008; Kilinc 2008). Significant changes in job-related motor performance tasks such as a 1RM lift and repetitive box lift have also been demonstrated (Kraemer, Mazzetti et al. 2001).

Similar to strength increases, changes in motor performance tests depend in part on the initial physical condition of the trainee, with smaller increases apparent with better initial physical fitness. Past training history, the type of weight training program, and the duration of training may also affect whether a change in motor performance occurs. The effect of the type of program on a motor performance task is shown by the following examples. Untrained women's vertical jump power and 40 yd sprint ability improved significantly more during six months of training with a multiple-set periodized program compared to a single-set-to-momentary-fatigue program (Marx et al. 2001). Similar results over nine months of training women collegiate tennis athletes have been shown: Vertical jump height and tennis serve velocity showed significant improvements with a multiple-set periodized program and no improvement with a single-set-to-momentary-fatigue program (Kraemer, Ratamess et al. 2000). Over nine months of training (Kraemer et al. 2003) women collegiate tennis athletes performing a multiple-set periodized program and a multiple-set nonperiodized program increased maximal strength similarly. However, the periodized program resulted in significantly greater increases in vertical jump, as well as serve, forehand, and backhand ball velocity. Thus, the type of program can affect whether significant increases in motor performance occur and the magnitude of those increases.

Other program variables may also affect the outcome on motor performance. For example, after weight training for five weeks with 20-second rest periods between sets (15- to 20RM), subjects experienced a significantly greater increase (12.5 vs. 5.4%) in repeat cycle sprint ability than did those training with 80-second rest periods (Hill-Hass et al. 2007). However, greater strength increases (3RM 45.9 vs. 19.6%) occurred in those taking the 80-second rest periods than did those taking the 20-second rest periods. Although conflicting results concerning significant changes in motor performance can be found, as a whole, research

supports the contention that DCER exercise can significantly improve motor performance ability.

Training smaller muscle groups may also affect motor performance. For example, significant increases in vertical jump and shot put ability occurred in college-age subjects after training only the toe and finger flexors over a 12-week period (Kokkonen et al. 1988). Dynamic resistance training of the finger flexors also increases rock climbing performance (Schweizer, Schneider, and Goehner 2007).

Many people assume that an increase in strength and power brought about by a training program can be usefully applied to a motor performance task. For this to occur, however, trainees must train all of the muscles involved in the motor performance task, especially the weakest muscles involved in the task, because they may limit the useful application of the strength and power from stronger muscle groups. Additionally, proper technique of the motor task must be trained, because technique may also limit the useful application of increased strength and power. This last point is supported by projects showing that direct practice, alone or combined with resistance training, increases standing long jump ability to a significantly greater extent than resistance training alone in previously untrained subjects (Schultz 1967), and strength training combined with sprint training results in greater changes in sprinting speed than either type of training alone (Delecluse et al. 1997).

Strength Changes

Strength increases in a large variety of muscle groups in both women and men from DCER training are well documented. Tables 2.3, 2.4, and 2.6 present changes in 1RM bench press and leg press ability in both sexes after short-term DCER training. Women demonstrate substantial increases in 1RM bench press ability; increases range from 8% in college tennis athletes after 36 weeks of training (Kraemer et al. 2000) to 47% in untrained women after 16 weeks of training (Hostler, Crill et al. 2001). Similarly, men experience strength increases ranging from 3% in college American football players after 10 weeks of training (Hoffman et al. 1990) to 44% in untrained men after 12 weeks of training (Allen, Byrd, and Smith 1976). Using 1RM as the testing criteria, women have demonstrated increases in leg press ability ranging from 8% in college tennis players after 36 weeks of training (Kraemer et al. 2000) to 148% in untrained women after 18 weeks of training (Staron et al. 1991). Increases in men's leg press ability range from 7% after 6 weeks of training (Stone, Nelson, et al. 1983) to 71% after 10 weeks of training (Allen, Byrd, and Smith 1976). The wide ranges in strength increases are probably related to differences in pretraining status, familiarity with the exercise tests, the duration of training, and the type of program.

Body Composition Changes

The normal changes in body composition as a result of short-term DCER exercise in both sexes are small increases in fat-free mass and small decreases in percent body fat (see table 3.3). The decrease in percent body fat is often due in large part to an increase in fat-free mass rather than a large decrease in fat mass. Many times these two changes occur simultaneously, resulting in little or no change in total body weight.

Safety Considerations

If DCER exercise is performed using free weights, appropriate spotting should be used. For machine DCER exercises, spotting is normally not needed. Because free weights must be controlled in three planes of movement, generally more time is needed to learn proper lifting technique, especially of multijoint or multi-muscle-group exercises, compared to a similar exercise performed using a machine.

Variable Resistance Training

Variable resistance equipment has a lever arm, cam, or pulley arrangement that varies the resistance throughout the exercise's range of motion. One possible advantage of variable resistance equipment is that it can match the increases and decreases in strength (strength curve) throughout an exercise's range of motion. This could result in the muscle exerting near-maximal or maximal force throughout the range of motion, resulting in maximal strength gains.

The three major types of strength curves are ascending, descending, and bell shaped (see figure 2.3). Although the ascending and descending strength curves shown in figure 2.3 are linear, generally they are curvilinear. In exercises such as the squat and bench press, which have an ascending strength curve, it is possible to lift more weight if

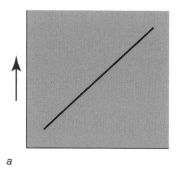

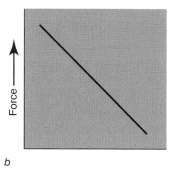

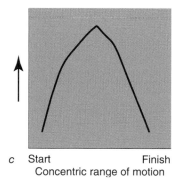

FIGURE 2.3 The three major types of strength curves are *(a)* ascending, *(b)* descending, and *(c)* bell shaped.

only the last half or last quarter of the concentric portion of a repetition is performed. If an exercise has a descending strength curve, it is possible to lift more weight if only the first half or first quarter of the concentric repetition phase is performed. An example of such an exercise is upright rowing. An exercise in which it is possible to lift more resistance if only the middle portion of the range of motion is performed has a bell-shaped strength curve. Arm curls, like many single-joint exercises, have a bell-shaped strength curve. To match the three major types of strength curves, variable resistance machines must be able to vary the resistance in three major patterns, which most types are not capable of doing (see the section Variable Variable Resistance later in this chapter). Additionally, because of variations in limb length, the point of attachment of the muscle's tendons to the bones, and torso size, it is difficult to conceive of one mechanical arrangement that would match all people's strength curves for a particular exercise.

Biomechanical research indicates that one type of cam variable resistance equipment does not match the strength curves of the elbow curl, multibiceps curl, chest fly, knee extension, knee flexion, and pullover exercises (Cabell and Zebras 1999; Harman 1983; Pizzimenti 1992). The equipment's ability to match the strength curve is especially ineffective at the extreme ranges of an exercise's range of motion (Cabell and Zebras 1999). A second type of cam equipment has been reported to match the strength curves of females fairly well (Johnson, Colodny, and Jackson 1990). However, for females the cam resulted in too great a resistance near the end of the knee extension exercise. The cam also provided too much resistance during the first half and too little during the second half of the elbow flexion and elbow extension exercises. The knee flexion machine matched females' strength curves well throughout the range of motion. The resistance curve of eight variable resistance knee extension machines from six manufacturers also poorly matched the strength curve of young men; the matching of the strength curve was highly variable from machine to machine and significantly less curvilinear than the actual isometric strength curve (Folland and Morris 2008). Thus, in general cam-type variable resistance equipment does not appear to match strength curves of exercises.

Number of Sets and Repetitions

Significant strength gains from short-term (4 to 18 weeks) variable resistance training have been demonstrated in a large variety of muscle groups with various combinations of sets and repetitions. Significant increases in strength have been shown with the following protocols (sets × repetitions):

- 1 × 6- to 10RM (Jacobson 1986)
- 1 × 7- to 10RM (Braith et al. 1993; Graves et al. 1989)
- 1 × 8- to 12RM (Coleman 1977; Hurley, Seals, Ehsani et al. 1984; Keeler et al. 2001;

Manning et al. 1990; Pollock et al. 1993; Silvester et al. 1984; Starkey et al. 1996; Westcott et al. 2001)
- 1 × 10- to 12RM (Peterson 1975)
- 1 × 12- to 15RM (Stone, Johnson, and Carter 1979)
- 2 × 10- to 12RM (Coleman 1977)
- 2 × 12 at 50% of 1RM (Gettman, Culter, and Strathman 1980)
- 2 or 3 × 8- to 10RM (LeMura et al. 2000)
- 3 × 6RM (Jacobson 1986; Silvester et al. 1984)
- 3 × 8- to 12RM (Starkey et al. 1996)
- 3 × 15RM (Hunter and Culpepper 1995)
- 6 × 15- to 20RM (Sale et al. 1990)
- 3 × 10RM for three weeks, 3 × 8RM for three weeks, and 3 × 6RM for six weeks (Boyer 1990)
- Four sets with increasing resistance and repetitions decreasing from eight to three in a half-pyramid program (Ariel 1977)

Variable resistance training has also been shown to increase maximal isometric strength throughout the full range of motion of an exercise (Hunter and Culpepper 1995). Thus, various combinations of sets and repetitions can cause significant strength increases.

Strength Changes

Substantial increases in strength have been demonstrated with variable resistance training. For example, after 16 weeks of training males demonstrated an increase of 50% in upper-body strength and 33% in lower-body strength (Hurley, Seals, Ehsani et al. 1984), and females demonstrated an increase of 29% in upper-body strength and 38% in lower-body strength (LeMura et al. 2000). Increases in bench press and leg press strength from variable resistance training are depicted in tables 2.3 and 2.4, respectively. Tests using variable resistance equipment and other types of muscle actions reveal that this type of resistance training can cause substantial increases in strength.

Variable Variable Resistance

One type of variable resistance equipment allows adjustment of the resistance curve of an exercise. **Variable variable resistance** equipment allows an exercise to be performed with an ascending, descending, and bell-shaped strength curves (see figure 2.4). The concept of this type of equipment is to force muscles to use more motor units at different points in the exercise's range of motion by using strength curves that do not match the strength curve of the exercise (e.g., using a bell-shaped and descending curve in addition to an ascending curve in an exercise that has an ascending strength curve). This type of equipment also offers the ability to decrease the force needed in a portion of an exercise's range of motion in which high force output is contraindicated, such as after some types of injuries. Women performing a total-body training program for 14 weeks of three sessions per week showed significant increases in 1RM strength and increased (dual-energy X-ray absorptiometry) lean soft tissue (see table 3.3) and decreased percent fat (Fleck, Mattie, and Martensen 2006). Training consisted of performing one set of 10 repetitions for each of the strength curves (bell-shaped, ascending, and descending) resulting in three sets of each exercise. Their 1RM strength increased significantly (between 25 and 30%) in the leg press, bench press, lat pull-down, and overhead press. Thus, this type of equipment

is effective in increasing strength and promoting body composition changes.

Motor Performance

Little information exists concerning changes in motor performance as a result of variable resistance training. American football players who participated in a combined program of in-season football training and total-body variable resistance strength training demonstrated small but greater mean improvements in the 40 yd sprint and vertical jump ability than a control group performing only the in-season football training program (Peterson 1975). Whether the changes were statistically significant or whether a significant difference existed between the groups was not addressed. Although this study showed a slightly greater increase in motor performance with variable resistance training, it offers little concrete evidence of variable resistance training effectiveness in terms of motor performance changes relative to other types of training.

A comparison of a cam-type variable resistance machine and an increasing lever arm–type variable resistance machine showed both types of equipment to increase motor performance (Silvester et

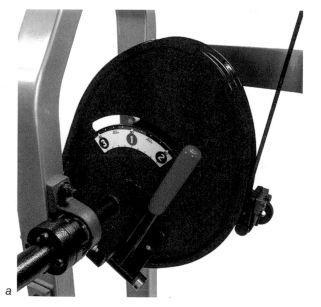

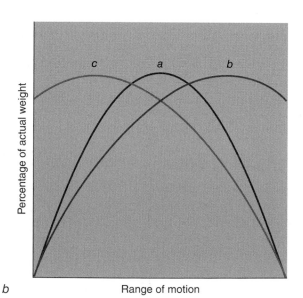

FIGURE 2.4 Variable variable resistance allows the strength curve of an exercise to be varied. (*a*) The handle on variable variable resistance machines rotates the starting position of the cam allowing switching among the three major types of strength curves. (*b*) The three major types of strength curves produced by moving the handle are the (*a*) bell-shaped, (*b*) ascending, and (*c*) descending curves.

Courtesy of Strive Fitness Inc., Cannonsburg, PA.

al. 1984). The cam-type group trained three days per week for six weeks followed by two days per week for five weeks. Participants did knee extensions immediately followed by leg presses and performed each exercise for one set of 12 repetitions to failure. The increasing lever arm–type group trained three days per week for the entire 11-week training period; they performed the leg press for one set of 7 to 10 repetitions followed by one set to concentric failure. No difference in static leg strength gains was demonstrated between the groups. The cam-type and lever arm–type groups increased their mean vertical jumps by 0.3 in. (0.76 cm) and 1.1 in. (2.8 cm), respectively. The increase in vertical jump shown by the lever arm–type group was significantly greater than the increase shown by the cam-type group. So motor performance can increase as a result of variable resistance training, and the increase depends in part on the training protocol, equipment used, or both.

Body Composition Changes

Significant increases in muscle thickness of the quadriceps and knee flexors (hamstrings) have been reported after variable resistance training (Starkey et al. 1996). Increases in fat-free mass and decreases in percent body fat also occur as a result of variable variable resistance training (Fleck, Mattie, and Martensen 2006). These changes in body composition are depicted in table 3.3 and are of the same magnitude as the changes that occur from DCER training.

Safety Considerations

As with all types of weight training machines, safety is not a major concern when using variable resistance or variable variable resistance machines, and a spotter is not normally necessary. Similarly, as with all weight training machines, care must be taken to ensure that the variable resistance machine fits the trainee properly and that the trainee is properly positioned on it. Without proper fit and positioning, proper exercise technique is impossible and risk of injury increases.

Isokinetic Training

Isokinetic refers to a muscular action performed at constant angular limb velocity. Unlike other types of resistance training, isokinetic training has no specified resistance to meet; rather, the velocity of movement is controlled. At the start of each movement, acceleration from 0 degrees per second takes place until the set velocity is achieved. After the set velocity is achieved, further acceleration is not possible and any force applied against the equipment results in an equal reaction force. The reaction force mirrors the force applied to the equipment throughout the range of movement of the exercise, until deceleration starts to occur at the end of the range of motion. It is theoretically possible for the muscle(s) to exert a continual maximal force throughout the movement's range of motion except where acceleration at the start and deceleration at the end of the movement occurs.

The majority of isokinetic equipment found in resistance training facilities allows concentric-only actions, although eccentric and coupled concentric–eccentric isokinetic actions (i.e., the same exercise movement performed in a concentric followed by an eccentric action) are possible on some isokinetic equipment. The emphasis here will be on concentric-only isokinetic training. Advantages of isokinetic training include the ability to exert maximal force throughout a large portion of an exercise's range of motion, the ability to train over a wide range of movement velocities, and minimal muscle and joint soreness. Another characteristic of many types of isokinetic equipment is that they allow only single-joint movements (knee extension, elbow flexion) in unilateral (one leg or arm) as opposed to bilateral (both arms or legs) actions. One major criticism of this type of training is that isokinetic muscle actions do not exist in the real world; this potentially limits the application of isokinetic training to daily life and sport activities.

Strength Changes

The vast majority of studies examining concentric-only isokinetic training have been of short duration (3 to 16 weeks); have examined strength changes of single-joint movements; and have tested for strength gains using isometric, DCER, eccentric-only isokinetic, and concentric-only isokinetic tests. As depicted in table 2.7, programs of 1 to 15 sets at various movement velocities and with various numbers of repetitions and sets cause significant increases in strength.

Significant gains in strength have also been achieved by performing as many repetitions as possible in a fixed period of time, as shown in the following studies:

TABLE 2.7 Isokinetic Training and Combinations of Sets and Repetitions That Cause Significant Gains in Strength

Reference	Sets × reps at degrees per second
Bond et al. 1996	1 × 12 at 15
Gur et al. 2002	1 × 12 at 30, 60, 90, 120, 150 and 180
Jenkins, Thackaberry, and Killian 1984	1 × 15 at 60 1 × 15 at 240
Lacerte et al. 1992	1 × 20 at 60 1 × 20 at 180
Moffroid et al. 1969	1 × 30 at 22.5
Knapik, Mawdsley, and Ramos 1983	1 × 50 at 30
Pearson and Costill 1988	1 × 65 at 120
Gettman, Culter, and Strathman 1980	2 × 12 at 60
Gettman et al. 1979	2 × 10 at 60 followed by 2 × 15 at 90
Farthing and Chilibeck 2003	2-6 × 8 at 30 2-6 × 8 at 180
Kelly et al. 2007	3 × 8 at 60
Higbie et al. 1996	3 × 10 at 60
Ewing et al. 1990	3 × 8 at 60 3 × 20 at 240
Tomberline et al. 1991	3 × 10 at 100
Morris, Tolfroy, and Coppack 2001	3 × 10 at 100
Gettman and Ayers 1978	3 × 15 at 90 3 × 15 at 60
Kanehisa and Miyashita 1983b	1 × 10 at 60 1 × 30 at 179 1 × 50 at 300
Blazevich et al. 2007	4-6 × 6 at 30
Seger, Arvidsson, and Thorstensson 1998	4 × 10 at 90
Colliander and Tesch 1990a	4 or 5 × 12 at 60
Coyle et al. 1981	5 × 6 at 60 5 × 12 at 300
Coyle et al. 1981	(6 sets total) 3 × 6 at 60 and 3 × 12 at 300
Cirello, Holden, and Evans 1983	5 × 5 at 60
Petersen et al. 1990	5 × 10 at 120
Mannion, Jakeman, and Willan 1992	6 × 25 at 240 5 × 15 at 60
Housh et al. 1992	6 × 10 at 120
Narici et al. 1989	6 × 10 at 120
Akima et al. 1999	10 × 5 at 120
Kovaleski et al. 1995	10 × 12 at 120 to 210
Cirello, Holden, and Evans 1983	5 × 5 at 60 15 × 10 at 60

- One set of 6 seconds at 180 degrees per second (Lesmes et al. 1978)
- One set of 30 seconds at 180 degrees per second (Lesmes et al. 1978)
- Two sets of 20 seconds at 180 degrees per second (Bell et al. 1992; Petersen et al. 1987)
- Two sets of 30 seconds at 60 degrees per second (Bell et al. 1991a)
- Two sets of 30 seconds at 120 or 300 degrees per second (Bell et al. 1989)
- One set of 60 seconds at 36 or 180 degrees per second (Seaborne and Taylor 1984)

Increases in strength have also been achieved by performing a set of maximal voluntary muscle actions until a given percentage of peak force could no longer be generated. One set continued until at least 60, 75, or 90% of peak force could no longer be generated at each velocity of 30, 60, and 90 degrees per second (Fleck et al. 1982) and until 50% of peak force could no longer be maintained during slow-speed training (one set each at a velocity of 30, 60, and 90 degrees per second) or fast-speed training (one set each at a velocity of 180, 240, and 300 degrees per second) (Smith and Melton 1981). All resulted in significant increases in strength.

Isokinetic **velocity spectrum training** has also resulted in significant strength gains. This type of training involves performing several sets in succession at various movement velocities. Velocity spectrum training can be performed with either the faster velocities or the slower velocities performed first. A typical fast-velocity spectrum exercise protocol is presented in table 2.8. A series of acute and short-duration (four-week) training studies (Kovaleski and Heitman 1993a, 1993b; Kovaleski et al. 1992) indicates that training protocols in which the fast-velocity sets are performed first result in greater power gains, especially at faster movement velocities, but not necessarily greater maximal torque gains across a range of movement velocities compared to protocols in which the slower movement velocities are performed first.

Velocity spectrum training (30 to 180 degrees per second at 30 degree per second intervals) in 41- to 75-year-olds resulted in significant concentric peak torque gains at 120 and 180 degrees per second, but not 60 degrees per second (Gur et al. 2002). The concentric velocity spectrum training also resulted in significant eccentric peak torque gains at 120 degrees per second, but not 60 and 180 degrees per second. Tables 2.3 and 2.4 include changes in strength of the bench press and leg press, respectively, after isokinetic training. Apparently, many combinations of sets, repetitions, and velocity of concentric-only isokinetic training can cause significant increases in strength.

Concentric-only isokinetic training can increase eccentric isokinetic strength (Blazevich et al. 2007; Seger, Arvidsson, and Thorstensson 1998; Tomberline et al. 1991). Although fewer studies have examined the effect of eccentric-only versus concentric-only isokinetic training, it is clear that both types of training can increase concentric and eccentric isokinetic strength (Blazevich et al. 2007; Higbie et al. 1996; Miller et al. 2006; Seger, Arvidsson, and Thorstensson 1998) at relatively slow velocities of 30 to 90 degrees per second. The majority of these studies indicate **contraction specificity;** in other words, the concentric training resulted in greater concentric strength gains, and vice versa. For example, concentric-only and eccentric-only training (knee extension, 90 degrees per second) have both been shown to increase concentric (14 vs. 2%) and eccentric (10 vs. 18%) strength significantly at the training velocity (Seger, Arvidsson, and Thorstensson 1998). Not all studies, however, consistently indicate a large contraction specificity (Blazevich et al. 2007).

Coupled eccentric–concentric isokinetic training (a movement performed in a concentric action followed by an eccentric action) also results in significant eccentric and concentric isokinetic strength gains (Caruso et al. 1997; Gur et al. 2002). Collectively, the preceding studies indicate that eccentric-only, concentric-only, and coupled eccentric–concentric isokinetic training result in significant eccentric and concentric isokinetic strength gains, and that eccentric-only and concentric-only training generally show contraction specificity.

TABLE 2.8 Typical Isokinetic Fast-Velocity Spectrum Training

Set	1	2	3	4	5	6	7	8	9	10
Velocity (degrees per second)	180	210	240	270	300	300	270	240	210	180
Reps	10	10	10	10	10	10	10	10	10	10

Number of Sets and Repetitions

Despite the vast quantity of research concerning the training effects of concentric-only isokinetic training, few studies have investigated the optimal training number of sets and repetitions. No difference in peak torque gains when training at 180 degrees per second between 10 sets of 6-second duration with as many repetitions as possible (approximately three), and two sets of 30-second duration with as many repetitions as possible (approximately 10) has been shown (Lesmes et al. 1978). A comparison of all combinations of 5, 10, and 15 repetitions at slow, intermediate, and fast velocities of movement showed no significant strength differences after training three days a week for nine weeks (Davies 1977). A comparison of 5 sets of 5 repetitions and 15 sets of 10 repetitions training at 60 degrees per second showed minimal differences (Cirello, Holden, and Evans 1983). Both groups improved strength significantly at all concentric test velocities ranging from 0 to 300 degrees per second; only one significant difference existed between the two groups: at 30 degrees per second the 15-set group showed greater gains than the 5-set group did. All three of these studies agree on at least one point: various numbers of repetitions per set and sets can result in significant increases in peak torque over short training durations. Additionally, three sets (60 degrees per second) result in significantly greater strength increases than one set at the same velocity (17 vs. 2%) when peak torque is tested at the training velocity (Kelly et al. 2007). Thus, similar to DCER training, multiple sets appear to result in significantly greater strength increases than one set.

Training Velocity

Previously cited studies firmly support the contention that concentric-only, eccentric-only, and coupled eccentric–concentric isokinetic training at a variety of velocities can result in increased strength. One question that has received some research attention is, What is the optimal concentric isokinetic training velocity—fast or slow? It is important to note that the answer may depend on the task the training is meant to improve. If strength at a slow velocity of movement is necessary for success, the optimal training velocity may be different from that for a task in which strength at a fast velocity of movement is necessary for success.

The question of optimal training velocity for concentric-only isokinetic training depends in part on the issue of velocity specificity, which states that strength increases due to training at a certain velocity are greatest at that velocity. The majority of research indicates that isokinetic training does have velocity specificity (Behm and Sale 1993), and that this specificity occurs even after very short (three sessions) training periods (Coburn et al. 2006). This means that greater strength gains are made at or near the training velocity; therefore, if strength at a fast velocity of movement is necessary, training should be performed at a fast velocity, and vice versa. Neural mechanisms, such as the selective activation of motor units, the selective activation of muscles, and the deactivation of co-contractions by antagonists, are generally believed to be the cause of velocity specificity (Behm and Sale 1993).

Other issues of optimal training velocity are to what extent velocity specificity exists and whether training at one velocity results in increased strength over a wide range of movement velocities. An early study indicated that two training velocities demonstrated some degree of velocity specificity (Moffroid and Whipple 1970). However, the faster training velocity demonstrated velocity specificity to a smaller extent and more consistent strength gains across the range of velocities at which strength was tested (see figure 2.5). It is important to note that both training velocities examined in this study were relatively slow. Another study showed that slow-speed training (four seconds to

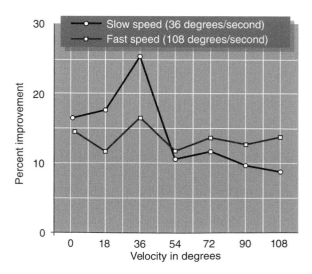

FIGURE 2.5 Percentage of change in peak torque due to slow- and fast-speed concentric-only isokinetic training.

Reprinted from M.T. Moffroid and R.H. Whipple, 1970, "Specificity of speed of exercise," *Physical Therapy* 50: 1695. ©1970 American Physical Therapy Association. Reprinted with permission.

complete one leg press repetition) resulted in a greater strength increase than fast-speed training (two seconds to complete one leg press repetition) (Oteghen 1975). However, the velocity at which strength was tested was undefined.

Several studies do provide more insight into the fast-versus-slow optimal concentric training velocity question. Training at velocities of 60, 179, and 300 degrees per second with 10, 30, and 50 maximal voluntary muscle actions per session, respectively, showed some advantage for the intermediate velocity (Kanehisa and Miyashita 1983b). All groups were tested for peak torque at a variety of velocities ranging from 60 to 300 degrees per second both before and after the training program. The varied number of repetitions at different training velocities limits general conclusions. However, the results indicate that an intermediate speed (179 degrees per second) may be the most advantageous for gains in average power across a range of movement velocities. Another study by Kanehisa and Miyashita (1983a) indicated velocity specific power gains after training at either 73 or 157 degrees per second.

Training at 60 and 240 degrees per second (Jenkins, Thackaberry, and Killian 1984) showed that peak torque of the 60-degrees-per-second group improved at all but the slowest and fastest velocities, whereas the 240-degree-per-second group improved significantly at all test velocities (see figure 2.6). No significant differences in

improvement between the two training groups were shown. However, because of the nonsignificant improvement at the 30-degrees-per-second and 300-degrees-per-second test velocities by the 60-degrees-per-second group, it could be concluded that the 240-degrees-per-second training resulted in superior overall strength gains.

A comparison of three velocities and with varying numbers of sets and repetitions indicates velocity specificity (Coyle et al. 1981). A slow-speed group trained at 60 degrees per second with five sets of six maximal muscular actions. A fast-speed group trained at 300 degrees per seconds with five sets of 12 maximal actions. A third group trained using a combination of slow and fast speeds, with two or three sets of six repetitions at 60 degrees per second and two or three sets of 12 repetitions at 300 degrees per second. Peak torque test results are presented in table 2.9. Each group showed its greatest gains at its specific training velocity, indicating that the velocity of training is in part dictated by the velocity at which peak torque increases are desired. However, substantial carryover to other velocities is also shown. This is especially apparent for velocities slower than the training velocity.

Some research suggests that there is little or no reason to favor a particular velocity when considering gains in strength. Training at 60 or 180 degrees per second results in equal gains in peak torque at 60, 120, 180, and 240 degrees per second (Bell et al. 1989; Lacerte et al. 1992). Additionally, training at 60 or 240 degrees per second results in equal isometric strength gains (Mannion, Jakeman, and

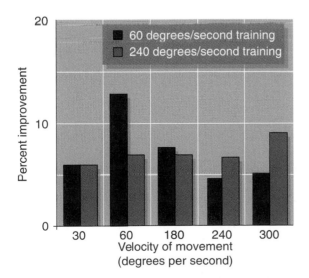

FIGURE 2.6 Percentage of change in peak torque with training at 60 degrees per second and 240 degrees per second.

Data from Jenkins, Thackaberry, and Killian 1984.

TABLE 2.9 **Percentage of Increases in Peak Torque Due to Isokinetic Training at Specific Velocities**

Testing velocity	Peak torque increases (%)		
PT/0	[Fast 23.6	Slow 20.3	Mixed] 18.9
PT/60	[Slow 31.8	Mixed 23.6	Fast] 15.1
PT/180	[Fast 16.8	Slow 9.2	Mixed] 7.9
PT/300	[Fast 18.5	Mixed] 16.1	Slow 0.9

PT/0-PT/300 = peak torque at 0 to 300 degrees per second; bracketed groups exhibit no statistically significant difference in peak torque.

Data from Coyle et al. 1981.

Willan 1992). All of these projects used a short training duration of no more than 16 weeks.

Collectively, the preceding studies indicate that, with concentric-only training, if gains in concentric strength over a wide range of velocities are desired, training should be at a velocity of somewhere between 180 and 240 degrees per second. Additionally, if the training goal is to maximally increase strength at a specific velocity, training should be performed at that velocity. However, because the majority of the studies used relatively slow training velocities in general, any comparisons between slow and fast speeds is in reality a comparison of two or more relatively slow concentric velocities. During many physical activities, angular limb velocities of greater than 300 degrees per second are easily achieved, making the application of conclusions to actual physical tasks tenuous.

Research concerning the optimal eccentric isokinetic training velocity is more limited. A study of two groups who trained eccentrically at 20 or 210 degrees per second revealed that overall strength gains at concentric and eccentric velocities of 20, 60, 120, 180 and 210 degrees per second were greater for those in the group that trained at 210 degrees per second (Shepstone et al. 2005). Similarly, training at 180 compared to 30 degrees per second resulted in greater overall strength gains at concentric and eccentric velocities of 30 and 180 degrees per second (Farthing and Chilibeck 2003). Both studies indicate that fast eccentric-only training results in greater strength gains than slow eccentric-only training does.

Velocity Specificity and Strength Carryover

Closely associated with the concept of velocity specificity is the question, To what extent do increases in strength carry over to velocities other than the training velocity? A previously discussed study (Moffroid and Whipple 1970) comparing concentric training at 36 and 108 degrees per second demonstrated that significant increases in peak torque carry over only at movement speeds below the training velocity (see figure 2.5). Similarly, a group that trained at 90 degrees per second demonstrated significant increases in peak torque at 90 and 30 degrees per second, but no significant increase in peak torque at 270 degrees per second (Seger, Arvidsson, and Thorstensson 1998). The

study illustrated in figure 2.6 indicates velocity specificity for slow (60 degrees per second) training and carryover below and above the training velocity, with less carryover as the velocity moves farther from the training velocity, while training at an intermediate velocity (240 degrees per second) results in carryover both below and above the training velocity. Another study testing concentric strength gains at 60 to 240 degrees per second (Ewing et al. 1990) suggests that there is carryover of peak torque gains at velocities above and below the training velocity. The carryover may be as great as 210 degrees per second below the training velocity and up to 180 degrees per second above the training velocity. Studies using training velocities of 60, 120, and 180 degrees per second indicate that significant gains in peak torque are made at all velocities from isometric to 240 degrees per second, but not necessarily at 300 degrees per second (Akima et al. 1999; Bell et al. 1989; Lacerte et al. 1992).

Collectively, the preceding studies indicate that significant gains in concentric peak torque may occur above and below the training velocity except when the training velocity is very slow (30 degrees per second) and that generally the greatest gains in strength are made at the training velocity. These studies all determined peak torque irrespective of the joint angle at which peak torque occurred. It might be questioned whether the torque actually increased at a specific joint angle and therefore a specific muscle length, an indication that the mechanisms controlling muscle tension at that length have been altered.

Peak torque of the knee extensors irrespective of joint angle at velocities from 30 to 300 degrees per second is slightly higher than joint-angle-specific torque at a knee angle 30 degrees from full extension (Yates and Kamon 1983). When subjects are grouped according to whether they have more or less than 50% type II muscle fibers, the two groups show no significant difference in the torque velocity curves for peak torque. For angle-specific torque, however, the torque velocity curves are significantly different between the two groups (Yates and Kamon 1983). This suggests that torque at a specific angle is influenced to a greater extent than peak torque by muscle fiber–type composition. Thus, comparisons of peak torque and angle-specific torque must be viewed with caution.

A comparison of training at 96 and 239 degrees per second determined torque at a specific joint angle (Caiozzo, Perrine, and Edgerton 1981). Figure 2.7 depicts the percentage of improvement that occurred at the testing velocities. The results indicate that when the test criterion is angle-specific torque, training at a slow velocity (96 degrees per second) causes significant increases in torque at faster velocities as well as at slower velocities, whereas training at a faster velocity (239 degrees per second) results in significant increases only at slower velocities close to the training velocity.

The results of research concerning concentric velocity specificity and carryover using peak torque and angle-specific torque as criterion measures are not necessarily contradictory (see figures 2.5, 2.6, and 2.7). All studies demonstrate that fast-velocity training (108 up to 240 degrees per second) results in significant increases in torque below the training velocity and in some cases above the training velocity. Differences in the magnitude (significant or insignificant) of carryover to other velocities may in part be attributed to the velocities that were defined as fast (108 up to 240 degrees per second). The preceding also indicates that slow-velocity training (36 to 96 degrees per second) causes significant carryover in torque below and above the training velocity. Generally, whether fast- or slow-velocity training is performed, carryover at velocities substantially faster than the training velocity are the least evident.

A previously cited comparison (Kanehisa and Miyashita 1983b) demonstrated that an intermediate training velocity (179 degrees per second) caused greater carryover of average power to a wider range of velocities both above and below the training velocity than did a slow (60 degrees per second) or fast (300 degrees per second) training velocity. Examinations of the changes in peak torque previously discussed indicate that training velocities in the range of 180 to 240 degrees per second result in carryover to velocities above and below the training velocity, but that the amount of carryover may decrease as the difference between the training and test velocity increases. The results indirectly support the contention that an intermediate concentric training velocity offers the best possible carryover to velocities other than the training velocity.

Research concerning the carryover of eccentric isokinetic training to velocities other than the training velocity is quite limited. Two previously described studies (Farthing and Chilibeck 2003; Shepstone et al. 2005) indicate that training with fast eccentric velocities (180 and 210 degrees per second) causes greater strength gains and carryover to velocities lower than the training velocity than slow eccentric velocities do (20 and 30 degrees per second). These studies did not test peak torque above the fast training velocity. So, as with concentric isokinetic training, strength increases due to eccentric isokinetic training carry over to velocities lower than the training velocity.

Body Composition Changes

Concentric-only isokinetic training has been reported to significantly increase muscle fiber cross-sectional area (Coyle et al. 1981; Ewing et al. 1990; Wernbom, Augustsson, and Thomee 2007) and total muscle cross-sectional area (Bell et al. 1992; Housh et al. 1992; Narici et al. 1989). However, nonsignificant changes in muscle fiber area (Akima et al. 1999; Colliander and Tesch 1990a; Costill et al. 1979; Cote et al. 1988; Seger, Arvidsson, and Thorstensson 1998) and total muscle cross-sectional area have also been shown (Akima et al. 1999; Seger, Arvidsson, and Thorstensson 1998). Increases of cross-sectional area in one muscle group (quadriceps) and not another (hamstrings) have also been reported after the same concentric-only isokinetic training program (Petersen et al. 1990). Additionally, concentric-only isokinetic training does result in an

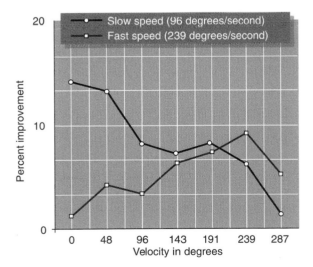

FIGURE 2.7 Percentage of changes in peak torque at a specific joint angle due to slow- and fast-speed concentric-only isokinetic training.

Data from Caiozzo, Perrine, and Edgerton 1981.

increase in fascicle angle (see chapter 3) indicating muscle hypertrophy (Blazevich et al. 2007).

Eccentric-only isokinetic training also increases muscle fiber cross-sectional area and total muscle cross-sectional area (Seger, Arvidsson, and Thorstensson 1998; Wernbom, Augustsson, and Thomee 2007). Additionally, fast eccentric isokinetic training (180 and 210 degrees per second) results in greater muscle and muscle fiber cross-sectional area increases than slow eccentric isokinetic training (20 and 30 degrees per second) and fast and slow (180 and 30 degrees per second) concentric isokinetic training (Farthing and Chilibeck 2003; Shepstone et al. 2005). Thus, concentric-only and eccentric-only isokinetic training can result in increased muscle fiber and muscle cross-sectional areas and so increased fat-free mass. However, these increases are not necessarily an outcome of all isokinetic training programs.

Changes in body composition as a result of concentric-only isokinetic training are included in table 3.3. These changes include increases in fat-free mass and decreases in percent fat and are of the same approximate magnitude as those induced by other types of training.

Motor Performance

Motor performance—specifically vertical jump ability (Augustsson et al. 1998; Blattner and Noble 1979; Oteghen 1975; Smith and Melton 1981), standing broad jump ability (Smith and Melton 1981), 40 yd sprint ability (Smith and Melton 1981), soccer ball kicking distance (Young and Rath 2011), and ball velocity of a tennis serve (Ellenbecker, Davies, and Rowinski 1988)—has been shown to improve with concentric-only isokinetic training. Power output during 6-second and 30-second maximal sprint cycling is also improved with concentric isokinetic training (Bell et al. 1989; Mannion, Jakeman, and Willan 1992). Functional ability (stair climbing, speed walking, rising from a chair) in people 41 to 75 years old is improved with both concentric-only and coupled concentric–eccentric isokinetic training, but more so with the latter (Gur et al. 2002). However, concentric-only training of the hip musculature (flexors and extensors, and abductors and adductors) for four weeks with training velocity increased weekly (60, 180, 300, and 400 degrees per second) did not result in significant changes in a rapid step test (Bera et al.

2007). This points out the potential disadvantage of isokinetic equipment generally allowing only the performance of single-joint exercises, which may not increase motor performance in some tasks. However, isokinetic training can improve motor performance.

Motor performance may be increased by fast-speed concentric isokinetic training more than by slow-speed training (Smith and Melton 1981). Training in the Smith and Melton study consisted of one set to 50% fatigue in peak torque at velocities of 180, 240, and 300 degrees per second for the fast-speed group and one set to 50% fatigue peak torque at velocities of 30, 60, and 90 degrees per second for the slow-speed group. The fast-speed and slow-speed groups improved, respectively, 5.4 and 3.9% in the vertical jump, 9.1 and 0.4% in the standing long jump, and −10.1 and +4.1% in the 40 yd sprint. However, increases in sprint cycling power output were shown not to be significantly different when isokinetic training was performed at 60, 180, or 240 degrees per second (Bell et al. 1989; Mannion, Jakeman, and Willan 1992). Thus, fast-speed isokinetic training may be more effective than slow-speed training for increasing some, but not all, motor performance tasks.

Other Considerations

Concentric-only isokinetic training has been reported to cause minimal muscle soreness after training (Atha 1981) and results in greater decreases in subjective evaluation of pain during everyday tasks than does coupled concentric–eccentric isokinetic training (Gur et al. 2002). Concentric isokinetic training may also result in significant strength gains (quadriceps) with three days of training (Coburn et al. 2006; Cramer et al. 2007), but such rapid increases may not be present in all muscle groups (e.g., elbow flexors and extensors; Beck et al. 2007). Such rapid strength gains may be useful in rehabilitation settings.

Because neither a free weight nor a weight stack has to be lifted in this type of training, the possibility of injury is minimal and no spotter is required. It is difficult to judge effort unless the machine has an accurate feedback system of either force generated or work performed that is visible to the exerciser. Furthermore, motivation may be a problem with some trainees because isokinetic equipment lacks the visible movement of a weight or weight stack.

Eccentric Training

Eccentric training (also called negative resistance training) refers to training with only the eccentric, or muscle lengthening, phase of a repetition or performing the eccentric phase with greater than the normal 1RM. Eccentric muscle actions occur in many daily activities such as walking down a flight of stairs, which requires the thigh muscles to perform eccentric muscle actions. During normal DCER training, when the weight is being lifted, the muscle shortens or performs a concentric action. When the weight is lowered, the same muscles that lifted the weight are active and lengthen in a controlled manner, or perform an eccentric action. If the muscles did not perform an eccentric action when the weight was lowered, the weight would fall as a result of the force of gravity.

Eccentric training can be achieved on many resistance training machines by lifting with both limbs a resistance greater than the 1RM of one arm or leg and then lowering it with only one limb. On some weight training machines it is also possible to perform the eccentric portion of repetitions with a resistance greater than that used in the concentric phase, but not necessarily more than that possible for 1RM. This type of training is termed **accentuated eccentric training** (sometimes called negative accentuated training). Some isokinetic machines also have an eccentric mode (isokinetic eccentric training was discussed earlier). Resistances heavier than 1RM may also be achieved with free weights by having spotters add more weight after the weight is lifted, having spotters apply resistance during the eccentric phase of a repetition, or having spotters help with the lifting of a resistance that is heavier than 1RM and then having the lifter perform the eccentric portion of the repetition without assistance. Weight release hooks (see figure 2.8) are also available to achieve a heavier resistance than 1RM with free weights (Doan et al. 2002; Moore et al. 2007).

Whenever eccentric training is performed, proper safety precautions should always be used, especially when using free weights or nonisokinetic machines. This is to avoid the temptation to use more weight than can be safely controlled during the eccentric portion of a repetition. Safety can be enhanced when performing eccentric training with some free weight exercises, such as the bench press and squat, by setting the pins of a power rack so they will catch the weight if needed at the lowest position of the exercise.

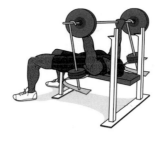

Weight release hooks hang from the bar during the eccentric phase of the lift, allowing for a heavier eccentric load.

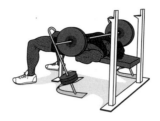

Weight release hooks pivot forward as the base of the device touches the ground and the hooks release from the bar just as the bar touches the lifter's chest (height of release is adjustable).

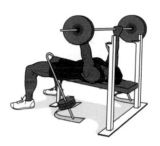

Weight release hooks are now cleared from the bar, and less weight is lifted concentrically than was lowered eccentrically.

FIGURE 2.8 Weight hooks can be used to increase the resistance during the eccentric phase of a repetition.

Adapted, by permission, from B.K. Doan et al., 2002. "The effects of increased eccentric loading on bench press." *Journal of Strength and Conditioning Research* 16:11.

Strength Changes

Normal DCER training of the legs with both a concentric and an eccentric action causes greater concentric and eccentric strength increases than performing concentric-only resistance training for the same number of repetitions (Dudley et al. 1991). Performing 50 or 75% of the repetitions with an eccentric phase results in greater increases in squat, but not bench press, ability than performing the same training program in a concentric-only manner (Häkkinen, Komi, and Tesch 1981). This indicates that an eccentric component during DCER training appears to be important, especially for the leg musculature.

Eccentric-only DCER training has been shown to increase maximal strength. For example, maximal eccentric 1RM significantly increased (29%) by training with three to five sets of six repetitions at 80% of the eccentric 1RM (Housh et al. 1998). A six-exercise total-body eccentric-only DCER program resulted in significant and similar 1RM increases (20-40%) when performed by previously untrained women with either 125 or 75% of the concentric 1RM, but no significant difference was shown between groups for strength gains (Schroeder, Hawkins, and Jaque 2004). Eccentric-only DCER training in seniors (74 years old) at 80% of the DCER 5RM increases isokinetic eccentric and isometric force capabilities, but not isokinetic concentric force capabilities (Reeves et al. 2009). Training in an eccentric-only manner with three sets of 120 to 180% of maximal isometric strength varied in a linear periodization style for three weeks significantly increased maximal isometric strength (Colduck and Abernathy 1997). Eccentric-only DCER training with six sets of five repetitions at 100% of 1RM significantly increased isometric and isokinetic strength at all velocities tested ranging from 60 to 360 degrees per second (Martin, Martin, and Morlon 1995).

Comparisons of DCER concentric-only and eccentric-only training indicate little difference between training modes. Two sets of 10 repetitions performed in a concentric-only manner at 80% of the normal 1RM or two sets of six repetitions performed in an eccentric-only fashion at 120% of the normal 1RM showed no difference in isometric or concentric-only 1RM increases (Johnson et al. 1976). Concentric-only and eccentric-only training for 20 weeks with four sets of 10 repetitions, at a contraction mode specific 10RM, demonstrated little advantage with either type of training (Smith and Rutherford 1995). No significant difference between training modes was demonstrated for isometric strength at 10-degree intervals of knee extension; however, the concentric-only mode did show significant increases in strength at a greater number of joint angles. Likewise, no significant differences were demonstrated for concentric isokinetic strength at velocities of movement ranging from 30 to 300 degrees per second; however, the eccentric-only mode demonstrated significant increases in strength at a greater number of velocities. It is important to note that in neither of the previously mentioned comparisons was eccentric maximal strength tested. However, the results indicate that DCER eccentric-only training does significantly increase isometric and concentric strength.

Comparisons of concentric-only and eccentric-only isokinetic training demonstrate conflicting results. Training at 60 degrees per second showed eccentric-only training to significantly increase isokinetic (60 degrees per second) eccentric strength to a greater extent than concentric-only training, with isometric and concentric isokinetic strength showing no significant difference between training modes (Hortobagyi et al. 1996). Training at 60 degrees per second either concentrically or eccentrically showed no significant difference in isokinetic (60 degrees per second) concentric or eccentric strength gains (Hawkins et al. 1999). Concentric-only training at 90 degrees per second demonstrated a greater number of significant increases in concentric and eccentric isokinetic strength at velocities of 30, 90, and 270 degrees per second than did eccentric-only training (Seger, Arvidsson, and Thorstensson 1998).

The studies mentioned indicate that eccentric muscle actions are needed to optimally increase muscle strength, especially when strength is measured in an eccentric manner. Although greater gains in eccentric strength have been shown with eccentric-only compared to DCER training (Reeves et al. 2009) and DCER eccentric-only compared to concentric-only training (Vikne et al. 2006), the majority of evidence indicates that eccentric-only training results in no greater gains in isometric, eccentric, and concentric strength than normal DCER training (Atha 1981; Clarke 1973; Fleck and Schutt 1985).

Accentuated eccentric training in which more resistance, but not necessarily more than the normal 1RM, is used in the eccentric phase of repetitions than in the concentric phase has received some study. This type of training is possible on some machines and with specialized devices that allow weight to be released from a barbell at the start of the concentric repetition phase. One practical question from a training perspective is, Does accentuated eccentric training result in greater strength gains than normal DCER training?

Accentuated eccentric DCER training has been shown to have an acute effect on strength in moderately trained males (Doan et al. 2002). When accentuated eccentric DCER repetitions are performed with 105% of the normal 1RM immediately before 1RM bench press attempts, 1RM significantly increases on average from 214 lb (97 kg) to 221 lb (100.2 kg). However, no acute effect on power was shown when jump squats at 30% squat 1RM were performed after repetitions using 30% of 1RM during the concentric phase and 20, 50, or 80% of 1RM during the eccentric repetition phase (Moore et al. 2007). Note that only the 50 and 80% 1RM eccentric resistances can be termed accentuated eccentric resistances. Contradicting these two previous studies, in the bench press, when accentuated eccentric DCER repetitions (105, 110, and 120% 1RM) are performed, no acute effect on maximal concentric strength, but an acute significant increase in concentric power, is shown (Ojastro and Hakkinen 2009).

Accentuated eccentric DCER training has been shown to increase strength to a greater extent than normal DCER training over seven consecutive training days (Hortobagyi et al. 2001). Normal training consisted of five or six sets of 10 to 12 repetitions at approximately 60% of 1RM. Accentuated eccentric training used the same numbers of repetitions and sets; however, during the eccentric portion of each repetition the resistance was increased 40 to 50%. Concentric 3RM and isokinetic (90 degrees per second) concentric strength gains were not significantly different between the two types of training. However, accentuated eccentric training resulted in significantly greater gains in eccentric 3RM (27 vs. 11%), isokinetic (90 degrees per second) eccentric, and isometric strength than the normal training did. Changes in electromyography (EMG) parameters paralleled the increases in strength, indicating that the majority of strength gains were related to neural adaptations, as would be expected over such a short training period.

Accentuated eccentric isokinetic training for 10 weeks demonstrated gains in concentric-only isokinetic (30 degrees per second) strength to be not significantly different from the gains from isokinetic training with both a concentric and an eccentric repetition phase (Godard et al. 1998). Training for both groups consisted of one set of 8 to 12 repetitions at 30 degrees per second. Resistance for the isokinetic training with both a concentric and an eccentric repetition phase was initially set at 80% of maximal concentric isokinetic torque. The accentuated eccentric isokinetic training followed the same training protocol, except that during the eccentric phase of each repetition, resistance was increased 40%. Unfortunately, no other strength measures were determined in this study.

A 12-week study of seniors does show that DCER eccentric accentuated training can be safely performed with six different machine exercises (Nichols, Hitzelberger et al. 1995). Training involved a higher percentage of 1RM to perform the eccentric compared to the concentric portions of repetitions respectively as follows: leg press, 57.5 and 50%; chest press, 70 and 50%; lat pull-down, 70 and 50%; seated row, 70 and 50%; fly, 70 and 60%; and shoulder press, 56.25 and 45%. All exercises were performed for three sets of 10 repetitions, except for the leg press, which was performed for four sets of 10 repetitions. Note that this accentuated eccentric system did not use more than the normal 1RM during the eccentric repetition phase. Compared to a training group that used the same resistance for an entire repetition and performed all exercises for three sets of 12 repetitions except for the leg press, which was performed for four sets of 12 repetitions, the only significant difference in predicted 1RM was in the shoulder press. For that exercise, the accentuated eccentric training resulted in a significantly greater increase (43.7 vs. 19.1%). Both training groups significantly improved in strength compared to a control group in the shoulder press, lat pull-down, and fly exercises, whereas only the accentuated eccentric system resulted in significant strength gains in the seated row. The results indicate that this accentuated eccentric system can be used safely in seniors, but that little advantage in strength gains is observed after 12 weeks of training.

Several accentuated eccentric studies have used resistances equal to or greater than the normal 1RM during the eccentric phase of repetitions. Young males with some resistance training experience training with either a traditional (four sets of 10 repetitions at 75% of 1RM) or DCER accentuated eccentric (three sets of 10 repetitions at 75% of 1RM concentric and 110-120% of 1RM eccentric repetition phase) program showed mixed results for 1RM strength gains (Brandenburg and Docherty 2002). The elbow flexors (preacher curl) showed similar gains in 1RM with traditional and accentuated eccentric training (11 vs. 9%). However, the elbow extensors (supine elbow extension) showed greater 1RM gains with accentuated eccentric training (24 vs. 15%). Untrained men after five weeks of training with either a traditional (four sets of six repetitions at 52.5% of 1RM) or an accentuated eccentric (three sets of six repetitions at 40% of 1RM concentric and 100% of

1RM eccentric repetition phases) program showed similar strength gains in the bench press and squat of approximately 10 and 22%, respectively (Yarrow et al. 2008). The use of these training resistances resulted in similar total training volume. Additionally, acute serum hormonal responses (growth hormone, testosterone) were similar between the two groups.

The preceding discussion indicates that when less-than-normal 1RM is used in accentuated eccentric training, there is no advantage in strength gains over traditional training. However, if greater-than-normal 1RM is used for accentuated eccentric training, greater 1RM gains in one muscle group (elbow extensors), but not another muscle group (elbow flexors), are apparent. Collectively, the preceding studies may indicate that for accentuated eccentric training to result in greater strength gains than traditional weight training, greater-than-normal 1RM must be used during the eccentric repetition phase. There is some support for this hypothesis (Schroeder, Hawkins, and Jaque 2004). Over 16 weeks, young women trained with six exercises. Training consisted of heavy negative-only (125% of 1RM for three sets of six repetitions) or light negative-only (75% of 1RM for three sets of 10 repetitions) training. Both groups significantly improved in 1RM in all six exercises (20-40%). The heavy negative-only training resulted in greater percentage gains in five of the six exercises, although these gains were not statistically significant. However, one exercise, the chest press, showed significantly greater gains in 1RM with the heavy negative-only training (65 vs. 40%), which indicates an advantage in maximal strength gains for the heavy negative-only training. Additionally, both groups significantly increased lean mass (dual-energy X-ray absorptiometry); however, the heavy negative-only training resulted in a significantly greater gain (0.9 vs. 0.7 kg, or 2 vs. 1.5 lb).

In summary, eccentric-only training does result in strength gains, and the gains may be greater than with normal training, although the majority of evidence shows no significant differences between eccentric-only and normal training. However, accentuated eccentric training of trained or moderately trained people does result in significant strength gains, especially when strength is determined in an eccentric manner, and it may be superior to normal resistance training when greater-than-normal 1RM is used in the eccentric

portion of repetitions. Not all muscle groups, though, may respond equally to accentuated eccentric DCER training.

Optimal Eccentric Training

Increases in strength have been reported following eccentric-only DCER training using the following:

- 120-180% of maximal isometric strength (Colduck and Abernathy 1997)
- 80% of the eccentric 1RM (Housh et al. 1998)
- 75% of concentric 1RM (Schroeder, Hawkins, and Jaque 2004)
- 100% of normal 1RM (Martin, Martin, and Morlon 1995)
- 120% of normal 1RM (Johnson et al. 1976)
- 125% of concentric 1RM (Schroeder, Hawkins, and Jaque 2004)
- 100% of 10RM (Smith and Rutherford 1995)
- 80% of 5RM (Reeves et al. 2009)
- 85-90% of 4- to 8RM (Vikne et al. 2006)

Increases in strength have also been shown using maximal isokinetic eccentric–only muscle actions (Hawkins et al. 1999; Hortobagyi et al. 1996; Seger, Arvidsson, and Thorstensson 1998). Accentuated eccentric DCER training using 40 to 50% more resistance than in the concentric phase of repetitions (Hortobagyi et al. 2001) and 75% of 1RM in concentric and 110 to 120% of 1RM in eccentric repetition phases (Brandenburg and Docherty 2002), and accentuated eccentric isokinetic training using 40% more resistance than in the concentric phase of repetitions (Godard et al. 1998), have also shown significant increases in strength. None of these studies, however, addressed what constitutes the optimal eccentric resistance to be used in eccentric training. Jones (1973) indicated the optimal resistance to be one that the trainee can lower slowly and stop at will. Using this definition, Johnson and colleagues (1976) claimed that a resistance of 120% of the DCER 1RM is the optimal eccentric resistance.

Previous studies have shown significant strength increases using greater than and less than 120% of the DCER 1RM. For example, eccentric strength depending on velocity of movement is greater than or at least equal to maximal isometric strength and up to 180% of maximal isometric strength (Colduck and Abernathy 1997). This may, however, be near the maximal resistance possible in eccentric training. If tension is applied rapidly or gradually to tetanized frog muscle, complete mechanical relaxation occurs at approximately 180 and 210%, respectively, of maximal voluntary contraction (Katz 1939). The optimal resistance to use in eccentric training has yet to be elucidated.

Another practical question concerning eccentric training is, How many repetitions need to be performed in a heavy eccentric or accentuated eccentric manner? One study (see the section on negative system training in chapter 6) indicates that as few as 25% of the total number of DCER repetitions need to be performed in an accentuated eccentric manner to bring about greater strength increases than normal DCER training (Häkkinen and Komi 1981). It is important to note that this project was performed on highly trained competitive Olympic weightlifters. Thus, results of these studies are applicable to highly trained resistance athletes.

Motor Performance and Body Composition Changes

Eccentric training and accentuated eccentric training can increase isometric, concentric, and eccentric strength. Thus, these types of training may increase motor performance ability. However, vertical jump ability has been shown to both increase (Bonde-Peterson and Knuttgen 1971) and remain unchanged (Stone, Johnson, and Carter 1979) with eccentric-only training. Tennis serve velocity has shown no change as a result of shoulder and arm musculature isokinetic eccentric training (Ellenbecker, Davies, and Rowinski 1988) and has shown a significant increase with isokinetic eccentric training, but the increase was not significantly different from that resulting from isokinetic-concentric training (Mont et al. 1994). Acutely accentuated eccentric training with up to 120% of 1RM used during the eccentric phase of a bench press does increase power in the concentric phase of a bench press (Ojastro and Häkkinen 2009), which indicates that accentuated eccentric training can increase motor performance. However, currently, the potential impact of eccentric training on motor performance is unclear.

Net muscle protein synthesis is a balance of protein synthesis and protein breakdown. Both eccentric-only and concentric-only muscle actions have been shown to increase muscle protein synthesis and increase muscle protein breakdown, resulting in an increase in net muscle protein synthesis in untrained subjects, with no difference by muscle action type (Phillips et al. 1997). Net protein synthesis rate has also been shown to significantly increase in both untrained and weight-trained people after an eccentric exercise bout of eight sets of 10 repetitions at 120% of DCER 1RM (Phillips et al. 1999). These results indicate that eccentric training can increase fat-free mass over time.

Increases in limb circumference and muscle cross-sectional area are usually associated with muscle hypertrophy. Limb circumferences increase with eccentric-only training (Komi and Buskirk 1972) and accentuated isokinetic eccentric training (Godard et al. 1998), but the increases are not different from those resulting from concentric or coupled concentric–eccentric training. Eccentric-only DCER has been shown to cause no significant change (Housh et al. 1998), an increase (Vikne et al. 2006) in muscle cross-sectional area, and a significant increase in muscle thickness (Reeves et al. 2009). While isokinetic eccentric-only training has been shown to significantly increase muscle cross-sectional area, concentric-only training shows no change (Hawkins et al. 1999; Seger, Arvidsson, and Thorstensson 1998), a significant increase (Higbie et al. 1996), and an increase in cross-sectional area not significantly different from eccentric-only training (Blazevich et al. 2007; Jones and Rutherford 1987).

DCER eccentric-only training increases type I and II muscle fiber cross-sectional area, whereas concentric-only training shows no change in these measures (Vikne et al. 2006). Isokinetic eccentric-only training has shown no significant change in type I and II muscle fiber cross-sectional area (Seger, Arvidsson, and Thorstensson 1998) and no significant change in type I, but a significant increase in type II, cross-sectional area (Hortobagyi et al. 1996). Isokinetic eccentric-only training has also shown a significant increase in muscle thickness (Farthing and Chilibeck 2003) and muscle fiber cross-sectional area in both type I and II fibers (Shepstone et al. 2005); greater increases in muscle size and type II fiber area are shown with fast compared to slow eccentric-only isokinetic training (210 vs. 20 and 180 vs. 30 degrees per second). Collectively, this information indicates that eccentric training can increase fat-free mass, but the increase may not be different from that resulting from other types of muscle actions or training.

Postexercise Soreness

A possible disadvantage of eccentric training, especially with greater than 1RM concentric strength or maximal eccentric actions, is the development of greater postexercise soreness, also termed **delayed-onset muscle soreness (DOMS)**, than that which accompanies isometric, DCER, or concentric-only isokinetic training (Fleck and Schutt 1985; Hamlin and Quigley 2001; Kellis and Baltzopoulos 1995). Additionally, women may (Sewright et al. 2008) or may not (Hubal, Rubinstein, and Clarkson 2008) be more susceptible to muscle damage and DOMS. DOMS generally begins approximately eight hours after eccentric exercise; it peaks two to three days after the exercise bout and lasts 8 to 10 days (Byrne, Twist, and Eston 2004; Cheung, Hume, and Maxwell 2003; Hamlin and Quigley 2001; Hubal, Rubinstein, and Clarkson 2007; Leiger and Milner 2001). Likewise, strength is decreased for up to 10 days after an eccentric exercise bout (Cheung, Hume, and Maxwell 2003; Leiger and Milner 2001). However, one bout of eccentric exercise appears to result in protection from excessive soreness due to another eccentric exercise session for a period of up to seven weeks in untrained or novice weight training people (Black and McCully 2008; Ebbeling and Clarkson 1990; Clarkson, Nosaka, and Braun 1992; Golden and Dudley 1992; Hyatt and Clarkson 1998; Nosaka et al. 1991) and possibly up to six months (Brughelli and Cronin 2007). Protection from excessive soreness due to another eccentric exercise bout may occur as early as 13 days after the first eccentric bout (Mair et al. 1995) and appears to occur even with low-volume eccentric exercise bouts (one set of six maximal eccentric actions for two sessions; Paddon-Jones and Abernathy 2001) and low-intensity eccentric training (40% maximal isometric force) repeated every two weeks (Chen et al. 2010). Additionally, performance of eccentric training at one velocity (30 degrees per second) results in a decrease in muscle soreness caused by performance of an exercise bout at another eccentric velocity (210 degrees per second) 14 days after the first exercise bout (Chapman et al. 2011).

Some information indicates that for excessive soreness to develop, the eccentric actions must be performed with a resistance greater than the concentric 1RM (Donnelly, Clarkson, and Maughan 1992), which can be accomplished with maximal eccentric actions because more force can be developed during an eccentric action than during a concentric action. However, little difference in the muscle damage immediately after exercise between maximal eccentric actions and eccentric actions performed with 50% of maximal isometric force has been shown (Nosaka and Newton 2002). Markers (i.e., creatine kinase, force recovery) of muscle damage indicate that maximal eccentric actions result in greater muscle damage two to three days postexercise than eccentric actions performed with 50% of maximal isometric force. Additionally, the performance of some eccentric actions before complete recovery from an eccentric exercise bout does not aid or hinder recovery from the initial eccentric exercise bout (Donnelly, Clarkson, and Maughan 1992; Nosaka and Clarkson 1995).

Light exercise for several days after an eccentric work bout may reduce muscle soreness slightly, although the effect is temporary (Cheung, Hume, and Maxwell 2003) and does not affect strength recovery (Saxton and Donnelly 1995). Moreover, stretching immediately before and immediately after an eccentric exercise bout does not affect muscle soreness or strength recovery (Cheung, Hume, and Maxwell 2003; Lund et al. 1998). Performance of another eccentric training bout three days after an initial training bout does not exacerbate soreness or decrease the rate of strength recovery and does not appear to affect muscle damage (Chen and Nosaka 2006). So performance of another eccentric exercise bout shortly after an initial bout has neither positive nor negative effects on recovery. After one to two weeks of eccentric training, the soreness appears to be no greater than that which follows isometric training (Komi and Buskirk 1972) or DCER training (Colduck and Abernathy 1997).

Some people seem to be prone to excessive muscle soreness and muscle fiber necrosis as a result of eccentric muscle actions. Forty-five percent of people experience a strength loss of 49% immediately after an eccentric exercise bout with a 33% strength loss still apparent 24 hours after an eccentric exercise bout (Hubal, Rubinstein, and Clarkson 2007). While as many as 21% of people exposed to an intense eccentric exercise bout (50 maximal eccentric actions) may not completely recover for 26 days, some require 89 days for complete recovery (Sayers and Clarkson 2001). Three percent of people may suffer from rhabdomyolysis after a strenuous eccentric exercise bout (Sayers et al. 1999). Rhabdomyolysis is the degeneration of muscle cells resulting in myalgia, muscle tenderness, weakness, swelling, and myoglobinuria (dark-color urine). This condition results in a loss of the muscles' ability to generate force and may last as long as seven weeks.

Why more soreness occurs after eccentric training than after normal DCER or concentric-only training is unclear. Electromyographic (EMG) activity can be less during an eccentric action than during a concentric action (Komi, Kaneko, and Aura 1987; Komi et al. 2000; Tesch et al. 1990), and eccentric actions rely more on type II muscle fibers than concentric actions do (Cheung, Hume, and Maxwell 2003; McHugh et al. 2002). This could lead to muscle fiber damage because fewer fibers are active exposing individual fibers to greater force, and because type II muscle fibers are more susceptible to damage than type I fibers are (Cheung, Hume, and Maxwell 2003).

Several factors are probably involved in causing the soreness and loss of strength following eccentric exercise (Byrne, Twist, and Eston 2004; Cheung, Hume, and Maxwell 2003; Hamlin and Quigley 2001). Factors such as edema, swelling, and inflammation are attractive explanations for the pain experienced several days after exercise (Clarkson, Nosaka, and Braun 1992; Stauber et al. 1990). As a result of muscle soreness, swelling, and stiffness, the voluntary activation of muscle is impaired, decreasing strength capabilities. Selective damage to the type II fibers, as described earlier, results in a decreased ability to generate force. Additionally, eccentric exercise results in the dilation of the sarcoplasmic reticulum, accompanied by a slowing of calcium release and uptake (Byrd 1992; Hamlin and Quigley 2001). These changes are transient, but they are related to decreased force production.

Damage to the sarcoplasmic reticulum also allows the influx of more calcium into muscle fibers. Calcium activates proteolytic enzymes, which degrade structures within muscle fibers (Z-disks, troponin, tropomyosin) and muscle fiber proteins by lysomal protease, which increases damage, edema, inflammation, and muscle soreness. Eccentric exercise may also result in a nonuniform distribution of sarcomere lengths:

Some sarcomeres rapidly stretch and become overextended resulting in insufficient overlap of the myofilaments and a failure to reintegrate the myofilaments upon relaxation. As a result, the still-functioning sarcomeres adapt to a shorter length, resulting in the muscle's length–tension curve shifting toward longer muscle lengths. The practical outcome of this is the inability to generate force when the muscle is at a short length.

Impaired muscle glycogen resynthesis, especially in type II fibers, is also evident after eccentric exercise, which suggests decreased recovery after eccentric exercise. Other factors such as muscle spasm and enzymes leaking out of the muscle fibers because of muscle membrane damage may also be involved in the loss of strength following eccentric exercise.

None of the preceding factors completely explains the soreness and loss of strength following eccentric exercise. For this reason it is likely that several or all of these factors are involved.

Repeated bouts of eccentric exercise may reduce sarcolemmal damage and hence the cascade of events resulting in muscle soreness. There are, however, other possible explanations of adaptations that can reduce the muscle damage and soreness from repeated exercise bouts. Repeated eccentric work bouts may result in an increased activation of type I muscle fibers and a concomitant decreased activation of type II fibers (Warren et al. 2000) to protect the type II fibers from damage. Eccentric training may also result in the addition of sarcomeres in series (Brockett, Morgan, and Proske 2001; Brughelli and Cronin 2007). This protects the muscle from microdamage because it allows the muscle fibers to be shorter at any given muscle length, thus avoiding the descending limb of the length–tension diagram or the decreased force capabilities at longer sarcomere lengths. The descending portion is the region of the length–tension diagram at which damage to sarcomeres may be most likely to occur. Although the exact explanation of the adaptations that protect against muscle soreness after repeated exercise bouts is unclear, some adaptation(s) do occur to protect muscle from soreness in successive exercise bouts.

Motivational Considerations

Some people derive great satisfaction from training with heavy resistances. Eccentric training for them is a positive motivational factor. However, the soreness that can accompany eccentric training, especially during the first week or two, can be a detriment to motivation.

Other Considerations

Because excessive soreness may accompany eccentric exercise, a program involving eccentric exercise should not be initiated immediately before a major competition. Similarly, eccentric exercise should be introduced progressively over several weeks to help reduce soreness and muscle damage (Cheung, Hume, and Maxwell 2003). The soreness and loss of strength due to eccentric training will decrease physical performance (Cheung, Hume, and Maxwell 2003). This may be especially true in rapid force development or power-type activities. For example, one-legged vertical jump height significantly decreased after an eccentric exercise bout and remained decreased for three to four days (Mair et al. 1995). A successive eccentric exercise bout four days after the initial bout resulted in the same decrease in vertical jump height immediately after the eccentric bout as that experienced after the initial eccentric bout. Although jump height recovered more quickly after the second eccentric bout, it did not reach baseline values until three to four days after the eccentric exercise bout. However, 13 days after the initial eccentric bout a successive eccentric bout resulted in no significant decrease in vertical jump height. These results indicate that caution must be used concerning the time frame in which eccentric training is initiated before a competition or a point in time when optimal physical performance is desired.

The incorporation of eccentric training is appropriate when a goal of the training program is to increase 1RM and bench press and squat ability. One factor that separates great from good powerlifters in the bench press and squat is the speed at which they perform the eccentric portion of the lift. Lifters who can lift heavier weights lower the resistance more slowly (Madsen and McLaughlin 1984; McLaughlin, Dillman, and Lardner 1977). This suggests that eccentric training may help lifters lower the resistance more slowly and maintain proper form while doing so.

Considerations for All Types of Training

Information for all of the training types discussed in this chapter indicates that multiple-set programs result in greater strength gains than single-set programs. However, most people, whether they are fitness enthusiasts or athletes, predominantly perform DCER and variable resistance training, although isometric, isokinetic, or eccentric training may also be incorporated into a training program. Guidelines for training have been developed, and although these guidelines could be applied to any training type, because the majority of research used to compile these guidelines concerned DCER and variable resistance training, they are generally more applicable to these types of training.

The majority of training studies and training programs used by fitness enthusiasts and athletes incorporate maximal voluntary muscle actions (MVMAs) at some point. This does not mean that a 1RM has to be performed; rather, it means that a set is performed to momentary concentric failure or sets are performed using RMs or close to RM resistances at some point in training, but not necessarily during all training sessions (see chapter 6, Sets to Failure Technique).

Berger and Hardage as early as 1967 demonstrated a need for MVMAs to bring about maximal strength gains. Sets to failure result in a significantly greater acute hormonal response (growth hormone, testosterone) compared to sets not to failure (Linnamo et al. 2005). However, during 16 weeks of training, sets not to failure resulted in lower resting blood cortisol levels and higher testosterone concentrations compared to training to failure; this indicates a more positive anabolic environment when training not to failure (Izquierdo et al. 2006). Training with sets to failure has shown no advantage for increasing maximal strength (1RM), and no advantage and an advantage for increasing local muscular endurance (Izquierdo et al. 2006; Willardson et al. 2008). Training with sets to failure also results in a change in exercise technique (bench press) as the repetitions in a set progress (Duffy and Challis 2007). Thus, no clear advantage of training with sets to failure has been shown. However, sets to failure have been proposed as a method for highly trained people to break through a training plateau (Willardson 2007a).

Because one-set programs do increase strength, it has been recommended that healthy adults interested in general fitness include a minimum of one set of 8 to 12 repetitions per set to improve muscular strength and power, that middle-aged and older adults perform 10 to 15 repetitions per set to improve strength, and 15 to 20 repetitions per set to improve muscular endurance, using at least one exercise for all major muscle groups in a weight training session (American College of Sports Medicine 2011). This recommendation is for healthy adults desiring fitness gains or maintenance of fitness and not for athletes or highly trained fitness enthusiasts. Guidelines (see table 7.2) for progressing resistance training programs suggest that different numbers of repetitions per set be used to emphasize different training outcomes, but that the person interested in general fitness or the advanced lifter progress to multiple-set programs (American College of Sports Medicine 2009). Although one set per exercise per training session may be appropriate as a short-term in-season program for some athletes, it is not recommended as a long-term program for athletes desiring optimal fitness gains. Multiple-set programs (American College of Sports Medicine 2009) as well as multiple-set periodized training programs result in greater strength and fitness gains than single-set programs do (Kraemer et al. 2000; Marx et al. 2001; McGee et al. 1992). Over the course of a training year or career, even small gains in strength, power, local muscular endurance, or body composition from performing multiple sets in a periodized fashion may result in greater performance increases than single sets would.

Meta-analyses (Rhea, Alvar, and Burkett 2002; Rhea et al. 2003; Peterson, Rhea, and Alvar 2004; Wolfe, LeMura, and Cole 2004) indicate that multiple sets performed by both trained and untrained people result in greater strength gains, especially during long-term training (6-16 weeks vs. 17-40 weeks), than single-set programs do. Additionally, multiple-set programs may be more important to bring about long-term gains in strength in trained compared to untrained people (Wolfe, LeMura, and Cole 2004). Conclusions from these meta-analyses are that three sets per muscle group result in greater strength gains than one set (Rhea, Alvar, and Burkett 2002), four sets per muscle group result in optimal maximal strength gains in both trained and untrained people (Rhea et al. 2003), four sets per muscle group result in optimal maximal strength gains in untrained people and trained nonathletes, and eight sets per muscle group result in optimal maximal strength gains in athletes (Peterson, Rhea, and Alvar 2005). A meta-analysis also concludes that multiple sets result in more hypertrophy than single sets do

(Krieger 2010). Thus, if maximal changes in body composition are desired, multiple-set programs are more appropriate than single-set programs.

Additionally, periodization of weight training may allow more frequent training sessions and the use of a higher total training volume compared to nonvaried training programs. In comparisons of a daily nonlinear periodized program (see chapter 7) and a single-set nonvaried program over six and nine months of training, the periodized program resulted in significantly greater strength, power, and motor performance changes, as well as more positive body composition changes, than the nonvaried programs did (Kraemer et al. 2000; Marx et al. 2001). However, total training volume performed by those in the periodized programs was substantially more (one set vs. multiple sets; Kraemer et al. 2000; Marx et al. 2001), and training frequency was greater (four vs. three sessions per week; Marx et al. 2001) than that performed by those in the nonvaried program. Thus, periodization of training may affect training volume, frequency, and intensity.

The greater training effect of multiple sets, the effects of various numbers of repetitions per set, and the effect of periodization on a training program has resulted in an American College of Sports Medicine (ACSM) *Progression models in resistance training for healthy adults* (2009). The ACSM recommends different training frequencies for people with varying resistance training experience as well as different numbers of sets and repetitions for increases in maximal strength, hypertrophy, power, and local muscular endurance (see table 7.2 for other recommendations and the recommendations for highly trained people from this position stand).

To improve strength, hypertrophy, or local muscular endurance, novices should train using a total-body program two or three days per week. Intermediate trainees should train either with a total-body program three days per week or with a split-body routine four days per week. Advanced lifters should train four to six days per week training a muscle group two days per week.

- Strength increases: Novice and intermediate trainees use 60 to 70% of 1RM for 8 to 12 repetitions per set for one to three sets per exercise; advanced trainees cycle training resistances between 80 and 100% of 1RM and use multiple sets per exercise.

• Hypertrophy: Novice and intermediate trainees use 70 to 85% of 1RM for 8 to 12 repetitions per set with one to three sets per exercise; advanced trainees cycle training between 70 and 100% of 1RM for 1 to 12 repetitions per set with three to six sets per exercise. The majority of training is devoted to 6- to 12RM resistances.

• Power increases: Power-type (Olympic lifts) or ballistic type (bench throws) resistance training should be incorporated into the typical strength training program using 30 to 60% of 1RM for one to three sets per exercise for upper-body exercises and 0 to 60% of 1RM for three to six repetitions per set for lower-body exercises. For advanced training, heavier resistances (85-100% of 1RM) may also be incorporated in a periodized manner using multiple sets (three to six) for one to six repetitions per set of power-type exercises.

• Muscular endurance: Novice and intermediate trainees should use light resistances for 10 to 15 repetitions per set; advanced trainees should use various resistances for 10 to 25 repetitions or more per set in a periodized manner.

Some of these recommendations need further research to elucidate more precisely the resistances, number of repetitions per set, and number of sets necessary to optimize training for a particular outcome.

Comparison of Training Types

Studies comparing the various types of resistance training are rare, and there are several difficulties in identifying the most beneficial type of training for a specific physiological adaptation. One issue is specificity of training and strength gains. When training and testing are performed using the same type of resistant equipment, a large increase in strength normally is demonstrated. If training and testing are performed on two different types of equipment, however, the increase in strength normally is substantially less and sometimes nonexistent. Ideally, strength should be tested using several types of muscular actions. This permits the examination of training specificity as well as carryover to other types of muscular actions.

Problems in comparison also arise in equating total training volume (i.e., sets and repetitions), total work (i.e., total repetitions × resistance × vertical distance the weight is moved), and the duration of a training session. These discrepancies

make it difficult to compare fairly and so prove the superiority of one resistance training type over another. Other study design difficulties that hinder the generalization of results to various populations include the training status of the subjects and the fact that some studies train only one muscle group. The application of results from training one muscle group or exercise to another muscle group or exercise can be difficult because muscle groups may not respond with the same magnitude or with the same time line of adaptations. Additionally, most comparisons train novice subjects with relatively short training durations (i.e., 10-20 weeks), which makes generalization to highly trained people and to long-term training (i.e., years) difficult.

Several of these difficulties are illustrated in one study (Leighton et al. 1967). Subjects trained twice a week for eight weeks using several isometric and DCER regimes. Two particular regimes were an isometric program consisting of one 6-second maximal voluntary muscle action and a DCER program using three sets of 10 repetitions progressing in resistance from 50 to 75% and finally to 100% of 10RM resistance. The isometric and DCER regimes resulted in a 0 and 9% increase in isometric elbow flexion force, respectively, and a 35 and 16% increase in isometric elbow extension force, respectively. Thus, depending on the muscle group tested, isometric and DCER training are both superior to the other training type in isometric strength gains. This same study also showed that a DCER cheat regime demonstrated a greater percentage of isometric strength gains in elbow flexion, elbow extension, and back and leg strength in a deadlift-type movement than the isometric regime and the DCER regime. The overall results are therefore ambiguous: isometric training is both inferior and superior to DCER training depending on the muscle group compared and the type of DCER regime. Testing specificity may also be of concern when comparing two types of resistance training of the same general type, such as DCER (see box 2.4).

Perhaps the most important factor when comparing training types is the efficacy of the training programs. Is each program optimal in bringing about physiological adaptations? If the answer to this question is no, any conclusions based on the studies' results must be viewed with caution. Despite the interpretation difficulties, however, some conclusions concerning comparisons of training types can be made, although virtually all

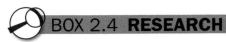

BOX 2.4 RESEARCH

Testing Specificity Between Two Types of DCER

Several types of machines can be classified as DCER. One is the traditional DCER machine that allows movement in only one plane of movement. Cable-type DCER machines allow some movement in all three planes of movement because of the use of the handles attached with cables to a pulley system. With this type of equipment, during a bench press the handles do not just move away from and toward the chest area; they can also move up and down and to the left and right to some extent. After eight weeks of training three days per week with three sets of 10 repetitions at 60% of machine-specific 1RM (Cacchio et al. 2008), the traditional machine training showed significant strength increases on both types of machines. However, significantly greater increases in 1RM strength on both types of machines were shown by training with the cable-type machine (see table 2.10).

TABLE 2.10 **Strength Increases on Cable and Traditional Machines**

Training machine type	1RM % increase on cable machine	1RM % increase on traditional machine
Cable	144*#	72*#
Traditional	34*	49*

* = significant increase pre- to posttraining; # = significant difference between training types.

Data from Cacchio et al. 2008.

The cable-type machine showed significantly greater increases than the traditional machine when the person was tested on both types of machines. But both types of machines showed testing specificity.

Cacchio, A., Don, R., Ranavolo, A., Guerra, E., McCaw, S.T., Procaccianti, R., Carnerota, F., Frascarell, M., and Santilli, V. 2008. Effects of 8-week strength training with two models of chest press machines on muscular activity pattern and strength. *Electromyography and Kinesiology* 18: 618-627.

comparisons of training modes warrant further study.

Isometric Versus Dynamic Constant External Resistance Training

Many comparisons of strength gains between isometric training and DCER training follow a pattern of test specificity. When isometric testing procedures are used, isometric training is superior (Amusa and Obajuluwa 1986; Berger 1962a, 1963b; Folland et al. 2005; Moffroid et al. 1969), and when DCER testing (1RM) is used, DCER training is superior (Berger 1962a, 1963c). However, it has also been shown that DCER training results in greater increases in isometric force than does isometric training (Rasch and Morehouse 1957). Isokinetic testing for increases in strength are inconclusive. When isokinetically tested at 20.5 degrees per second, both isometric and DCER training improved peak torque 3% (Moffroid et al.

1969). Another comparison demonstrated a 13% increase in peak torque for isometric training and a 28% increase for DCER training (the velocity of isokinetic testing was not reported; Thistle et al. 1967). No significant difference in isokinetic peak torque increases at several velocities (45, 150, and 300 degrees per second) due to isometric training at four different joint angles compared to DCER training has been shown (Folland et al. 2005).

A review of the literature concludes that well-designed DCER programs are more effective than standard isometric programs for increasing strength (Atha 1981). Isometric training at one joint angle and DCER training through a restricted range of motion (knee extension, 80 to 115 degrees; knee flexion, 170 to 135 degrees) both increase power with no significant difference between training regimes (Ullrich, Kleinder, and Bruggemann 2010); this indicates that both training modes can increase motor performance. However, isometric training at one joint angle does not consistently increase dynamic motor performance (see Isometric Training earlier in chapter), whereas DCER training can increase dynamic motor performance.

It is not surprising, then, that motor performance is improved to a greater extent by DCER training than by isometric training at only one joint angle (Brown et al. 1988; Campbell 1962; Chu 1950). Thus, if an increase in motor performance is desired, DCER training would be a better choice than isometric training at one joint angle. Both types of training can result in muscle hypertrophy, and currently there is no information favoring either one for muscle hypertrophy (Wernbom, Augustsson, and Thomee 2007).

Isometric Versus Variable Resistance Training

The authors are aware of no studies that directly compare isometric and variable resistance training. However, it can be hypothesized that strength gains may follow a specificity of testing pattern similar to comparisons of isometric and DCER. It can also be hypothesized that because no improvement in motor performance has been reported from isometric training at one joint angle (Clarke 1973; Fleck and Schutt 1985), and because improvement in motor performance has been shown with variable resistance training (Peterson 1975; Silvester et al. 1984), variable resistance training may be superior to isometric training in this parameter. Thus, if an increase in motor performance is desired, variable resistance training would be a better choice than isometric training at one joint angle.

Isometric Versus Concentric Isokinetic Resistance Training

Comparisons of isometric and concentric isokinetic training for the most part follow a pattern of test specificity. However, direct comparisons have used only relatively slow-velocity isokinetic training (up to 30 degrees per second). Isometric training is superior to isokinetic training at 22.5 degrees per second for increasing isometric strength (Moffroid et al. 1969). Isometric force of the knee extensors at knee angles of 90 and 45 degrees increased 17 and 14%, respectively, with isometric training and 14 and 24%, respectively, with isokinetic training. Similarly, knee flexor isometric strength at knee angles of 90 and 45 degrees increased 26 and 24%, respectively, with isometric training and 11 and 19%, respectively, with isokinetic training. The isometric training demonstrated superior isometric force improvements over the isokinetic training in three of these four tests. However, isokinetic training of the elbow extensors at 30 degrees per second resulted in greater increases in isometric force than isometric training did (Knapik, Mawdsley, and Ramos 1983).

Isokinetic training is superior to isometric training in the development of isokinetic torque (Moffroid et al. 1969; Thistle et al. 1967). For example, knee extensor strength for isokinetic and isometric training increased 47 and 13%, respectively (Thistle et al. 1967). Another comparison reported that isokinetically and isometrically trained groups increased 11 and 3%, respectively, in knee extension peak torque at 22.5 degrees per second. For knee flexion the increases in peak torque were 15 and 3%, respectively, at 22.5 degrees per second (Moffroid et al. 1969). Thus, the phenomenon of test specificity is evident in the strength increases that result from both isometric and isokinetic training.

Training isometrically at one joint angle results in no improvement in motor performance (Clarke 1973; Fleck and Schutt 1985), whereas improvements in motor performance have been achieved with isokinetic training (Bell et al. 1989; Blattner and Noble 1979; Mannion, Jakeman, and Willan 1992). Thus, it can be hypothesized that isokinetic training is superior to isometric training at one joint angle for improving motor performance. Both modes of training can result in significant increases in muscle hypertrophy, although little information indicates the superiority of one mode over the other (Wernbom, Augustsson, and Thomee 2007).

Isometric Versus Eccentric Resistance Training

The comparisons made in this section are between isometric training and eccentric training with free weights or normal resistance training machines. Measured isometrically, isometric and eccentric training show no difference in strength gains. A comparison of training the elbow flexors and knee extensors either only isometrically or only eccentrically shows little difference between training types (Bonde-Peterson 1960). All trainees performed 10 maximal five-second actions per day. The isometric training showed the following improvements in isometric strength: elbow flexion, 13.8% for males and 1% for females; knee extension, 10% for males and 8.3% for females. The eccentric training showed the following improvements in isometric strength: elbow flexion, 8.5% for males and 5% for females; knee extension, 14.6% for males and 11.2% for females. Thus, there may be no significant difference between these two types of training with regard to increasing isometric strength.

The same conclusion was reached after training subjects' knee extensors three times per week for six weeks (Laycoe and Marteniuk 1971). The isometric and eccentric training improved isometric knee extension force 17.4 and 17%, respectively. Other studies also report no difference in strength gains between these two training methods (Atha 1981).

Reviews conclude that isometric training at one joint angle does not result in increased motor performance (Clarke 1973; Fleck and Schutt 1985), whereas the effect of eccentric training on motor performance is unclear, with increases (Bonde-Peterson and Knuttgen 1971) and no change (Ellenbecker, Davies, and Rowinski 1988; Stone, Johnson, and Carter 1979) in motor performance shown. Thus, the superiority of one of these training types over the other in terms of motor performance increases is unclear.

Dynamic Constant External Resistance Versus Variable Resistance Training

Comparisons of strength increases as a result of DCER and variable resistance training are equivocal. After 20 weeks of training, variable resistance training demonstrated a clear superiority over DCER training in 1RM free weight bench press ability (Ariel 1977). DCER and variable resistance training produced gains of 14 and 29.5%, respectively. Another bench press comparison demonstrated a specificity of training (Boyer 1990); both training types showed significantly greater increases in 1RM over the other type when tested on the type of equipment on which training was performed. Further information concerning these studies is presented in table 2.3.

Leg press strength shows test specificity for these two types of training. After 10 weeks of training, a variable resistance group increased 27% when tested with variable resistance equipment and 7.5% when tested with DCER methods

(Pipes 1978). Conversely, a group trained with DCER improved 7.5% when tested on variable resistance equipment and 28.9% when tested with DCER methods. Three other exercises tested and trained in the study demonstrated a similar test specificity pattern. Likewise, after 12 weeks, DCER training significantly improved DCER and variable resistance leg press ability by 15.5 and 17.1%, respectively (Boyer 1990), whereas variable resistance training significantly improved DCER and variable resistance leg press ability by 11.2 and 28.2%, respectively. Both groups showed a significantly greater increase than the other group when tested on the type of equipment on which subjects trained. More information concerning these studies is presented in table 2.4.

After a five-week program, DCER training was found to be superior to variable resistance training in producing strength gains determined by DCER testing (Stone, Johnson, and Carter 1979). No difference between the two types of training was shown when tested for variable resistance strength improvements.

After 10 weeks of training, variable resistance training and DCER training resulted in no significant difference in isometric knee extension strength gains at multiple knee angles (Manning et al. 1990). Another comparison (Silvester et al. 1984) supports the conclusion that these two training types result in the same gains in isometric strength. Collectively, this information indicates no clear superiority of either training type over the other in terms of strength gains.

Silvester and colleagues (1984) demonstrated that both DCER (free weight) and increasing lever-arm variable resistance training result in significantly greater increases in vertical jump ability than does cam-type variable resistance training. Thus, the superiority of either training type over the other may be explained in part by the type of variable resistance equipment or the training program used.

Table 3.3 indicates that body composition changes from these two types of training are of the same magnitude. A 10-week (Pipes 1978) and a 12-week (Boyer 1990) comparative study demonstrated no significant difference between DCER and variable resistance training in changes of percent fat, fat-free mass, total body weight, and limb circumferences. Thus, body composition changes with these two types of training are similar.

Concentric Versus Eccentric Resistance Training

Concentric and eccentric training can both be performed isokinetically or using DCER equipment. A review of comparative studies indicates no significant difference in strength gains between concentric and eccentric training when the training is performed using DCER equipment (Atha 1981).

For example, strength gains tested with DCER elbow curls, arm presses, knee flexions, and knee extensions after six weeks of training are not significantly different between these two training types (Johnson et al. 1976). Concentric training consisted of two sets of 10 repetitions at 80% of 1RM, and eccentric training consisted of two sets of six repetitions at 120% of 1RM. Moreover, after 20 weeks of training little advantage in isometric or isokinetic strength gains was shown for either concentric or eccentric DCER training (Smith and Rutherford 1995). It should be noted that maximal eccentric strength was not determined in either of the aforementioned studies. However, eccentric-only DCER training has also shown similar concentric 1RM strength gains (14 vs. 18%), but significantly greater eccentric 1RM strength gains (26 vs. 9%) compared to concentric-only DCER training (Vikne et al. 2006).

A comparison of three DCER squat types of training has been done (Häkkinen and Komi 1981): concentric-only training in which only the concentric repetition phase was performed, concentric–eccentric training in which primarily the concentric phase of repetitions with some eccentric phases of repetitions was performed, and eccentric–concentric training that consisted primarily of the eccentric phase and some concentric phases of repetitions. Those training with both eccentric and concentric actions made significantly greater gains in 1RM squat ability (approximately 29%) than those training with concentric actions only (approximately 23%). This suggests that both eccentric and concentric actions may be necessary to bring about maximal strength gains. This conclusion is supported by a 20-week training comparison in which normal DCER training was compared to concentric-only DCER training (O'Hagan et al. 1995a). Note that a direct comparison of concentric-only and eccentric-only training cannot be made from these studies.

Concentric and eccentric resistance training have also been compared using isokinetic muscle actions. Short-term training periods have shown no significant difference between concentric-only and eccentric-only isokinetic training for maximal concentric, eccentric, or isometric strength increases (Hawkins et al. 1999; Komi and Buskirk 1972).

However, contraction mode specificity has also been shown when training with isokinetic concentric-only and eccentric-only actions. After short-term training periods (6-20 weeks) eccentric-only and concentric-only isokinetic training at 30 to 100 degrees per second generally result in both concentric and eccentric strength gains (Blazevich et al. 2007; Farthing and Chilibeck 2003; Higbie et al. 1996; Hortobagyi et al. 1996; Miller et al. 2006; Seger, Arvidsson, and Thorstensson 1998; Tomberline et al. 1991). The majority of these studies demonstrate contraction mode specificity, although it is not always present. Training at 30 degrees per second, concentric-only and eccentric-only training resulted in concentric peak torque increases of 24 and 16% and eccentric peak torque increases of 36 and 39%, respectively (Blazevich et al. 2007). The difference in concentric peak torque increases between concentric-only and eccentric-only training was significant, whereas the difference in eccentric peak torque was not. Some information also favors fast eccentric-only training for strength gains. Fast eccentric-only training (180 and 210 degrees per second) results in greater strength gains than slow eccentric-only (20 and 30 degrees per second) and fast and slow (180 and 30 degrees per second) concentric-only isokinetic training (Farthing and Chilibeck 2003; Shepstone et al. 2005).

The effect isokinetic concentric-only and eccentric-only training of the shoulder internal and external rotators has on tennis serve velocity (a motor performance) task is inconclusive. Six weeks of training with six sets of 10 repetitions at velocities ranging from 60 degrees per second to 210 degrees per second (velocity spectrum training) demonstrated that eccentric but not concentric training significantly increases serve velocity (Ellenbecker, Davies, and Rowinski 1988). Another comparison of six-week training regimes of concentric-only and eccentric-only with eight sets of 10 repetitions at velocities ranging from 90 to 180 degrees per second (velocity spectrum training) demonstrated that both eccentric and concentric training significantly increases serve velocity, but there was no significant difference between training types (Mont et al. 1994).

As discussed in the section on eccentric training, although eccentric training does bring about increases in motor performance and changes in body composition, the changes appear not to be significantly different from those resulting from other types of muscle actions or training types. Postexercise soreness is a potential disadvantage of eccentric-only training, especially during the first several weeks of training. Thus, eccentric-only training should be incorporated slowly into a training program to minimize muscle soreness. Both concentric-only and eccentric-only isokinetic training, as discussed in the section on isokinetic training, can increase muscle and muscle fiber cross-sectional area indicating that both can affect body composition by increasing fat-free mass.

Dynamic Constant External Resistance Versus Isokinetic Resistance Training

Studies comparing DCER and concentric-only isokinetic resistance training indicate no clear superiority of either type over the other. After eight weeks of training, the isokinetic torque of the knee extensors due to isokinetic training increased 47.2%, whereas DCER training resulted in an increase of 28.6% (Thistle et al. 1967). Daily training of the knee extensors and flexors for four weeks demonstrated that isokinetic and isometric strength gains with isokinetic training (22.5 degrees per seconds) are superior to those with DCER training (Moffroid et al. 1969). The isokinetic and DCER training resulted in increases of 24 and 13%, respectively, in isometric knee extension force and 19 and 1%, respectively, in isometric knee flexion force. Isokinetic peak torque at 22.5 degrees per seconds with the isokinetic and DCER training increased 11 and 3%, respectively, in knee extension and 16 and 1%, respectively, in knee flexion.

In contrast to the previously mentioned studies, DCER training was demonstrated to be superior to isokinetic training in producing strength and power gains (Kovaleski et al. 1995). Subjects separated into the two training types trained the knee extensors three days per week for six weeks with 12 sets of 10 repetitions. The isokinetic training consisted of using velocities of movement ranging from 120 degrees per second to 210 degrees per

second in a velocity spectrum training protocol. The DCER training consisted of using 25% of peak isometric force during the first week with the resistance increased (5 Newton meters) weekly. The DCER training resulted in greater peak DCER power than the isokinetic training did and greater peak isokinetic power at velocities of 120, 150, 180, and 210 degrees per second than the isokinetic training did. DCER and isokinetic training have also shown testing specificity (Pearson and Costill 1988). After eight weeks, DCER and isokinetic training demonstrated 32 and 4% increases, respectively, in 1RM strength tested in a DCER fashion. The isokinetic and DCER training resulted in 12 and 8% increases, respectively, in isokinetic force at 60 degrees per second and 10 and 1% increases, respectively, at 240 degrees per second, indicating testing specificity.

Training the elbow flexors for 20 weeks with either a hydraulic isokinetic device or resistance training machine favored the resistance training machine for muscle cross-sectional area and 1RM (87 vs. 43% increase) (O'Hagan et al. 1995a). However, no significant difference between increases in type I and II muscle fiber area were shown. The hydraulic isokinetic machine did allow variability in the velocity of movement (35-51 degrees per second).

A biomechanical comparison of free weight and isokinetic bench pressing indicates some similarity (Lander et al. 1985). Subjects performed a free weight bench press at 90 and 75% of their 1RM and maximal isokinetic bench presses at a velocity of movement corresponding to their individual movement velocities during their 90 and 75% free weight bench presses. No significant difference in maximal force existed between the isokinetic bench press and the 90% or the 75% of 1RM free weight bench press. This indicates that free weights may affect muscles in a manner similar to isokinetic devices, at least in the context of force production, during the major portion of an exercise movement.

DCER and isokinetic training increase motor performance ability similarly. A comparison of two-legged leg press training for five weeks demonstrated no significant difference in one-legged jumping ability (ground reaction force; Cordova et al. 1995).

Both modes of training increase muscle and muscle fiber cross-sectional area, and changes in body composition with DCER and isokinetic training are of the same magnitude. See table 3.3 for information concerning comparative changes in percent fat, fat-free mass, and total body weight.

Isokinetic Versus Variable Resistance Training

Comparisons of isokinetic and variable resistance training demonstrate testing specificity. A comparison of slow- and fast-speed concentric-only isokinetic training with variable resistance training of the knee extensors and flexors showed testing specificity (Smith and Welton 1981). Slow-speed concentric-only isokinetic training consisted of one set until peak torque declined to 50% at velocities of 30, 60, and 90 degrees per second. Fast-speed isokinetic training followed the same format as the slow-speed training, except that the training velocities were 180, 240, and 300 degrees per second. Variable resistance training initially

consisted of three sets of 10 repetitions at 80% of 10RM with resistance increased as strength increased. Figures 2.9 and 2.10 present the results of this study. In measures of strength, the isokinetic training demonstrated a relatively consistent pattern of test speed specificity. The variable resistance training demonstrated consistent increases in knee flexion, irrelevant of the test criterion, but knee extension showed large increases in isometric force only. In leg press ability the variable resistance and slow-speed isokinetic training showed similar and larger gains than the fast-speed isokinetic training. Another comparison (see table 2.4) of changes in leg press strength also clearly illustrated testing specificity between these two types of training (Gettman, Culter, and Strathman 1980).

Figure 2.10 compares the motor performance benefits of isokinetic and variable resistance training. Fast-speed isokinetic training demonstrated greater increases in all three motor performance

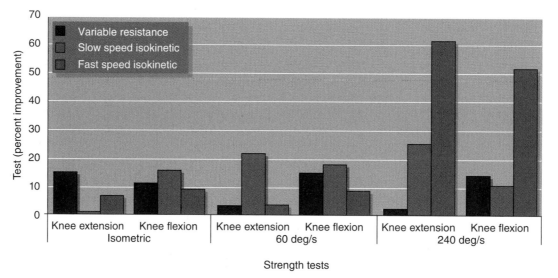

FIGURE 2.9 Isokinetic versus variable resistance training: strength changes with training.

Data from Smith and Melton 1981.

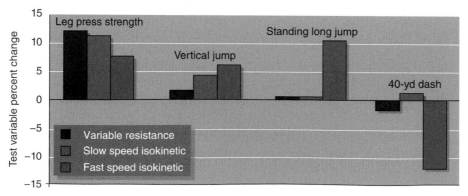

FIGURE 2.10 Isokinetic versus variable resistance: motor performance changes with training.

Data from Smith and Melton 1981.

tests than the other two types of training, whereas the variable resistance and slow-speed isokinetic training groups showed similar changes in the motor performance tests. The training protocols used by all three groups were described previously (Smith and Melton 1981). These results indicate that fast-speed isokinetic training may be superior to slow-speed isokinetic and variable resistance training in the context of motor performance improvement.

Body composition changes due to isokinetic and variable resistance training are presented in table 3.3. Although minimal data are available, these two training types appear to bring about similar changes in body composition.

Summary

The information presented in this chapter concerning types of resistance training and changes in strength, muscle hypertrophy, body composition, motor performance, training frequency, number of sets, number of repetitions per set, and test specificity should be considered in the design of all resistance training programs. The next chapter discusses the physiological adaptations to resistance training.

SELECTED READINGS

Atha, J. 1981. Strengthening muscle. *Exercise and Sport Sciences Reviews* 9: 1-73.

Behm, D.G., and Sale, D.G. 1993. Velocity specificity of resistance training. *Sports Medicine* 15: 374-388.

Blazevich, A.J., Cannavan, D., Coleman, D.R., and Horne, S. 2007. Influence of concentric and eccentric resistance training on architectural adaptation in human quadriceps muscles. *Journal of Applied Physiology* 103: 1565-1575.

Brughelli, M., and Cronin, J. 2007. Altering the length-tension relationship with eccentric exercise implications for performance and injury. *Sports Medicine* 37: 807-826.

Byrne, C., Twist, C., and Eston, R. 2004. Neuromuscular function after exercise-induced muscle damage: Theoretical and practical implications. *Sports Medicine* 34: 149-69.

Cheung, K., Hume, P.A., and Maxwell, L. 2003. Delayed onset muscle soreness treatment strategies and performance factors. *Sports Medicine* 33: 145-164.

Clarke, D.H. 1973. Adaptations in strength and muscular endurance resulting from exercise. *Exercise and Sport Sciences Reviews* 1: 73-102.

Fleck, S.J., and Schutt, R.C. 1985. Types of strength training. *Clinics in Sports Medicine* 4: 150-169.

Hortobagyi, T., Devita, P., Money, J., and Barrier, J. 2001. Effects of standard and eccentric overload strength training in young women. *Medicine & Science in Sports & Exercise* 33: 1206-1212.

Kraemer, W.J., Mazzetti, S.A., Ratamess, N.A., and Fleck, S.J. 2000. Specificity of training modes. In *Isokinetics in the human performance*, edited by L.E. Brown. Champaign, IL: Human Kinetics.

McDonagh, M.J.N., and Davies, C.T.M. 1984. Adaptive response of mammalian skeletal muscle to exercise with high loads. *European Journal of Applied Physiology* 52: 139-155.

Wernbom, M., Augustsson, J., and Thomee, R. 2007. The influence of frequency, intensity, volume and mode of strength training on whole muscle cross-sectional area in humans. *Sports Medicine* 37: 225-264.

Physiological Adaptations to Resistance Training

After studying this chapter, you should be able to

1. understand the basic components of exercise metabolism and how they contribute and adapt to differing exercise stimuli,

2. describe the anatomy and physiology of skeletal muscle, as well as the mechanisms of adaptation specificity to exercise,

3. explain the role of the nervous system in muscle actions, control, and adaptations to exercise,

4. describe the size principle and understand how it reflects and fundamentally determines functional and metabolic aspects of exercise as well as adaptations,

5. explain changes in body composition that would be expected with different forms of exercise training, and the time course of such changes,

6. discuss the complexity and importance of resistance exercise responses and adaptations of the major anabolic and catabolic hormones, and how this relates to program design,

7. understand the connective tissue adaptations to resistance exercise, and

8. describe the acute responses and chronic adaptations of the cardiovascular system to resistance exercise, at rest and during exercise.

Adaptations to a resistance training program are related to the physical demands placed on the neuromuscular system and the associated physiological systems needed to perform a training session. The physiological process by which the body responds to exercise is called adaptation. Interestingly, each physiological variable adapts on a unique time line (e.g., nervous system versus protein accretion in muscle) and in a specific manner related to the specific type of exercise program—thus, the term **exercise specificity.** Choices made for each of the acute program variables (see chapter 5) result in specific workout or training sessions with their own physiological demands. Various numbers of motor units, which are made of up a motor neuron and its associated muscle fibers, are recruited to create the force needed to lift a weight or perform a resistance exercise in a training session. The choices made within the different acute program variable domains affect how muscle fibers are recruited and what physiological systems will be needed to support the activated motor units. Thus, the physiological support of the activated motor units defines the acute physiological responses to the resistance exercise performed in a workout and with repeated use the specific adaptations associated with training. This is why understanding motor unit recruitment and muscle fiber types is important for understanding adaptations to training.

The acute program variable choices result in the engagement of other physiological systems, such as the cardiovascular, immune, and endocrine systems, to meet the demands of the training session and aid in the recovery process that follows. Recovery after each workout is vital to the adaptation process. Remodeling and repair processes in muscle and other tissues contribute to the accumulated long-term adaptations, such as increased muscle fiber size and decreased resting blood pressure.

An immediate change that occurs to support the demands of the workout, such as an increase in heart rate, is called an acute physiological response. For example, when performing a circuit weight training workout with rest periods of 60 seconds between sets and exercises, the heart rate response pattern will be much different from that resulting from a "heavy day" (95% of 1RM) with rest periods of five to seven minutes. The heart rate increase needed to support a circuit weight training program is much greater than that needed to support a heavy lifting protocol. Workout design choices (e.g., use of shorter rest periods) determine the needed acute physiological support (e.g., higher heart rate for short-rest circuit training). However, these same choices also dictate the rate and magnitude of increases in strength, power, and muscle hypertrophy with training. The acute response also includes the physiological recovery responses immediately after a session, such as the repair and remodeling of tissues. Thus, chronic adaptations to any training program are the accumulated effects of the acute physiological demands of each workout over time.

The body's response to long-term exposure to exercise stimuli results in adaptations to better meet the demands of exercise and reduce the stress of the exercise challenge. Program progression and overload are needed to adequately stress the physiological systems to result in continued adaptation. Over the course of a long-term training program, adaptations occur at different rates and plateaus can occur (i.e., little or no improvements in some physiological functions such as blood pressure response or in anatomical structures such as muscle fibers). When this happens, the training program needs to be evaluated to make sure adequate variation, rest, and recovery are provided to optimize the training program. As we will see later, mistakes in training leading to nonfunctional overreaching or even overtraining can cause pos-itive adaptations to cease. Adaptations can take place within days of training (e.g., changes in the isoforms of myosin ATPase; Staron et al. 1994) or continue to make small improvements with years of training (e.g., muscle size increases in elite weightlifters; Häkkinen, Pakarinen et al. 1988c). However, eventually, each physiological function or structure will reach a maximum adaptation to the training program based on the trainee's inherent genetic potential.

Ultimately, adaptations to training determine whether a resistance training program is effective and whether the trainee is capable of a higher level of physiological function, performance, or both. The extent of an adaptation to a resistance training program depends on the person's starting fitness level and inherent genetic potential and the length of training (see figure 3.1). This chapter provides an overview of the physiological adaptations to resistance training.

Physiological Adaptations

Before we discuss adaptations to resistance training, let's examine what exactly is meant by physiological adaptation. First, if a person has never trained the squat exercise, the change in the first several weeks in 1RM strength will be dramatic (e.g., 50% improvement). However, after the person has progressively trained this exercise for a long period of time, the strength gains will be smaller for each successive month of training. This is because the potential for adaptation in this exercise, or physiological function, has reached close to its genetic ceiling. In other words, the **window of adaptation**, or how large of an adaptation is possible, is now much smaller as a result of prior training (Newton and Kraemer 1994). With six months of training, trained people make less than a third of the strength gains that untrained people make in only 12 weeks (Häkkinen 1985). In highly trained athletes, the physiological mechanisms that mediate strength gains (e.g., nervous system and muscle fiber adaptations) are highly developed. Unless there is some increase in physiological potential, such as natural growth and development from 16 to 20 years (i.e., the genetic potential has not yet been realized), improvements, though possible, will be slow. Thus, fitness gains or adaptations do not take place at a constant rate throughout a training program (American College of Sports Medicine 2009). For the average person the most

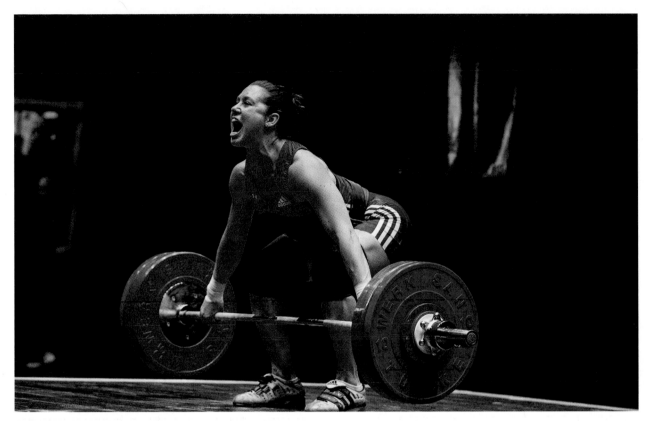

FIGURE 3.1 Elite Olympic weightlifters require years of training to reach their full genetic potential.
Kelly Kline/Icon SMI

dramatic increases in strength occur during the first six months of training; to reach one's genetic potential, more sophisticated resistance training programs are needed (American College of Sports Medicine 2009).

Bioenergetics

Bioenergetics refers to the sources of energy for bodily functions including muscle activity. Such general terms as **aerobic** (energy production with oxygen) and **anaerobic** (energy production without the immediate need for oxygen) have become popular among fitness enthusiasts, coaches, and athletes. The two major sources of anaerobic energy are the phosphocreatine system and anaerobic glycolysis; the source of aerobic energy is oxidative phosphorylation. Knowledge of these energy sources and their interactions with each other is necessary for planning a resistance training program that will optimally condition a person for a particular sport or activity. Each sport or activity has a unique energy demand and profile. Resistance training enhances primarily anaerobic and to some extent aerobic metabolism. It is important to understand that the bioenergetic demands are specific to the neuromuscular recruitment demands because those demands change throughout an activity. Thus, each activity demands different percentages of the three energy systems depending on the specific physiological demands for the muscles involved in producing force or power. Understanding the bioenergetics of any activity or sport is vital to the development of the needs analysis (see chapter 5) in the exercise prescription and program development processes.

ATP, the Energy Molecule

The source of energy for muscle activation is the adenosine triphosphate molecule, or ATP. The main functional components of ATP are adenosine, ribose, and three phosphate groups. When ATP is broken down to adenosine diphosphate (ADP; the adenosine molecule now has only two attached phosphates) and a free phosphate molecule (P_i), energy is released. ATP is used for many physiological functions including crossbridge movement, in which it helps to mediate pulling the actin filaments across the myosin filaments to shorten the muscle fiber. ATP is the immediate energy source for muscular actions (see figure 3.2). However, all three major energy systems supply ATP in different ways.

The adenosine triphosphate–phosphocreatine (ATP-PC) energy system (also called the phosphagen system; see the section that follows) is important for muscle actions (whether concentric shortening, eccentric elongation, or isometric action). When adenosine triphosphate (ATP) breaks down to adenosine diphosphate (ADP) as a result of the hydrolysis of one of the phosphates from the ATP molecule, energy is produced and is used in muscle actions. Important in muscle is the reverse reaction of adding an inorganic phosphate (P_i) to ADP; energy provided from the hydrolysis of a phosphate molecule from phosphocreatine (PC) results in creatine (Cr) and Pi providing the energy to resynthesize (add a phosphate molecule to ADP) to make ATP, which again is needed for muscle contractions. Each bioenergetic reaction is mediated by an enzyme (ATPase and creatine phosphokinase, respectively), as shown in figure 3.2. Both reactions are reversible as indicated by the dual-direction arrows.

Adenosine Triphosphate–Phosphocreatine (ATP-PC) Energy System

Stored within muscle and ready for immediate use to supply energy to the muscle are two compounds that work together to make energy quickly available—ATP and PC. Phosphocreatine is similar to ATP in that it also has a phosphate

group attached with a high-energy bond. In PC the inorganic phosphate group is bound to a creatine molecule. Phosphocreatine provides a convenient mechanism to help maintain ATP concentrations. When ATP is broken down to ADP and Pi, energy is released. This energy is needed to support muscular actions (see the section Sliding Filament Theory later in this chapter). However, when PC is broken down to Cr and Pi, the resulting energy is used to recombine ADP and Pi to create ATP (see figure 3.2). The rebuilt ATP can then be again broken down to ADP and Pi and the energy again used to continue a specific muscle action. The energy released from the breakdown of PC cannot be used to cause muscle shortening because PC does not bind to the myosin crossbridges (again, see the Sliding Filament Theory section later in this chapter).

ATP and PC are stored within the muscle fiber in the sarcoplasm, which is the fluid compartment of the muscle fiber. However, intramuscular stores of ATP and PC are limited, which limits the amount of energy that the ATP-PC system can produce. In fact, in an all-out exercise bout, the energy available from the ATP-PC system (phosphagen energy) will be exhausted in 30 seconds or less (Meyer and Terjung 1979). Although it is attractive to associate the depletion of intramuscular ATP and PC with a singular cause of fatigue, such as an inability to perform two repetitions with a true 1RM weight, several factors make this sole association unlikely (Fitts 1996). ATP does not show a correlation to force declines, and PC decreases show a different time course than force decreases. This indicates that other factors also contribute to the elusive cause of fatigue, yet a depletion in the rate of ATP energy supply to the muscle will limit force and power production.

Although not shown in figure 3.2, when ATP is broken down to ADP, a hydrogen ion results, which partially contributes to the increased acidity of the muscle but is only one source of hydrogen ions with exercise stress. Thus, an imbalance between ATP use and resynthesis can contribute to an increase in acidity, which is associated with fatigue. Another factor associated with fatigue is an increase in P_i that is not bound to creatine, which also increases with an imbalance between ATP use and resynthesis.

Although decreased ATP concentrations do occur with fatiguing exercise, they may not be the sole cause of fatigue. One advantage of this energy

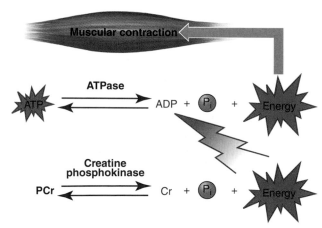

FIGURE 3.2 The production of energy, mediated by ATPase and creatine phosphokinase.

system is that the energy is immediately available for use in the muscle. A second advantage is that the ATP-PC system has a large power capacity; that is, it can provide the muscle with a large amount of ATP energy per second to support repetitive myosin crossbridge interactions with actin due to its immediate availability at the site of the crossbridge interactions in the sarcoplasm.

Because of the characteristics of the ATP-PC energy system, it is the primary source of energy for short-duration, high-power, and high-force events or resistance exercises. It supplies the major portion of energy to the muscles for such activities as a maximal lift, the shot put, the high jump, and the 40 yd (36.7 m) dash. One of the reasons for continued heavy breathing after an intense short-duration exercise bout or competition (e.g., between interval sprints or wrestling periods, respectively) is that the muscular stores of ATP and PC must be replenished aerobically if the ATP-PC system is to be used again for such training or competition. The success of creatine supplementation to enhance the PC pool (resulting in greater availability of energy, thereby improved explosive and repeated high-intensity performances, including high-power and high-force resistance workouts) underscores the importance of this energy system for these types of conditioning activities and sports (Rawson and Volek 2003; Volek et al. 1999).

Anaerobic Glycolytic Energy System

Glycolysis, a metabolic pathway that uses a sequence of reactions to produce ATP, uses only carbohydrate as an energy substrate. Carbohydrate in the form of glucose can be obtained from the bloodstream or from glycogen stored in the muscle. Glycogen is made up of a long chain of glucose molecules that can be broken down to provide glucose, which can enter the glycolytic reactions. Glycogen stored in the liver is broken down as needed to help maintain blood glucose concentrations. In a series of enzymatic reactions, glucose is broken down into two pyruvate molecules resulting in the energy necessary to make ATP. The energy released from splitting each glucose molecule produces a net gain of two ATP molecules if the glucose comes from the blood and three ATP molecules if the glucose comes from intramuscular glycogen. The pyruvate is then enzymatically converted into lactic acid. Note that no oxygen is needed for these reactions; if the pyruvate is converted into lactic acid, the process is called anaerobic glycolysis. Thus, many people also term this energy system the "lactic acid system."

Anaerobic glycolysis and its role in human metabolism during exercise is still an area of important research (Brooks 2010). A major research question is, Does a relationship between lactate generation and acidosis exist? The active area of research is whether the H^+ ions resulting in acidity are derived more from ATP hydrolysis or lactate generation. Recently, scientists have suggested that lactate acidosis does occur and is related to the production of H^+ ions and decreases in pH (Marcinek, Kusmerick, and Conley 2010). Yet, the role of lactate in causing fatigue directly is more controversial because of its circumstantial association with the production of H^+ ions and increased acidity (Robergs, Ghiasvand, and Parker 2004). It may well be that the reduction of ATP turnover rates may be the ultimate fatigue mechanism. Additionally, with intense exercise, an increase in the intramuscular lactate concentration and an increase in PCO_2 results in an increase in H^+, which contributes to a decrease in pH. However, the reduction in pH due to increased H^+ production does decrease enzyme function and other factors related to fatigue. These effects can influence the fatigue associated with various resistance exercise protocols and impact training adaptations.

The extreme fatigue and nauseous feeling after several sets of a 10RM squat with only a minute of rest between sets is associated with the buildup of lactate. The breakdown of lactic acid in the muscle to lactate and its associated hydrogen ions causes concentrations of these compounds to increase in the muscle and blood. While not causal, lactate is associated with fatigue and reduction in the force muscle is capable of producing (Hogan et al. 1995). With severe exercise, blood pH can go from a resting level of 7.4 to as low as 6.6 (Gordon et al. 1994; Sahlin and Ren 1989). This increase in hydrogen ions and decrease in pH are thought to be major contributors to fatigue by decreasing the release of Ca^{++} from the sarcoplasmic reticulum (see the section Sliding Filament Theory later in the chapter). The breakdown of intramuscular lactate concentration with intense exercise along with an increase in PCO_2 results in an increase in H^+, which contributes to a decrease in pH. This increase in acidity and a decrease in pH can cause problems with chemical reactions in the metabolic cycles of the energy systems and slow the production of ATP molecules. For example, the inhibition of key glycolytic enzymes such as phosphofructokinase, which is a rate-limiting enzyme, can slow down glycolysis with reductions in pH (Gordon, Kraemer, Pedro et al. 1991). This can interfere with the chemical processes of the muscle cell, including the processes of producing more ATP (Trivedi and Dansforth 1966) and altering membrane ion (sodium and potassium) permeability. This in turn results in hyperpolarization, which inhibits glycolysis through the allosteric regulation of enzyme function, and the binding of Ca^{++} to troponin (Nakamaru and Schwartz 1972). Thus, exercise protocols that produce high concentrations of blood lactate are associated with high levels of fatigue and acidic conditions (e.g., short-rest circuit weight training protocols), but the actual cause of fatigue is still not clear due to the many different sites (e.g., central inhibition and muscle tissue damage) that can influence a loss of force or power production.

Despite the side effects of lactate accumulation, the anaerobic glycolytic energy system (also called the glycolytic or lactic acid energy system) can produce a greater amount of energy than the ATP-PC system can and is 100 times faster than the aerobic energy system (discussed next) in producing ATP energy. The amount of energy that can be obtained from this system is limited, however, by the side effects of increased acidity. Anaerobic glycolysis cannot supply the muscle with as much energy per second as the ATP-PC system can and therefore is not as powerful. Thus, as one starts to rely more and more on glycolysis and less on the ATP-PC system, muscular power decreases. The anaerobic energy system is a major supplier of ATP in all-out exercise bouts lasting from approximately one to three minutes (Kraemer et al. 1989). Such bouts may include high-intensity sets at 10- to 12RM with very short rest periods (30 to 60 seconds) or a 400 m sprint.

Another side effect of the glycolytic anaerobic energy system is pain when the lactate and hydrogen ion concentrations are high enough to affect nerve endings. In addition, nausea and dizziness can occur with short-rest, high-intensity resistance exercise protocols (Kraemer, Noble et al. 1987). Heavy breathing continues after completion of these types of exercise bouts. This is in part due to the need to remove the accumulated lactate from the body. Resistance training has been shown to specifically improve anaerobic capacity without affecting oxidative metabolism (LeBrasseur, Walsh, and Arany 2011).

Aerobic, or Oxidative, Energy System

The aerobic (or oxidative) energy system has received a lot of attention for many years. The major goal of jogging, swimming, cycling, and aerobic dancing is to improve cardiorespiratory fitness, which is analogous to improving oxidative phosphorylation. This energy system uses oxygen in the production of ATP and is therefore called an aerobic energy system.

The aerobic energy system can metabolize carbohydrate, fat (fatty acids), and protein, but significant amounts of protein are not normally metabolized (see figure 3.3). However, during long-term starvation and long exercise bouts, especially during the last minutes of exercise, significant amounts of protein (5-15% of total energy) can be metabolized to produce energy (Abernathy, Thayer, and Taylor 1990; Dohm et al. 1982; Lemon and Mullin 1980; Tarnopolsky, MacDougall, and Atkinson 1988). Normally, at rest, the body derives one-third of the needed ATP from metabolizing carbohydrate and two-thirds from fat. As exercise intensity increases, the body undergoes a gradual change to metabolizing more and more carbohydrate and less and less fat. During maximal physical exercise the muscle is metabolizing nearly 100% carbohydrate if carbohydrate stores are sufficient (Maresh et al. 1989, 1992).

Aerobic metabolism of the glucose from intramuscular glycogen or glucose from the blood begins in the same manner as it does in anaerobic glycolysis. In this system, however, as a result of the presence of sufficient oxygen, the pyruvate is not converted into lactic acid, but enters into two long series of chemical reactions called the Krebs cycle and the electron transport chain. These series of reactions produce carbon dioxide, which is expired at the lungs, and water. The water is produced by combining hydrogen molecules with the oxygen that was originally taken into the body via the lungs. Thirty-eight molecules of ATP can be produced by aerobically metabolizing 1 glucose molecule from the blood and 39 from a glucose molecule obtained from intramuscular glycogen. The aerobic metabolism of fatty acids does not have to start with glycolysis. Fatty acids can go

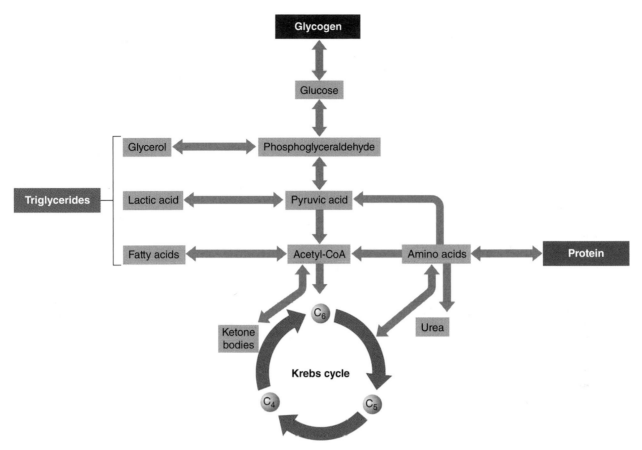

FIGURE 3.3 Carbohydrate, fatty acids, and amino acids can all be aerobically metabolized. However, the entrance into aerobic metabolism varies among these substrates based on availability and the intensity of exercise.

through a series of reactions called beta oxidation and then enter directly into the Krebs cycle. The products of fatty acid metabolism are similarly water, carbon dioxide, and ATP. Interestingly, protein in the form of amino acids can enter aerobic metabolism by being transformed into pyruvate or directly at several other places (acetyl-Co-A or the Krebs cycle). No matter where amino acids enter metabolism, they must first be deaminated (i.e., remove the amine group from an amino acid).

The maximal amount of energy per unit of time that can be produced via aerobic metabolism is lower than that produced by the ATP-PC and anaerobic glycolytic energy systems and depends on how much oxygen the body can obtain and use. If a plateau of oxygen consumption can be determined, it is called maximal oxygen consumption ($\dot{V}O_2$max). This is typically determined via a treadmill exercise test. However, when a plateau of 30 seconds to a minute is not seen in the measurement of oxygen consumption, the highest value is used, and it is typically then called peak

oxygen consumption ($\dot{V}O_2$peak). Cycle ergometer and lifting tasks usually produce only a single peak measurement. Maximal aerobic power ($\dot{V}O2$peak or $\dot{V}O2$max) is the maximal amount of oxygen the body can obtain and use per unit of time. It is usually expressed either in absolute terms as liters of oxygen per minute (L · min–1) or in relative terms as milliliters of oxygen per kilogram (2.2 lb) of body mass per minute (mL · kg–1 · min–1). When expressed in absolute terms (L · min–1), it does not take into account body mass. A larger person might be expected to use more oxygen per minute solely as a result of body size. Expressing oxygen consumption, either submaximal or maximal on a per body mass basis ($\dot{V}O_2$max = mL · kg^{-1} · min^{-1}) places everyone on a scale relative to body mass. In this way, comparisons can be made among people with varying amounts of body mass.

The aerobic energy system is less powerful than either of the two anaerobic energy–producing systems (ATP-PC and glycolytic/lactic acid). The aerobic energy system cannot produce enough ATP per second to allow the performance of maximal intensity exercise, such as a 1RM lift or a 400 m sprint. On the other hand, this system, because of the abundance of carbohydrate and fatty acids and the lack of by-products that can immediately inhibit performance, can supply virtually an unlimited amount of ATP over a long period of time. Therefore, it is the predominant energy source for long-duration, submaximal activities (e.g., a 10K run). In addition, this energy system contributes a moderate to high percentage of the ATP during activities composed of high-intensity exercise interspersed with rest periods or high-intensity activities lasting longer than about 25 seconds, such as interval run training and wrestling. These activities result in very high blood lactate levels ranging from 15 to 22 mmol $\cdot$ L^{-1} (Serresse et al. 1988). In these conditioning activities, both aerobic and anaerobic energy systems are needed at different times during the activity but the aerobic system predominates during the recovery period or between rounds or intervals to help with the recovery of ATP energy molecules. During many activities one system may provide the majority of energy (e.g., the aerobic system during a marathon), but all energy systems contribute some of the energy during all activities. The percentage of contribution from each system can change as the demands of the activity (e.g., running up a steep hill during a marathon) or the muscles involved change.

Replenishing the Anaerobic Energy Systems

After an intense exercise bout, the anaerobic energy systems must be replenished so it can be used again at a later time. Interestingly, the anaerobic energy sources are replenished by the aerobic energy system. After cessation of an anaerobic activity, heavy breathing continues for a period of time even though physical activity is no longer taking place. The oxygen taken into the body, above the resting value, is used to replenish the two anaerobic energy sources. This extra oxygen has been referred to as an oxygen debt or now more commonly called excess postexercise oxygen consumption (EPOC). Aerobic fitness does aid in replenishing the anaerobic energy stores (Tomlin and Wenger 2001). Replenishing both the ATP-PC and the anaerobic glycolytic energy systems needs to be accomplished after an intense exercise bout if

these systems are to be optimally recovered for later use, such as the next interval in a sprint training workout, next set in a resistance workout, or the next round in a wrestling match.

Replenishing the ATP-PC Energy System

Immediately after an intense exercise bout, there is a several-minute period of very heavy, rapid breathing. The oxygen taken into the body above normal resting oxygen consumption is used to aerobically produce ATP in excess of what is required at rest. Part of this excess ATP is immediately broken down to ADP and Pi; the energy released is used to combine Pi and creatine back into PC. Part of the excess ATP is simply stored as intramuscular ATP. This rebuilding of the ATP and PC stores is accomplished in several minutes (Hultman, Bergstrom, and Anderson 1967; Karlsson et al. 1975; Lemon and Mullin 1980). This part of EPOC has been referred to as the alactacid portion of the oxygen debt.

The half-life of the alactacid portion of the oxygen debt has been estimated to be approximately 20 seconds (DiPrampero and Margaria 1978; Meyer and Terjung 1979) and as long as 36 to 48 seconds (Laurent et al. 1992). Half-life means that within that time period 50%, or half, of the alactacid debt is repaid. So within 20 to 48 seconds, 50% of the depleted ATP and PC is replenished; in 40 to 96 seconds, 75% is replenished; and in 60 to 144 seconds, 87% is replenished. Thus, within approximately 2 to 4 minutes the majority of the depleted ATP and PC intramuscular stores are replenished. Clearly, short rest resistance programs that use only one minute or less of rest result in incomplete recovery of the ATP-PC energy system and thereby place more demands on the anaerobic energy system contributing to the high blood concentrations of lactate (e.g., 10-20 mmol $\cdot$ L^{-1}) with such workout protocols.

If activity is performed during the alactacid portion of the oxygen debt, the rebuilding of the ATP and PC intramuscular stores will take longer. This is because part of the ATP generated via the aerobic system has to be used to provide energy to perform the activity. An understanding both of the alactacid portion of the oxygen debt and of the rebuilding of the ATP-PC energy system is important when planning a training program that involves short-duration, high-intensity exercise, such as heavy sets of an exercise. The ATP-PC energy system is the most powerful and is therefore the major source of energy for maximal lifts and heavy sets. Several minutes of rest must be allowed between heavy sets and maximal lifts to replenish the ATP and PC intramuscular stores; otherwise, they will not be available for use in the next heavy set. If sufficient recovery time is not allowed between heavy sets or maximal lifts, the lift or set either will not be completed for the desired number of repetitions or it will not be completed with the desired speed or proper technique.

Recovery of the Lactacid Portion of the Energy Debt System

The aerobic energy system is also, in part, responsible for removing accumulated lactate from the body. Approximately 70% of the accumulated lactic acid is aerobically metabolized during this portion of EPOC, 20% is used to synthesize glucose, and 10% is used to synthesize amino acids. The energy produced from the metabolism of lactic acid is used by tissues.

The relationship between the lactacid portion of the oxygen debt and lactate removal has been questioned (Roth, Stanley, and Brooks 1988); however, many tissues of the body can aerobically metabolize lactate. Skeletal muscle active during an exercise bout (Hatta et al. 1989; McLoughlin, McCaffrey, and Moynihan 1991), skeletal muscle inactive during an exercise bout (Kowalchuk et al. 1988), cardiac muscle (Hatta et al. 1989; Spitzer 1974; Stanley 1991), the kidneys (Hatta et al. 1989; Yudkin and Cohen 1974), the liver (Rowell et al. 1966; Wasserman, Connely, and Pagliassotti 1991), and the brain (Nemoto, Hoff, and Sereringhaus 1974) can all metabolize lactate. The half-life of the lactacid portion of the oxygen debt is approximately 25 minutes (Hermansen et al. 1976). Thus, approximately 95% of the accumulated lactic acid is removed from the blood in 1 hour and 15 minutes. Many sporting events use this information to determine the minimal rest needed between events or matches (e.g., track events or wrestling matches in a tournament).

If light activity (walking, slow jogging) is performed after a workout, the accumulated lactate is removed more quickly than if complete rest follows the workout (Hermansen et al. 1976; Hildebrandt, Schutze, and Stegemann 1992; McLoughlin, McCaffrey, and Moynihan 1991; Mero 1988).

When light activity is performed after the activity, a portion of the accumulated lactate is aerobically metabolized to supply some of the needed ATP to perform the light activity. It also appears that accumulated lactate is removed from the blood more quickly when the light activity is performed by the muscles active during the exercise bout and not by the muscles that were inactive during the exercise bout (Hildebrandt, Schutze, and Stegemann 1992). The light activity must be below the person's lactic acid threshold, or the exercise intensity below which a significant increase in blood lactate occurs. In aerobically untrained people, the lactic acid threshold is approximately 50 to 60% of peak oxygen consumption; in highly trained endurance athletes, it may be 80 to 85% of peak oxygen consumption. So, as aerobic fitness increases, so does the lactic acid threshold.

Light activity between sets during a weight training workout has been shown to be beneficial. Pedaling a bike at 25% of peak oxygen consumption during rest periods of four minutes between six sets of squats (85% of 10RM) results in a lower blood lactate compared to pedaling at 50% of peak oxygen consumption or resting quietly (Corder et al. 2000). Additionally, at the end of a workout during which a bike was ridden at 25% of peak oxygen consumption, more repetitions were performed in a set to volitional fatigue (65% of 10RM) than during other types of rest periods.

A higher maximal oxygen consumption is beneficial in recovery; quicker recovery of heart rate and blood lactate concentration occurred after performing four sets of 15 repetitions at 60% of 1RM and four sets of 10 repetitions at 75% of 1RM than after performing four sets of four repetitions at 90% of 1RM (Kang et al. 2005). The blood lactate concentration was lower after the sets at 90% of 1RM than after the other sets, which may account for the lack of a higher maximal oxygen consumption being a factor related to recovery after the sets at 90% of 1RM.

The preceding information indicates that it may be prudent for weightlifters and anaerobic-type athletes to maintain at least average aerobic fitness to aid in recovery between anaerobic exercise bouts, such as sets during weight training sessions. Yet, this does not mean that intense long-distance running (i.e., road work) or long intervals in a training program are required because these may be detrimental to force and power development (see chapter 4). Lower-volume, higher-intensity short sprint intervals can bring about the needed aerobic fitness. Additionally, light exercise can aid recovery between sets in a weight training workout if the rest periods are of sufficient length. Because of this, experts recommend light activity rather than complete rest, if practical, between sets in which lactate accumulation occurs, such as short-rest-period programs and circuit weight training.

Interaction of the Energy Systems

Although one energy system may be the predominant energy source for a particular activity, such as the ATP-PC energy system for a maximal lift or the aerobic energy system for running a marathon, as mentioned earlier, all three systems supply a portion of the ATP needed by the body at all times. Thus, the ATP-PC energy system is operating even when the body is at rest, and the aerobic energy system is operating during a maximal lift. Even at rest some lactate is being released by muscles into the blood (Brooks et al. 1991). During a marathon, even though the majority of energy is supplied by the aerobic energy system, a small percentage of the needed energy is supplied by the ATP-PC and anaerobic glycolytic energy systems.

As the duration and intensity of activity changes, the predominant energy system also changes. At one end of the spectrum are activities such as a maximal lift, the shot put, and a 40 yd sprint (see box 3.1). The ATP-PC energy system supplies the vast majority of energy for these activities. The anaerobic energy systems supply the majority of the energy for activities such as sets of 20 to 25 repetitions with no rest between sets or exercises in a circuit program, three sets of 10RM with one-minute rest periods, or 200 m sprints. The

aerobic energy system supplies the majority of the needed ATP for long duration continuous exercise beyond 2 to 3 minutes and for endurance events such as a 5K run. However, all three systems are still producing some energy at all times; the percentage of contribution of the systems to the total energy varies.

There is no point at which one energy system provides the majority of ATP energy for an activity. Shifts in the percentage of contribution from each system are based on the intensity and duration of the activity. Also, muscles may be under different metabolic demands, and the differential use of energy systems is based on the type and number of motor units activated to meet the intensity and duration demands of the activity. For example, as a marathon runner climbs a steep hill and lactate accumulates in the body, the anaerobic systems will contribute more energy to the performance of the activity at that point because the leg and arm muscles will have greater energy demands than running on the flat.

Bioenergetic Adaptations

Increases in the enzyme activities of an energy system can lead to more ATP production and use per unit of time, which could lead to increases in physical performance. Enzyme activity of the ATP-PC energy system (e.g., creatine phosphokinase and myokinase) has been shown to increase in humans after isokinetic training (Costill et al. 1979) and traditional resistance training (Komi et al. 1982; Thorstensson, Hulten et al. 1976), and in rats after isometric training (Exner, Staudte, and Pette 1973). In two isokinetic training regimes the enzymes associated with the ATP-PC energy system

 ## BOX 3.1 RESEARCH

Energy Sources During High-Intensity, Short-Duration Activity

Energy systems other than the ATP-PC system supply energy during high-intensity, short-duration activity. Even during very short high-intensity activity, all three energy systems supply some portion of the needed energy (Spencer et al. 2005). For example, during a three-second cycling sprint, approximately 3, 10, and 87% of the needed energy is obtained from aerobic metabolism, anaerobic glycolysis, and the ATP-PC energy system, respectively. Although it is clear that the ATP-PC system supplies the vast majority of the energy needed for this activity, the other two systems contribute.

Spencer, M., Bishop, D., Dawson, B., and Goodman, C. 2005. Physiological and metabolic responses of repeated-sprint activities specific to field-based team sports. *Sports Medicine* 35: 1025-1044.

showed significant increases of approximately 12% in legs trained with 30-second bouts and insignificant changes in legs trained with 6-second bouts (Costill et al. 1979). According to these findings, enzymatic changes associated with the ATP-PC energy system are linked to the duration of the exercise bouts; the changes do not take place with exercise bouts of six seconds or less. However, little change, no change, or a decrease in enzymes (creatine phosphokinase and myokinase) associated with the ATP-PC energy system have also been observed after resistance training (Tesch 1992; Tesch, Komi, and Häkkinen 1987).

A significant increase was also observed in phosphofructokinase (PFK), the rate-limiting enzyme associated with the glycolysis of 7 and 18%, respectively, in the 6-second- and 30-second-trained legs discussed earlier (Costill et al. 1979). Neither leg showed a significant increase in a second enzyme (lactate dehydrogenase) associated with the anaerobic energy system. Other glycolytic enzymes have also shown increases, decreases, and no change with training. The enzyme phosphorylase has been shown to increase after 12 weeks of resistance training (Green et al. 1999). The enzymes PFK, lactate dehydrogenase, and hexokinase have also been shown to be unaffected by, or to decrease after, heavy resistance exercise training (Green et al. 1999; Houston et al. 1983; Komi et al. 1982; Tesch 1987; Tesch, Thorsson, and Colliander 1990; Thorstensson, Hulten et al. 1976).

The preceding results suggest that the type of resistance program affects the enzymatic adaptations. In addition, most studies showing no change or a decrease in enzyme activity also reported significant muscle **hypertrophy,** or an increase in individual muscle fiber size. This indicates that enzyme activity may increase in response to resistance training, but it may not change or decrease if the subsequent training produces significant muscle hypertrophy. A reduction in enzyme concentration per unit of muscle mass or enzyme dilution can occur. Thus, the type of lifting protocol and the magnitude of muscle hypertrophy affect the adaptations of the enzymes associated with the ATP-PC and anaerobic glycolytic energy systems.

Increases in the activity of enzymes associated with aerobic metabolism have been reported with isokinetic training in humans (Costill et al. 1979), isometric training in humans (Grimby et al. 1973), and isometric training in rats (Exner, Staudte, and Pette 1973). Enzymatic changes associated with the aerobic energy system may also depend on the duration of the exercise bout (Costill et al. 1979). However, enzymes involved with aerobic metabolism obtained from pooled samples of weight-trained muscle fibers have not demonstrated increased activity (Tesch 1992), have been shown to decrease with resistance training (Chilibeck, Syrotuik, and Bell 1999), and have been shown to be lower in lifters than in untrained people (Tesch, Thorsson, and Essen-Gustavsson 1989). Bodybuilders using high-volume programs, short rest periods between sets and exercises, and moderate-intensity training resistances have been shown to have higher citrate synthase, an enzyme of the Krebs cycle, and more activity in type II fibers (fast twitch) than lifters who train with heavier loads and take longer rest periods between sets (Tesch 1992). This demonstrates the influence of short rest periods on oxidative enzymes where shorter rest between sets places a higher demand on the aerobic system. However, because bodybuilders typically perform aerobic exercise as well as resistance training, this cross-sectional data should be viewed with caution as the stimulus for the changes in the aerobic enzymes may arise from multiple exercise stimuli. Again, the type of program design (e.g., rest period lengths) may influence the magnitude of enzyme changes in the muscle.

Myosin ATPase, an enzyme associated with all three energy systems and one that breaks down ATP to supply energy for muscle shortening, has shown only minor changes in pooled muscle fibers (Tesch 1992). The fact that various types of myosin ATPase exist and are altered with strength training may indicate that the absolute concentration is not as important as the type of ATPase.

Enzymatic changes associated with any of the three energy systems depend on the acute program variables. Normal heavy resistance programs appear to have a minimal effect on enzyme activities over time. However, a training program that minimizes hypertrophy and targets specific energy systems will most likely result in increased enzyme activities.

Muscle Substrate Stores

One adaptation that can lead to increased physical performance is an increase in the substrate available to the three energy systems. In humans, after five months of strength training, the resting intramuscular concentrations of PC and ATP are elevated 28 and 18%, respectively (MacDougall et al. 1977), although this finding is not supported by other studies (Tesch 1992). The resting PC-to-inorganic-phosphate ratio has been shown to increase after five weeks of resistance training (Walker et al. 1998). However, cross-sectional information shows that in athletes with a significant amount of hypertrophy, PC and ATP concentrations are not increased (Tesch 1992).

A 66% increase in intramuscular glycogen stores was shown after resistance training for five months (MacDougall et al. 1977). Bodybuilders have been shown to have approximately a 50% greater concentration of glycogen than untrained people (Tesch 1992). However, muscle glycogen content has also been shown to not change with resistance training (Tesch 1992). Several research studies have also shown that blood glucose levels do not change significantly during resistance training sessions (Keul et al. 1978; Kraemer et al. 1990). Whether an increase in PC and ATP occurs with resistance training may depend on pretraining status, the muscle group examined, and the type of program. However, it is clear that skeletal muscle glycogen content can increase as a result of resistance training and that blood glucose concentrations do not decrease during resistance training. This indicates that at least during one training session carbohydrate availability for the anaerobic energy system is not a limiting factor to performance.

The aerobic energy system metabolizes glucose, fatty acids, and some protein to produce ATP. Intramuscular glycogen stores can be increased through strength training. The enhancement of triglyceride (fat) stores in muscles after resistance training, however, remains equivocal, as decreases in and no difference from normal triglyceride content in the muscles of trained lifters have been reported (Tesch 1992). Increased lipid content has been observed in the triceps, but not in the quadriceps, after training (Tesch 1992). Thus, muscle groups may respond differently as to how they store and use triglyceride depending upon their use (i.e., whether activated as part of a motor unit needed to perform the exercise) in an exercise or training program. Although dietary practices and the type of program may affect triglyceride concentrations, we can speculate that because most resistance training programs are anaerobic, intramuscular triglyceride concentrations are minimally affected by resistance training unless it is accompanied by significant body mass or fat mass loss.

Skeletal Muscle Fibers

Skeletal muscle fibers are unique as cells in that they are multinucleated. Because of this characteristic, the protein that makes up the muscle fiber is under the control of different nuclei throughout the fiber. The portion of a fiber under the control of one nucleus is termed a **myonuclear domain**; different portions of the muscle fiber are controlled by different individual nuclei (Hall and Ralston 1989; Hikida et al. 1997; Kadi et al. 2005; Pavlath et al. 1989) (see figure 3.4). **Satellite cells** are small cells with no cytoplasm that are found in skeletal muscle between the basement membrane and the sarcolemma or cell membrane of the muscle fiber (see the section Satellite Cells and Myonuclei later in this chapter). Even more interesting is the fact that unless the number of nuclei is increased through mitotic division of satellite cells, muscle proteins, which are needed for hypertrophy to occur, may not be able to be added to the muscle fiber (Hawke and Garry 2001; Staron and Hikida 2001). Therefore, the greater the hypertrophy of the muscle fiber, the greater the need for satellite cells to divide to supply myonuclei to control more myonuclear domains (Hall and Ralston 1989). Increases in the pool of myonuclei that result from satellite division may well begin before hypertrophy or significant protein accretion in muscle fibers occurs (Bruusgaard et al. 2010). In addition, people with higher numbers of satellite cells prior to training may be more capable of greater muscle hypertrophy (Petrella et al. 2008).

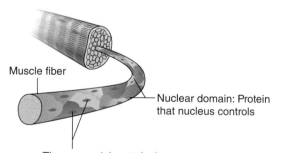

Muscle fiber

Nuclear domain: Protein that nucleus controls

The myonuclei contain the cell's DNA machinery and receive the molecular signaling from hormones and other molecules to synthesize proteins.

FIGURE 3.4 Each myonucleus controls a given amount of muscle protein, called the nuclear domain. If a muscle fiber increases in size, more myonuclei are needed to keep the nuclear domains a similar size.

Skeletal muscle is a heterogeneous mixture of several types of muscle fibers. Quantification of the biochemical and physical characteristics of the various muscle fibers has led to the development of several muscle fiber histochemical classification systems (Pette and Staron 1990). Although these classification systems appear similar, they are different. The characteristics of the **type I** (slow-twitch) and **type II** (fast-twitch) muscle fibers are shown in table 3.1. The most popular classification system used in the literature today is the myosin ATPase typing system.

Figure 3.5 shows how muscle fiber types are classified using the histochemical **myosin ATPase staining method.** Myosin ATPase is the enzyme that is intimately involved in the cleaving of ATP to ADP, Pi, H+, and energy and is vital to the rate of crossbridge cycling. It is found in the heads of the myosin crossbridges. This classification system is possible because different types (isoforms) of myosin ATPase are found in the various muscle fiber types. Different pH conditions result in dif-ferent staining intensities of the muscle fiber types. Myosin ATPase is an enzyme very specific to the cycling speed of myosin heads on the actin active sites; thus, it provides a functional classification representative of a muscle fiber's functional ability without the actual determination of "twitch speed."

The most common method of obtaining a muscle sample in humans is the **muscle biopsy** (see figure 3.6). A hollow stainless steel needle is used to obtain about 100 to 400 mg of muscle tissue, typically from a thigh, calf, or arm muscle. The sample is removed from the needle, processed, and then frozen. The muscle sample is then cut (sectioned) into consecutive (serial) sections and placed on cover slips for histochemical assay to determine the various muscle fiber types (Staron et al. 2000). Other variables, such as the glycogen content of the fibers, receptor numbers, mitochondria, capillaries, and other metabolic enzymes, can also be analyzed from a serial section of the biopsy sample.

Of great importance to the histochemical muscle fiber typing procedure is the fact that serial sections from the same muscle are placed into each of the preincubation baths, which consist of an alkaline (pH 10.4) and two acid (pH 4.6 and 4.3) baths, before the rest of the histochemical assay. Ultimately, after the assay is completed, a muscle fiber is typed by comparing its color under each of the pH conditions (see figure 3.7).

TABLE 3.1 Some of the Primary Muscle Fiber Type Classification Systems

Classification system	Theoretical basis
Red and white fibers	View of fiber color; the more myoglobin (oxygen carrier in a fiber), the darker or redder the color.
Fast twitch and slow twitch	Based on the speed and shape of the muscle twitch with stimulation. Fast-twitch fibers have higher rates of force development and a greater fatigue rate than slow-twitch fibers.
Slow oxidative, fast oxidative glycolytic, fast glycolytic	Based on metabolic staining and the characteristics of oxidative and glycolytic enzymes.
Type I and type II	Stability of the enzyme myosin ATPase under various pH conditions. The enzyme myosin ATPase has differ-ent forms, some of which result in quicker enzymatic reactions for ATP breakdown and thus higher cycling rates for that fiber's actin–myosin interactions.

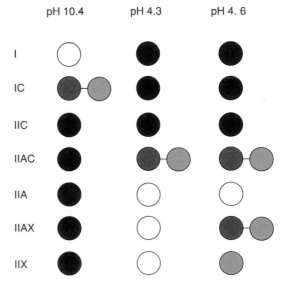

FIGURE 3.5 Myosin ATPase staining nomenclature for determining type I and type II muscle fiber types.

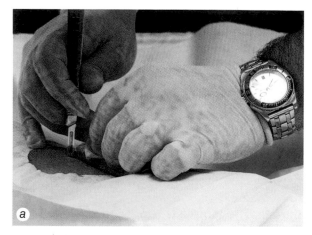

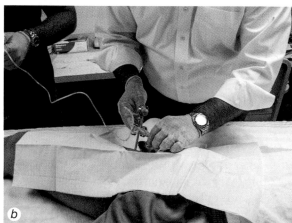

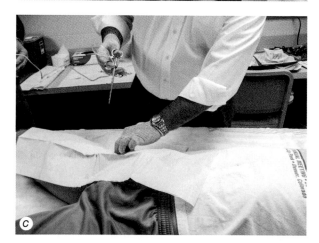

FIGURE 3.6 Obtaining a muscle biopsy involves anesthetizing the surface area and *(a)* making a small incision in the skin and subcutaneous fat tissue. *(b)* The biopsy needle is inserted into the incision and suction is provided by a syringe connected via tubing; the biopsy needle is used to obtain a small portion of muscle (100-400 mg). *(c)* The needle is removed, and the muscle sample is then frozen for subsequent analyses.

Courtesy of Dr. William J. Kraemer, Department of Kinesiology, University of Connecticut, Storrs, CT.

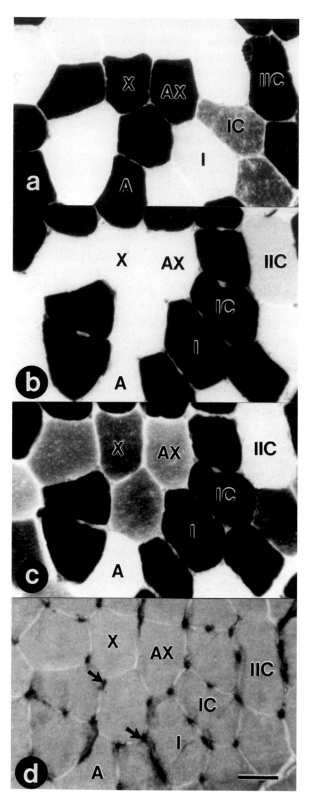

FIGURE 3.7 Myosin ATPase–stained muscle fibers demonstrating types I, IIa, IIax, and IIx fibers: *(a)* pH 4.3, *(b)* pH 10, and *(c)* pH 4.6 indicate fibers that stain slightly differently in different serial sections of the same pH. *(d)* The black dots around the fibers are capillaries.

Courtesy of Dr. Robert S. Staron, Ohio University, Athens, OH.

In the classification system presented in figure 3.5, muscle fibers are classified as type I or type II. In addition, various muscle fiber subtypes (also called hybrids) can also be determined in both of the general type I and type II categories. The type I fiber is the most oxidative. Starting at the top and progressing toward the bottom in figure 3.5, each succeeding fiber type becomes less oxidative than the previous one. In figure 3.7 the fiber subtypes can be seen in the muscle fibers after myosin ATPase histochemical staining. Fiber subtypes are highly related to the type of myosin heavy chain contained in the muscle's structure (Fry, Kraemer, Stone et al. 1994; Staron et al. 1991). In this way they are also related to the rate at which the crossbridges can be cycled, and therefore to "twitch speed."

Functional abilities have been associated with the classifications of fiber types because type II (white, fast twitch, fast oxidative glycolytic, and fast glycolytic) and type I (red, slow twitch, and slow oxidative) fibers have different metabolic and contractile properties. Table 3.2 shows that type II fibers are better adapted to anaerobic exercise, whereas type I fibers are better adapted to aerobic exercise.

Type II fibers are suited to the performance of high-intensity, short-duration exercise bouts as evidenced by their biochemical and physical characteristics (see table 3.2). Examples of such exercise bouts are a 40 yd sprint (36.6 m), a 1RM lift, and sets with heavy resistance (2- to 4RM). These fiber types have a high activity of myofibrillar ATPase, the enzyme that breaks down ATP and releases the energy to cause fiber shortening. Type II fibers are able to shorten with a faster contraction speed and have fast relaxation times. Thus, they can develop force in a short period of time or have a high power output. Type II fibers rely predominantly on anaerobic sources to supply the energy necessary for muscle activation. This is evidenced by their high levels of ATP and PC intramuscular stores, as well as their high glycolytic enzyme activity. Type II fibers have a low aerobic capability as evidenced by their low intramuscular stores of triglyceride, low capillary density, low mitochondria density, and low aerobic enzyme activity. The fact that type II fibers rely predominantly on anaerobic sources for ATP and have low capabilities to supply ATP aerobically makes them highly susceptible to fatigue. Type II fibers are suited to short-duration activities that require high power output.

Type I fibers are more suited to endurance (aerobic) activities. These fibers have high levels of aerobic enzyme activity, capillary density, mitochondrial density, and intramuscular triglyceride stores, and low fatigability. Type I fibers are ideal for low-intensity, long-duration (endurance) activities, such as long-distance running and swimming and high numbers of repetitions in a set with light weights.

TABLE 3.2 Characteristics of Type I and Type II Muscle Fibers

Characteristic	Type I	Type II
Force per cross-sectional area	Low	High
Myofibrillar ATPase activity (pH 9.4)	Low	High
Intramuscular ATP stores	Low	High
Intramuscular PC stores	Low	High
Contraction speed	Slow	Fast
Relaxation time	Slow	Fast
Glycolytic enzyme activity	Low	High
Endurance	High	Low
Intramuscular glycogen stores	No difference	No difference
Intramuscular triglyceride stores	High	Low
Myoglobin content	High	Low
Aerobic enzyme activity	High	Low
Capillary density	High	Low
Mitochondrial density	High	Low

Several subtypes of type I and type II fibers have been demonstrated. Type IIa fibers possess good aerobic and anaerobic characteristics, whereas type IIx (the former name was type IIb, but new genetic studies showed this type is not typically found in human muscle so these fibers were renamed and called type IIx) fibers possess good anaerobic characteristics, but poor aerobic characteristics (Essen et al. 1975; Staron, Hagerman et al. 2000; Staron, Hikida, and Hagerman 1983). It now appears that the type IIx fibers may in fact be just a pool of unused fibers (with low oxidative ability) that upon recruitment start a shift or transformation to the type IIa fiber type (Adams et al. 1993; Staron et al. 1991, 1994). Dramatic reductions in the IIx fiber type occur with heavy resistance training, which supports such a theory (Kraemer, Patton et al. 1995). In humans, type IIc fibers occur infrequently (less than 3% of all fibers), but these are more oxidative than type IIa and type IIx fibers in several biochemical characteristics. Type IIax fibers represent a hybrid (i.e., a combination of type IIa and IIx fiber types) and are a transition phase going to more or less oxidative fiber types.

The type I muscle fiber has only one subtype, Ic. There are very few type Ic fibers, usually less than 5% of the total, and they are a less oxidative (aerobic) form of the type I fiber. With resistance training or some types of anaerobic training, type Ic fibers may make small increases in number because of the lack of increased oxidative stress with these types of training.

Type II muscle fiber subtypes represent a continuum from the least oxidative type IIx to the more oxidative type IIc. The larger array of type II muscle fiber subtypes allows for a greater transformation among type II fiber subtypes with physical training (Ingjer 1969; Staron, Hikida, and Hagerman 1983; Staron et al. 1991, 1994). A number of older studies that did not use a full spectrum of fiber type profiles indicated that a fiber transformation may occur between the type I and type II fibers with exercise training (Haggmark, Jansson, and Eriksson 1982; Howald 1982). However, it now appears that the changes occur only within the subtypes of type I or type II fibers and that these early studies most likely were in error as a result of a lack of histochemical subtyping of all muscle fiber subtypes (Pette and Staron 1997). Thus, fiber type transformation occurs within the major fiber types of I and II, but not between types I and II (see box 3.2).

Sliding Filament Theory

How muscles contract remained a mystery until an interesting theory was proposed in the middle of the 20th century. In 1954 two papers were published simultaneously in the journal *Nature*. Papers by A.F. Huxley and R. Niedergerke and by H.E. Huxley and E.J. Hansen provided the first fundamentally important insights into how muscles shortened. These scientists explained that muscle shortening was associated with the sliding of two protein filaments over each other (i.e., myosin and actin filaments) without these filaments themselves changing significantly in length. When the **sarcomere** (the smallest length of muscle capable of developing force and shortening; see

---

 BOX 3.2 PRACTICAL QUESTION

Can Intense Resistance Training Convert Type I Fibers Into Type II Fibers?

The quick answer is no! Early studies that examined muscle fiber types using a limited histochemical profile showed slight increases in the percentage of type I or type II fibers following either endurance or heavy resistance training; this was most likely due to misclassified fibers. Under normal physiological circumstances, leading experts in muscle physiology agree that type I to type II muscle fiber changes, or vice versa, do not occur, but resistance training can increase fiber size and force production. Conversely, endurance training has been shown to decrease type I muscle fiber size and show little or no changes in type II muscle fiber size. So training may alter the percentage of a muscle's cross-sectional area that is in a certain fiber type (e.g., hypertrophy of type II fibers), which increases the percentage of an intact muscle's cross-sectional area that is type II, but the percentage of fibers that are type II is not changed.

figure 3.8) shortens, myosin filaments remain stationary while myosin heads pull the actin filaments over the myosin filaments, resulting in the actin filaments sliding over the myosin filaments. By the turn of the 21st century, a host of findings on the dynamics of muscle contraction had been demonstrated, but interestingly, the basic theory remained intact (A.F. Huxley 2000). The contractile proteins are held in a very tight relationship by the noncontractile proteins, which make up an extensive type of basket weave to keep the protein filaments of the sarcomere in place.

An understanding of the structural arrangement of skeletal muscle is needed to understand the **sliding filament theory** of muscular activation. Skeletal muscle is called striated muscle because the arrangement of proteins in the muscle gives it a striped, or striated, appearance under a microscope (see figure 3.9). Muscle fibers are composed of sarcomeres stacked end to end. At rest, several

distinct light and dark areas create striations within each sarcomere. These light and dark areas are the result of the arrangement of the actin and myosin filaments, the major proteins involved in the contractile process. In the contracted (fully shortened) state, there are still striations, but they have a different pattern. This change in the striation pattern occurs as a result of the sliding of the actin over the myosin protein filaments.

A sarcomere runs from one Z-line to the next Z-line. At rest there are two distinct light areas in each sarcomere: the H-zone, which contains no actin but does contain myosin, and the I-bands located at the ends of the sarcomere, which contain only actin filaments. These two areas appear light in comparison to the A-band, which contains both actin and myosin filaments.

As the sarcomere shortens, the actin filaments slide over the myosin filaments. This causes the H-zone to seem to disappear as actin filaments

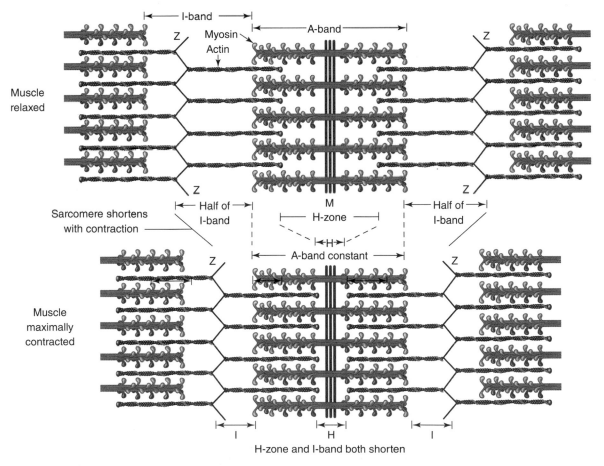

FIGURE 3.8 Sarcomere demonstrating the sliding filament theory: As the actin and myosin filaments slide over each other, the entire sarcomere shortens, but the lengths of the individual actin and myosin filaments do not change.

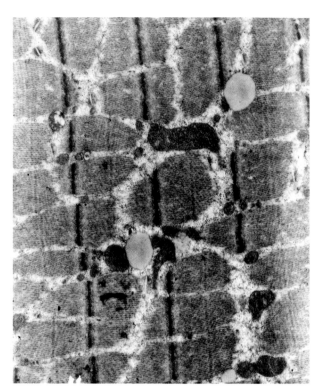

FIGURE 3.9 Electron micrograph of human skeletal muscle from the lateral head of the gastrocnemius showing the sarcomere and associated bands and organelles.
Courtesy of Dr. William J. Kraemer, Department of Kinesiology, University of Connecticut, Storrs, CT.

slide into it and give it a darker appearance. The I-bands become shorter as the Z-lines come closer to the ends of the myosin filaments. When the sarcomere relaxes and returns to its original length, the H-zone and I-bands return to their original size and appearance.

Phases of Muscle Action

Since the sliding filament theory was originally proposed in the 1950s, many newer studies have discovered how the protein filaments of muscle interact (for a review, see A.F. Huxley 2000). At rest, the projections or crossbridges of the myosin filaments touch the actin filaments, but cannot interact to cause shortening. The actin filament has active sites on it that the myosin crossbridges can interact with to cause shortening. At rest, however, the active sites are covered by tropomyosin, to which troponin is also attached. These two important regulatory proteins are associated with the actin filament (see figure 3.10).

In the resting state the myosin heads are cocked and ready to swivel or ratchet upon interaction with the active site on the actin filament. Upon electrical activation of a motor unit (discussed later), the result is the release of the neurotransmitter acetylcholine, or ACh, into the neuromuscular junction. ACh binds with postjunctional receptors on the muscle and causes an ionic electrical current to run down the T-tubules and throughout the sarcoplasmic reticulum, a membranous structure that surrounds each muscle fiber. This causes the energy-mediated Ca^{++} pump in the sarcoplasmic reticulum to stop, releasing large concentrations of Ca^{++} **into the sarcoplasm of the muscle.** The released Ca^{++} binds to the troponin molecule, which is attached to the tropomyosin protein of the actin filament. This triggers a change in the troponin structure, which then pulls on the tropomyosin protein taking it out of its groove within the actin filaments. This exposes the active sites on the actin filament. The blocking of the active sites by tropomyosin is called the steric blocking model. With the active site now exposed, the myosin crossbridges can make contact with the active sites on the actin filament. Contraction, or shortening of the sarcomere, can now take place. The heads of the crossbridge of the myosin filament now attach to the active sites on the actin filament. Attached, the heads of the myosin filament pull and swivel, or ratchet, the actin filament a short distance inward toward the center of the sarcomere. At this point another ATP molecule that is proximate to these heads and derived from the energy systems binds to the myosin heads and activates the enzyme myosin ATPase that is located in the heads of the myosin crossbridges. This results in the breakdown of the ATP molecule, releasing energy and helping to again "cock" the myosin crossbridge head and make it ready to interact with a new actin active site closer to the Z-line as a result of the inward movement of the filament. The process of breaking contact with one active site and binding to another is termed recharging. This process pulls the actin over the myosin, causing the sarcomere to shorten.

The tilt of the crossbridge has been generally accepted as producing all of the force generation in muscle, but recent studies implicate a much more complicated series of steps in the movement of the crossbridge and possible roles for other factors such as nonmyosin proteins and temperature (for a detailed review, see A.F. Huxley 2000). Upon contact with a new active site, the myosin head again swivels. This causes the actin to slide farther over the myosin, resulting in the shortening of the sarcomere. This cyclical (or "ratcheting") process is

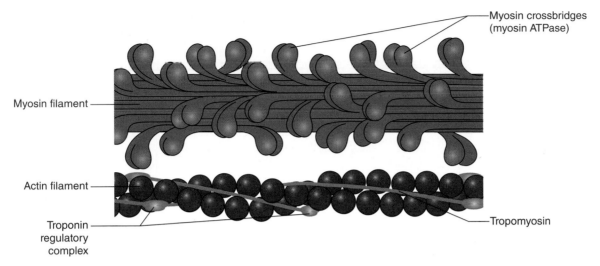

FIGURE 3.10 Schematic of a myosin and actin filament. The active sites are located on the actin filament underneath the tropomyosin and troponin regulatory proteins.

repeated until either the sarcomere has shortened as much as possible or the muscle relaxes. In an isometric muscle action, the heads of the myosin crossbridge remain in the same place interacting with the same active site while producing force at that range of motion, but no movement occurs. Eccentrically, as the muscle lengthens, myosin crossbridges interact or grab hold of each active site producing more force as the speed of the eccentric action increases (see the later discussion of the force velocity curve). However, the exact molecular dynamics of this muscle action are still unclear and continue to be an area of scientific research in muscle physiology and molecular biology.

ATPase breaks down the new ATP, causing the crossbridge head to be cocked and ready for inter-action with a new active site. Relaxation of the muscle occurs when the electrical impulse from the motor cortex in the brain stops sending action potentials down the alpha motor neuron. As a result, the secretion of the ACh neurotransmitter stops. This triggers the startup of the Ca^{++} because of the lack of electrical interference, and once again Ca^{++} is actively pumped back into the sarcoplasmic reticulum. This pump mechanism also requires energy from the breakdown of ATP to function. With no Ca^{++} bound to the troponin, it assumes its original shape and allows tropomyosin to fall back into its groove within the actin filament covering the active sites. The crossbridges of the myosin filament now have no active sites to interact with, and movement stops. With the relaxation of a motor unit and its alpha motor neurons, muscle activity stops. The muscle remains in the shortened position it finds itself in when neural activations stops unless it is passively pulled to a lengthened position by gravity or an outside force, such as an antagonistic muscle.

Length–Tension (Force) Curve

The **length–tension (force) curve** (see figure 3.11) demonstrates that there is an optimal length at which muscle fibers generate maximal force. The amount of force developed depends on the number of myosin crossbridges interacting with active sites on the actin. At different lengths different numbers of crossbridges are attached to the actin filament. At the optimal length, there is the potential for maximal crossbridge interaction and thus maximal force. Below this optimal length, less tension is developed during activation because with excessive shortening actin filaments overlap and thus interfere with each other's ability to contact the myosin crossbridges. Less crossbridge contact with the active sites on the actin results in a smaller potential to develop tension.

At lengths greater than optimal, less overlap of the actin and myosin filaments occurs. This results in less of a potential for crossbridge contact with the active sites on the actin. Thus, if the sarcomere's length is greater than optimal, less force can be developed.

The length–tension curve indicates that some prestretch of the muscle before initiation of a contraction will increase the amount of force gen-erated. Many everyday and sporting activities do

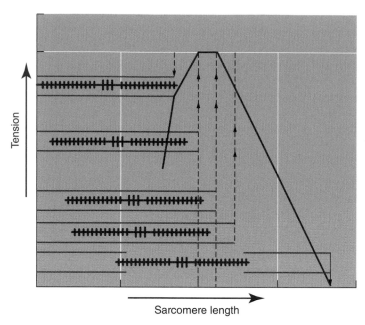

FIGURE 3.11 There is an optimal length at which a sarcomere develops maximal tension (force). At lengths less than or greater than optimal, less tension is developed.

involve a prestretch. For example, every time the knee slightly bends before extending while walking, the quadriceps muscle is prestretched. Some powerlifters attempt to use a prestretch by pulling their shoulders back (adducting the scapulas) and stretching the pectoral muscles before performing the bench press.

Adaptations to Muscle Fibers

One of the most prominent adaptations to a resistance training program is the enlargement of muscles. Today, sport scientists, athletes, personnel trainers, and coaches all agree that a properly designed and implemented strength training program leads to muscle growth. This growth in muscle size has been thought to be primarily due to muscle fiber hypertrophy, or an increase in the size of the individual muscle fibers (Kraemer, Fleck, and Evans 1996; MacDougall 1992; Schoenfeld 2010).

Muscle fiber **hyperplasia,** or an increase in the number of muscle fibers, has also been proposed as a mechanism for increasing the size of muscle. The concept of hyperplasia after resistance training in humans has not been directly proven because of methodological difficulties (e.g., one cannot take out the whole human muscle for examination), but it has been shown in response to various exercise protocols in birds and mammals (for reviews, see Antonio and Gonyea 1994; MacDougall 1992).

Hypertrophy

An increase in muscle size has been observed in both animals and humans. In laboratory animals, muscle growth has occurred as a result of hypertrophy alone (Bass, Mackova, and Vitek 1973; Gollnick et al. 1981; Timson et al. 1985). Increased muscle size in strength-trained athletes has been attributed to hypertrophy of existing muscle fibers (Alway 1994; Alway et al. 1989; Haggmark, Jansson, and Svane 1978). This increase in the cross-sectional area of existing muscle fibers is attributed to the increased size and number of the actin and myosin filaments and the addition of sarcomeres within existing muscle fibers (Goldspink 1992; MacDougall et al. 1979), although it has been suggested that an increase in noncontractile proteins also occurs (Phillips et al. 1999). This is reflected by an increase in myofibrillar volume after resistance training (Luthi et al. 1986; MacDougall 1986). Interestingly, extreme muscle hypertrophy may actually reduce myofibrillar volume (MacDougall et al. 1982).

Not all muscle fibers undergo the same amount of hypertrophy. The amount of hypertrophy depends on the type of muscle fiber and the pattern of recruitment (Kraemer, Fleck, and Evans 1996). Muscle fiber hypertrophy has been demonstrated in both type I and type II fibers after resistance training (McCall et al. 1996). However, conventional weight training in humans (Gonyea and Sale

1982) and animals (Edgerton 1978) appears to increase the size of type II muscle fibers to a greater degree than type I muscle fibers (Kraemer, Patton et al. 1995). Hypertrophy is a result of the balance between protein degradation and synthesis. It occurs when either degradation is decreased or synthesis is increased. However, differences in the two muscle fiber types are related to the magnitude of increase in synthesis or the decrease in degradation of protein synthesis that is simultaneously going on. The greater hypertrophy of type II fibers may be due to differences in protein accretion mechanisms in the two fiber types; type I fibers depend on a greater reduction in protein degradation, whereas type II fibers increase synthesis to a greater extent, facilitating hypertrophy.

However, it may be possible to selectively increase either the type II or the type I muscle fibers depending on the training regimen. Powerlifters and weightlifters who train predominantly with high intensity (i.e., heavy resistances) and lower volume (i.e., small number of sets and repetitions) have been shown to have type II fibers with a mean fiber area of 9,300 µm² in the vastus lateralis (Tesch, Thorsson, and Kaiser 1984). Conversely, bodybuilders who train at certain phases of their contest preparation phase with a slightly lower intensity but a higher volume have been shown to have type II fibers with a mean fiber area of 6,200 µm² in the same muscle (Tesch and Larson 1982).

In addition, bodybuilders have been shown to possess a lower total percentage of type II fiber area in the vastus lateralis than Olympic weightlifters and powerlifters do (50 vs. 69%, respectively) (Tesch and Larson 1982).

Powerlifters and weightlifters who lift much heavier resistances than are typical of bodybuilders exhibit greater hypertrophy in type II muscle fibers than do bodybuilders, who appear to exhibit equal increases in the size of both fiber types (Fry 2004). Thus, the high-intensity, low-volume training of Olympic weightlifters and powerlifters may more selectively increase type II fibers than the lower-intensity, higher-volume training of bodybuilders as a result of the stimulus of the more prolific signaling and neurological mechanisms that are operational in this fiber type (Folland and Williams 2007; Schoenfeld 2010).

The increase in muscle fiber size can be seen by examining a group of muscle fibers under a microscope after they have been stained using the myosin ATPase method at pH 4.6. In figure 3.12, a sample obtained from a woman's vastus lateralis (quadriceps muscle) is shown before (a) and after (b) an eight-week heavy resistance training program. The fibers are cut in cross-section; the darkest ones are the type I fibers, the intermediate ones are type IIx, and the white ones are type IIa muscle fibers. This woman obviously increased the size of all of her muscle fibers with heavy resistance

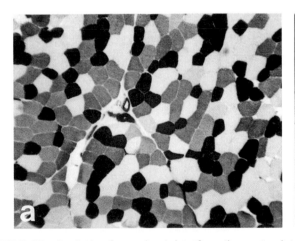
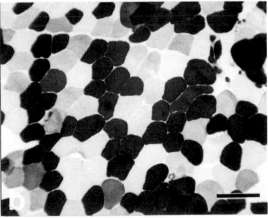

FIGURE 3.12 Analysis of samples taken from the vastus lateralis muscle before (a) and after (b) eight weeks of high-intensity resistance training. The muscle fibers have been cut in cross-section and assayed for myosin adenosine triphosphatase (mATPase) activity following pre-incubation at pH 4.6. The darkest fibers are type I, the light fibers are type IIa, and the intermediate fibers are type IIx. Note the increase in the size of the fibers (hypertrophy) and the decrease in the number of intermediate stained fibers posttraining.

Bar = 200 µm.

Courtesy of Dr. Robert S. Staron, Ohio University, Athens, Ohio.

training, especially the type II muscle fibers. The larger cross-sectional area increase (hypertrophy) pre- to posttraining of the type II fibers can easily be seen. Muscle hypertrophy is one of the hallmarks of training adaptations to heavy resistance training protocols. However, the individual muscle fiber must be recruited to see protein accretion and such fiber size increases.

Adaptations in muscle fibers with heavy resistance training must be viewed from both a quality and quantity (of the contractile proteins) perspective (i.e., actin and myosin). With the initiation of a heavy resistance training program, changes in the types of muscle proteins (e.g., myosin heavy chains) start to take place within a couple of workouts (Staron et al. 1994). As training continues, the quantity of contractile proteins starts to increase as muscle fibers develop increased cross-sectional areas. To demonstrate a significant amount of muscle fiber hypertrophy, a longer period of training time (more than eight workouts) is needed to increase the contractile protein content in all muscle fibers. During the early phases of training, typically, changes in protein quality (changes in myosin ATPase isoforms, going from IIx to IIax or IIa), but not very large changes in muscle fiber size or the whole muscle, occur.

Muscle hypertrophy gives the lifter a potential advantage for producing greater force, but not contraction velocity if the hypertrophy of the muscle is too great. However, what constitutes excessive hypertrophy is unclear because of the many anatomical differences among people (e.g., limb lengths).

The **pennation angle** of muscle fibers is defined as the angle at which muscle fibers attach to their tendon in relation to the direction of pull of the tendon (see figure 3.13). In pennate muscles pennation angle increases to a certain extent with resistance training; for example, 5% after nine weeks of resistance training (Erskine et al. 2010). Too much of an increase in the pennation angle might be unfavorable for force production because, as pennation angle increases, the muscle fibers are not pulling directly in line with the line of pull of the tendon. The pennation angle of the triceps brachii in bodybuilders is significantly greater than that in untrained men (33 vs. 15 degrees for long head, 19 vs. 11 degrees for short head), which is due directly to the impressive hypertrophy needed for bodybuilding success (Kawakami, Abe, and Fukunaga 1993). It has also been reported that the pennation angles of the long head of the triceps (21.4 vs. 16.5 degrees), medial aspect of the gastrocnemius (23.6 vs. 21.3 degrees), and lateral aspect of the gastrocnemius (15.4 vs. 13.5 degrees) were greater in sumo wrestlers than in untrained men (Kearns, Abe, and Brechue 2000). An increase in pennation angle of the triceps brachii from 16.5 to 21.3 degrees after 16 weeks of resistance training has been reported with training (Kawakami et al. 1995). Resistance training for 14 weeks increases the pennation angle of the vastus lateralis from 8 to 10.7 degrees in addition to an 18.4% increase in type II muscle fiber area (Aagaard et al. 2001). In addition, a correlation between muscle angle of pennation and muscle volume ($r = .622$) has been observed (Aagaard et al. 2001), as have significant correlations between muscle thickness and pennation angle in some (triceps long head and gastrocnemius medialis) but not other (vastus lateralis) muscles of elite powerlifters (Brechue and Abe 2002).

An increase in pennation angle is due to an increase in muscle size. However, as pennation angle increases, force per cross-sectional area of muscle may decrease. The impact of pennation angle on the force per cross-sectional area is shown in a comparison of bodybuilders' and weightlifters' force in an elbow extensor movement. The bodybuilders had a significantly lower ratio of force to

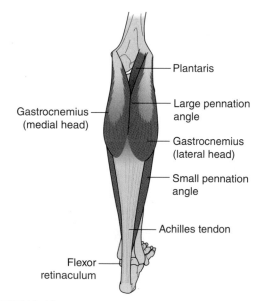

FIGURE 3.13 Pennation angle is determined by the angle at which muscle fibers attach to their tendon. An increase in pennation angle occurs with muscle hypertrophy and may decrease force production per cross-sectional area of muscle.

cross-sectional area than the weightlifters had, as well as a larger pennation angle. This indicates that a larger pennation angle is associated with lower force relative to the muscle's cross-sectional area (Ikegawa et al. 2008). Thus, very excessive hypertrophy that affects the pennation angles of the muscles could potentially limit force production.

There appears to be a limit to how much the pennation angle of a muscle can increase. Some scientists have suggested that with extreme hypertrophy, such as that attained by bodybuilders or some other athletes, a plateau exists in pennation angle after which an increase in fascicle length may limit individual fiber pennation angle (Kearns, Abe, and Brechue 2000). That is, an increase in the number of sarcomeres in a series has been proposed to limit changes in pennation angle (Kearns, Abe, and Brechue 2000). American football players (Abe, Brown, and Brechue 1999), sumo wrestlers (Kearns, Abe, and Brechue 2000), and sprinters (Kumagai et al. 2000) have longer fascicle lengths (both absolute and relative to limb length) of the triceps, vastus lateralis, and gastrocnemius muscles than untrained men do. In addition, increased fascicle length has been implicated for increasing the force per cross-sectional area of muscle and the velocity of contraction. Faster sprinters (e.g., 10.0-10.9 s in 100 m) have greater fascicle length and smaller angles of pennation in comparison to slower sprinters (11.0-11.7 s in 100 m) (Kumagai et al. 2000). Although genetic predisposition cannot be ruled out, it appears that either the addition of sarcomeres in a series or an increase in sarcomere length may occur when a certain threshold of hypertrophy or a critical level of pennation angle has been reached (Kearns, Abe, and Brechue 2000). In general, pennation angle increases with hypertrophy, but may have a maximal value after which sarcomeres in a series are added. This limits the increase in pennation angle.

Hyperplasia

Hyperplasia was first implicated as an adaptive strategy for muscle enlargement in laboratory animals (Gonyea 1980; Ho et al. 1980). Critics of these studies claimed that methods of evaluation, damage to the muscle samples, and degenerating muscle fibers accounted for the observed hyperplasia. However, a few later studies attempting to correct for such problems still demonstrated increases in muscle fiber number (Alway et al. 1989; Gonyea et al. 1986).

Several studies comparing bodybuilders and powerlifters concluded that the cross-sectional area of the bodybuilders' individual muscle fibers was not significantly larger than normal, yet these athletes possessed larger muscles than normal (MacDougall et al. 1982; Tesch and Larsson 1982). This indicates that these athletes have a greater total number of muscle fibers than normal, and hyperplasia may account for this increase. However, it has also been shown that bodybuilders possessed the same number of muscle fibers as untrained people, but had much larger muscles (MacDougall et al. 1984). This finding indicated that the large muscle size of bodybuilders is due to hypertrophy of existing muscle fibers rather than hyperplasia.

In a 12-week training study of men using both magnetic resonance imaging (MRI) and biopsy techniques to examine hypertrophy and the possible increase in muscle fibers after a heavy resistance program, some evidence for hyperplasia in the biceps muscle was shown, despite hypertrophy accounting for the greatest portion of muscle enlargement (McCall et al. 1996). A study of hyperplasia in cats indicated that for hyperplasia to occur, the exercise intensity must be sufficient to recruit fast-twitch muscle fibers (type II fibers) (Gonyea 1980). It is possible that only high-intensity resistance training can cause hyperplasia and that type II muscle fibers may be targeted for this type of adaptation. Powerlifters have been shown to have higher numbers of myonuclei, satellite cells, and small-diameter fibers expressing markers for early myogenesis, thereby indicating hyperplasia (Kadi et al. 1999). These effects appear to be enhanced by anabolic steroid use (Kadi et al. 2000), which potentially demonstrates an additional mechanism, because more myonuclei means a greater number of androgen receptors available for interaction, in the case of steroid-enhanced muscle growth.

Although limited data support hyperplasia in humans, there are indications that it can occur as a result of resistance training. Because of these conflicting results, this topic remains controversial; further research on elite competitive lifters may help to resolve the controversy. Although hyperplasia in humans may occur, it is not be the primary adaptational mechanism of most muscle fibers to resistance overload. It might represent an adaptation to resistance training when certain muscle fibers reach a theoretical upper limit in size. It might be theorized that very intense long-term training may make some type II muscle fibers primary candidates for such an adaptational response. However, if hyperplasia does occur, it may account for only a very small portion (e.g., 3 to 5%) of the increase in muscle size.

Protein Synthesis

Muscle hypertrophy is the result of an increase in protein synthesis, a decrease in protein degradation, or a combination of both. Protein synthesis increases after an acute bout of resistance exercise. When the amount of protein synthesized exceeds that which is degraded, then net protein accretion is positive and hypertrophy can occur. Hypertrophy in type II muscle fibers appears to involve primarily an increase in the rate of protein synthesis, whereas hypertrophy in type I muscle fibers appears to involve primarily a decrease in the rate of degradation (Goldspink 1992) (see discussion on degradation and synthesis of protein).

When Tarnopolsky and colleagues examined (1991) total-body protein synthesis during resistance exercise, they observed no changes. However, total-body measurements do not reflect changes at the individual muscle or muscle fiber levels. When measured in the biceps brachii and the vastus lateralis, protein synthesis is significantly elevated up to 48 hours postexercise (Chesley et al. 1992; MacDougall, Tarnopolsky et al. 1992, 1995; Phillips et al. 1997). Protein synthesis can be elevated by 112, 65, and 34%, respectively, at 3, 24, and 48 hours post–resistance exercise (Phillips et al. 1997). In addition, the protein degradation rate was elevated by only 31, 18, and 1% at these same time points, indicating that muscle protein balance was elevated 23 to 48% over the 48-hour postexercise time period.

With heavy resistance training the integrated mixed muscle (i.e., all fibers) fractional synthetic rate was similar between rest and acute resistance exercise (five sets at 85% of 1RM to failure in the unilateral leg press and knee extension with the other limb acting as a within-subject control), but specific myofibrillar fractional synthetic rate was higher in the resistance-exercised thighs than in those of untrained subjects (Gasier et al. 2012). Collectively, the preceding studies indicate that resistance training can acutely increase protein synthesis in response to the activation of motor units to produce force.

Training status plays a role in the post–resistance exercise change in protein synthesis. Phillips and colleagues (1999) compared the fractional rate of protein synthesis and degradation in resistance-trained (at least five years of experience) and untrained men. Interestingly, this comparison showed that the rate of protein synthesis four hours postexercise was higher in untrained men than in trained men (118 vs. 48%, respectively). However, the rate of breakdown was also higher in the untrained men leading to a similar net protein balance of 37 and 34%, respectively, for the untrained and trained men. The investigators suggested that chronic resistance training reduces muscle damage, and consequently protein degradation, which would increase net protein synthesis.

Amino acid transport across the cell membrane and consequent uptake by skeletal muscle is important for enhancing protein synthesis. An increase in amino acid transport of 60 to 120% occurs (depending on the amino acid) in the three hours after resistance exercise workouts (Biolo, Fleming, and Wolfe 1995). Interestingly, arterial amino acid concentrations did not change; rather, a 90% increase in muscle blood flow accounted for much of the increase in amino acid transport.

Growing evidence demonstrates the importance of blood flow in protein synthesis and muscle hypertrophy. Studies that have restricted blood flow and used light loading during resistance exercise (thereby increasing the concentrations of metabolites and the anaerobic nature of the exercise stimulus) have shown hypertrophy increases comparable to those that occur with heavier loading. This demonstrates the importance of blood flow or anabolic hormone/metabolite accumulation, or both, during resistance training to bring about adaptations (Rooney, Herbert, and Balwave 1994; Shinohara et al. 1998; Smith and Rutherford 1995; Yasuda et al. 2010).

Kaatsu training (also called blood flow restriction training), in which occlusion occurs as a result of restricting blood flow to target muscle groups and light resistances are used (e.g., 20% of 1RM) has gained popularity (see Vascular Occlusion in chapter 6) because of its apparent effects on strength and hypertrophy (Yasuda et al. 2010). Although a potential tool in weight training, safety issues have been noted as a result of its limited use in long-term studies and the presence of hypoxia, oxidative stress, and potential problems with edema (Loenneke et al. 2011). This may explain in part the efficacy of bodybuilding programs for increasing muscle hypertrophy using moderate loading and high volumes of work with short rest intervals to increase the metabolites in muscle.

Muscle protein synthesis after resistance exercise depends heavily on amino acid availability, the timing of protein intake, and insulin concentrations in addition to other factors such as hormones (e.g., GH, testosterone, IGF-I, MGF), mechanical stress, and cellular hydration. The acute increases in protein synthesis appear to be influenced by changes at the nuclear level. This includes mechanisms not related to the RNA signaling such as enhancing ribosome biogenesis, increasing the abundance of translation initiation factors, or both changes occurring simultaneously (Baar and Esser 1999; Jefferson and Kimball 2001). When insulin concentrations are elevated after resistance exercise (either by glucose intake or insulin infusion), the exercise-mediated acceleration of protein breakdown is reduced and synthesis rates are not significantly increased, thereby resulting in a net protein accretion of approximately 36% (Biolo et al. 1999; Roy et al. 1997).

It is interesting to note that insulin increases have occurred after a resistance training session when followed by postexercise carbohydrate supplementation (Williams et al. 2002). After resistance exercise, protein synthesis rate stimulated by amino acid intake is doubled when coinciding with increases in muscle blood flow (Biolo et al. 1997). This effect may be greater when amino acids are taken before a workout to optimize amino acid delivery and transport during the workout as a result of greater blood flow (Tipton et al. 2001). These results indicate a potential ergogenic effect of glucose and amino acid intake before or directly after resistance exercise to maximize protein synthesis and recovery. The majority of studies demonstrate that protein (primarily essential amino acids) and whey protein taken before and after a resistance exercise workout enhance muscle hypertrophy, and that training and recovery from resistance exercise improve muscle protein synthesis (Hulmi, Lockwood, and Stout 2010).

A model of protein metabolism during resistance exercise has been proposed (Tipton and Wolfe 1998): (1) resistance exercise stimulates protein synthesis, (2) intracellular amino acid concentrations are reduced, (3) decreased amino acid concentrations stimulate protein breakdown and transport of amino acids into the muscle cell, (4) increased availability of amino acids further stimulates protein synthesis, and (5) tissue remodeling occurs. Therefore, it appears that optimal protein intake, especially of essential amino acids, is crucial to optimizing recovery and performance as well as subsequent adaptations to resistance training (Volek 2004).

Structural Changes in Muscle

Structural changes refers to the size, number, or distance between structures within muscle. Structural changes can affect the function of muscle. Even though myofilament number increases with resistance training, the myofibrillar packing distance (i.e., the distance between myosin or other protein filaments) and the length of the sarcomere appear to remain constant after six weeks to six months of resistance training (Claassen et al. 1989; Erskine et al. 2011; Luthi et al. 1986; MacDougall 1986). However, fascicle length may increase with resistance training (see the section on hypertrophy) and has been significantly correlated with fat-free mass in elite male powerlifters (Brechue and Abe 1986). The ratio of actin to myosin filaments does not change after six weeks of resistance training (Claassen et al. 1989). The relative volume of the sarcoplasm, T-tubules, and other noncontractile tissue does not appear to change significantly as a result of resistance training (Alway et al. 1988, 1989; Luthi et al. 1986; MacDougall et al. 1984; Sale et al. 1987). Thus, although increases in myofilament number take place, the spatial orientation of the sarcomere appears to remain unchanged after resistance training. With training sarcomeres are added in parallel, contributing to the increase in muscle cross-sectional area and fat-free mass, but how the sarcomere functions is unchanged.

Structural changes do, however, occur within skeletal muscle as a result of resistance training. The sodium–potassium ATPase pump activity, which maintains sodium and potassium ion gradients and membrane potential, has been shown to increase by 16% after 11 weeks of resistance training (Green et al. 1999). In healthy young people few structural changes occur, but in the elderly resistance training appears to attenuate some of the age-related declines in muscle morphology. Resistance training has been shown to attenuate the age-related decreases in tropomyosin (Klitgaard et al. 1990), the maximal rate of sarcoplasmic reticulum calcium uptake (Hunter et al. 1999), sarcoplasmic reticulum calcium ATPase activity (Hunter et al. 1999; Klitgaard, Aussoni, and Damiani 1989), and calsequestrin concentrations

(Klitgaard, Aussoni, and Damiani 1989). These changes were not observed in younger populations (Green, Goreham et al. 1998; Green, Grange et al. 1998; Hunter et al. 1999; McKenna et al. 1996). These data indicate the importance of resistance training for limiting the age-related reductions in muscle structure and performance.

Noncontractile structural proteins and scaffolding proteins (i.e., dystrophin-associated protein complex [DAPC]) link the intracellular and extracellular structures and are important to the stability and transmission of forces in the sarcomere and the muscle. This transmission of forces is also important for signaling within muscle (e.g., stimulation of the **mammalian target of rapamycin** (mTOR), an important protein for signaling cell growth and protein synthesis). Progressive heavy resistance training for 16 weeks did increase various proteins in the DAPC and showed similar effects in both older and younger men. However, the increase in stress-induced mitogen-activated protein kinases (MAPK) in older men only might be one reason the magnitude of muscle fiber hypertrophy was dramatically lower in older men than in younger men after 16 weeks of training (Kosek and Bamman 2008).

Muscle Fiber Type Transition

The quality of protein refers to the type of protein, such as the type of ATPase, found in the contractile machinery. The type of protein has the ability to change the functional profile of muscle (Pette and Staron 2001). Much of the resistance training research focuses on the myosin molecule and the examination of fiber types based on the use of the histochemical myosin adenosine triphosphatase (mATPase) staining activities at different pHs,

which was discussed earlier. Changes in muscle mATPase fiber types also give an indication of associated changes in the myosin heavy chain (MHC) content (Fry, Kraemer, Stone et al. 1994). We now know that a continuum of muscle fiber types exist and that transformation (e.g., from type IIx to type IIa) within type II fibers is a common adaptation to resistance training (Adams et al. 1993; Kesidis et al. 2008; Kraemer, Fleck, and Evans 1996; Kraemer, Patton, et al. 1995; Staron et al. 1991, 1994).

As soon as type IIx muscle fibers are stimulated as a result of motor unit activation, they appear to start a process of transformation toward the type IIa profile by changing the quality of proteins and expressing different numbers or percentages of the muscle fiber types using the mATPase histochemical analysis of muscle. Figure 3.14 shows the transformation process that occurs with heavy resistance training in the muscle fiber subtypes moving toward the type IIa subtype. With exercise training, one cannot transform muscle fibers from type II to type I, or vice versa. Thus, muscle fiber type changes appear to be predominantly related to changes only within the type I or type II fiber type profile specifically (for reviews, see Kraemer, Fleck, and Evans 1996; Staron and Johnson 1993).

Both men and women training with a high-intensity resistance protocol twice a week for eight weeks showed fiber type transformation. The protocol focused on the thigh musculature with heavy multiple sets of 6- to 8RM on one training day and 10- to 12RM on the other training day per week for several exercises (squat, leg press, and knee extension). Two-minute rest periods were used to allow for adequate rest between sets and exercises and induce hormonal changes with the exercise protocol (Staron et al. 1994). Maximal dynamic strength increased over the eight-week training

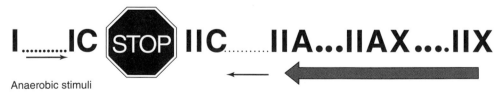

Anaerobic stimuli

Resistance exercise stimuli

FIGURE 3.14 When recruited as part of the needed motor units to lift a weight, type II fibers start a transformation process in the direction of the type IIa fibers with a very small (<1%) number of fibers going to type IIc. A very small number of type I fibers go to type Ic (<1%) with anaerobic training. However, the type II fibers do not transform into type I fibers. Changes in myosin ATPase isoforms and myosin heavy chain proteins underlie this process. Ultimately, when all motor units are recruited in a conditioning program, the trainee ends up with type I and type IIa muscle fibers. Transitions between type I and type II fiber types do not typically occur.

period without any significant changes in muscle fiber size or fat-free mass in the men or the women. This supported the concept that neural adaptations are the predominant mechanism in the early phase of training. However, it also demonstrated that changes also occur in the quality of the contractile proteins during the early phase of training because a significant decrease in the percentage of type IIx fibers was observed in women after just two weeks of training (i.e., four workouts) and in the men after four weeks of training (i.e., eight workouts). Over the eight-week training program (16 workouts), the type IIx muscle fiber types decreased from 21 to about 7% of the total muscle fibers in both men and women. The alteration in the muscle fiber types was supported by myosin heavy chain (MHC) analyses. This study established the time course in both men and women of specific muscular adaptations of the myosin ATPase proteins that start their transition from type IIx to type IIa in the early phase of a resistance training program in which strength increases may occur with or without muscle fiber hypertrophy. Heavier loading is typically associated with muscle fiber hypertrophy in the early phase of training (1 to 10RM), whereas light lifting (20RM and higher) shows little if any changes in both adult men and women (Campos et al. 2002, Schuenke et al. 2012; Schuenke, Herman and Staron 2013). A key factor in these results is that the stimulation of motor units with heavy weights produces a much higher electrical depolarization charge (Hz) than light weights, and it is this high Hz that runs through the low-threshold motor units that contributes to increased hypertrophic training effects as seen in these studies.

It is not known to what extent muscle fiber remodeling contributes to muscle strength; however, gradual increases in the number and size of myofibrils and perhaps conversions of type IIx fibers to type IIa fibers might contribute to increased force production. In addition, changes in hormonal factors (testosterone and cortisol) are correlated with such changes in the muscle fibers (e.g., the percentage shift in type IIa) and may help to mediate such adaptations. Many other changes that are taking place during muscle fiber remodeling in the early phase of training may influence when hypertrophy is initiated. Thus, the quality of the protein type in the remodeling of muscle may be an important aspect of muscular development, especially in the early phases of resistance training.

Longer-duration heavy-resistance training also results in changes in the quality of protein as well as cross-sectional area size. Skeletal muscle was examined in women who trained for 20 weeks, detrained for 2 weeks, and then retrained for 6 weeks (Staron et al. 1991). Increases in muscle fiber cross section were seen with training. The percentage of type IIx fibers decreased from 16 to 0.9%. This study also demonstrated that short detraining periods result in muscle fibers (especially type II) starting to return to pretraining values for muscle fiber cross-sectional areas and starting to transition from type IIa back to type IIx fibers. In addition, it was demonstrated that retraining resulted in a quicker change in muscle size and transition back to type IIa fibers than when starting from the untrained condition. Thus, changes with retraining after a period of detraining occur faster than when starting from the untrained state.

A series of studies using the same subject population examined the effect of resistance training on muscle strength, morphology, histochemical responses, and MHC responses (Adams et al. 1993; Dudley et al. 1991; Hather, Mason, and Dudley 1991). Three groups of men trained for 19 weeks. One group (CON/ECC) trained using both concentric and eccentric muscle actions in a "normal" resistance training program of four to five sets of 6 to 12 repetitions. A second group (CON) trained with only concentric actions for four to five sets of 6 to 12 repetitions, and a third group (CON/CON) used concentric-only actions but for 8 to 10 sets of 6 to 12 repetitions. Thus, the third group performed twice the training volume as the second group as they did more CON repetitions. All groups showed significant gains in strength and an increase in the percentage of type IIa fibers with an accompanying decrease in the percentage of type IIx fibers. Increases in type I fiber area occurred only in the CON/ECC group, and type II fiber area increased in both the CON/ECC and CON/CON groups. Capillaries per unit muscle fiber area increased only in the CON/CON and CON groups. The changes in type II fiber myosin ATPase subtypes were paralleled by an increase in myosin heavy chain MHCIIa and a decrease in the myosin heavy chain MHCIIx. The combined results of these studies indicate that hypertrophy, type II fiber type transformation, and capillaries per unit fiber area are all affected by the type of muscle action or repetition style as well as training volume. Thus, fiber type transitions occur with resistance training but appear to be predominantly limited to changes within the subtypes of type II fibers.

Myoglobin Content

The content of muscle myoglobin, a molecule that transports oxygen from the cell wall to the mitochondria, may decrease after strength training (Tesch 1992). How this decrease affects the muscle fibers' metabolic capabilities for aerobic exercise remains speculative. The initial state of training as well as the specific type of program and magnitude of hypertrophy may influence the effect of resistance training on myoglobin content. Examining resistance training programs in men that used either low intensity and short rest periods or heavy resistance and long rest periods showed that both programs maintained muscle myoglobin content concomitant with increases in muscle size and strength after two months of training. Oxygen-carrying capacity from capillaries to mitochondria was not adversely affected with either type of program even when the diffusion distance was increased as a result of hypertrophy (Masuda et al. 1999).

Capillary Supply

An increased number of capillaries in a muscle helps support aerobic metabolism by increasing the potential blood supply to the active muscle and the surface area where gas exchange can take place between blood and the muscle fiber. Following eight weeks of training with four sets of either a heavy resistance training load (3- to 5RM zone), a moderate resistance training load (9- to 11RM zone), or a light resistance training load (20- to 28RM zone), the only increase in capillaries per fiber was in the type IIa fibers with the moderate resistance training. This change resulted in an increase in capillary number and the number of capillaries per cross-sectional area of tissue or density in only this fiber type (Campos et al. 2002). Although capillary density in total was maintained with the moderate and heavy training zones despite increases in muscle fiber hypertrophy, this demonstrated that capillary number per fiber mirrored the increase in muscle fiber size. Interestingly, the light resistance training zone resulted in no muscle fiber hypertrophy or increase in capillaries per fiber, resulting in no significant change in capillary density. So, training intensity or volume, or both, may affect whether capillary number or density changes.

With typical resistance training (three sets of 10 repetitions) over 12 weeks, significant increases in the numbers of capillaries in type I and type II fibers were observed (McCall et al. 1996). However, because of fiber hypertrophy, no changes in capillaries per fiber area or per area of muscle were shown. Improved capillarization has been observed with resistance training of untrained subjects (Frontera et al. 1988; Hather et al. 1991; Staron et al. 1989; Tesch 1992). It has also been demonstrated that with different types of training (i.e., combinations of concentric and eccentric muscle actions), capillaries per unit area and per fiber increased significantly in response to heavy resistance training even with hypertrophy resulting in increased fiber areas. As with the selective hypertrophy of type II fibers shown by some studies, any increase in capillaries appears to be linked to the intensity and volume of resistance training (Campos et al. 2002; Hather et al. 1991). However, the time course of changes in capillary density appears to be slow because studies show that 6 to 12 weeks may not stimulate capillary growth beyond normal untrained levels (Tesch 1992; Tesch, Hjort, and Balldin 1983).

Powerlifters and weightlifters exhibit no difference from nonathletic people in the number of capillaries per muscle fiber. However, as a result of muscle hypertrophy, these same athletes have less capillary density than nonathletic people (Tesch, Thorsson, and Kaiser 1984). Conversely, a higher number of capillaries than normal surrounding the type I muscle fibers in the trapezius muscles of elite powerlifters has been shown (Kadi et al. 1999). The capillary density was higher for control subjects in the type IIa muscle fibers, indicating that hypertrophy increases capillary diffusion distances in some type II fibers. Bodybuilding training may promote increased capillarization as a result of a higher training volume (Schantz 1982) and also greater metabolic demands because of short-rest training protocols (Kraemer, Noble et al. 1987). This indicates that bodybuilding training that exerts a greater hypoxic stimulus may stimulate capillary development. An increase in capillary density may facilitate the performance of low-intensity weight training by increasing the blood supply to the active muscle.

Thus, capillarization can be increased with resistance training, but any change may depend on the acute program variables: Intensity, volume, and rest period length are important considerations for stimulating changes. However, the time required for this adaptation to take place may be 12 weeks or longer. An increase in the number of capillaries can be masked by muscle hypertrophy resulting in no change in number of capillaries per fiber area or capillary density. A high-volume program using moderate intensity (8- to 12RM zone) may cause capillarization to occur, whereas low-volume programs with heavy resistance may not. Thus, periodized training programs in which resistance loads are varied over a training cycle and both moderate and heavy resistances are used provide for the inclusion of workouts that can address any need for increased capillarization. Finally, it is very important to remember that only muscle fibers that are part of motor units stimulated as a result of training will show an adaptive response.

Mitochondrial Density

In a fashion similar to capillaries per muscle fiber, mitochondrial density has been shown to decrease with resistance training as a result of the dilution effects of muscle fiber hypertrophy (Luthi et al. 1986; MacDougall et al. 1979). The observation of decreased mitochondrial density is consistent with the minimal demands for oxidative metabolism placed on the musculature during most resistance training programs. Twelve weeks of resistance training results in significantly increased type I and II muscle fiber cross-sectional areas of 26 and 28%, respectively (Chilibeck, Syrotuik, and Bell 1999). The analysis of mitochondria demonstrated that strength training resulted in similar reduced density in both the subsarcolemmal and intermyofibrillar mitochondria as a result of the dilution effect caused by muscle fiber hypertrophy. However, interestingly, resistance training has not been shown to inhibit the development of maximal oxygen consumption capacity, suggesting that mitochondrial responses in muscle as a result of resistance training do not negatively affect oxidative capacity. Ten weeks of resistance training (multiple sets of 12 repetitions at 80% of 1RM) or endurance training (two weekly continuous sessions at 75% of maximal heart rate [HRmax] and one session of three sets of interval training at 95% of HRmax on a cycle ergometer) in adults demonstrated similar adaptations in key mitochondrial quality markers increasing

the relative capacity for fatty acid oxidation and tissue-specific respiratory capacity (e.g., increase in the tissue-specific enzymes glutamate, malate, succinate, octanoylcarnitine). This indicates good mitochondrial health with either type of training program (Pesta et al. 2011). Although resistance training shows a decrease in mitochondrial density due to the dilution of the analysis (i.e., per a specific area measurement) as a result of muscle hypertrophy, this effect depends on the type of resistance program and requires further study to better understand its functional outcomes, absolute mitochondrial number, and cellular effects.

Satellite Cells and Myonuclei

Satellite cells are small cells with no cytoplasm that are found in skeletal muscle between the basement membrane and the sarcolemma, or cell membrane, of the muscle fiber. Satellite cells can differentiate into myoblasts and fuse into existing fibers to help in the repair process, acting as a type of stem cell. Importantly, they may also provide daughter nuclei to replace damaged nuclei or add new nuclei to maintain myonuclear domain size during the hypertrophy process of protein accretion with training. These processes are important for the repair and remodeling of muscle fibers after damage or to accommodate the hypertrophy that is produced by resistance training. Increased numbers of satellite cells and myonuclei may indicate cellular repair and the formation of new muscle cells.

Investigations into the role and adaptive ability of myonuclei have been extensive over the past 15 years as the appreciation of their importance to muscle fiber function and repair has grown. The newest theory is that myonuclei increase before any hypertrophy takes place and that during a detraining period they are maintained and remain in an elevated concentration for three months in detrained mouse muscle, thereby mediating muscle memory (see box 3.3) (Bruusgaard et al. 2010). This may also mediate the rapid retraining of muscle fiber size and strength seen in formally trained people (Staron et al. 1991). This rapid improvement may be due to the previously increased concentrations of satellite cells that still exist in detrained muscle for a long period of time (Bruusgaard et al. 2010).

Early on in the study of myonuclei, scientists demonstrated that the number of myonuclei in

BOX 3.3 RESEARCH

Muscle Memory

The ability to make quicker adaptations upon retraining a skeletal muscle has been called muscle memory. Back in 1991 investigators at Ohio University examined a group of untrained women who trained for 20 weeks, then detrained for 30 to 32 weeks, and then retrained for 6 weeks (Staron et al. 1991). Another group of untrained women performed only a six-week training program that was identical to the retraining program of the other group. The previously trained group made faster transitions from type IIx to type IIa fibers upon retraining. They also made quicker gains in cross-sectional muscle fiber size when compared to the women who were just beginning a resistance training program. However, the underlying reasons for this were not clear.

In 2010, a research team from the University of Oslo gave some insight into why this more rapid gain in muscle hypertrophy was achieved during retraining (Bruusgaard et al. 2010). Key to this discovery was not only the role satellite cells play in providing myoblasts for microtear repair, but also the daughter myonuclei they contribute, which allows for an increase in muscle fiber size while maintaining the number of nuclei per area of muscle protein, or the size of the myonuclear domain. They found that while new myonuclei are produced with training, old nuclei are not lost for up to three months in a mouse model after the overload stimulus is removed. From a life cycle perspective, this translates into several months in a human. This allows for a larger pool of myonuclei in the muscle allowing for a more rapid expansion of muscle fiber size as a result of more nuclei ready to take on the added increases in muscle proteins or the increased size and number of myonuclear domains. So, muscle memory may be due to this pool of old myonuclei that have been preserved for a long time after training has ceased, thereby allowing for a more rapid hypertrophic response to retraining.

Bruusgaard, J.C., Johansen, I.B., Egner, I.M., Rana, Z.A., and Gundersen, K. 2010. Myonuclei acquired by overload exercise precede hypertrophy and are not lost on detraining. *Proceedings of the National Academy of Sciences* 107: 15111-15116.

Staron, R.S., Leonardi, M.J., Karapondo, D.L., Malicky, E.S., Falkel, J.E., Hagerman, F.C., and Hikida, R.S. 1991. Strength and skeletal muscle adaptations in heavy-resistance-trained women after detraining and retraining. *Journal of Applied Physiology* 70: 631-640.

type II fibers was much higher in elite powerlifters than in control subjects. This allowed for maintenance of the myonuclear domain size and satellite cells contributing nuclei to fibers showing early myogenesis and possible formation of new fibers (Kadi et al. 1999). Ten weeks of heavy resistance training can induce changes in the number of myonuclei and satellite cells in women's trapezius muscles (Kadi and Thornell 2000). A 36% increase occurred in the cross-sectional area of muscle fibers. The hypertrophy of muscle fibers was accompanied by an approximately 70% increase in myonuclear number and a 46% increase in the number of satellite cells. Myonuclei number was positively correlated to satellite cell number, indicating that a muscle with an increased concentration of myonuclei contains a correspondingly higher number of satellite cells. The authors suggested that the acquisition of additional myonuclei appears to be required to support the enlargement of the multinucleated muscle cells after 10 weeks of strength training. Increased satellite cell content suggests that mitotic divisions of satellite cells produce daughter cells that become satellite cells. With moderate gains in muscle hypertrophy, no addition of myonuclei seems to occur, and with detraining, an increase in satellite cell number was maintained for only 60 days (Kadi et al. 2004). Because myonuclei in mature muscle fibers are not able to divide, the authors suggested that the incorporation of satellite cell nuclei into muscle fibers resulted in the maintenance of a constant nuclear-to-cytoplasmic ratio or that the nuclear domain size was maintained. It has been postulated that satellite cells may not have to be stimulated to provide additional daughter myonuclei until the hypertrophy of the muscle fiber exceeds about 25%. Alternatively, those with higher pretraining levels of myonuclei may have a greater potential for muscle hypertrophy.

The pattern of motor unit recruitment (discussed next) and the amount of muscle tissue recruited determines whether cellular and whole muscle changes occur. When enough muscle is affected, fat-free mass increases in the resistance-trained person. The amount of muscle mass gained and fiber transformed consequent to a resistance training program will also be affected by the person's genetic potential. In the future, long-term resistance training studies lasting several years with associated muscle biopsies will be needed to understand the cellular adaptations that take place after most of the muscle's morphological changes have been made during the first three to six months of training.

The Motor Unit

The first step in any adaptation to a resistance training program is to activate the muscles needed to produce force and lift a weight. For a muscle to be activated, neural innervation is necessary. The **motor unit** is composed of an alpha motor neuron and all the muscle fibers it innervates (see figure 3.15). The activation of motor units is what

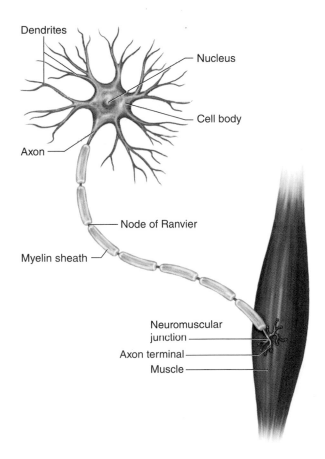

Dendrites

Nucleus

Cell body

Axon

Node of Ranvier

Myelin sheath

Neuromuscular junction

Axon terminal

Muscle

FIGURE 3.15 An alpha motor neuron and the muscle fibers it innervates are called a motor unit.

causes the muscle fibers to contract. The motor unit is controlled by the nervous system and is fundamental to the body's ability to provide just the right amount of force to achieve a desired movement. Each muscle fiber is innervated by at least one alpha motor neuron. The smaller the number of muscle fibers in a motor unit, the smaller the amount of force that motor unit can produce when activated. The number of muscle fibers in a motor unit is highly variable and depends on the muscle's function. For example, in muscles that stretch the lens of the eye, motor units may contain from 1 or 2 up to 10 muscle fibers, whereas the vastus lateralis muscle of the thigh has a much greater range (some motor units contain over 1,000 muscle fibers). Outside of some very small muscles that control very fine movement, as in the example of eye musculature, the typical motor unit contains about 100 muscle fibers. The number of motor units in a muscle also varies. Large muscles typically have more motor units than small muscles do. However, muscles used in movements requiring fine control of force production will have a large number of motor units compared to muscles that do not. The number of fibers a person has in a given muscle in part determines the potential for gains in muscle size and strength.

As discussed in part previously, muscle function is controlled by the nervous system and starts when impulses called action potentials are sent from the higher brain centers in the central nervous system—more specifically, from the motor cortex down the spinal cord and then out to the periphery via the alpha motor neuron. Understanding motor unit recruitment is paramount to understanding the specificity of resistance exercise and training.

The central nervous system consists of more than 100 billion nerve cells. Neurons are involved in many more physiological functions (e.g., pain perception, brain functions, sweating) than just stimulating muscle to contract, and therefore come in many shapes and sizes. But it is the alpha motor neurons that control muscle contraction and produce movement in the human body. Figure 3.15 is a schematic of a motor unit consisting of an alpha motor neuron and its associated muscle fibers. All neurons have three basic components: dendrites, somas (cell bodies), and axons. Typically, dendrites receive information, the soma processes the information, and axons send the information out to other neurons or target cells such as muscle fibers. An alpha motor neuron has relatively short dendrites and a long axon that carries action potentials from the central nervous system to the muscle.

Axons may be covered with a white substance high in lipid content called the myelin sheath. The myelin sheath is sometimes even thicker than the axon itself and is composed of multiple layers of this lipid substance. Nerve fibers possessing a myelin sheath are referred to as myelinated nerve fibers; those lacking a myelin sheath are called unmyelinated nerve fibers. The myelin sheath is created and maintained by Schwann cells. In a typical nerve there are about twice as many unmyelinated fibers as myelinated fibers. The smaller unmyelinated fibers typically are found between myelinated fibers. The myelin insulates the action potential as it travels down the axon. This helps prevent impulses from being transferred to neighboring fibers. The myelin sheath does not run continuously along the length of the axon but is segmented with small spaces about 2 to 3 micrometers (μm) in length where the membrane of the axon is exposed. These spaces occur about every 1 to 3 mm along the length of the axon and are termed nodes of Ranvier.

The movement of ions, or charged molecules, causes the action potential to move down the membrane of an axon or dendrite. The impulse in an axon causes the release of chemicals called neurotransmitters into the synapse (between neurons) or neuromuscular junction (the synapse between a neuron and a muscle fiber). The neurotransmitter binds to receptors on the dendrite of another nerve cell or a target tissue, such as a muscle fiber, which initiates a new electrical impulse. This new impulse then travels down the dendrite, or in the case of muscle fibers, initiates muscle action. In the case of the motor unit, electrical stimuli for voluntary actions originate in the motor cortex and travel down the nervous system neuron to neuron until they reach the neuromuscular junction.

Neuromuscular Junction

The **neuromuscular junction** is the morphological structure that acts as the interface between the alpha motor neuron and the muscle fiber. Figure 3.16 is a schematic of the neuromuscular junction. All neuromuscular junctions have five common features: (1) a Schwann cell that forms a cap over the axon; (2) an axon terminal ending in a synaptic knob that contains the neurotransmitter acetylcholine (ACh) and other substances needed for metabolic support and function, such as ATP, mitochondria, lysosomes, and glycogen molecules; (3) a junctional cleft or space; (4) a postjunctional membrane that contains ACh receptors; and (5) junctional sarcoplasm and cytoskeleton that provide metabolic and structural support.

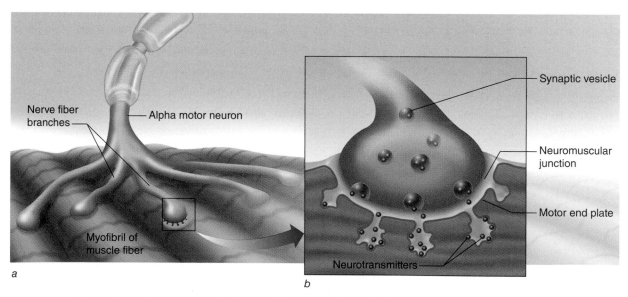

FIGURE 3.16 An alpha motor neuron activates multiple muscle fibers (a) that end at a neuromuscular junction (b) where neurotransmitter acetylcholine (ACh) molecules are released into the neuromuscular junction and bind on the postjunctional receptors to complete the muscle fiber activation process.

When an impulse reaches the end of the neuron side of the neuromuscular junction, it causes the release of ACh. ACh is the primary stimulatory neurotransmitter for a motor neuron, and it is stored within the synaptic vesicles in the terminal ends of the axon. Approximately 50 to 70 ACh-containing vesicles are found per μm^2 of nerve terminal area. When the action potential reaches the axon terminal, calcium channels on the membrane of the synaptic knob open, causing the uptake of calcium ions (Ca^{++}). The increase in Ca^{++} concentration causes the release of ACh from the vesicles. The ACh diffuses from the prejunctional membrane across the synaptic cleft (about 50 nm wide) between the pre- and postjunctional membranes to the postsynaptic membrane.

On the postjunctional side of the neuromuscular junction, the ACh binds to receptors located on the postjunctional membrane. The postjunctional membrane is a specialized part of the muscle cell's membrane and has junctional folds and ACh receptors. If enough ACh becomes bound to the postjunctional membrane receptors, the permeability of the membrane will increase and create a conducted ionic electrical current with Ca^{++} as the ion predominantly involved. This postsynaptic ionic current, or electrical impulse, is what initiates muscle action. The muscle fiber will continue to be activated as long as a sufficient amount of ACh is bound to the postsynaptic membrane receptors.

The ACh is eventually destroyed by the enzyme acetylcholinesterase found at the base of the junctional folds of the junctional cleft. Destruction of ACh stops the stimulus needed for muscle fiber activation. The majority of by-products produced from the breakdown of ACh by acetylcholinesterase are taken up by the presynaptic membrane and used to produce new ACh.

Why is ACh needed at the neuromuscular junction? Why can't the ionic current of the neuron simply be conducted to the membrane surrounding the muscle fiber and thus stimulate muscle actions? Because the neuron is very small compared to a muscle fiber, the ionic current it conducts is insufficient to be directly transferred to the muscle fiber's membrane and to stimulate the fiber sufficiently to cause a muscle action. ACh is needed to cause an ionic current of sufficient strength (threshold) to be conducted by the muscle fiber's membrane and initiate muscle action. Figure 3.17 is a micrograph of a motor

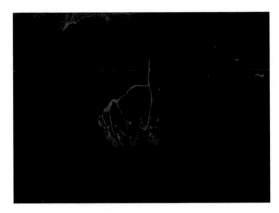

FIGURE 3.17 Neuromuscular junction with the presynaptic nerve terminal branches in green and postsynaptic ACh receptor clusters in red.

Courtesy of Dr. Michael Deschenes, Department of Kinesiology, The College of William and Mary, Williamsburg, VA.

end plate showing several structural aspects of the neuromuscular junction (Deschenes et al. 1993).

Conduction of Impulses

A nervous impulse or action potential is conducted in the form of electrical energy. When no impulse is being conducted, the inside of the neuron has a net negative charge, compared to the outside of the neuron, which has a net positive charge. This arrangement of the positive and negative charges is termed the resting membrane potential. It is attributable to the distribution of molecules with electrical charges, or ions, and the impermeability of the resting cell membrane to these ions. Sodium (Na^+) and potassium (K^+) ions are the major molecules responsible for the membrane potential. Na^+ ions are predominantly located outside the neuron's cell membrane. K^+ ions are located mainly inside the neuron. There are, however, more Na^+ ions on the outside of the neuron than K^+ on the inside of the neuron, giving the inside a less positive or net negative charge as compared to the outside of the neuron.

When an impulse is being conducted down a dendrite or an axon, the cell membrane of the neuron becomes permeable to both Na^+ and K^+ ions. If a membrane is permeable to ions, they tend to move down their concentration gradient from areas where they are highly concentrated to areas where they are less concentrated. First, Na^+ ions move into the neuron giving the inside a plus charge compared to the outside of the neuron. This is termed depolarization and lasts for only a brief period of time (milliseconds) because the membrane becomes permeable to K^+ ions. This results in K^+ ions leaving the interior of the membrane so that the interior of the membrane once again has a net negative charge relative to the exterior. This is termed repolarization. The periods of permeability to both Na^+ and K^+ ions are very brief so that relatively few ions actually move from the exterior to the interior, and vice versa. An energy-dependent pumping system called the Na^+-K^+ pump is needed to maintain and restore the resting membrane potential after an impulse has been conducted. This pump actively removes Na^+ ions from the interior of the neuron and moves K^+ ions from the exterior to the interior of the neuron. This quickly restores the K^+ and Na^+ back to the interior and exterior of the membrane, respectively, and the axon or dendrite to its original resting membrane potential in which there is a net negative charge on the inside. This entire series of events is termed an action potential and is repeated each time a neuron conducts a nervous impulse.

The type of nervous conduction is related to whether the nerve is myelinated or unmyelinated. Myelinated nerves conduct their impulses using what is called saltatory conduction, and unmyelinated nerves use a conduction process called local conduction. The movement of the ions producing an action potential remains the same (as described earlier) for either type of conduction. In myelinated nerves the nodes of Ranvier allow the action potential to jump from node to node using saltatory conduction (*saltatory* means "to jump"). A significant amount of ions cannot move through the thick myelin sheath, but can easily move through the membrane at the nodes of Ranvier because of the low resistance to ionic current there. Saltatory conduction has two advantages. First, it allows the action potential to make jumps down the axon, thereby increasing the velocity of nerve transmission by five- to fiftyfold. Saltatory conduction results in the action potentials moving at a velocity of 60 to 100 m per second. Second, it conserves energy because only the nodes depolarize, which reduces the energy needed to reestablish the resting membrane potential.

Conversely, unmyelinated nerve fibers use a local circuit of ionic current flow to conduct the action potential along the entire length of the nerve fiber. A small section of the nerve fiber membrane depolarizes, the continuation of local circuit ionic current flow causes membrane depolarization to continue, and the action potential travels down the entire length of the nerve fiber. The velocity of this type of nerve impulse conduction is much slower than that of myelinated nerve fibers, ranging from 0.5 to 10 m $\cdot$ s^{-1}.

The neuron's diameter in part also determines the impulse conduction velocity. In general, the greater the diameter of a nerve fiber, the greater the conduction velocity. In myelinated nerve fibers, the impulse velocity increases approximately with the increase in the fiber diameter. In unmyelinated nerve fibers, the velocity of the impulse increases with the square root of the fiber diameter. Thus, as fiber diameter increases, the conduction velocity of myelinated fibers increases substantially more than that of unmyelinated fibers. The faster velocities of the larger myelinated fibers, such as the ones that innervate skeletal muscle, produce more rapid stimulation of muscle actions, but have higher thresholds for recruitment. Typically, type II skeletal muscle fibers are innervated by larger-diameter axons than type I muscle fibers. Thus, motor units made up of type I fibers are typically recruited first because of the lower electrical recruitment thresholds of their neurons. Typically, motor units made up of type II fibers are recruited after those made up of type I fibers because their larger axons require more stimulation before they will carry an action potential. The recruitment by the amount of electrical activation needed (low versus higher electrical thresholds) to stimulate a motor unit is one sizing factor in the concept of the size principle of motor unit recruitment discussed next.

Motor Unit Activation and the Size Principle

The size principle is important for understanding motor unit recruitment (Duchateau and Enoka 2011). A motor unit is composed of either all type I or all type II muscle fibers (Hodson-Tole and Wakeling 2009). However, the number of muscle fibers in each type of motor unit can vary, as previously discussed. For quite some time it has been recognized that the cross-sectional area of muscle fibers can also vary given that some type I muscle fibers are larger than some type II fibers (Burke et al. 1974). Yet force production demands are the key element in the outcome of a guided recruitment pattern. The neurons innervating type I fibers are recruited first in a muscle action followed by the neurons innervating type II (type IIa toward type IIx). Thus, the order of recruitment is normally type I first and then type II if more force than the type I motor units can generate is needed. There is, however, some integration or overlap between the last of the type I fibers recruited and the first of the type II fibers recruited and the last of the type IIa (least fatigable type II fibers) and the first of the more fatigable type II fibers (IIax–IIx) recruited.

The muscle fibers in a motor unit are not all located adjacent to each other but are spread out in the muscle in what are called microbundles of about 3 to 15 fibers. Thus, adjacent muscle fibers are not necessarily from the same motor unit. Because of the dispersement of fibers in a motor unit, when a motor unit is activated, the entire muscle appears to be activated because movement occurs. However, not all motor units of the muscle were activated if the force is not maximal.

Probably one of the most important concepts to keep in mind in the area of exercise training is that only the motor units that are recruited to produce force will be subject to adaptational changes with exercise training. Furthermore, that recruitment is very specific to the external demands of the exercise. Thus, motor unit recruitment is of fundamental importance in the prescription of resistance exercise.

Activated motor units stay facilitated, or primed, for another contraction for a short time after use, which is very important for subsequent muscle contractions. That is, maximal or near-maximal contractions elicit a postactivation potentiation for muscle contractions occurring within several seconds to a few minutes of a high-intensity contraction (Hamada et al. 2000). This potentiation is more prominent in type II muscle fibers (Hamada et al. 2000) and is believed to render muscle fibers more sensitive to calcium (due to phosphorylation of myosin regulatory light chains). Postactivation potentiation has important ramifications for muscular performance and the recruitment of muscle fibers during exercise because it can result in slightly greater force production (see Complex Training, or Contrast Loading, System in chapter 6).

Another important concept is the **all or none law.** This law states that when a threshold level for electrical activation is reached for a specific motor unit, all of the muscle fibers in that motor unit are activated. If the threshold is not reached, then none of the muscle fibers in that motor unit are activated. Although this holds true for individual motor units, whole muscles, such as the biceps, are not governed by the all or none law. Force generation of a muscle is increased with the recruitment of more motor units, and if all motor units in a muscle (or as many motor units as possible) are recruited, maximal force is produced. The ability to recruit individual motor units makes possible very fine control of the force produced in a movement or isometrically. Motor units and their associated muscle fibers that are not activated generate no force and move passively through the range of motion made possible by the activated motor units. Without such a phenomenon of graded force production, there would be very little control of the amount of force the whole muscle could generate and therefore poor control of body movements.

The all or none law provides one way to vary the force produced by a muscle. The more motor units within a muscle that are stimulated, the greater the amount of force that is developed. In other words, if one motor unit is activated, a very small amount of force is developed. If several motor units are activated, more force is developed. If all of the motor units in a muscle are activated, maximal force is produced by the muscle. This method of varying the force produced by a muscle is called multiple motor unit summation. The activation of motor units is based on the force production needs of the activity. For example, a person might activate only a small number of motor units to perform 15 repetitions using 10 lb (4.5 kg) for an arm curl, because the resistance may only represent about 10% of maximal strength. Therefore, a small number of muscle fibers can provide the force needed for performing the exercise. Conversely, a 100 lb (45.4 kg) arm curl, which represents a 1RM, would require all of the available motor units to produce maximal force.

Gradations of force can also be achieved by controlling the force produced by one motor unit. This is called wave summation. A motor unit responds to a single nerve impulse by producing a "twitch." A twitch (see figure 3.18) is a brief period of muscle activity producing force, which is followed by relaxation of the motor unit. When two impulses conducted by an axon reach the neuromuscular junction close together, the motor unit responds with two twitches. The second twitch, however, occurs before the complete relaxation from the first twitch. The second twitch summates with the force of the first twitch, producing more total force. This wave (twitch) summation can continue until the impulses occur at a high enough frequency that the twitches are completely summated. Complete summation is called tetanus and is the maximal force a motor unit can naturally develop.

The order in which motor units are recruited in most cases is relatively constant for a particular movement (Desmedt and Godaux 1977; Hodson-Tole and Wakeling 2009). According to the **size principle** for the recruitment of motor neurons, the smaller motor units, or what are called low-threshold (i.e., low electrical level needed for activation) motor units, are recruited first. Low-threshold motor units are composed of type I muscle fibers. Then, progressively higher-threshold motor units are recruited based on the increasing demands of the activity (Chalmers 2008). The higher-threshold motor units are composed of type II fibers. Heavier resistances (e.g., 3- to 5RM) require the recruitment of higher-threshold motor units more so than lighter resistances (e.g., 12- to 15RM). However, lifting heavier resistances will (according to the size principle) start with the recruitment of low-threshold motor units (type I) and progressively recruit more motor units until enough are recruited to produce the needed force (see figure 3.19).

Different motor units have different numbers of muscle fibers and different cross-sectional areas of muscle fibers, which leads to a variety of graded force production capabilities. Each muscle has different types and numbers of motor units, and not all people have the same array of motor units available to them. For example, an elite distance runner does not have large numbers of type II motor units.

It has long been speculated that exceptions to the size principle may occur in very high-velocity (ballistic) movements and at high power outputs using highly trained movement patterns. In other words, under these conditions the normal recruitment pattern of progressing from low-threshold to high-threshold motor units would be replaced by a pattern of inhibiting low-threshold motor units so that high-threshold motor units can be recruited first. In other species this is seen with escape (a fish's tail flick to change direction) and catching movements (e.g., the flick of a cat's paw to knock a prey down). To date, the concept remains theoretical because lower-threshold type I motor units have always been shown to be recruited before high-threshold type II motor units even in high-force activities (Chalmers 2008). The more likely way a person could more quickly recruit high-threshold motor units would be to decrease the activation threshold of type I motor units thereby lessening the time to the recruitment of higher-threshold type II motor units (Duchateau and Enoka 2011). How resistance training would affect this mechanism remains unclear.

The determining factor of whether to recruit high- or low-threshold motor units is the total amount of force or power necessary to perform the muscular action. If a large amount of force or power is necessary either to move a heavy weight slowly or to move a light weight quickly, high-threshold motor units will be recruited. The higher-threshold motor units are composed of

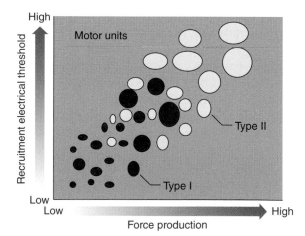

FIGURE 3.19 The size principle of motor unit activation. In this theoretical diagram representing potential motor units in a skeletal muscle, each circle represents a motor unit with a given number of muscle fibers associated with it. The brown circles represent type I motor units, and the off-white circles represent type II motor units. The larger the circle, the higher the number of muscle fibers contained within the motor unit.

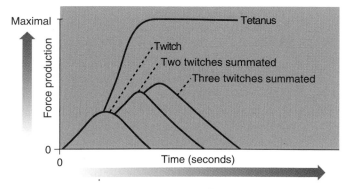

FIGURE 3.18 Gradations in force of one motor unit caused by wave summation.

type II muscle fibers and typically contain a higher number of muscle fibers than lower-threshold motor units do. Thus, their recruitment results in higher force or power production.

The size principle order of recruitment ensures that low-threshold motor units are predominantly recruited to perform lower-intensity, long-duration (endurance) activities. Higher-threshold motor units are used only to produce higher levels of force, which result in greater strength or power. Additionally, the higher-threshold motor units' neurons recover more quickly (i.e., experience faster repolarization), allowing them to be activated more quickly in repeated actions than lower-threshold motor units are. So, although the high-threshold type II motor units fatigue quickly, the ability of their neurons to recover quickly makes them ideal for repeated high-force, short-duration activities.

The size principle order of recruitment helps to delay fatigue during submaximal muscle actions because the high-threshold, highly fatigable type II motor units are not recruited unless high levels of force or power are needed. Likewise, the early recruitment of the lower-threshold predominantly type I fibers, which are less prone to fatigue, also helps to delay fatigue. Higher-threshold motor units would only be recruited when low force levels are needed if enough total work was performed to dramatically reduce glycogen stores in the lower-threshold motor units. However, this has not been typically observed with resistance exercise protocols. When the force production needs are low to moderate, motor units can be alternately recruited to meet the force demands (asynchronous recruitment). This means that a motor unit may be recruited during the first repetition with a light weight and not during the second, but again in the third. This ability to rest motor units when submaximal force is needed also helps to delay fatigue.

Recruitment order is important from a practical standpoint for several reasons. First, to recruit type II fibers to achieve a training effect in these fibers, the exercise must be characterized by heavy loading, high power output demands, or both. Second, the order of recruitment is fixed for many movements including resistance exercise (Desmedt and Godaux 1977). If the body position is changed, however, the order of recruitment can also change and different motor units will be recruited (Grimby and Hannerz 1977; Lusk, Hale, and Russell 2010;

Matheson et al. 2001). The order of recruitment can also change for multifunctional muscles from one movement or exercise to another (Grimby and Hannerz 1977; Harr Romey, Denier Van Der Gon, and Gielen 1982; Nozaki 2009). The magnitude of recruitment of different portions of the quadriceps is different for the performance of a leg press than it is for a squat (Escamilla et al. 2001), and from one type of quadriceps exercise to another (Matheson et al. 2001; Trebs, Brandenburg, and Pitney 2010). Likewise, the magnitude of recruitment of various abdominal muscles is different from one abdominal exercise to another (Willett et al. 2001). This does not mean that type II motor units are recruited before type I motor units, but that the order in which type I motor units are recruited and the order in which type II motor units are recruited varies. Variation in the recruitment order and magnitude of recruitment of different muscles and motor units may be one of the factors responsible for strength gains being somewhat specific to particular exercises. The variation in recruitment order provides some evidence to support the belief held by many strength coaches that a particular muscle must be exercised using several movement angles or exercises to be developed completely.

Like fiber typing, the motor unit profile can differ from person to person. Variations also occur from muscle to muscle. However, some muscles, such as the abdominal muscles, are similar in every person in that lower-threshold motor units predominate. Differences in the numbers and types of muscle fibers results in the differences in force and power capabilities from person to person. With aging, due to preferential loss of type II motor units, the motor unit profiles of many muscles are now predominantly composed of mostly low-threshold motor units made up of type I muscle fibers. This limits power and force production, and the loss of strength is a classic problem with aging (see chapter 11). However, even with the loss of muscle fibers, the size principle of motor unit recruitment still holds true in older people (Fling, Knight, and Kamen 2009). The type, number, and size of muscle fibers in the motor unit dictate the functional abilities of individual motor units and consequently muscle strength and power.

Proprioception

Length and tension within muscles and tendons are continually monitored by specialized sensory receptors located within the muscles and tendons called **proprioceptors.** The length and tension of the muscles acting at a joint determine the joint's position. Thus, if the muscle length acting on a joint is known, the joint's position is also known, and changes in the joint's position can be monitored. The information proprioceptors gather is constantly relayed to conscious and subconscious portions of the brain and is important for motor learning (Hutton and Atwater 1992). Proprioception is also important for static and dynamic balance. Balance training has been used as an adjunct to resistance training to enhance sport-specific skills or prevent falls in older adults (Hrysomallis 2011). Proprioceptors keep the central nervous system constantly informed of movements or series of movements.

Muscle Spindles

The two functions of **muscle spindles** are to monitor the stretch or length of the muscle in which they are embedded and to initiate a contraction to reduce the stretch in the muscle (see figure 3.20). The stretch reflex is attributed to the response of muscle spindles.

Spindles are located in modified muscle fibers and therefore are arranged parallel to normal muscle fibers. The modified muscle fibers containing spindles, called intrafusal fibers, are composed of a stretch-sensitive central area, or sensory area, embedded in a muscle fiber capable of contraction. If a muscle is stretched, as in tapping the patellar tendon to initiate the knee-jerk reflex or by a force, the spindles are also stretched. The sensory nerve of the spindle carries an impulse to the spinal cord; here the sensory neuron synapses with alpha motor neurons. The alpha motor neurons relay a nerve impulse causing activation of the stretched muscle and its agonists. In addition, other neurons inhibit the activation of antagonistic muscles to the stretched muscle. The stretched muscle shortens, and the stretch on the spindle is relieved. Per-

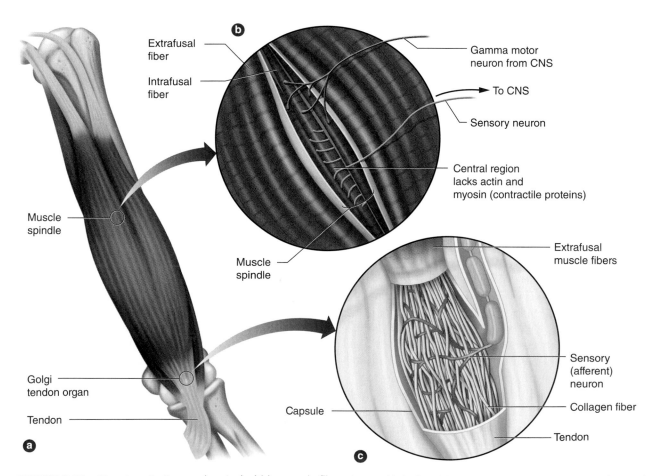

FIGURE 3.20 Muscle spindles are located within muscle fibers termed intrafusal fibers. Golgi tendon organs are located in tendons. These proprioceptors monitor the stretch on muscle fibers and the tension developed by a muscle.

forming strength training or plyometric exercises with prestretching takes advantage of this stretch reflex (i.e., stretch-shortening cycle). This reflex is one explanation for the greater force output after prestretching a muscle.

Gamma motor neurons innervate the end portions of the intrafusal fibers, which are capable of shortening. Stimulation of these end portions by the central nervous system regulates the length and therefore the sensitivity of the spindles to changes in the length of the extrafusal fibers. Adjustments of the spindles in this fashion enable the spindle to more accurately monitor the length of the muscles in which they are embedded.

Golgi Tendon Organs

Golgi tendon organs' main functions are to respond to tension or force within the tendon and, if it becomes excessive, to relieve that tension (see figure 3.20). Because these proprioceptors are located within the tendons of muscles, they are in a good location to monitor the tension developed by muscles.

The sensory neuron of a Golgi tendon organ travels to the spinal cord. There it synapses with the alpha motor neurons both of the muscle whose tension it is monitoring and of the antagonist muscles. As an activated muscle develops tension, the tension within the muscle's tendon increases and is monitored by the Golgi tendon organs. If the tension becomes so great that damage to the muscle or tendon is possible, inhibition of the activated muscle occurs and activation of the antagonist muscle(s) is initiated. The tension within the muscle is thus alleviated, avoiding damage to the muscle or tendon.

This protective function is not foolproof. It may be possible through resistance training to learn to disinhibit the effects of the Golgi tendon organs. The ability to disinhibit this protective function may be responsible in part for some neural adaptations and injuries that occur in maximal lifts by highly resistance-trained athletes.

Nervous System Adaptations

The nervous system is complex, and with emerging technologies we are just beginning to understand some of the mechanisms involved with its adaptations to resistance exercise (Carroll et al. 2011). Given the very intimate interaction between the nervous system and skeletal muscle, we typically talk about the neuromuscular system because both neural and hypertrophic adaptations occur in response to resistance training (Folland and Williams 2007). Figure 3.21 presents a theoretical overview of the basic interactions and relationships among components of the neuromuscular system.

The neuromuscular recruitment process begins when a message is developed in the higher brain centers. This is transmitted to the motor cortex, where the stimulus (i.e., an action potential) for muscle activation is transmitted to a lower-level controller (spinal cord or brain stem). From there, the message is passed to the motor neurons of the muscle and results in a specific pattern of motor unit activation. Via various feedback loops information is sent back to the brain. This process can help modify force production as well as provide communication with other physiological systems such as the endocrine, cardiovascular, and respiratory systems. The external demands for motor unit recruitment dictate the magnitude and extent of the involvement of other physiological systems to support the motor unit activation. The high and low brain level commands can be modified by feedback from both the peripheral sensory neurons and the high-level central command controller.

Adaptations in the communications among the various parts of the neuromuscular systems can be observed with resistance training. Differences in neural activation as a result of different resistance training programs can produce different types of adaptations, such as increases in strength with little change in muscle size (Campos et al. 2002; Ploutz et al. 1994).

When muscle attempts to produce the maximal force possible, typically all or as many as possible of the available motor units are activated. As discussed earlier, the activation of motor units is influenced by the size principle (Duchateau and Enoka 2011). This principle is based on the observed relationship between motor unit twitch force and recruitment threshold (Desmedt 1981; Duchateau and Enoka 2011; Hodson-Tole and Wakeling 2009). Force can be increased by recruiting more motor units; however, an increase in motor unit firing rate or wave summation also increases force. These two factors result in a continuum of voluntary force in the muscle (Henneman, Somjen, and Carpenter 1985). Not only does maximal force production require the recruitment of all motor units including the high-threshold motor units,

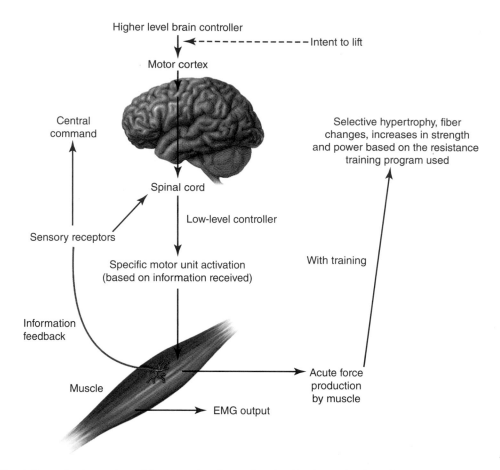

Higher level brain controller

Intent to lift

Motor cortex

Central command

Selective hypertrophy, fiber changes, increases in strength and power based on the resistance training program used

Spinal cord

Low-level controller

Sensory receptors

With training

Specific motor unit activation (based on information received)

Information feedback

Muscle

Acute force production by muscle

EMG output

FIGURE 3.21 A theoretical overview of the neural pathways involved in the activation of and sensory feedback for muscle.

but also these motor units must be recruited at a firing rate high enough to produce maximal force (Sale 1992). Some have theorized that untrained people may not be able to voluntarily recruit the highest-threshold motor units or maximally activate their muscles, but this ability is also related to the resistance and velocity of movement (Carroll, Riek, and Carson 2001; Dudley et al. 1990; Sale 1992). Thus, part of the training adaptation is developing the ability to recruit all motor units in a specific exercise movement, and this in part may be related to reducing the neural inhibition to maximal force production both centrally and peripherally (Folland and Williams 2007).

Other neural adaptations also take place (Carroll, Riek, and Carson 2001; Folland and Williams 2007). Activation of antagonists is reduced in some movements resulting in increased measurable force of the agonists. The activation of all motor units in all of the muscle(s) involved in a movement is coordinated or optimized to result in maximal force or power. Neuromuscular adaptations result in better movement coordination with both maximal and submaximal force production. The coordination of motor units and the muscles involved is affected by the speed and type of muscle action. The central nervous system is also capable of limiting force via inhibitory mechanisms, which may be protective. Thus, training may result in changes in the order of fiber recruitment in both the agonists and antagonists or reduced inhibition, which may help in the performance of certain types of muscle actions.

Muscle Tissue Activation

New technologies have been developed and will continue to help in our understanding of the morphological and neural adaptations with resistance exercise (Carroll et al. 2011). Magnetic resonance imaging (MRI), for example, allows the visualization of whole muscle groups. Activated muscle can be observed via changes in images before and after exercise. For example, MRI images show that muscle activation can be directly related to force development from muscle actions evoked by both voluntary and surface electromyostimulation (Ploutz et al. 1994). A representative MRI image before and after multiple sets of 10RM leg press exercises is shown in figure 3.22.

Strength can increase as a result of neural adaptations despite only small changes in muscle hypertrophy, especially over the first few months of training. MRI techniques have been used to demonstrate this phenomenon (Conley et al. 1997; Ploutz et al. 1994). In one study that is representative of this phenomenon, training was performed two days a week using a single-knee extension exercise of only the left thigh musculature with three to six sets of 12 repetitions (Ploutz et al. 1994). One-repetition maximum (1RM) strength increased by 14% over the training period in the trained left thigh musculature and 7% in the right untrained thigh musculature. The left quadriceps femoris muscle cross-sectional area increased by 5%, and the right demonstrated no changes. This indicated that neural factors influenced much

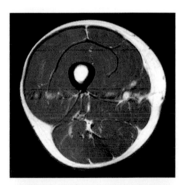

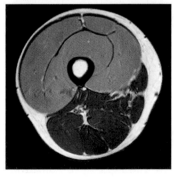

FIGURE 3.22 T2-weighted image of the mid-thigh before (pre) and after (post) knee extension exercise (five sets of 10 repetitions at 80% of 1RM). The lighter color of the postexercise condition demonstrates the amount of activation and exactly where the most activation occurred.

Courtesy of Dr. Jill Slade, Department of Radiology, Michigan State University, East Lansing, MI.

of the improvement in 1RM strength, especially of the right untrained thigh, because the amount of muscle hypertrophy was limited.

Another concept that was demonstrated in the preceding studies was that, after training, fewer motor units were needed to lift the pretraining weights. Thus, a training effect can be seen in the early phase of training in which a greater amount of force can be developed per cross-sectional area of muscle. Thus, if progressive resistance training is not used to recruit more motor units after this initial training adaptation, a plateau or limited progress in strength will be observed. In other words, progressively demanding more from a muscle via progressive resistance training and periodization is vital for adaptations to be made. This can be achieved by using heavier resistances for a specific number of repetitions or performing fewer repetitions with heavier resistances, both of which would activate more motor units.

The current data also give insights as to why a classic modification of the progressive overload concept—specifically, periodized training in which variations in resistances and exercise volume are used—may in fact provide recovery for certain muscle fibers. With increasing muscle strength over the course of a training program, the use of heavy, moderate, and light resistances promotes recovery by not heavily recruiting specific muscle fibers on light and moderate training days. Yet the increased stress per cross-sectional unit area of activated muscle could potentially elicit a physiological stimulus for strength gains and tissue growth (Ploutz et al. 1994). The heavy training days would maximally activate the available musculature, but by alternating the intensities over time, overtraining, or a lack of recovery, could be minimized (Fry, Allemeier, and Staron 1994; Fry, Kraemer, Stone et al. 1994; Kraemer and Fleck 2007). Such periodized training manipulations have been found to be important, especially as fitness or training level increases.

Changes in the Neuromuscular Junction

The study of morphological changes in the nervous system of humans with heavy resistance training is difficult because muscle biopsies cannot be used to obtain the needed neuromuscular junctions (NMJ). Animal models have been used and have provided initial insights into the adaptability of NMJ with varying intensities of exercise (Deschenes et al. 1993). Both high- and low-intensity exercise running by rats produced an increased area of the NMJ in the soleus. Although NMJ hypertrophic responses were observed in both groups, the high-intensity group showed more dispersed, irregularly shaped synapses, and the low-intensity group showed more compact, symmetrical synapses. The high-intensity training group also exhibited a greater total length of NMJ branching when compared to the low-intensity and control groups. Thus, it might be hypothesized that heavy resistance exercise training would also produce morphological changes in the NMJ. These changes may be of much greater magnitude than those resulting from endurance training because of the differences in required amount of neurotransmitter needed for the recruitment of high-threshold motor units.

Using a resistance training ladder climbing model, which resembles resistance training, rats either participated in a seven-week resistance training program or served as untrained controls. After training, the NMJs of soleus muscles, which

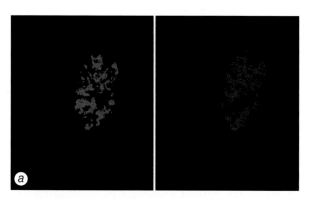
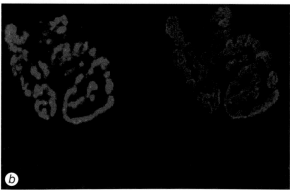

FIGURE 3.23 Micrograph of the neuromuscular junction before (a) and after (b) training with increases in areas both pre- and postneuromuscular junctional areas.

Courtesy of Dr. Michael R. Deschenes, Department of Kinesiology, The College of William and Mary, Williamsburg, VA.

in the rat are composed primarily of type I fibers, were visualized with immunofluorescent techniques (see figure 3.23), and muscle fibers were stained histochemically. The results indicated that resistance training significantly increased end plate perimeter length (15%) and area (16%) and significantly enhanced the dispersion of ACh receptors within the end plate region. Pre- and postsynaptic area modifications to ladder exercise were highly related, or in other words, the NMJ area in the presynaptic and postsynaptic membranes showed similar changes (Deschenes et al. 2000). No significant alterations in muscle fiber size or fiber type were detected. These data indicate that the stimulus of ladder training was sufficiently potent to remodel NMJ structure in type I muscle fibers, and that this effect cannot be attributed to muscle fiber hypertrophy or any changes in the muscle's fiber type profile using myosin ATPase histochemical analysis. This disconnect between the changes in the muscle fibers and the NMJ has also been observed with endurance training in the rat model. Interestingly, it was demonstrated that aging negatively affects the remodeling process of the NMJs to endurance exercise training (Deschenes, Roby, and Glass 2011). Yet with higher levels of overload stress in a rat model using unilateral synergist ablation to overload the plantaris and soleus hindlimb muscles, it was shown that aging did not modify the sensitivity of the NMJ remodeling (Deschenes et al. 2007). Therefore, the complexity of the remodeling processes in the NMJ appears to involve both the type and intensity of exercise and can be influenced by aging if endurance exercise is the training modality.

Time Course of Neural Changes: Initial Gains in Strength

Over the past several decades it has become clear that quick initial gains in strength can occur over the first two or three months of resistance training. The predominant theory is that these gains are dramatically influenced by the initial neural adaptations (Moritani 1992; Moritani and DeVries 1979, 1980; Sale 1992). After a resistance training program there can be weak relationships between increases in strength and changes in muscle cross-sectional area (Ploutz et al. 1994), limb circumference (Moritani and DeVries 1979, 1980), and muscle fiber cross-sectional area (Costill et al. 1979; Ploutz et al. 1994; Staron et al. 1994), indicating that other factors are responsible for gains in strength. In one study, isometric training produced a 92% increase in maximal static strength but only a 23% increase in muscle cross-sectional area (Ikai and Fukunaga 1970). On the basis of this kind of evidence, scientists have theorized that neural factors have an influence on muscular force production (Carroll, Riek, and Carson 2001). Such neural factors are related to the following processes: increased neural drive (i.e., the recruitment and rate of firing) to the muscle, increased synchronization of the motor units, increased activation of agonists, decreased activation of antagonists, the coordination of all motor units and muscle(s) involved in a movement, and the inhibition of the muscle protective mechanisms (i.e., Golgi tendon organs). However, other factors may also play a larger role than previously thought; for example, initial protein accretion and the quality of protein changes in muscle might also contribute to the initial increases in force production (Folland and Williams 2007).

The quality of protein (e.g., alterations in the type of myosin heavy chains and the type of myosin ATPase enzymes) does change in the first weeks of training (two to eight weeks) and may influence initial strength gains. Women and men have been shown to significantly shift myosin ATPase toward the type IIa fiber type from type IIx within two and four weeks of resistance training, respectively. Thus, the quality of protein starts to very quickly shift in the initial phase of heavy resistance training (Staron et al. 1994). Strength gains during this time are much greater than what can be explained by changes in muscle hypertrophy, at the individual fiber or whole muscle levels. Significant muscle fiber hypertrophy has been shown to require more than 16 workouts (Staron et al. 1994). Thus, not only neural factors but also the quality of protein may affect initial strength gains.

The response of muscle to training in the first two months depends on the intensity and volume of resistance exercise used in the program. Increases in muscle cell hypertrophy have been seen in as little as eight weeks with moderate to heavy loading (Campos et al. 2002). Higher training volume might more quickly enhance the hypertrophy of muscle in the early phases (one to eight weeks) of training thereby enhancing the hypertrophic contribution to strength and power gains (Campos et al. 2002; Cannon and Cafarelli 1987; Carolyn and Cafarelli 1992; Thorstensson,

Karlsson et al. 1976). However, strength gains in the first few weeks of a resistance training program appear to be predominantly related to neural and protein quality adaptations. Protein accretion and muscle hypertrophy of the motor units recruited eventually contribute to strength and power gains.

Neural Drive

Neural drive (a measure of the number and amplitude of nervous impulses) to a muscle can be investigated using integrated electromyogram (EMG) techniques (Häkkinen and Komi 1983; Kamen, Kroll, and Ziagon 1984; Moritani and DeVries 1980; Sale et al. 1983; Thorstensson, Karlsson et al. 1976). EMG techniques measure the electrical activity within the muscle and nerves and indicate the amount of neural drive to a muscle. In one of these studies, eight weeks of dynamic constant external resistance weight training caused a shift to a lower level in the EMG-activity-to-muscular-force ratio (Moritani and DeVries 1980). Because the muscle produced more force with a lower amount of EMG activity, more force production occurred with less neural drive. Calculations predicted a 9% strength increase due to training-induced hypertrophy; in actuality, however, strength increased 30%. It is believed that this increase in strength beyond that expected from hypertrophy resulted from the combination of the shift in the EMG-to-force ratio and the 12% increase in maximal EMG activity. This and other research supports the idea that an increase in maximal neural drive to a muscle increases strength. Thus, less neural drive is required to produce any particular submaximal force after training; consequently, there is either an improved activation of the muscle or a more efficient recruitment pattern of the muscle fibers. However, some studies have demonstrated that improved activation of the muscle does not occur after training (McDonagh, Hayward, and Davies 1983).

Additional motor units can be recruited after strength training (Sale et al. 1983). As a mechanism to increase force production, this process assumes that the person is not able to activate simultaneously all motor units in a muscle before training. However, because this may be true for some muscles but not for others, such a mechanism may not occur for all muscles or resistances (Belanger and McComas 1981).

Another neural factor that could cause increased force production is increased synchronization of motor unit firing, which has been observed after strength training (Felici et al. 2001; Milner-Brown, Stein, and Yemin 1973). Synchronization of motor units results in an increase in EMG activity (65 to 130%) and an increase in force fluctuations (Yao, Fuglevand, and Enoka 2000). Additionally, synchronization is more prevalent during high-intensity contractions (Kamen and Roy 2000). However, this concept has been questioned as a mechanism causing strength increases (Duchateau, Semmler, and Enoka 2006). During submaximal force production increased synchronization of motor units is actually less effective in producing force than asynchronous activation of motor units (Lind and Petrofsky 1978; Rack and Westbury 1969). Average force produced by synchronization with stimulations of 5 to 100% of maximum was not different from that produced by asynchronous firing (Yao, Fuglevand, and Enoka 2000). Thus, it is unclear whether greater synchronization of motor units produces greater force. Increased synchronization does, however, result in greater force fluctuations in simple isometric tasks (Carroll, Riek, and Carson 2001). This could decrease the steadiness of a muscle action, which could be detrimental to performance in some activities.

Training has been shown to increase the period of time in which all motor units can be active from several to 30 seconds (Grimby, Hannerz, and Hedman 1981). An adaptation of this type may not cause an increase in maximal force, but it does aid in maintaining force for a longer period of time. During maximal voluntary muscle actions, the high-threshold type II motor units normally do not reach the stimulation rates required for complete tetanus to occur (DeLuca et al. 1982). If the stimulation rate to these high-threshold motor units were increased, the actual force production would also increase. Although neural adaptations clearly can increase strength, exactly how all of the neuronal mechanisms interact to bring about strength increases is not completely elucidated. Also, high variability may exist among people concerning the neural mechanisms enhancing force production (Folland and Williams 2007; Timmons 2011).

Inhibitory Mechanisms

The inhibition of muscle action by reflex protective mechanisms, such as the Golgi tendon organs, has been hypothesized to limit muscular force production (Caiozzo, Perrine, and Edgerton 1981; Wickiewicz et al. 1984). The effect of these inhibitory mechanisms can be partially removed by hypnosis. A classic study showed that force developed during maximal forearm flexion by untrained people could increase 17% under hypnosis indicating that there was a potential inhibition to produce maximal force (Ikai and Steinhaus 1961). In the same study, the force developed by highly resistance-trained people under hypnosis was not significantly different from the force developed in the normal conscious state. The investigators concluded that inhibition may be a protective mechanism and that resistance training results in a reduction in the amount of inhibition when performing maximal efforts. These protective mechanisms appear to be especially active when large amounts of force are developed, such as maximal force development at slow speeds (Caiozzo, Perrine, and Edgerton 1981; Dudley et al. 1990; Wickiewicz et al. 1984).

Information concerning protective mechanisms has several practical applications. Many resistance training exercises involve action by the same muscle groups of both limbs simultaneously, or bilateral actions. The force developed during bilateral actions is less by 3 to 25% than the sum of the force developed by each limb independently, especially during fast contraction velocities (Jakobi and Chilibeck 2001; Ohtsuki 1981; Secher, Rorsgaard, and Secher 1978). The difference between the force developed during bilateral action and the sum of the force developed by each limb independently is called **bilateral deficit** and is associated with reduced motor unit stimulation of mostly fast-twitch motor units (Jakobi and Chilibeck 2001; Vandervoot, Sale, and Moroz 1984). The reduced motor unit stimulation could be due to inhibition by the protective mechanisms and subsequently less force production. Training with bilateral actions reduces bilateral deficit (Secher 1975), thus bringing bilateral force production closer to the sum of unilateral force production or greater. Although bilateral exercise reduces the bilateral deficit, the performance of unilateral, or one-limb, exercises may be important to equate limb strength in both limbs. Unilateral exercises can be performed using dumbbells, medicine balls, cable exercises, and some types of weight machines.

In computer modeling experiments of maximal countermovement vertical jumping, a difference of 10% for strength in one leg can be compensated for biomechanically by shifting the load requirements between each limb force and power production so that the vertical jump height is essentially not affected by the differential between the limbs in strength (Yoshioka et al. 2010). The same result was observed for the squat jump; the strong leg compensated for the weaker one in the performance of the jump (Yoshioka et al. 2011). However, how such limb asymmetry in strength affects other single-joint movements and multi-directional movements important in sport skills remains unclear. The acute hormonal response is also different between bilateral and unilateral exercises. The acute growth hormone and insulin responses are greater in bilateral exercise than in unilateral exercise, but the cortisol response is not (Migiano et al. 2010). The acute blood lactate response is also greater, but these differences are probable due to 52% more work being performed with the bilateral exercise. Ensuring that both unilateral and bilateral exercises are performed when needed should be part of any complete resistance training program design.

Knowledge of the neural protective mechanisms may be useful in the expression of maximal strength. Neural protective mechanisms appear to have their greatest effect in slow-velocity, high-resistance movements (Caiozzo, Perrine, and Edgerton 1981; Dudley et al. 1990; Wickiewicz et al. 1984). A resistance training program in which the antagonists are activated immediately before performance of the exercise is more effective in increasing strength at low velocities than a program in which precontraction of the antagonists is not performed (Caiozzo et al. 1983). The precontraction may in some way partially inhibit the neural self-protective mechanisms, thus allowing a more forceful action. Precontraction of the antagonists can be used to both enhance the training effect and inhibit the neural protective mechanisms during a maximal lift. For example, immediately before a maximal bench press, forceful actions of the arm flexors and muscles that adduct the scapula (i.e., pull the scapula toward the spine) should make possible a heavier maximal bench press than no precontraction of the antagonists.

Neural Changes and Long-Term Training

Neural adaptations may also play a major role in mediating strength gains in advanced lifters. Over two years of training, minimal changes in muscle fiber size have been observed in competitive Olympic weightlifters, but strength and power increased (Häkkinen et al. 1988c). EMG data demonstrated that voluntary activation of muscle was enhanced over the training period. Thus, even in advanced resistance-trained athletes, the mechanisms of strength and power improvement may be related to neural factors because hypertrophy in highly trained muscles may be limited. However, the subjects in this investigation were competitive weightlifters who compete in body mass classification groups, and gains in muscle mass may not necessarily enhance their competitive advantage. Furthermore, the types of programs used by Olympic weightlifters are primarily related to strength and power development and associated hypertrophy of muscle fibers in the muscles trained (Garhammer and Takano 1992; Kraemer and Koziris 1994). Other types of programs for bodybuilders or other athletes may have some similar program goals related to power development, but they must also be designed to meet muscle mass needs, specific sport performance needs, or both. Thus, training goals and specific protocols may play a key role in the neural adaptation to resistance training in highly trained athletes.

The classic representation of the relationship for the dynamic interplay between neural and muscle hypertrophy factors causing strength increases is shown in figure 3.24 (Sale 1992). The time course of these changes is highly individualistic and affected by many factors, such as the number of muscle fibers, neural adaptations, sex, and the training program. In this conceptualized time course, neural factors explain the majority of strength increases in the early phases of training (e.g., first several weeks to months). Protein quality also starts to change early in training, but significant fiber cross-sectional changes due to protein accretion are not observed early in training. After several weeks muscle fiber size increases and starts to theoretically contribute more to strength increases as a result of the increase in the whole muscle's cross-sectional area. As hypertrophy reaches an upper limit, neural mechanisms may again explain further gains in strength. However, this time line of adaptations is highly dependent on the program design, the initial training level, and the training level achieved. Therefore, such a theoretical time line can only act as a guideline for expected adaptations.

It is interesting to note that increases in muscle fiber cross-sectional area range from about 20 to 40% in most training studies. Few studies have training periods long enough to increase muscle fiber size beyond this level. Muscle fiber cross-sectional area changes do not necessarily reflect the magnitude of changes in the whole muscle cross-sectional area determined by image systems (MRI, CAT scans). This lack of relationship may be related to the possible need for several exercises or training angles to optimally stimulate the entire cross-sectional area of a whole muscle, whereas changes in a specific fiber may be brought about by only one exercise (Ploutz et al. 1994). Nevertheless, eventually, strength and power gains derived from "progressively and properly" loaded and activated musculature appear to be bounded by a genetic upper limit of neuromuscular adaptation (Häkkinen 1989).

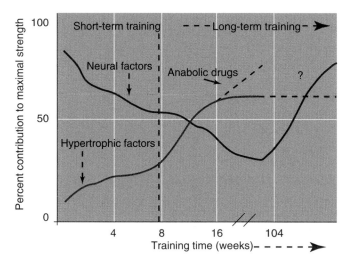

FIGURE 3.24 The dynamic interplay of neural and hypertrophic factors resulting in increased strength during short- and long-term training periods.

Force–Time and Force–Velocity Curves

The force–time and force–velocity curves are important when examining forms of weight training, such as power training, plyometric training, and isokinetic training. Changes in these curves depend on neural, protein quality, and muscle size changes with training. With strength training, ideally, the skeletal muscle **force–time curve**, which depicts force increases with increasing time of muscle activation, moves up and to the left (see figure 3.25). An optimal training type configu-

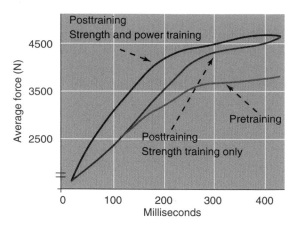

FIGURE 3.25 Response of the force–time curve for the squat movement to various types of resistance training programs.

ration (e.g., periodization) is needed to achieve changes in all portions of the force–velocity curve. Typically, periodized training strategies that address each of the components of the power equation (i.e., force and velocity) are used to cause the strength and power increases needed to change the force–time curve.

When only maximal strength training using heavy resistance at relatively slow velocities is performed, maximal strength is increased, but little change occurs in the early portions of the force–time curve. This means that force developed in the first 100 to 200 milliseconds of a maximal muscle contraction changes very little. If strength along with power training, using such power exercises as plyometrics, Olympic lifts, or squat jumps, are performed, then force in the first portion of the force–time curve increases as do maximal force levels. Increases in the first portion of the force–time curve are important for many sport activities because the time to develop force is limited. For example, limited time is available to develop force during foot contact when sprinting.

The **force–velocity curve** depicts maximal force capabilities with changes in velocity (see figure 3.26). As the velocity of movement increases, the maximal force a muscle can produce concentrically decreases. This is empirically true. If an athlete is asked to perform a jump squat with a high percentage of 1RM, the weight will move very slowly. But if the same athlete is asked to perform a jump squat with 30% of 1RM, the bar moves faster. Maximal velocity of shortening occurs when no resistance (weight) is being moved or lifted. Concentric maximal velocity is determined by the maximal rate

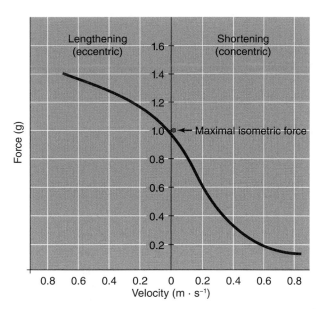

FIGURE 3.26 The force–velocity curve depicts the maximal force as velocity of concentric and eccentric muscle actions changes. Note that maximal force in any eccentric action is greater than force in an isometric or concentric muscle action.

at which crossbridges can be formed and broken with the active sites on the actin filament. Thus, a high percentage of type II fibers results in a faster contraction velocity and moves the force–velocity curve to the left and up.

Conversely, as the velocity of movement increases, the force that a muscle can develop eccentrically actually increases. This is thought to be due to the elastic component of muscle. However, the actual explanation for such a response remains unclear. It is interesting to note that eccentric force at even low velocities is higher than the highest concentric force or isometric force. Such high force development when using maximal eccentric muscle actions has been related to muscle damage in untrained people. However, it has been demonstrated that muscle exposed to repeated eccentric actions can adapt, and the damage per training session is reduced in successive training sessions (Clarkson and Tremblay 1988; Gibala et al. 2000; Howatson and van Someren 2008; Mair et al. 1995). Interestingly, maximal eccentric force is not achieved at the percentages of 1RM normally used for resistance training. Although concentric training causes changes in the eccentric portion of the force–velocity curve, greater force increases occur in the concentric portion of the curve with concentric training (see the discussion of isoki-

netics in chapter 2). Conversely, eccentric training results in greater changes in the eccentric portion of the force–velocity curve. Therefore, inclusion of both the concentric and eccentric components in a repetition, as in normal weight training, is vitally important to any resistance training program if changes in both the concentric and eccentric portions of the force–velocity curve are desired.

The information concerning velocity at which training is performed points to four important conclusions (see the discussion of isokinetics in chapter 2). First, if the training program prescribes the use of only one velocity of movement, it should be an intermediate velocity. Second, any training velocity increases strength within a range above and below the training velocity. Third, velocity-specific training may be needed for optimal performance in some sports. Fourth, ideally, a periodized program with varying resistance loads will improve the entire force–velocity curve. Finally, more research is needed to distinguish between the effects of neural factors and the effects of changes within the muscle fibers on the changes in the force–velocity curve.

Body Composition Changes

Body composition changes do occur in short-term resistance training programs (6 to 24 weeks). Table 3.3 depicts the changes in body composition due to various training programs. Normally, the body is divided into two compartments when examining body composition. The terms *lean body mass* (LBM) and *fat-free mass* (FFM) are often used interchangeably. However, the two terms do have different definitions. Lean body mass refers to essential fat plus all nonfat tissue, and fat-free mass refers to only all nonfat tissue. Essential fat is the fat necessary for normal body functions. It is not possible to have 0% fat. Fat stores are needed to pad the heart, kidneys, and other vital organs; they also serve as the structural components of membranes and as fuel stores for energy. With the commonly used means to determine body composition (hydrostatic weighing, skinfolds, dual-energy X-ray absorptiometry), it is not possible to differentiate between essential fat and nonessential fat, so fat-free mass is actually what is being determined. Fat weight is the weight of fat contained in the body. Total body weight equals fat-free mass plus fat weight. For the purpose of comparison, fat weight is frequently expressed as

TABLE 3.3 Changes in Body Composition Due to Weight Training

Reference	Sex	Changes based on type of training							
		Type of training	Length of training (weeks)	Days of training per week	Intensity of available % 1RM/ Set and repetitions performed if no % then RM resistance and repetitions	Number of exercises	Total weight (kg)	LBM (kg)	% fat
Withers et al. 1970	F	DCER	10	3	40-55% of 1RM/ 1 set of repetitions for 30 sec	10	+0.1	+1.3	−1.8
Withers et al. 1970	M	DCER	20	3	Intensity 40-55% of 1RM/ 1 set of repetitions for 30 sec	10	+0.7	+1.7	−1.5
Fahey and Brown 1973	M	DCER	9	3	2 exercises 5 sets × 5 reps 2 exercises 3 sets × 5 reps 1 exercise 5 sets × 1 or 2 reps	5	+0.5	+1.4	−1.0
Brown and Wilmore 1974	F	DCER	24	3	8 wk = 1 × set of 10, 8, 7, 6, 5, 4 reps 16 wk = 1 set of × 10, 6, 5, 4, 3reps	4	−0.4	+1.0	−2.1
Mayhew and Gross 1974	F	DCER	9	3	2 sets × 10 reps	11	+0.4	+1.5	−1.3
Misner et al. 1974	M	DCER	8	3	1 set × 3-8 reps	10	+1.0	+3.1	−2.9
Peterson 1975	M	VR	6	3	1set × 10-12 reps	20	—	−0.8	+0.6
Coleman 1977	M	IT	10	3	2 sets × 8- to 10RM reps	11	+1.7	+2.4	−9.1
Coleman 1977	M	VR	10	3	1 set × 10- to 12RM reps	11	+1.8	+2.0	−9.3
Gettman and Ayres 1978	M	IK (60°/sec)	10	3	3 sets × 10-15 reps	7	−1.9	+3.2	−2.5
Gettman and Ayres 1978	M	IK (120°/sec)	10	3	3 sets × 10-15 reps	7	+0.3	+1.0	−0.9
Wilmore et al. 1978	F	DCER	10	2	2 sets × 7-16 reps	8	−0.1	+1.1	−1.9
Wilmore et al. 1978	M	DCER	10	2	2 sets × 7-16 reps	8	+0.3	+1.2	−1.3
Gettman et al. 1979	M	DCER	20	3	50% of 1RM, 6 wk = 2 sets × 10-20 reps 14 wk = 2 sets × 15 reps	10	+0.5	+1.8	−1.7
Gettman et al. 1979	M	IK	8	3	4 wk = 1 set × 10 reps at 60°/sec 4 wk = 1 set × 15 reps at 90°/sec	9	+0.3	+1.0	−0.9
Gettman et al. 1980	M	VR	20	3	2 sets × 12 reps	9	−0.1	+1.6	−1.9
Gettman et al. 1980	M	IK (60°/sec)	20	3	2 sets × 12 reps	10	−0.6	+2.1	−2.8
Hurley Seals, Ehsani et al. 1984a	M	VR	16	3 or 4	1 set × 8- to 12RM	14	+1.6	+1.9	−0.8
Hunter 1985	F	DCER	7	3	3 sets × 7-10 reps	7	−0.9	+0.3	−1.5
Hunter 1985	F	DCER	7	4	2 sets × 7-10 reps	7	+0.7	+0.7	−0.5
Hunter 1985	M	DCER	7	3	3 sets × 7-10 reps	7	+0.6	+0.5	−0.2
Hunter 1985	M	DCER	7	4	2 sets × 7-10 reps	7	0	+0.5	−0.9
Crist et al. 1988	M and F	DCER	6	5	—	—	+1.0	+2.0	−3.0

| | | | | | Changes based on type of training | | | | |
Reference	Sex	Type of training	Length of training (weeks)	Days of training per week	Intensity of available % 1RM/ Set and repetitions performed if no % then RM resistance and repetitions	Number of exercises	Total weight (kg)	LBM (kg)	% fat
Bauer, Thayer, and Baras 1990	M and F	SSC	10	3	4-7 sets × 20 sec for continuous reps	—	0	+1.0	−3.0
Staron et al. 1991	F	DCER	20	2	1 day/wk 3 sets × 6- to 8RM 1 day/wk 3 sets × 10- to 12RM	3	+2.0	+6.0	−4.0
Staron et al. 1989	F	DCER	18	2	3 sets × 6-8 reps	4	0	+1.0	−1.0
Pierce, Rozenek, and Stone 1993	M	DCER	8	3	3 wk 3 sets × 10RM 3 wk 3 sets × 5RM 2 wk 2 sets × 10RM	10	+1.0	+1.0	−4.0
Butts and Price 1994	F	DCER	12	3	1 set × 8- to 12RM	12	−0.1	+1.3	−2.2
Staron et al. 1994	M	DCER	8	2	First 4-wk cycle warm-up 6- to 8RM Second 4-wk cycle warm-up 10- to 12RM	3	+0.7	+1.8	−2.1
Staron et al. 1994	F	DCER	8	2	Training Cycle 1 warm-up 6- to 8RM Training Cycle 2 warm-up 10- to 12RM	3	+1.3	+2.4	−2.9
Hennessy and Watson 1994	M	DCER	8	3	2-6 sets × 1-10 reps	7	+2.9	+3.7	−1.4
Kraemer 1997	M	DCER	14	3 3	1 set × 8-10 RM 2-5 sets × 8-10 RM	10 9	+1.4 +4.3	+2.7 +8.2	−1.5 −4.3
Kramer, J.B. et al. 1997	M	DCER	14	3	3 sets × 10 reps 3 sets × 1-10 reps 1 set × 8-12 reps	4 4 4	+1.5 +0.3 +0.2	+1.1 +0 +0.4	+0.2 +0.2 −0.1
Hoffman and Kalfeld 1998	F	DCER	13	4 days/wk for 3 wks 1 day/wk	3 wk 3-4 sets × 8-12 RM	4-6	+2.6	+3.1	−2.1
McLester et al. 2000	M and F	DCER	12	1	3 sets × 3-10 reps	9	+0.4	+1.0	−0.6
McLester et al. 2000	M and F	DCER	12	3	1 set × 3-10 reps	9	+3.5	+4.6	−1.2
Mazzetti et al. 2000	M	DCER	12	2-4	2-4 sets × 3-12 reps	7 or 8	+4.1	+1.4	+2.1
Kraemer, Keuning, Ratamess 2001	F	DCER	12	3	2 or 3 sets × 10 RM	10	−1.0	+3.6	−5.3
Kraemer Mazzetti 2001	F	DCER	36	2 or 3	1 set × 8-12RM	14	—	+1.0	−2.5
Kraemer, Mazzetti et al. 2001	F	DCER	36	4	2-4 sets × 3-5RM 2-4 sets × 8-10RM 2-4 sets × 12-15RM	12	—	+3.3	−4.0
Lemmer et al. 2001	M	AR	24	3	Upper body 1 set × 15RM lower body 2 sets × 15RM	8	+0.2	+2.0	−1.9

>continued

TABLE 3.3 >*continued*

		Changes based on type of training							
Reference	Sex	Type of training	Length of training (weeks)	Days of training per week	Intensity of available % 1RM/ Set and repetitions performed if no % then RM resistance and repetitions	Number of exercises	Total weight (kg)	LBM (kg)	% fat
Lemmer et al. 2001	F	AR	24	3	Upper body 1 set × 15RM lower body 2 sets × 15RM	8	+2.5	+1.9	+0.4
Marx et al. 2001	F	DCER	24	3	1 set × 8- to 12RM	10	—	+1.0	−2.5
Marx et al. 2001	F	DCER	24	4	2-4 sets × 3-5RM 2-4 sets × 8-10RM 2-4 sets × 12-15RM	7-12	—	+3.3	−6.7
Campos et al. 2002	M	DCER	8	2 for first 4 wk 3 for second 4 wk	4 sets × 3-5RM	3	+2.3	—	—
Campos et al. 2002	M	DCER	8	2 for first 4 wk 3 for second 4 wk	3 sets × 9-11RM	3	+1.7	—	—
Campos et al. 2002	M	DCER	8	2 for first 4 wk 3 for second 4 wk	2 sets × 20-28RM	3	+1.3	—	—
Kemmler et al. 2004	F	DCER	29	2	1 set × 65-90%	11	—	—	—
Kemmler et al. 2004	F	DCER	29	2	2-4 sets × 65-90% of 1RM	11	—	—	—
Galvao and Taaffe 2005	M and F	DCER	20	2 and fewer	1 set × 8 reps	7 upper	−0.1	+0.5	−0.6
Galvao and Taaffe 2005	M and F	DCER	20	2	3 sets × 8 reps and lower	7 upper	0	+0.7	−1
Ibañez et al. 2005	M	DCER	16	Min 2 day elapsed between 2 and 4 consecutive days	First 8 wk 2-4 sets × 10-15 res (50-70% of 1RM) Second 8 wk 3-5 sets × 5-6 reps (70-80% of 1RM) 3 or 4 sets × 6-8 reps (30-50% of 1RM)	2 leg extension 5 main muscle groups	−0.5	+1.8	−1.8%
Ades et al. 2005	F	DCER	5	3	1 set × 10 reps 2 sets × 10 reps	8-1	0	−0.6	—
Fleck, Mattie, and Martensen 2006	F	VRVR	14	3	3 × 10	11	−0.4	2.0	−1.2
Brooks et al. 2006	Sex (male/ female) ST 21/10 Control 19/12	AR	16	3	Wk 1-8: 3 sets × 8 reps at 60-80% of 1RM wk 10-14: 3 sets × 8 reps at 70-80% of 1RM	5	—	+1.1	—

					Changes based on type of training				
Reference	Sex	Type of training	Length of training (weeks)	Days of training per week	Intensity of available % 1RM/ Set and repetitions performed if no % then RM resistance and repetitions	Number of exercises	Total weight (kg)	LBM (kg)	% fat
Ronnestad et al. 2007	M	DCER	11	3	Wk 1 and 2: 3 sets × 10 reps upper 1 set × 10 reps upper Wk 3 and 4: 3 sets × 8 reps upper 1 set × 8 reps lower Wk 5-11: 3 sets × 7 reps upper 1 set × 7 reps lower	8	+1.8%	—	–7.5
Ronnestad et al. 2007	M	DCER	11	3	Wk 1 and 2: 3 sets × 10 reps lower 1 set × 10 reps upper Wk 3 and 4: 3 sets × 8 reps lower 1 set × 8 reps upper Wk 5-11: 3 sets × 7 reps lower 1 set × 7 reps upper	8	+3.6%	—	–12
Henwood et al. 2008	M and F	DCER	24	2	3 sets × 8 reps at 75% of 1RM	6	+1.5	–0.8	—
Henwood et al. 2008	M and F	DCER	24	2	1 set × 8 reps at 45% of 1RM 1 set × 8 reps at 50% of 1RM 1 set × ≥8 reps at 75% of 1RM	5	+1.2	–0.6	—
Benson et al. 2008	M and F	DCER	8	2	2 sets × 8 reps	11	+1.5	+1.4	–0.3
McGuigan et al. 2009	M and F	DCER	8	3	Training Cycle 1: 3 sets × 10 reps Training Cycle 2: 3 sets × 10-12 reps Cycle: 3 sets × 3-5 reps	7 7 7	+1.1	+1.7	–1.2
Benton et al. 2011	F	DCER	8	3 nonconsecutive	3 sets × 8-12 reps	8	+1.4	+1.3	+0.2
Benton et al. 2011	F	DCER	8	4 consecutive	3 sets × 8-12 reps	6 upper or 6 lower	+0.7	+0.7	+0.1

AR = air resistance; DCER = dynamic constant external resistance; IK = isokinetic; SSC = stretch-shortening cycle; ST = strength training; VR = variable resistance; VVR = variable variable resistance.

a percentage of total body weight or percent body fat (% fat). For example, if a 100 kg (220 lb) athlete is 15% fat, his fat-free mass, fat weight, and total body weight are related as follows:

$$\text{Fat weight} = 0.15 \times 100 \text{ kg} = 15 \text{ kg}$$
$$\text{Fat-free mass} = \text{total body weight} - \text{fat weight}$$
$$= 100 \text{ kg} - 15 \text{ kg} = 85 \text{ kg}$$

Normally, the goals of a strength training program are to increase fat-free mass and decrease fat weight and percent fat. Increases in fat-free mass are normally viewed as mirroring increases in muscle tissue weight. Strength training induces decreases in percent fat and increases in fat-free mass (see table 3.3). Total body weight, for the most part, shows small increases over short training periods. This occurs in both men and women using dynamic constant external resistance (DCER), variable resistance (VR), and isokinetic (IK) training with programs involving a variety of combinations of exercises, sets, and repetitions. Because of the variation in the numbers of sets, repetitions, and exercises and relatively small body composition changes, it is impossible to reach concrete conclusions concerning which program is optimal for decreasing percent fat and increasing fat-free mass. However, several studies report significantly greater changes in body composition with high-volume, multiple-set programs compared to low-volume, single-set programs (Kraemer et al. 2000; Marx et al. 2001) and suggest that periodized programs can result in greater changes in body composition than nonperiodized programs (Fleck 1999).

Although some studies report larger increases in fat-free mass, the largest increases consistently reported are a little greater than 3 kg (6.6 lb) in approximately 10 weeks of drug-free training. This translates into a fat-free mass increase of 0.3 kg (0.66 lb) per week. When larger gains in fat-free mass are shown, factors such as the trainees going through a natural growth period may be the cause. The very large gains in body weight that some coaches desire for their athletes during the off-season are unlikely to be muscle mass unless the athletes are young and going through a growth period.

Table 3.4 summarizes the results of studies investigating percent fat in bodybuilders and Olympic

TABLE 3.4 Percent Fat of Advanced Strength-Trained Athletes

Reference	Caliber of athletes	Percent fat
Men		
Fahey, Akka, and Rolph 1975	OL—national and international	12.2
Tanner 1964	OL—national and international	10.0
Sprynarova and Parizkova 1971	OL—national and international	9.8
Fry et al. 1994	OL—national and international	8.9
Katch et al. 1980	OL and PL—national and international	9.7
McBride et al. 1999	OL—national PL—national	10.4 8.7
Fahey, Akka, and Rolph 1975	PL—national and international	15.6
Dickerman, Pertusi, and Smith 2000	PL—national and international (record holder case study)	14.0
Fry, Kraemer, Stone, et al. 1994	OL—junior national	5.0
Katch et al. 1980	BB—national	9.3
Zrubak 1972	BB—national	6.6
Fahey, Akka, and Rolph 1975	BB—national and international	8.4
Pipes 1979	BB—national and international	8.3
Bamman et al. 1993	BB—regional (12 weeks pre) BB—regional (competition)	9.1 4.1
Manore, Thompson, and Russo 1993	BB—international	6.9
Kleiner, Bazzarre and Ainsworth 1994	BB—national	5.0
Withers et al. 1997	BB—national (10 weeks precompetition) BB national (competition)	9.1 5.0
Too et al. 1998	BB—regional (competition)	4.1
Maestu et al. 2010	BB—national and international	9.6-6.5*
Women		
Freedson et al. 1983	BB—national and international	13.2
Walberg-Rankin, Edmonds, and Gwazdauskas 1993	BB—regional	12.7
Kleiner, Bazzarre, and Ainsworth 1994	BB—national	9.0
Alway 1994	BB—national and international	13.8
Alway 1994	BB—national	18.7
Van der Ploeg et al. 2001	BB—local (12 weeks precompetition) BB—local (competition)	18.3 12.7
Stoessel et al. 1991	OL—national and international	20.4
Fry et al. 2006	OL—national and international	6.4

OL = Olympic lifters; PL = powerlifters; BB = bodybuilders.

* 9.6% = training; 6.5% = precompetition.

weightlifters and powerlifters. Average percent fat of these highly resistance-trained males ranged from 4.1 to 15.6%, whereas female bodybuilders demonstrated an average of 6.4 to 20.4%. For the bodybuilders, these values significantly decreased as the competition day approached. All of these values are lower than the average percent fat of college-age males and females of 14 to 16% and 20 to 24%, respectively. Highly resistance-trained athletes are therefore leaner than average people of the same age.

It should be noted, however, that the average off-season percent fat of most of the depicted groups of male athletes is above the fat levels of 3 to 5% for men and 12 to 14% for women needed to maintain normal bodily function (Frish and McArthur 1974; Heyward and Wagner 2004; Sinning 1974). However, several of the groups did approach the minimal fat levels needed to maintain normal bodily function, and a few were at these percent fat levels. The fat levels women need to maintain normal bodily function may be higher than those for men to ensure normal functioning of the reproductive cycle (Frisch and McArthur 1974; Heyward and Wagner 2004). Additionally, when people approach or reach essential fat levels and are losing total body weight, a large portion of the weight they lose is fat-free mass. This is true even in highly weight-trained people such as bodybuilders, who continue to weight train while losing total body weight and fat weight (Too et al. 1998; Withers et al. 1997). Essential fat levels, therefore, are not to be viewed as ideal or target fat levels for athletes.

Hormonal Systems in Resistance Exercise and Training

The endocrine system is part of a complex and interactive signaling system mediating a host of physiological processes both at rest and in response to the recruitment of motor units with exercise stress. Many hormone actions are subtle, but without them, normal physiological function would not be possible. The basic function of a hormone is to send a signal to a target tissue via its receptor. With resistance exercise, motor units recruited dictate the amount of muscle activity and in turn the need for various hormones to support the acute homeostatic demands as well as the eventual needs for repair and recovery from the

exercise stress-induced damage leading to long-term adaptations in muscle and other tissues.

In classic terms, the endocrine system involves a **hormone** molecule secreted from a gland into the blood, which is transported to a target cell where it binds to a receptor delivering a signal to the cell (e.g., epinephrine released from the adrenal medulla interacts with beta-2 receptors in the muscle). The system in which a hormone is released from a cell and binds to the receptor of another cell is called the **paracrine system** (e.g., adipocytes releasing leptin to interact with other fat cells); the system involved when a hormone is released from a cell and interacts with the same cell is called the **autocrine system** (e.g., muscle fibers releasing a splice variant of IGF-I, or mechano growth factor, to interact with the same muscle fiber that released it). Thus, hormones can interact with the cells of the body in a number of ways. The close association of hormones to the nervous system makes the neuroendocrine system potentially one of the most important physiological systems related to resistance training adaptations. The overall systematic interface of hormones with target cells, primarily muscle cells, is shown in figure 3.27.

Hormones are signaling molecules that send messages to target cell receptors by binding to them. Depending on the state of the receptor, the signal may or may not be transmitted because the hormone may or may not bind with the receptor. Receptors are either upregulated, meaning that they will accept a hormonal signal and there is an increase in the maximum binding capacity, or they are downregulated, meaning that they will not accept a hormonal signal because of decreased binding capacity or the fact that they are already saturated with that hormone. Based on any of the preceding binding conditions the hormonal signal is either increased, decreased, or nonexistent. Furthermore, almost all hormones have multiple target cells and are involved with multiple physiological systems. The types of hormones and the ways they can interact with target tissue make the actions of hormones diverse (Kraemer 1988, 1992a, b, 1994; Kraemer and Ratamess 2005; Norris 1980).

It is well established that resistance exercise causes a release of hormones in the classic sense as well as by autocrine and paracrine release mechanisms. Furthermore, these release mechanisms are sensitive to the acute program variables that create various resistance exercise workouts. Sex and

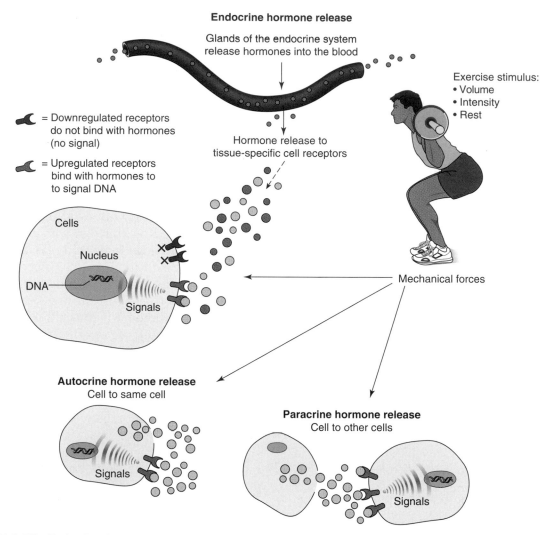

Endocrine hormone release

Glands of the endocrine system release hormones into the blood

Exercise stimulus:
• Volume
• Intensity
• Rest

= Downregulated receptors do not bind with hormones (no signal)

= Upregulated receptors bind with hormones to to signal DNA

Hormone release to tissue-specific cell receptors

Cells

Nucleus

DNA

Signals

Mechanical forces

Autocrine hormone release
Cell to same cell

Signals

Paracrine hormone release
Cell to other cells

Signals

FIGURE 3.27 Endocrine interactions with cells. Resistance exercise stimulates the body's endocrine response by causing the release of hormones. These hormones interact with various cell receptors. Hormonal signals come from the endocrine, paracrine, and autocrine mechanisms and interact with the cell's DNA, resulting in the hormone's signal for either an increase or decrease in protein synthesis.

training level may also modulate the magnitude of a hormonal response. It is apparent that the endocrine release of hormones is sensitive to the following characteristics created by varying combinations of the acute program variables:

• Amount of muscle mass recruited
• Intensity of the workout
• Amount of rest between sets and exercises
• Volume of total work

In addition to the acute program variables, other physiological mechanisms may contribute in varying degrees to the observed changes in peripheral blood concentrations of hormones, acute responses to resistance training, and chronic adaptations. These include the following:

• Fluid volume shifts: Body fluid tends to shift from the blood to the cells as a result of exercise. This shift can increase hormone concentrations in the blood without any change in secretion from endocrine glands. It has been hypothesized that regardless of the mechanism of increase, such concentration changes increase the possibility of receptor interaction.

• Amount of synthesis and amount of hormones stored in glands: These factors can affect the release of, and therefore the concentration of, a hormone in the circulation.

• Tissue (especially liver) clearance rates of a hormone: Hormones circulate through various tissues and organs (the liver is one of the major processing organs in the body). The liver does break down, or degrade, some hormones. Time delays of the hormone being available to a target tissue are seen as the hormone goes through the circulation in the liver and other tissues (e.g., lungs). The clearance time of a tissue keeps the hormone away from contact with target receptors in other parts of the body or can degrade it, making it nonfunctional.

• Hormonal degradation (i.e., breakdown of the hormone): Each hormone has a specific half-life. In other words, each hormone is available to bind with receptors only for a specific amount of time before it is degraded.

• Venous pooling of blood: Blood flow back to the heart is slowed by the pooling of blood in the veins; the blood is delayed in the peripheral circulation as a result of intense muscle activity (i.e., muscle contractions greater than 45% of maximal). Thus, blood flow must recover during intervals when muscle activity is reduced. Blood pooling can increase the concentrations of hormones in the venous blood and also increase the time of exposure to target tissues.

• Interactions with binding proteins in the blood: Hormones bind with specialized proteins in the blood that help with their transport. **Free hormones** (i.e., those hormones that exist in the blood not bound to a binding protein) and bound hormones interact differently with tissue. Ultimately, the free hormone typically interacts with the membrane or other cellular or nuclear receptors, although recent investigations show that aggregates of hormones, hormones bound to a binding protein or hormone dimer (i.e., two of the same hormone bound together), can also interact with some receptors. So the conceptualization of hormone binding has now started to evolve beyond the "free hormone hypothesis" where it was once thought that only hormones not bound to a binding protein can bind to a receptor and signal the genetic machinery.

• Receptor interactions: All of the previously mentioned mechanisms interact to produce a certain concentration of a hormone in the blood, which influences the potential for interaction with the receptors in target tissue. Receptor interaction is also affected by receptor affinity for a hormone and receptor density in the target cells. These factors all interact and result in the number of hormonal signals sent to the cell nucleus by the hormone, a hormone–receptor complex, or secondary messenger systems.

Another factor that can affect a hormone's measured blood concentration is the timing of obtaining a blood sample. For example, increases in serum total testosterone are evident when blood is sampled during and immediately after training protocols that use large-muscle-group exercises (e.g., deadlift). When blood is sampled four hours or more after exercise, other factors, such as diurnal variations (normal fluctuations in hormone levels throughout the day) or recovery phenomena can affect the hormone's concentration in the blood (see figure 3.28).

Resistance training can acutely (Kraemer et al. 1990, 1991; Kraemer, Dziados et al. 1993; Kraemer, Fleck et al. 1993) increase circulating concentrations of hormones, but hormones are differentially sensitive to different types of acute program variables. The endocrine system plays an important support function for adaptational mechanisms, ultimately with continued training resulting in enhanced muscular force production (Kraemer 1988, 1992a, 1992b; Kraemer et al. 1991, 1992a, 1992b). However, the hormonal responses to resistance exercise are highly integrated with nutritional status, acute nutritional intake, training status, and other external factors (e.g., stress, sleep, disease) that affect the remodeling and repair processes of the body. Regulation of blood glucose concentrations, fluid regulation, body temperature control, blood vessel diameter control, brain function, and mineral metabolism are just a few of the physiological functions regulated

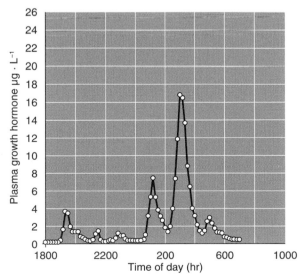

FIGURE 3.28 Example of a circadian rhythm pattern of immunoreactive (22 kD) growth hormone.

Courtesy of Dr. William J. Kraemer, Department of Kinesiology, University of Connecticut, Storrs, CT.

or mediated by hormonal actions during exercise. Once a resistance exercise session is completed, the body's hormonal systems help to mediate the repair and remodeling processes in tissues disrupted or damaged; this involves the modulation of anabolic and catabolic responses in cells and tissues affected by the exercise session. While some have called for a requiem on the measurement of hormonal concentrations in the blood, this approach is illogical as such data represent one step in the biocompartmentation for signaling molecules for target cells and provide insights as to overt responses. What is needed is proper understanding of context and interpretation of the results and understanding of the binding characteristics of the target cells and tissues.

Both the endocrine glands and tissues improve their structure and function to cope with the physiological demands of resistance training. Table 3.5 provides a summary of the major hormones and their actions.

Hormonal Responses and Adaptations

Again, beyond maintaining normal homeostasis in cells and tissues, hormones act as signal molecules and respond to support the demands of motor unit recruitment for movement. Organs such as skeletal muscle, bone, and connective tissue are the ultimate target cells of most resistance training programs. However, with resistance exercise stress, every system that is called on to support a homeostatic response during exercise or is involved with recovery from exercise experiences a training effect, including the endocrine glands themselves. As an example, the adrenal medulla release of epinephrine in highly trained athletes performing maximal levels of exercise is greater than that in untrained people; this results in a higher blood concentration in trained athletes, which facilitates high levels of cardiovascular function (Kraemer et al. 1985).

The endocrine system can be activated in response to an acute resistance exercise stress or be altered after a period of chronic resistance training. The mechanisms that mediate acute homeostatic changes typically respond to acute resistance exercise stress with a sharp increase or decrease in hormonal concentrations, to regulate a physiological function such as protein metabolism or immune cell activation. Many adaptations occur within the endocrine, paracrine, and autocrine systems and are often hard to distinguish from each other. These changes are temporally related to changes

in the target organs and the tolerance of exercise stress. However, factors other than exercise stress can also affect the endocrine system. For example, serum testosterone decreases with the ingestion of protein or a meal indicating an increased uptake by the androgen receptor. The potential for adaptation is great because of the many sites and mechanisms that can be affected. Thus, the interpretation of circulating concentrations must be done with care and considering the physiological context of an increase or a decrease in blood concentrations at rest or following exercise. For example, increases in a hormone can be an important signal for the upregulation of a receptor followed by a decrease in the circulatory concentrations. Thus, the interpretation of blood concentrations must consider the context of the demands of the exercise and other external factors (e.g., nutrition, environment). Physical stress can increase a hormonal concentration in the blood, but that does not mean that all target tissues will be affected. Because of the many differences in circulatory profusion and specific motor unit recruitment demands (e.g., less for endurance exercise and more for heavy resistance exercise), the hormonal signals and receptor interactions can be quite different despite a similar concentration in the blood. However, to summarily discount even small increases or decreases in the hormonal responses to a stress as trivial or without meaning belies the true complexity and evolutionary development of a highly responsive and active hormonal system to cope with physiological demands. The responses of the neuroendocrine system are one of the primary mediators of adaptations to resistance training.

Anabolic and Catabolic Hormones

The primary anabolic hormones involved in muscle tissue growth and remodeling discussed in this section are testosterone, growth hormone(s), and insulin-like growth factors (IGF). Insulin also plays a key role, but it does not appear to be operational in normal ranges of protein metabolism (Wolfe 2000). Cortisol plays a major catabolic role and is also a vital hormone beyond this function. Likewise, thyroid hormones are vital (i.e., without them, chemical reactions cannot occur normally) to the biochemical and metabolic reactions regulated by other hormones (Greenspan 1994).

Testosterone

Historically, **testosterone**, a major androgenic-anabolic hormone, has been attributed with

TABLE 3.5 Selected Hormones of the Endocrine System and Their Functions

Endocrine gland	Hormone	Some important functions
Testes	Testosterone	Stimulates development and maintenance of male sex characteristics; promotes growth; interacts with satellite cell function; increases protein anabolism.
Anterior pituitary	Growth hormone(s)	Stimulates insulin-like growth factor release from liver; interacts with adipocytes; increases protein synthesis; promotes growth and organic metabolism.
	Adrenocorticotropin (ACTH)	Stimulates glucocorticoid release from adrenal cortex.
	Thyroid-stimulating hormone (TSH)	Stimulates thyroid hormone synthesis and secretion.
	Follicle-stimulating hormone (FSH)	Stimulates growth of follicles in ovaries, seminiferous tubules in testes, and ova, as well as sperm production.
	Luteinizing hormone (LH)	Stimulates ovulation and secretion of sex hormones from ovaries and testes.
	Prolactin (LTH)	Stimulates milk production in mammary glands; maintains corpora lutea; and stimulates secretion of progesterone.
	Melanocyte-stimulating hormone	Stimulates melanocytes, which contain the dark pigment melanin.
Posterior pituitary	Antidiuretic hormone (ADH)	Increases contraction of smooth muscle and reabsorption of water by kidneys.
	Oxytocin	Stimulates uterine contractions and release of milk by mammary glands.
Adrenal cortex	Glucocorticoids	Inhibit or retard amino acid incorporation into proteins (cortisol, cortisone); stimulate conversion of protein into carbohydrate; maintain normal blood sugar level; conserve glucose; promote fat metabolism.
	Mineralcorticoids	Increase or decrease sodium–potassium metabolism; increase (aldosterone, deoxycorticosterone) body fluid.
Adrenal medulla	Epinephrine	Increases cardiac output; increases blood sugar, glycogen breakdown, and fat mobilization; stimulates muscle force production.
	Norepinephrine (10%)	Similar to epinephrine and also controls constriction of blood vessels; approximately 90% of norepinephrine comes from the sympathetic nervous system as a neurotransmitter.
	Proenkephalins (e.g., peptide F, E,)	Analgesia, enhance immune function.
Thyroid	Thyroxine	Stimulates oxidative metabolism in mitochondria and cell growth.
	Calcitonin	Reduces blood calcium phosphate levels.
Pancreas	Insulin	Causes glycogen storage; aids in the absorption of glucose.
	Glucagon	Increases blood glucose concentrations.
Ovaries	Estrogens	Develop female sex characteristics; exert system effects such as growth and maturation of long bones.
	Progesterone	Develops female sex characteristics; maintains pregnancy; develops mammary glands.
Parathyroids	Parathyroid hormone	Increases blood calcium; decreases blood phosphate.

significant influences on anabolic functions in the human body, especially males (Bricourt et al. 1994; Kraemer 1988:Vingren et al. 2010). After secretion, testosterone is transported to target tissues bound to a transport protein, termed sex hormone–binding globulin, after which it associates with a membrane-bound protein or cytosolic receptor, is activated, and subsequently migrates to the cell nucleus where interactions with nuclear receptors take place. This results in protein synthesis. When normal hypothalamic hormones were blocked from producing luteinizing hormone, which resulted in testosterone deprivation or lowering testosterone to minimal detectable concentrations in young men during a resistance training program, strength development was thwarted despite the fact that other anabolic signaling systems remained intact (Kvorning et al. 2006, 2007). This finding demonstrates the dramatic importance of normal testosterone concentrations in developing muscle force production capabilities in men.

In men several factors appear to influence the acute serum concentrations of total testosterone (free plus bound to sex hormone–binding globulin). The magnitude of increase during resistance exercise has been shown to be affected by the muscle mass involved and exercise selection (Volek et al. 1997), exercise intensity and volume (Kraemer et al. 1990, 1991; Raastad, Bjoro, and Hallen 2000; Schwab et al. 1993), nutrition intake as protein, carbohydrate supplementation (Kraemer, Volek et al. 1998), and training experience (Kraemer, Fleck et al. 1999). Large-muscle-mass exercises such as Olympic lifts (Kraemer et al. 1992), the deadlift (Fahey et al. 1976), and the jump squat (Volek et al. 1997) have been shown to produce significant elevations in testosterone. In addition, variation in the training stimulus may be important in causing increases in serum testosterone (Hickson, Hidaka et al. 1994). The elevation in testosterone under fasted conditions acts as a signal along with the Hz generated by the external load and motor unit activations. When examined under fed conditions, testosterone decreases in the blood due to the uptake by muscle cells via increased binding to androgen receptors in the activated tissue.

Not all resistance exercise protocols increase testosterone. This may be due to sampling in the fed state (protein and some carbohydrate), low volume and intensity, longer rest periods, lack of enough activated muscle tissue to affect androgen receptor binding, or a lack of needed physical stress (e.g., adrenergic response) to stimulate release. For example, knee extensions can develop quadriceps strength, but if this is the only exercise in the workout, a circulatory increase in testosterone may not be seen because of the dilution of the small amounts secreted into the larger blood supply. Many studies are limited by measuring testosterone at only one time point, but collectively they indicate independently or in various combinations that the following exercise variables can acutely increase serum testosterone concentrations in men after resistance exercise workouts:

- Large-muscle-group exercises (e.g., deadlift, power clean, squat)
- Heavy resistance (85 to 95% of 1RM)
- Moderate to high volume of exercise, achieved with multiple sets, multiple exercises, or both
- Short rest intervals (30 seconds to 1 minute)

The majority of studies show that women typically do not demonstrate an exercise-induced increase in testosterone consequent to various forms of heavy resistance exercise (Bosco et al. 2000; Consitt, Copeland, and Tremblay 2001; Häkkinen and Pakarinen 1995; Kraemer, Fleck et al. 1993; Stoessel et al. 1991). However, studies have also shown that women can show small acute increases of testosterone in response to resistance exercise (Kraemer et al. 1991; Kraemer, Fleck et al. 1993; Nindl, Kraemer, Gotshalk et al. 2001). The testosterone response may vary with individual women, because some women are capable of greater adrenal androgen release. Significant elevations in resting serum testosterone due to resistance training has been shown; the response was greater with higher-volume, periodized, and multiple-set training than with a single-set program during six months of training (Marx et al. 2001). The type of resistance training program (i.e., volume, number of sets, intensity) may affect the magnitude of change in testosterone after a workout. A study with greater statistical power as a result of a large sample size showed smaller postexercise increases in testosterone after a resistance exercise workout in women (Nindl, Kraemer, Gotshalk et al. 2001). Thus, the inconsistent increases of testosterone in women may be due to small increases and the low number of participants in study samples or ineffective resistance exercise stressors.

Androgen concentrations in women are an inheritable trait, which suggests that some women are more capable of developing lean tissue mass and strength than other women are. This may be due to a greater number of muscle fibers in some women as a result of the influence of testosterone during embryonic development and cellular differentiation. These hypotheses require further investigation (Coviello et al. 2011), but they indicate that the response of testosterone to training may depend on a variety of factors, and that some women may show a testosterone response to exercise that is higher than that shown by most women.

Adrenal androgens other than testosterone may play a greater role in women than men considering women's low concentrations of testosterone. At rest, women typically have higher concentrations of androstenedione than men do. In programs consisting of four exercises for three sets to failure with 80% of 1RM and two-minute rest intervals, acute increases in circulating androstenedione of 8 to 11% occur in both men and women, respectively (Weiss, Cureton, and Thompson 1983). However, androstenedione is significantly less potent than testosterone. Few studies have examined the acute response of testosterone precursors to resistance exercise. To date little is known about the effect of acute increases in androstenedione on muscle strength increases and hypertrophy.

Changes in androgen receptors are also an important consideration in the testosterone response to resistance exercise. Using a rat model, investigators found that in the soleus, a predominantly type I muscle, androgen receptors were downregulated, whereas in the extensor digitorum longus, a predominantly type II muscle, androgen receptors were upregulated in response to resistance training. This indicates a possible fiber-specific response to resistance exercise of androgen receptors (Deschenes et al. 1994). Powerlifters who use anabolic steroids have a much higher expression of androgen receptors in their muscles compared to nonsteroid users (Kadi et al. 2000). This was most likely due to the pharmacological effects of the exogenous anabolic drug on skeletal muscle. Additionally, androgen receptor expression in neck muscles was higher than that in thigh muscles, which indicates a difference in the receptors in different muscles. Eccentric loading results in an increase of the mRNA for androgen receptors 48 hours after exercise, indicating that acute changes in receptors might be related to signaling protein synthesis in the repair process in muscle tissue (Bamman et al. 2001). So, resistance exercise may upregulate or downregulate androgen receptor content in a fiber- or muscle-specific manner, and the androgen receptor response after exercise may be related to repair processes.

Training volume may have an impact on receptor down- or upregulation. Comparing one set of 10RM to six sets of 10RM in the squat, investigators observed significant elevations in serum testosterone with the multiple-set protocol, but not the single-set protocol. One hour after the session no changes in the androgen receptor content in the thigh muscle with the single-set protocol were shown, but a decrease in androgen receptor content was observed with the multiple-set protocol, indicating that the volume of exercise affects the androgen receptor response (Ratamess et al. 2005). The decrease in androgen receptors with the multiple-set protocol requires further explanation. It has been postulated that the first response after exercise in androgen receptors is a stabilization or no change followed by a decrease in androgen receptor content leading to a rebound or an upregulation of the androgen receptors, which results in an increase in the maximum binding capacity (Kraemer and Ratamess 2005; Ratamess et al. 2005; Vingren et al. 2010). Therefore, the response of androgen receptors depends on when the androgen receptor content is measured, and the receptor response may depend on the testosterone response and dictate the pattern of changes in the biocompartment of blood.

To determine whether higher levels of testosterone could augment the response of the androgen receptor with resistance exercise, subjects performed resistance exercise of the upper body, which increased testosterone concentrations in the blood, prior to performing heavy knee extension exercise versus just doing the heavy knee extension exercise with normal resting testosterone concentrations. Androgen receptor content was augmented with the prior resistance exercise demonstrating that increased circulating concentrations of testosterone stimulate upregulation of androgen receptors (Spiering et al. 2009). A similar study using leg exercise to increase testosterone (as well as growth hormone) prior to arm exercise showed enhanced development of arm musculature and strength compared to arm exercise in which anabolic hormones were not elevated prior to the arm exercise (Rønnestad, Nygaard, and Raastad 2011). This indicates the possibility that an interplay exists between the testosterone concentration and receptor response to resistance exercise that results in the anabolic response to exercise.

Training status may also affect the testosterone and receptor response in both men and women. Highly strength-trained men and women show increases in total and free testosterone in response to resistance exercise, albeit women show 20- to 30-fold lower values. However, in women androgen receptors increased more quickly in the receptor stabilization phase and showed downregulation followed by upregulation of the androgen receptors within one hour. The men were still in the downregulation phase as previously noted at one hour postexercise (Vingren et al. 2009). This indicates that the time course of receptor down- and upregulation may be different between the sexes. Additionally, glucocorticoid receptor numbers in both sexes did not change. However, because the women showed a higher postexercise cortisol concentrations, the glucocorticoid receptors in women may have been saturated. Owing to the catabolic roles played by cortisol in muscle and its interference with the androgen receptor binding at the gene level, the interpretation of these findings is unclear.

Nutritional status may affect the testosterone and receptor response to exercise. Most studies have measured the testosterone response in a fasted state. Consuming protein and carbohydrate results in decreased blood testosterone concentrations compared to no caloric consumption; this was hypothesized to be due to the uptake of testosterone by the skeletal muscle's androgen receptors (Chandler et al. 1994; Kraemer, Volek et al. 1998). To test this hypothesis, scientists had subjects perform a resistance exercise workout (four sets of 10RM of squat, bench, bent-over row, and shoulder press) twice, separated by one week. After each experimental training session they ingested either a water placebo or a shake consisting of 8 kcal · kg^{-1} · body mass^{-1}, consisting of 56% carbohydrate, 16% protein, and 28% fat (Kraemer, Spiering et al. 2006). Testosterone decreased from resting values during the recovery, whereas androgen receptors increased when the shake was ingested. The androgen receptor response was greater with the shake ingestion than with water ingestion. From this it appears that protein and carbohydrate intake augments the androgen receptor upregulated response. This might be one reason for the value of the use of protein and carbohydrate supplementation before and after a resistance training workout.

The previous information concerns acute responses or short-term resistance training in generally untrained or moderately trained people. Over the course of two years of training, increases in resting serum testosterone concentrations do occur in elite weightlifters (Häkkinen et al. 1988c). This was concomitant to increases in follicle-stimulating hormone and luteinizing hormone, which are the higher brain regulators of testosterone production and release. Such changes may help augment the neural adaptations that occur for strength gain in highly trained power athletes. The

testosterone changes showed remarkable similarities to the patterns of strength changes; however, the ratio of sex hormone–binding globulin to testosterone mirrored strength changes even more closely. It is interesting to hypothesize that in athletes with little adaptive potential for changes in muscle hypertrophy (i.e., highly trained strength athletes), changes in testosterone cybernetics may be a part of a more advanced adaptive strategy for increasing the force capabilities of muscle via neural factors. This may reflect the interplay of various neural and hypertrophic factors involved in mediating strength and power changes as training time is extended into years.

Growth Hormone(s)

Growth hormone (GH) appears to be involved with the growth process of skeletal muscle and many other tissues in the body (Kraemer et al. 2010). Furthermore, its role in metabolism also seems diverse. Additionally, GH has positive effects on growth, which is important for the normal development of a child. However, it also appears to play a vital role in the body's adaptation to the stress of resistance training. The main physiological roles attributed to growth hormone are as follows:

- Decreases glucose use in metabolism
- Decreases glycogen synthesis
- Increases amino acid transport across cell membranes
- Increases protein synthesis
- Increases the use of fatty acids in metabolism
- Increases lipolysis (fat breakdown)
- Increases the availability of glucose and amino acids
- Increases collagen synthesis
- Stimulates cartilage growth
- Increases the retention of nitrogen, sodium, potassium, and phosphorus by the kidneys
- Increases renal plasma flow and glomerular filtration
- Promotes compensatory renal hypertrophy

How can one 191 amino acid polypeptide be responsible for so many functions? The answer is that GH is not one hormone but a part of a complex superfamily of GH variants, aggregates, and binding proteins (for more detail, see Kraemer et al. 2010). The goal of this discussion is to review the GH response to resistance training. GH is secreted by the anterior pituitary gland. However, because it is not one hormone but a heterogeneous GH superfamily of molecules, this complicates our understanding of the response to resistance exercise and adaptations to exercise.

The GH superfamily includes many different isoforms, variants, or aggregates of the 191 amino acid GH hormone that is genetically produced in the anterior pituitary gland. There are many examples of over 100 different possible modifications of the original GH hormone. You could have a splice variant called the 20 kD mRNA splice variant, which has amino acids removed from the 22 kD polypeptide; or disulfide-linked homodimers (i.e., two 22 kD GH bonded together) and heterodimers (i.e., two GH isoforms bonded together, 22 kD and 20 kD, or 22 kD and a GH-binding protein); glycosylated GH; high-molecular-weight oligomers (i.e., multiple GH and binding proteins forming a high-molecular-weight protein); receptor-bound forms of GH; and hormone fragments resulting from proteolysis (Baumann 1991a). There are also two GH-binding proteins, one with high and the other with low affinity, which act as receptors for the external domain of the peptide receptor complex, which binds to GH or other GH isoforms and helps create higher-molecular-weight aggregates along with GH isoforms binding to GH isoforms. The high-affinity GHBP does increase with resistance exercise, but does not appear to be affected by resistance training (Rubin et al. 2005). Thus, the complexity of growth hormone secretions from the anterior pituitary gland are complex (Kraemer et al. 2010).

The actions of many members of the GH superfamily are not clearly understood. However, given their complex nature and numerous physiological actions, their responses to exercise may be different. Additionally, some of the effects of the GH hormones on lipid, carbohydrate, and protein metabolism; longitudinal bone growth; and skeletal muscle protein turnover may be controlled by different GH isoforms (Hymer et al. 2001; Rowlinson et al. 1996).

The concept that different members of the GH family may have different responses to exercise and that understanding the GH response is complicated is shown by the following examples. The effects of acute heavy resistance exercise on biologically active circulating GH in young women measured via immunoassay (22 kD) versus bioassay (>22 kD) techniques are different

(Hymer et al. 2001). For example, the acute effect of resistance exercise was to significantly increase the lower-molecular-weight GH isoforms (30-60 kD and <30 kD) when measured by the immunoassay (Strasburger et al. 1996), but not in the classic rat tibial line bioassay. Clearly, these two assays are not measuring the same members of the GH superfamily or are not identical in their sensitivity when measuring GH. Meanwhile, acute circulatory increases have been observed in men for bioactive GH (>22 kD) using the tibial line bioassay (McCall et al. 2000). This indicates that the GH response may be different depending on the assay used to measure the response. Thus, if not all assays for GH are measuring the same GH molecule, the interpretation of such results must be related to the type of assay that is being used. Historically, the majority of studies have measured GH using only immunoassays that determine only the responses and adaptations of the 22 kD GH polypeptide. Recent studies have shown that this may not represent the most biologically active GH form in the body. Therefore, future research needs to consider the complex pituitary control of the physiological response and adaptation of GH and the superfamily members.

The complexity of growth hormones' response or adaptation to exercise is shown by the following examples. Identified over a decade ago, a small peptide called tibial line peptide (about 5 kD) was discovered in human plasma and human postmortem pituitary tissue (Hymer et al. 2000). It is not part of the GH or IGF superfamilies of polypeptides, but it does control the growth of the growth plate in bone. However, because interaction with other tissues appears possible, it may be important in the response and adaptation to resistance training.

The main circulating isoform of GH is the 22 kD polypeptide hormone. This hormone is also the most common GH measured. However, other spliced fragments, including 22 kD missing residues 32-46 or missing residues 1-43 and 44-191 making 5- and 17 kD, respectively, have been identified. The distribution of 22 kD GH, and non-22 kD isoforms varies in human blood and is thought to be due to varying metabolic clearance rates, circulating binding proteins, and the formation of GH fragments in peripheral tissues (Baumann 1991b). Interestingly, the resting concentrations of bioactive GH aggregates are dramatically higher than those of the 22 kD isoform (e.g., resting concentrations of 22 kD isoform about 5 to 10 μg · L^{-1} versus bioactive aggregate GHs about 1,900 to

2,100 µg · L^{-1}) suggesting that the aggregate bioactive GH isoforms may have a much larger potential for tissue interactions. The presence and possible biological roles of these isoforms and aggregates of the GH superfamily of polypeptides in the control of fat metabolism and growth-promoting actions make the role of the primary 22 kD monomer less clear (Kraemer et al. 2010).

Blood circulation changes with exercise, and the effects of recombinant GH administration have been examined to try to understand the effects of GH (Hymer et al. 2000, 2001; McCall et al. 2000; Wallace et al. 2001). Historically, these effects of GH have been investigated through the examination of the 22 kD immunoreactive polypeptide or recombinant form (Nindl et al. 2003). Although not yet completely understood, some of the effects of GH are thought to be mediated by stimulating the cell-released insulin-like growth factors (IGFs; see the section Insulin-Like Growth Factors later in this chapter) via autocrine, paracrine, and/or endocrine mechanisms (Florini, Ewton, and Coolican 1996; Florini et al. 1996). Although the exact binding interactions with skeletal muscle remain unknown, some information indicates that GH does bind to skeletal muscle receptors in pigs (Schnoebelen-Combes et al. 1996). Moreover, exogenous GH administration in children and adults who are GH deficient has been shown to increase muscle mass and decrease body fat (Cuneo et al. 1991; Rooyackers and Nair 1997). This information suggests the obvious conclusion that GH plays a significant anabolic role in skeletal muscle growth and that these effects of GH on skeletal muscle appear to have both direct and indirect influences.

Training adaptations are likely mediated by GH's ability to increase muscle protein synthesis and decrease protein breakdown (Fryburg and Barrett 1995). Also, GH is known to stimulate the release of available amino acids for protein synthesis in vivo, as well as the release of other growth factors (e.g., IGF-I) from muscle cells, thereby implicating GH in recovery and tissue repair (Florini, Ewton, and Coolican 1996). Moreover, it has been shown that increases occur in circulating GH concentrations during or after heavy resistance exercise (or both) in men (Kraemer et al. 1990), women (Kraemer, Fleck et al. 1993), and the elderly (Kraemer, Häkkinen et al. 1998). This indicates that increased GH secretion and its associated enhanced potential for receptor interactions helps to improve muscle size, strength, and power consequent to heavy resistance exercise. The increased secretion may also be associated with the repair and remodeling of muscle tissue after resistance exercise.

Human 22 kD GH has been shown to increase during resistance exercise and 30 minutes postexercise; greater values are associated with greater muscle mass involvement to perform the exercise (Kraemer et al. 1992), increased exercise intensity (Pyka, Wiswell, and Marcus 1992; Vanhelder, Radomski, and Goode 1984), increased exercise volume (Häkkinen and Pakarinen 1993; Kraemer, Fleck et al. 1993), and shorter rest periods between sets (Kraemer et al. 1990, 1991; Kraemer, Patton et al. 1995). However, because not all resistance training programs produce a significant elevation in serum 22 kD GH concentrations, a threshold volume and intensity may be needed for increases to occur (Vanhelder, Radomski, and Goode 1984). The exercise-induced increase of the 22 kD GH has been significantly correlated with the magnitude of type I and type II muscle fiber hypertrophy (r = .62-.74) after resistance training (McCall et al. 1999). This indicates that the 22 kD GH in some way affects fiber hypertrophy.

Increased resistance exercise volume generally increases the acute GH response. Moderate- to high-intensity programs high in total work using short rest periods appear to have the greatest effect on the acute 22 kD GH response compared to conventional strength or power training using high loads, low repetitions, and long rest intervals in men (Kraemer et al. 1990, 1991) and women, although the resting concentrations of GH are significantly higher in women (Kraemer, Fleck et al. 1993). The effect of volume on the GH response is shown by the fact that 20 repetitions of 1RM in the squat produces only a slight increase in GH, whereas a substantial increase in GH was shown after 10 sets of 10 repetitions with 70% of 1RM (Häkkinen and Pakarinen 1993). Multiple-set protocols have elicited greater GH responses than single-set protocols in both sexes (Craig and Kang 1994; Gotshalk et al. 1997; Mulligan et al. 1996). The preceding indicates that programs moderate in intensity but high in total work or volume using short rest intervals may elicit the greatest acute increase in 22 kD GH concentrations probably as a result of high metabolic demands.

The effect of high metabolic demands on 22 kD GH release is supported by high correlations between blood lactate and serum GH concentrations (Häkkinen and Pakarinen 1993), and it has been proposed that the H+ accumulation associated with lactic acidosis may be a primary factor influencing 22 kD GH release (Gordon et al. 1994). This finding is supported by an attenuated GH response after induced alkalosis during high-intensity cycling (Gordon et al. 1994). Hypoxia, breath holding, increased acidity, and increased protein catabolism have all been reported to increase 22 kD GH release and may affect the release of higher-molecular-weight GH aggregates as well. Thus, the metabolic demands of resistance exercise play a significant role in blood GH concentrations.

Factors other than training volume and intensity may also affect the GH response to exercise. The GH response to acute resistance exercise is significantly greater when using conventional concentric–eccentric repetitions compared to concentric-only repetitions (Kraemer, Dudley et al. 2001). This indicates that the 22 kD GH is sensitive to the specific type of muscle actions used during resistance training. As with testosterone, the ingestion of carbohydrate and protein affects the GH response. For example, carbohydrate and protein supplementation prior to exercise and two hours after exercise results in a decreased GH level in the blood (Chandler et al. 1994).

Training experience may also affect the GH response. Increased training experience in men results in an increased 22 kD GH response during and after resistance exercise (Kraemer et al. 1992). A greater acute increase in resistance-trained women than in untrained women performing the same workout has also been observed (Taylor et al. 2000). However, training results in an increased ability to lift greater resistances, which may affect the magnitude of exertion and, thus, GH response. Therefore, increased training experience may increase the acute 22 kD GH response to resistance exercise.

Although the acute response of GH to resistance exercise is an increase, resting concentrations appear to be less sensitive to exercise. The resting concentrations of 22kD GH in elite Olympic lifters show little change with years of training (Häkkinen, Pakarinen et al. 1988c). Additionally, no changes in resting 22 kD GH concentrations have been observed in several training studies (Kraemer, Häkkinen et al. 1999; Marx et al. 2001; McCall et al. 1999). However, alterations in the aggregate

bioactive GH may be what is altered in the resting state with training (Kraemer, Nindl et al. 2006). This may be due to the interactive effects of various GH molecules, aggregates, and variants with training. Little change in resting GH values indicates that the acute response of GH to resistance exercise may be the most prominent mechanism for interacting with target tissue receptors leading to adaptations, as the hormonal signal is higher with exercise stress for the receptor.

The acute and chronic responses of GH variants may differ. With six months of performing a linear periodized resistance training program, women's resting concentrations of the higher-molecular-weight GH variants, measured with a GH bioassay, increased. However, resting concentrations of the smaller 22 kD isoforms measured with immunoassays showed no significant changes. With an acute resistance exercise stress (six sets of 10RM), the GH aggregates greater than 60 kD showed no significant change pretraining, but demonstrated a significant exercise-induced increase after a six-month training period with a whole-body heavy resistance program. This was in contrast to the immunoassay results of the 22 kD isoforms, which increased pretraining and posttraining in response to the resistance exercise–induced stress; this response significantly increased in magnitude with six months of resistance training (Kraemer, Nindl et al. 2006). Thus, it appears that chronic training affects the resting concentrations of the large GH aggregates, which have dramatically higher concentrations than the smaller 22kD GH isoform concentrations. Meanwhile, the acute exercise response in untrained people increases only the smaller GH variants. However, after training, both the higher- and lower-molecular-weight GHs increase acutely in response to resistance exercise (Kraemer et al. 2010).

Interestingly, stronger untrained women have demonstrated higher resting concentrations of the higher-molecular-weight GH aggregates (measured via bioassay) than weaker women do (Kraemer, Rubin et al. 2003). High concentrations of lactic acid, reflective of lower pH in the blood, during and after an exercise protocol may limit the creation of the larger aggregates of GH. It is theorized that this is due to low pH, which disrupts the function of the pH-sensitive heat shock proteins required for the organization of the chaperone proteins needed to organize the smaller GH isoforms into the larger aggregate GH molecules within the chromaffin secretory granules of the pituitary gland (Kraemer et al. 2010). This shows that there is indeed a complex regulation of various GH isoforms both at rest and in response to the acute stress of exercise.

Growth hormone is also sensitive to a circadian rhythm. A measurement of typical 22 kD GH one hour after resistance exercise (high volume, 50 sets, total-body training) performed at 3:00 p.m. and throughout the night revealed some change. GH was significantly elevated up to 30 minutes postexercise. The 22 kD GH is secreted in pulses throughout the day resulting in increases and decreases. The area under the time curve of these pulses indicates whether changes in release have occurred. The maximum GH concentrations and pulse amplitudes were lower overnight after the high-volume, high-intensity resistance exercise protocol, although the total concentrations were similar to no exercise. This was evident throughout the early to middle segments of the night (i.e., 6:00 p.m. to 3:00 a.m.). However, from 3:00 a.m. to 6:00 a.m., the mean GH concentrations were greater in the resistance exercise condition (Nindl, Hymer et al. 2001). This demonstrates that heavy resistance exercise modified the pulse pattern of GH secretion during the night; the adaptational implications of such changes, however, are unclear.

Collectively, the preceding studies indicate that GHs do respond to resistance exercise and may affect the adaptation to resistance exercise, such as muscle fiber hypertrophy. However, the various acute responses and those due to long-term training of the GH superfamily's many members make understanding their role in adaptation to resistance exercise complicated.

Insulin-Like Growth Factors

Over the past 10 years a host of studies have been undertaken to learn about **insulin-like growth factors** (IGF-I and IGF-II) and their six binding proteins. It appears that they may be a salient biomarker for monitoring health, fitness, and training status and reflect nutritional status as well (Nindl and Pierce 2010; Nindl, Kraemer, Marx et al. 2001). Now called a superfamily of polypeptides, they have many physiological functions. Insulin-like growth and insulin-like growth factor–binding proteins (IGFBPs) (-1, -2, -3, -4, -5, and -6) are produced and secreted by the liver (Florini, Ewton, and Coolican 1996; Frost and Lang 1999). IGF can also be produced by other cells including

skeletal muscle; a splice variant of IGF-I, known as mechano growth factor (MGF), is released from skeletal muscle with the stimulation of a stretch or contraction. This variant of IGF-I acts in an autocrine fashion on the same muscle cell from which it is released (Matheny, Nindl, and Adamo 2010).

IGFs are small polypeptide hormones (70 and 67 amino acid residues for IGF-I and -II, respectively) that are secreted as they are produced and are not stored in large quantities in any organ or tissue. Similar to insulin, as well as other peptide hormones, IGFs are synthesized as a larger precursor peptide that is posttranslationally processed into the final IGF-I or -II molecule. Because of their structural similarities, the IGFs can bind to insulin receptors, and vice versa. Two IGF receptor types have been identified: type 1 and type 2. The binding affinities or the strength of binding among these molecules and their receptors are as follows: IGF-I binds type 1 > type 2 > IR (insulin receptor); IGF-II binds type 2 > type 1 > IR; and insulin binds IR > type 1 (Thissen, Ketelslegers, and Underwood 1994). The interaction of IGF-I with these receptors in skeletal muscle stimulates the mTOR signal cascade, which mediates increases in protein synthesis.

Insulin-like growth factor I directly interacts with skeletal muscle and is involved with resistance training adaptations. Its release is stimulated by muscle contraction and tissue damage. IGF-I and MGF from the muscle are released with contraction, and liver-synthesized IGF is also thought to be released as a result of exercise-stimulated GH release from the pituitary and its interaction with liver cells. It was thought for a long time that GH effects were mediated by IGF release, but now we understand that GHs also have their own direct interaction with target tissues per the preceding discussion. Nevertheless, the cybernetics of IGF interactions with GH and skeletal muscle is a topic of intense study. Other factors, such as nutritional status and insulin levels, have also been shown to be important signal mechanisms for IGF release. Although the liver is thought to be responsible for the majority of circulating IGFs, they are known to be produced by many other tissues and cells, including muscle (Goldspink 1999; Goldspink and Yang 2001). Support for autocrine and paracrine actions of the IGFs in muscle adaptational processes arise from the results of several studies that have shown significant hypertrophic effects of local IGF infusion directly into rat muscle (Adams and

McCue 1998) and human skeletal muscle (Fryburg 1994, 1996; Fryburg et al. 1995; Russell-Jones et al. 1994). Thus, the primary actions of the local IGFs on skeletal muscle do not appear to be influenced greatly by GH; other factors (e.g., mechanical loading, stretch) may be more important for local IGF production and release (Adams 1998).

IGFs are found in various biocompartments and have the greatest concentration in the transdermal fluid that bathes skeletal muscle (Scofield et al. 2011) Thus, the translation of IGF-I to various receptors in muscle requires a transit from the blood to the transdermal fluid that bathes the muscle cells to the receptors for signal interactions. Nearly all IGFs (IGF-I and IGF-II) in circulation, and some IGFs in tissues (muscle), are bound to IGF-binding proteins (IGFBPs). These IGFBPs help transport the IGFs in the bloodstream, regulate IGF availability by prolonging their half-lives in blood (~12-15 hours), control their transport out of circulation, and localize IGFs to tissues (Collett-Solberg and Cohen 1996). Also, IGFBPs diminish the hypoglycemic potential of IGFs by limiting the concentrations of free IGF molecules in circulation (DeMeyts et al. 1994; Zapf 1997).

After an initial increase, IGF-binding protein elements tend to decrease beginning within hours after a heavy resistance exercise bout. Circulating concentrations of the acid–labile subunits begin to decrease two hours after a heavy resistance exercise bout and are still lower than controls after 13 hours postexercise (Nindl et al. 2001). Long-term resistance training can increase the resting concentration of IGF-I in men (Borst et al. 2001; Kraemer, Aguilera, et al. 1995). Long-term studies in women have also shown elevations in resting IGF-I, particularly with high-volume training (Koziris et al. 1999; Marx et al. 2001). In addition, the increase in resting IGF-I was significantly greater with a high-volume, multiple-set program than it was with a single-set circuit-type program (Marx et al. 2001).

Thus, it appears that the volume and intensity of training are important for chronic IGF-I adaptations and that the IGF system undergoes adaptations with training that in turn improve the ability of the circulating IGFs to interact with skeletal muscle for cell growth and repair. Such adaptations in the endocrine actions of the IGFs on skeletal muscle could theoretically be mediated by, or simply complement, the autocrine and paracrine actions of the IGFs.

A specific splice variant of IGF-I isoform (also known as mechano growth factor) is expressed by skeletal muscle in response to stretch, loading, or both (Bamman et al. 2001; Goldspink 1998; Goldspink and Yang 2001; Perrone, Fenwick-Smith, and Vandenburgh 1995). It has been thought that it may play an important role in muscle hypertrophy (Goldspink, Wessner, and Bachl 2008). Bamman and colleagues (2001) have shown that mechanical loading of human muscle (i.e., resistance exercise) results in increased muscle, but not serum, IGF-I. Whether any further homeostatic increases are possible may well depend on the resting concentrations of IGF (Nindl, Alemany, Tuckow et al. 2010).

The eccentric component of resistance exercise appears to be a potent stimulus for the production and release of local growth factors in skeletal muscle (Kraemer, Dudley et al. 2001). The results from this study also showed that the expression of skeletal muscle IGF-I mRNA in humans was greater after an eccentric than after a concentric bout of heavy squat exercise. Together, these data appear to emphasize the importance of mechanical loading–induced IGF isoforms for mediating muscle mass adaptations to resistance training. Perhaps such eccentric load–induced growth factors play a less significant role in explosive or maximal concentric strength and power development. This may explain why many bodybuilding-type resistance training programs that emphasize higher volume (sets and repetitions) and slower, more controlled exercise movements (especially eccentric) are used more often for producing gains in muscle size, but not necessarily for strength and power performance.

Insulin

Insulin stimulates a wide variety of signaling pathways related to the use of metabolic substrates and can influence protein synthesis (Ho, Alcazar, and Goodyear 2005). Its ability to stimulate an increase in skeletal muscle protein has been recognized in pathological conditions since the 1940s when people with type 1 diabetes (i.e., insulin-dependent) first began using insulin therapy to help regulate their blood glucose. However, whether this increase in skeletal muscle protein in humans is due to increased protein synthesis, a decrease in protein degradation, or a combination of both remains unclear (Rooyackers and Nair 1997; Wolfe 2000). A typical change with acute exercise is a decrease in insulin. However, nutritional intakes (low carbohydrate vs. high carbohydrate plus protein) may play a role in stimulating insulin release after a training session compared to fasting conditions (Baty et al. 2007; Kraemer, Volek et al. 1998). Adding protein to a low-carbohydrate drink enhances muscle tissue repair and reduces soreness, suggesting that although carbohydrate may be important for the insulin signal, it is the protein intake that allows for the needed amino acids for muscle repair and remodeling (Baty et al. 2007). When insulin has the most dramatic effects on protein synthesis remains unclear, but it may be only during times of very low or very high levels of protein synthesis (Farrell et al. 2000; Szanberg et al. 1997).

In normal daily life, resting insulin concentrations induce a low-level suppressive effect on protein degradation via reduced ATP-dependent ubiquitin proteolysis. However, acute exercise in the fasted state typically results in lower circulating concentrations of insulin; the inhibitory effects of insulin on lysosomal protein degradation are reduced and protein degradation increases transiently. Basal concentrations of insulin are not regulated by normal basal serum glucose concentrations (e.g., 80-100 mg $\cdot$ dL^{-1}) and have been shown to be lowered with regular strength training (Miller, Sherman, and Ivy 1984), with overreaching (unpublished data from Dr. Kraemer's laboratory), and in bodybuilders with large muscle mass (Szczypaczewska, Nazar, and Kaciuba-Uscilko 1989). Thus, the role of insulin in resistance training adaptations and protein accretion resulting in muscle hypertrophy in humans remains speculative.

Cortisol as a Primary Catabolic Hormone

Cortisol, like all hormones, is a chemical signal that has a temporal time frame in which to deliver a message to target cells that have the appropriate upregulated receptors with which the hormone can interact. Cortisol is considered a primary catabolic hormone and is involved in the inflammatory response to exercise and protein degradation. Increases in cortisol should not be thought of as bad or good but rather as a response to the stressors imposed. However, increased cortisol concentrations that do not return to normal (i.e., 100-450 nmol $\cdot$ L^{-1}) do suggest a problem with stress homeostasis. Cortisol is important in the context of both the acute exercise and chronic training

response because it affects not only skeletal muscle, but also connective tissue.

Adrenocortical steroid hormones, such as cortisol, were originally given the name glucocorticoids because of their effects on intermediary metabolism. This is because in the fasted state, cortisol helps to maintain blood glucose by stimulating gluconeogenesis from amino acids and to peripherally release metabolic substrates, both of which are catabolic processes. In adipose cells cortisol stimulates lipolysis, and in muscle cells it increases protein degradation and decreases protein synthesis, resulting in a greater release of lipids and amino acids into the circulation, respectively (Hickson and Marone 1993). Another important role of the glucocorticoids is in the local and systemic inflammatory mechanisms related to cytokine-mediated cortisol secretion via the hypothalamic-pituitary-adrenal axis (reviewed by Smith 2000). Perhaps the most notable function of the glucocorticoids, however, is their various roles in the body's response to stressful stimuli (e.g., injury, surgery, physical activity). Although evidence supporting other related concepts is increasing, Hans Selye's original general adaptation syndrome (i.e., that the stress-induced secretion of glucocorticoids enhances and mediates stress responses) remains a topic of study (Pacak et al. 1998; Sapolsky, Romero, and Munck 2000; Selye 1936). Overall, the importance of the glucocorticoids to strength and power adaptations is related to their catabolic effects on skeletal muscle. These catabolic effects are greater in type II than in type I muscle fibers (Kraemer, Staron et al. 1998).

The catabolic actions are mediated by many different cellular signaling mechanisms and are regulated by a complex integration of permissive, suppressive, stimulatory, and preparative actions that work together to help maintain (or reestablish) a homeostatic cellular environment and ultimately prevent any lasting deleterious effects of an acute stress on the body (Sapolsky, Romero, and Munck 2000). Resistance exercise can be thought of as a microtrauma that can lead to local acute inflammation, chronic inflammation, systemic inflammation, and the activation of the hypothalamic-pituitary-adrenal axis and the subsequent rapid increase in circulating cortisol concentrations for tissue repair and remodeling (Fragala et al. 2011a; Smith 2000; Spiering et al. 2008b). It is important to note that adaptation to resistance training involves microtrauma or breakdown of muscle tissue followed by the repair and remodeling to a stronger and larger muscle fiber and eventually intact muscle.

Glucocorticoids are released from the adrenal cortex in response to exercise. Of these, cortisol accounts for approximately 95% of all glucocorticoid activity (Guyton 1991). Cortisol and adrenocorticotropic hormone (ACTH) significantly increase during an acute bout of resistance exercise (Guezennec et al. 1986; Häkkinen, Pakarinen et al. 1988a, 1988b; Kraemer et al. 1992; Kraemer, Dziados et al. 1993; Kraemer, Fleck et al. 1999; Kraemer, Fleck, and Evans 1996; Kraemer, Noble et al. 1987). The response is similar between men and women who perform the same resistance training protocol (Häkkinen and Pakarinen 1995). Cortisol secretion responds quite rapidly to various stresses (e.g., exercise, hypoglycemia, surgery), typically within minutes. The acute increase of cortisol to resistance exercise is greatest with high-intensity, short-rest protocols (i.e., over 1,000 nmol · L^{-1}) and may reflect the acute metabolic response to resistance exercise. Such increases can contribute to muscle degradation. Although most inflammatory and blood-glucose regulatory actions of glucocorticoids may be directly associated with these rapid responses, changes in muscle protein turnover are mostly controlled by the classic steroid hormone–binding mechanism. Like testosterone, cortisol binds to a cytoplasmic receptor and activates a receptor complex so that it can enter the nucleus, bind specific hormone response elements on DNA, and act directly at the level of the gene. By doing this, cortisol alters the transcription and subsequent translation of specific proteins, but these processes take hours to days to complete. Cortisol can also block the regulatory element of testosterone, thereby in part blocking testosterone's anabolic signal, which is another way cortisol acts as a catabolic hormone.

As with other hormones, the biological activity of glucocorticoids is regulated by the percentage of freely circulating hormone. About 10% of circulating cortisol is free, whereas approximately 15% is bound to albumin and 75% is bound to corticosteroid-binding globulin. The primary pathway for cortisol secretion begins with the stimulation of the hypothalamus by the central nervous system, which can occur as a result of hypoglycemia, the flight or fight response, or exercise.

Cytokine-mediated cortisol release is implicated in high-volume and high-intensity exercise (especially eccentric muscle actions) and occurs as a result of microtrauma injury to the muscle tissue that causes the infiltration of white blood cells, such as neutrophils and monocytes, into the tissue (Fragala et al. 2011a; Smith 2000). The monocytes can then be activated in the circulation or in the tissues, where they remain and become macrophages. Both circulating monocytes and tissue macrophages are immune cells capable of secreting hundreds of different cytokines that mediate local and systemic inflammatory processes. Interleukin-1 and interleukin-6 (IL-1 and IL-6) are proinflammatory cytokines secreted by activated monocytes (or macrophages) that are known to activate the hypothalamic-pituitary-adrenal axis (Kalra, Sahu, and Kalra 1990; Path et al. 1997). These cytokines interact with receptors on the hypothalamus and cause the sequential secretion of corticotropin-releasing hormone (CRH), ACTH, and cortisol from the hypothalamus, anterior pituitary, and adrenal cortex, respectively (Kraemer and Ratamess 2005; Smith 2000).

At each level of interaction (e.g., neutrophils to monocytes to cytokines to other cytokines to hypothalamus), all of these responses can be amplified, but the magnitude(s) will ultimately depend on the severity of the initial microtrauma. Severity of the microtrauma for exercise refers to intensity. Severe inflammatory responses appear to occur only after severe injury, trauma, infection, very high-intensity resistance exercise, or very high-volume endurance training, and thus are implicated in the overtraining syndrome (Fry and Kraemer 1997; Smith 2000; Stone et al. 1991). However, daily exercise training is also associated with local and systemic cytokine responses at different levels, depending on the intensity of the exercise (Moldoveanu, Shephard, and Shek 2001).

Recently, it has been shown that skeletal muscle glucocorticoid receptors are saturated before and after exercise in highly resistance-trained men and women; increases in receptors on immune cells follow acute exercise. Therefore, interference with testosterone binding and also inhibition of the activity of immune cells important for tissue remodeling and adaptation to exercise are two mechanisms that can promote a catabolic effect (Fragala et al. 2011a, 2011b, 2011c; Spiering et al. 2008a; b; Vingren et al. 2010). In addition, blocking cell signaling (mTOR system) in the muscle for protein synthesis, apart from testosterone effects, has also been observed. Therefore, a series of mechanisms that are engaged by cortisol can result in decreased muscle protein accretion, especially when its concentration dramatically increases beyond normal concentration in the blood (e.g., >700 nmol $\cdot$ L^{-1}) (Spiering et al. 2008a).

Interestingly, programs that elicit the greatest cortisol response also elicit the greatest acute GH and lactate responses. Significant correlations between blood lactate and serum cortisol ($r = .64$) have been reported (Kraemer, Patton et al. 1989). In addition, acute elevations in serum cortisol have been significantly correlated ($r = .84$) to 24-hour postexercise markers of muscle damage (i.e., serum creatine kinase concentrations) (Kraemer, Dziados, et al. 1993).

Metabolically demanding resistance training protocols (i.e., high volume, moderate to high intensity, with short rest periods) have shown the greatest acute cortisol response (Häkkinen and Pakarinen 1993; Kraemer, Noble et al. 1987, Kraemer and, Dziados 1993); little change was shown with conventional strength and power training. For example, performing eight sets of a 10RM leg press exercise with one-minute rest periods between sets elicited a significantly greater acute cortisol response than the same protocol using three-minute rest periods (Kraemer et al. 1996). These acute increases may be part of the muscle tissue remodeling process. However, one aspect of successful training may be whether cortisol concentrations return to normal resting values in 24 hours following a training session.

Resting cortisol concentrations generally reflect long-term training stress. Chronic resistance training does not appear to produce consistent changes in resting cortisol concentrations because no change (Fry, Kraemer, Stone et al. 1994; Häkkinen et al. 1990; Häkkinen, Pakarinen et al. 1987; Häkkinen, Pakarinen et al. 1988c; Häkkinen, Pakarinen, and Kallinen 1992; Kraemer et al. 2002), decreases (Alen et al. 1988; Häkkinen, Pakarinen et al. 1985c; Kraemer, Staron et al. 1998; Marx et al. 2001; McCall et al. 1999), and increases (Häkkinen and Pakarinen 1991; Kraemer, Patton et al. 1995) have been reported during normal strength and power training and during overreaching in men and women. Nevertheless, greater reductions in resting serum cortisol after 24 weeks of strength training compared to power training have been shown (Häkkinen, Pakarinen, et al. 1985c).

A comparison in women of periodized multiple-set resistance training to single-set training over six months showed that only the higher-volume training resulted in a significant reduction in resting serum cortisol (Marx et al. 2001). A decrease in resting concentration of serum cortisol has been shown by the third week of a 10-week program of periodized resistance training in elderly people with sufficient rest between sessions (Kraemer, Häkkinen et al. 1999). In animals resting cortisol concentrations may explain most of the variance (~60%) in muscle mass changes (Crowley and Matt 1996). Thus, any chronic adaptations or changes in resting cortisol concentrations are involved with tissue homeostasis and protein metabolism, whereas the acute cortisol response appears to reflect metabolic stress (Florini 1987).

Testosterone-to-cortisol (T/C) ratios have been used as a measure of overall muscle protein accretion. This ratio most likely has been overvalued and is really a very general marker of the secretion of these hormones and not a marker of muscle tissue response and the many receptors that interact with testosterone and cortisol (See box 3.4). The use of this ratio came from early studies that used various ratios of cortisol and testosterone concentrations in the blood to estimate the anabolic status of the body during prolonged resistance training or with overtraining (Fry and Kraemer 1997; Häkkinen 1989; Häkkinen and Komi 1985c; Stone et al. 1991). Older studies have shown changes in the T/C ratio during strength and power training, and this ratio has been positively related to physical performance (Alen et al. 1988; Häkkinen and Komi 1985c). Stressful training (overreaching) in elite Olympic weightlifters has been shown to decrease the T/C ratio (Häkkinen, Pakarinen et al. 1987). Periodized, higher-volume programs have been shown to produce a significantly greater increase in the T/C ratio than low-volume, single-set programs (Marx et al. 2001). However, an animal study in which the T/C ratio was manipulated to investigate muscle hypertrophy reported that the T/C ratio was not a useful indicator of tissue anabolism (Crowley and Matt 1996).

The T/C ratio and/or free testosterone-to-cortisol ratios are the ratios most used to indicate the anabolic/catabolic status during resistance training. Thus, an increase in testosterone, a decrease in cortisol, or both, would indicate increased tissue anabolism. However, this appears to be an oversimplification and is at best only a gross indirect measure of the anabolic/catabolic properties of

BOX 3.4 **RESEARCH**

Influence of Hormones on Gains in Muscle Size and Strength

The importance of hormones to gains in muscle size and strength is controversial. To investigate this controversy, a group from Norway used a unique study design to see whether, in fact, the concentrations of circulating hormones affect muscle size and strength increases (Rønnestad, Nygaard, and Raastad 2011). Subjects performed four sessions per week of unilateral strength training for the elbow flexors for 11 weeks. In one training protocol performed two times per week, a leg press exercise was performed prior to performing exercises for the elbow flexors of one arm. In a second protocol, also performed two times per week, no leg press exercise was performed prior to training the elbow flexors of the other arm. Serum testosterone and growth hormone were significantly increased as a result of performing the leg press exercise prior to the elbow flexor exercise. Thus, one arm's elbow flexors were trained when exposed to increased hormones in the circulation. Both arms increased in biceps curl 1RM and power at 30 and 60% of the 1RM. However, the percentage of increase in these measures favored the arm trained after the leg press was performed. Additionally, only the arm trained with the prior leg press exercise, which elevated anabolic hormones, demonstrated a significant increase in muscle cross-sectional area at all levels of the biceps. Thus, it appears that the signals from circulating hormones augment muscle tissue growth and repair, indicating that the order of exercise might play an important role. Therefore, a resistance training protocol that uses large-muscle-group exercises first stimulates larger increases in anabolic hormone in the circulation compared to small-muscle-group exercises. This may facilitate improved physiological signaling for growth when small muscle group exercises are performed.

Rønnestad, B.R., Nygaard, H., and Raastad, T. 2011. Physiological elevation of endogenous hormones results in superior strength training adaptation. *European Journal of Applied Physiology* 111: 2249-2259.

skeletal muscle and should be used very cautiously, if at all (Fry and Kraemer 1997; Vingren et al. 2010). Blood variables at a single temporal point in time should not be correlated with any accumulating variable over time, such as strength or muscle size, because the complex interaction with receptors and hormone alterations in the blood do not adequately reflect the composite effects of signaling from hormones. For example, if uptake of testosterone is high because of increases in androgen receptor binding and blood testosterone goes down, but cortisol stays the same, one could interpret this to mean that there is a predominance of catabolism when in fact anabolism is dramatically going up (Kraemer, Spiering et al. 2006; Vingren et al. 2009). Although cortisol represents the primary catabolic influence on muscle, how useful T/C ratios are for indicating anabolic/catabolic status remains unclear.

Connective Tissue

It has been known for some time that physical activity increases the size and strength of ligaments, tendons, and bone (Fahey, Akka, and Rolph 1975;

Stone 1992; Zernicke and Loitz 1992). Recently, it has become apparent that resistance training that properly loads the musculoskeletal system can increase bone and tendon characteristics.

The acute variables of programs that change bone and tendon characteristics are not fully understood. However, it appears that heavy loading is vital for connective tissue changes, especially bone. These fundamental features of a program have been known for some time (Conroy et al. 1992). Bone is very sensitive to mechanical forces such as compression, strain, and strain rate (Chow 2000). Such forces are common in resistance training (especially with multiple-joint structural exercises) and are affected by the type of exercise, the intensity of the resistance, the number of sets, the rate of loading, the direction of forces, and the frequency of training. The majority of resistance training studies do show some positive effect on bone mineral density (Layne and Nelson 1999). However, bone has a tendency to adapt much more slowly (e.g., 6 to 12 months are needed to see a change in bone density) than muscle does (Conroy et al. 1992). A meta-analysis has confirmed that the most effective intervention for improving bone mineral density appears to be high-force exercise (Howe et al. 2011).

As the skeletal muscles become stronger and can lift more weight, the ligaments, tendons, and bones also adapt to support greater forces and weights. This concept is supported by significant correlations between muscle cross-sectional area and bone cross-sectional area in Olympic weightlifters with a mean training experience of five years (Kanehisa, Ikegawa, and Fukunaga 1998). This indicates that long-term participation in weightlifting results in increased bone and muscle cross-sectional areas.

Bone mineral density (BMD) increases as a result of resistance training, provided sufficient intensity and volume are performed (Kelley, Kelley, and Tran 2001) (see table 3.6). In a cross-sectional study, elite junior weightlifters 14 to 17 years old who had been training for over a year had significantly higher bone density in the hip and femur regions than did age-matched control subjects (Conroy et al. 1993). Even more impressive was that these young lifters had bone densities higher than those of adult men. In addition, bone density continued to increase over the next year of training (unpublished data). The importance of high impulse factors in sport along with heavy resistance training to cause changes in bone has also been observed in other young athletes (Emeterio et al. 2011).

A previous world-record holder in the squat (1RM greater than 469 kg, or 1,034 lb) demonstrated an average BMD of 1.86 g · cm^{-2} for the lumbar spine, which is the highest BMD reported to date (Dickerman, Pertusi, and Smith 2000). Significantly greater lumbar spine and whole-body BMD between young male powerlifters and controls have also been shown (Tsuzuku, Ikegami, and Yabe 1998). In addition, a significant correlation was found between lumbar spine BMD and powerlifting performance. High-intensity resistance training in young men results in greater increases in BMD , whereas no significant BMD differences between the low-intensity training group and the control group were shown except at the trochanter region (Tsuzuku et al. 2001). It appears that heavy resistance training is needed to see improvements in BMD. Meta-analysis indicates that resistance training can increase BMD (approximately 2.6%) at skeletal sites stressed by the training (Kelley, Kelley, and Tran 2000). The effect, however, may be age dependent: People older than 31 show significant effects, whereas people younger than 31 show no significant effects if bone density is in normal ranges (Kelley, Kelley, and Tran 2000).

Resistance training is effective for increasing BMD in women of all ages. Similar to the male powerlifter described earlier, two female U.S. National Age Group Champions have very high BMD (Walters, Jezequel, and Grove 2012). These women, 49 and 54 years of age, had lumbar, femoral, and total-body BMDs well above normal for their age; the 54-year-old lifter had mean lumbar spine (1-3), femoral, and total-body BMDs of 1.44, 1.19 and 1.34 g · cm^{-2}, respectively, the greatest reported to date for a Caucasian of this

TABLE 3.6 Bone Mineral Density Values for the Spine and Proximal Femur

Site	Bone mineral density (g · cm^{-2})		[% comparison to adult reference data] (% comparison to matched anatomical controls)
	Junior lifters	Controls	
Spine	1.41 ± 0.20*#	1.06 ± 0.21	[113%] (133%)
Femoral neck	1.30 ± 0.15*#	1.05 ± 0.12	[131%] (124%)
Trochanter	1.05 ± 0.13*	0.89 ± 0.12	ND (118%)
Ward's triangle	1.26 ± 0.20*	0.99 ± 0.16	ND (127%)

Values are means ± 1 SD. * $P \le$ .05 from corresponding control data, # $P \le$ .05 from corresponding adult reference data. ND = no reference data available.

Adapted, by permission, from B.P. Conroy et al., 1993, "Bone mineral density in elite junior weightlifters," *Medicine and Science in Sports and Exercise* 25(10): 1105.

age. Fifteen months of resistance training of adolescent girls (14-17 years old) demonstrated leg strength increases of 40% and a significant increase in BMD of the femoral neck (1.035 to 1.073 g · cm^{-2}) (Nichols, Sanborn, and Love 2001). Meta-analysis showed that resistance training had a positive effect on the BMD at the lumbar spine of all women and at the femur and radius sites for postmenopausal women (Kelley et al. 2001) and that high-impact exercise including resistance training increases BMD of the lumbar spine and femoral neck in premenopausal women (Martyn-St. James and Carrol 2010). The positive effects of multiple-set strength training performed three times a week in older women was demonstrated by a significant improvement in bone density at the intertrochanter hip site (Kerr et al. 2001). This study demonstrated the effectiveness of a progressive strength program in increasing BMD at the clinically important hip site and in elderly women who are vulnerable to osteoporosis.

Although the evidence that resistance training can positively affect BMD is compelling, significant changes in BMD may not occur with all resistance training programs. This is probably due to the possible differences the acute program variables may have on changes in BMD. Because of the need for mechanical stress on bone for adaptation to occur, it is recommended that three to six sets with 1- to 10RM resistances of multiple-joint exercises be used with one to four minutes of rest between sets for optimal bone loading; more rest should be used with heavier resistances.

Physiological adaptations to ligaments and tendons after physical training do occur and may aid in injury prevention. Physical activity causes increased metabolism, thickness, weight, and strength of ligaments (Staff 1982; Tipton et al. 1975). Damaged ligaments regain their strength at a faster rate when physical activity is performed after the damage has occurred (Staff 1982; Tipton et al. 1975). Both the attachment site of a ligament or tendon to a bone and the muscle–tendinous junction are frequent sites of injury. With endurance-type training, the amount of force necessary to cause separation at these areas increases in laboratory animals (Tipton et al. 1975). Human tendon fibroblasts subjected to mechanical stretch in vitro show increased secretion patterns of growth factors (Skutek et al. 2001), indicating that stretch may have a positive effect on tendon and ligament

tissue by cell proliferation, differentiation, and matrix formation.

Increasing the strength of the ligaments and tendons can help prevent damage to these structures caused by the muscle's abilities to lift heavier weights and develop more force. These structures also appear to hypertrophy somewhat more slowly than muscle. After 8 and 12 weeks of resistance training of the plantar flexors and knee extensors, muscle size and strength increased significantly with no increase in tendon cross-sectional area (Kubo et al. 2001; Kubo, Kanehisa, and Fukunaga 2002). However, resistance training resulted in significant increases in tendon stiffness. The authors concluded that the training-induced changes in the internal structures of the tendon (e.g., the mechanical quality of collagen) accounted for the changes in stiffness and that increases in tendon cross-sectional area may take longer than 12 weeks. This may be a factor in anabolic steroid–induced musculotendinous injuries, because it has been hypothesized that large increases in muscle size and strength (and consequent training loads) may occur too rapidly to allow adequate connective tissue adaptation. Interestingly, it has been shown that tendon size and strength can be improved with heavy resistance training in a relatively short period of time (e.g., months), and differential changes can occur along the long axis of the tendon. This may indicate the importance of the exercise choices and ranges of motion used (Kongsgaard et al. 2007; Magnusson et al. 2007). For example, patellar tendon cross-sectional area increased 7% with 12 weeks of resistance training (Ronnestad, Hansen, and Raastad 2012a). The extent of changes in tendon is not as dramatic in women, which may be related to hormonal differences between the sexes and the impact of these differences on tendon adaptations (Magnusson et al. 2007).

The **connective tissue sheaths** that surround the entire muscle (epimysium), groups of muscle fibers (perimysium), and individual muscle fibers (endomysium) may also adapt to resistance training. These sheaths are of major importance in the tensile strength and elastic properties of muscle and form the framework that supports an overload on the muscle. Compensatory hypertrophy induced in the muscle of laboratory animals also causes an increase in the collagen content of these connective tissue sheaths (Laurent et al. 1978; Turto, Lindy, and Halme 1974). The relative amount of connective tissue in the biceps brachii of bodybuilders does not differ from that of age-matched control subjects (MacDougall et al. 1985; Sale et al. 1987), and male and female bodybuilders possess similar relative amounts of connective tissue as control subjects (Alway, MacDougall et al. 1988). Thus, the connective tissue sheaths in muscle appear to increase with training so that the same ratio between connective and muscle tissue is maintained.

Resistance training has been found to increase the thickness of hyaline cartilage on the articular surfaces of bone (Holmdahl and Ingelmark 1948; Ingelmark and Elsholm 1948). One major function of hyaline cartilage is to act as a shock absorber between the bony surfaces of a joint. Increasing the thickness of this cartilage could facilitate the performance of this shock absorber function. In summary, bone, tendon, and other types of connective tissue appear to adapt to resistance training, but to a lesser extent and at a slower rate than muscle tissue.

Cardiovascular Adaptations

Similar to skeletal muscle, cardiac muscle also undergoes adaptations to resistance training. Likewise, other aspects of the cardiovascular system, such as the blood lipid profile, also demonstrate adaptations. Adaptations and acute responses of the cardiovascular system to resistance training are especially important when weight training is performed by some special populations, such as seniors and those undergoing cardiac rehabilitation. As with all adaptations to resistance training, the response depends in part on training volume and intensity.

Some of the cardiovascular system's adaptations brought about by resistance training, as well as other forms of physical conditioning, resemble the adaptations to hypertension, such as increased ventricular wall thickness and chamber size. When examined closely, however, the adaptations to hypertension and those to resistance training are different. As an example, with hypertension, ventricular wall thickness increases beyond normal limits. With weight training, this rarely occurs and is not evident when examined relative to fat-free mass, whereas with hypertension wall thickness increases are evident even when examined relative to fat-free mass. Differences in cardiac adaptations have resulted in the use of the terms *pathological*

hypertrophy to refer to the changes that occur with hypertension and other pathological conditions and *physiological hypertrophy* to refer to the changes that occur with physical training.

Cardiovascular adaptations are caused by the training stimulus to which the cardiovascular system is exposed. Endurance training brings about different cardiovascular adaptations than resistance training does. In general, these differences are caused by the need to pump a large volume of blood at an elevated blood pressure during endurance exercise, whereas during resistance training a relatively small volume of blood is pumped at an elevated blood pressure. This difference between endurance and resistance training results in different cardiovascular adaptations.

Training Adaptations at Rest

Resistance training can affect virtually all of the major aspects of cardiovascular function (see tables 3.7 and 3.8). Changes in cardiac morphology, systolic function, diastolic function, heart rate, blood pressure, lipid profile, as well as other indicators of disease risk, decrease the overall risk of disease. For example, men who perform a minimum of 30 minutes of resistance training per week decrease their overall risk of coronary heart disease by 23% compared to sedentary men (Tanasescu et al. 2002). Other adaptations due to weight training also reduce the risk of disease. Perhaps surprisingly, men who are in the lowest third for maximal strength (bench press and leg press) have a significantly greater risk of dying from any cause and cancer compared to men who are in the upper third for maximal strength (Ruiz et al. 2008). Maximal strength was inversely associated with all-cause mortality in both normal-weight and overweight men, and with cancer mortality in overweight men. A significant age-adjusted trend was shown for death rate per 10,000 person years of 33, 26, and 21 in normal-weight men and 42, 26, and 34 in overweight men in the lowest, middle, and upper third for maximal strength. These observations are probably not related to maximal strength per se, but to other factors related to maintaining maximal strength.

Resting heart rates of junior and senior competitive bodybuilders, powerlifters, and Olympic lifters range from 60 to 78 beats per minute (Adler et al. 2008; Colan et al. 1985; D'Andrea, Riegler et al. 2010; Fleck and Dean 1987; George et al. 1995;

TABLE 3.7 Chronic Resting Cardiovascular Adaptations From Resistance Exercise

Cardiovascular indicator	Adaptation
Heart rate	No change or small decrease
Blood pressure	
Systolic	No change or small decrease
Diastolic	No change or small decrease
Stroke volume	
Absolute	Small increase or no change
Relative to BSA	No change
Relative to LBM	No change
Cardiac function	
Systolic	No change
Diastolic	No change
Lipid profile	
Total cholesterol	No change or small decrease
HDL-C	No change or small increase
LDL-C	No change or small decrease
Total cholesterol/HDL-C	No change or small decrease

BSA = body surface area (m^2); LBM = lean body mass (kg); HDL-C = high-densitylipoprotein cholesterol; LDL-C = low-density lipoprotein cholesterol.

TABLE 3.8 Cardiac Morphology Adaptations at Rest Due to Resistance Training

		Relative to	
	Absolute	BSA	FFM
Wall thickness			
Left ventricle	Increase or no change	No change	No change
Septal	Increase or no change	No change	No change
Right ventricle	Increase or no change	No change	No change
Chamber volume			
Left ventricle	No change or slight increase	No change or slight increase	No change or slight increase
Right ventricle	No change or slight increase (?)	No change or slight increase (?)	No change or slight increase (?)
Atrial	No change or slight increase (?)	No change or slight increase (?)	No change or slight increase (?)
Left ventricular mass	Increase or no change	No change	No change

BSA = body surface area (m^2); FFM = fat-free mass (kg); ? = minimal data.

Haykowsky et al. 2000; Smith and Raven 1986). The vast majority of cross-sectional data indicate that the resting heart rates of highly strength-trained athletes are not significantly different from those of sedentary people (Fleck 1988, 2002). However, the resting heart rates of male Olympic weightlifters have been reported to be lower (60 vs. 69 beats per minute) than those of sedentary people (Adler et al. 2008), whereas the resting heart rates of master-level powerlifters has been reported to be 87 beats per minute, which was significantly higher than those of age-matched control subjects (Haykowsky et al. 2000). Not surprisingly, the resting heart rates of strength-trained athletes (bodybuilding, weightlifting, martial arts, windsurfing) is significantly higher (69 vs. 52 beats per minute) than those of aerobically trained athletes (long- and middle-distance swimmers and runners, soccer players, basketball players) (D'Andrea, Riegler et al. 2010).

The majority of short-term (up to 20 weeks) longitudinal studies report significant decreases of approximately 4 to 13% and small nonsignificant decreases in resting heart rate (Fleck 2002; Karavirta et al. 2009). The mechanism causing a decrease in resting heart rate after weight training is not clearly elucidated. However, decreased heart rate is typically associated with a combination of increased parasympathetic and decreased sympathetic cardiac tone. Some cardiovascular responses to isometric actions resemble responses to typical weight training activity. During low-level isometric actions (30% of maximal voluntary contraction), both autonomic branches show increased activity (Gonzalez-Camarena et al. 2000). Thus, a decrease in resting heart rate, when it does occur as a result of weight training, may not be due to an increase in parasympathetic cardiac tone and a decrease in sympathetic cardiac tone, but rather to the increased activity of both autonomic branches.

Blood Pressure

The majority of cross-sectional data clearly demonstrate that highly strength-trained athletes have average resting systolic and diastolic blood pressures (Byrne and Wilmore 2000; Fleck 2002). However, significantly above-average (Snoecky et al. 1982), and less-than-average (Adler et al. 2008; Smith and Raven 1986) resting blood pressures in weightlifters have also been reported. Not surprisingly, strength-trained athletes (bodybuilding, weightlifting, martial arts, windsurfing) have higher resting blood pressures than aerobically trained athletes (long- and middle-distance swimmers and runners, soccer players, basketball players) (D'Andrea, Riegler et al. 2010).

Short-term training studies have shown both significant decreases and nonsignificant changes in both systolic and diastolic resting blood pressure. Meta-analyses conclude that resistance training can significantly decrease systolic (3 to 4.55 mmHg) and diastolic (3 to 3.79 mmHg) blood pressure (Cornelissen and Fagard 2005; Fargard 2006; Kelley 1997; Kelley and Kelley 2000) or results in a nonsignificant decrease (3.2 mmHg) in systolic blood pressure (Fagard 2006). This results in approximately a 2 to 4% decrease in systolic and diastolic blood pressure. The decrease in blood pressure may be greater in those with hypertension, but additional studies including only hypertensive people are needed. Although such small decreases may seem trivial, they have been associated with a decreased risk for stroke and coronary heart disease (Kelley and Kelley 2000). Thus, resistance training can result in significant decreases in resting blood pressure.

Stroke Volume

Stroke volume is the amount of blood pumped per heartbeat. An increase in resting stroke volume is viewed as a positive adaptation to training and is often accompanied by a decrease in resting heart rate. No difference (Brown et al. 1983; Dickhuth et al. 1979) between highly strength-trained males and normal people in absolute stroke volume have been reported, as have greater values (Fleck, Bennett et al.1989; Pearson et al. 1986) in highly strength-trained people and greater values in weightlifters (Adler et al. 2008) than in normal people. Absolute stroke volume of any group of strength-trained athletes is typically less than that of aerobically trained athletes (D'Andrea et al. 2010). Increased absolute stroke volume, when present, appears to be due to a significantly greater end diastolic left ventricular internal dimension and a normal ejection fraction (Adler et al. 2008; Fleck 1988). A meta-analysis indicates that the caliber of athlete may influence absolute stroke volume: National- and international-caliber athletes have a greater absolute stroke volume than lesser-caliber athletes (Fleck 1988). Although a few comparisons between highly resistance-trained people and normal people show a significantly greater stroke volume relative to body surface area in the strength-trained people, the majority of comparisons show no significant difference between these two groups in stroke volume relative to body surface area (Fleck 2002). When a significant difference in stroke volume relative to body surface area is shown, the difference generally becomes nonsignificant when expressed relative to fat-free mass (Fleck 2002; Fleck, Bennett et al. 1989). A meta-analysis of stroke volume relative to body surface area demonstrates no difference by caliber of athlete (Fleck 1988). Thus, the greater absolute stroke volume in some national- and international-caliber highly strength-trained athletes may be explained in part by body size. The preponderance of cross-sectional data indicates weight training to have no or little effect on absolute stroke volume or stroke volume relative to body surface area or fat-free mass. This conclusion is supported by studies reporting no change in absolute resting stroke volume after the performance of a short-term weight training program (Camargo et al. 2008; Lusiani et al. 1986).

Blood Lipid Profile

Literature reviews report that resistance-trained male athletes have normal, higher-than-normal, and lower-than-normal high-density lipoprotein cholesterol (HDL-C), low-density lipoprotein cholesterol (LDL-C), total cholesterol (TC), and TC-to-HDL-C ratio (Hurley 1989; Kraemer, Deschenes, and Fleck 1988; Stone et al. 1991). Meanwhile, literature reviews on training studies suggest that resistance training has little or no effect on the lipid profile in adults (Braith and Stewart 2006; Williams et al. 2007). However, a meta-analysis indicates that resistance training does have small but significant effects on the blood lipid profile in both adult men and women (Kelley and Kelley 2009a). This meta-analysis indicates that resistance training significantly decreases TC by 2.7%, LDL-C by 4.6%, total triglyceride (TG) by 6.4%, and TC-to-HDL-C ratio by 11.6%. However, high-density lipoprotein cholesterol was not significantly affected (+1.4%).

The blood lipid profile response to resistance training varies substantially, and this variation is in part due to differences in resistance training program intensity and volume. Associations indicated by the meta-analysis and previous research support this contention. The meta-analysis indicates an inverse relationship between decreases in TC and TC-to-HDL-C ratio and greater dropout rates in training studies, which could be indicative of more difficult weight training programs. This is supported by another indication of the meta-analysis and some previous studies. The meta-analysis indicated an association between increased training intensity and greater decreases in LDL-C, whereas previous studies indicate that weight training volume may have some effect on the lipid profile. Bodybuilders have been reported to have lipid profiles similar to those of runners. Powerlifters, on the other hand, have lower HDL-C and higher LDL-C concentrations than runners when body fat, age, and androgen use (which has been shown to depress HDL-C concentrations) are accounted for (Hurley et al. 1987; Hurley, Seals, Hagberg et al. 1984). Over 12 weeks of training, middle-aged men showed the greatest positive changes in the

lipid profile during the program's highest training volume phase (Blessing et al. 1987; Johnson et al. 1982). Thus, weight training volume and intensity may both affect blood lipid profile.

Most studies examining the effect of weight training on the lipid profile can be criticized. Limitations of the studies include inadequate control of age, diet, and training program; the use of only one blood sample in determining the lipid profile; the lack of a control group; not controlling for changes in body composition; and short duration. An acute increase in HDL-C and a decrease in total cholesterol occur 24 hours after a 90-minute resistance exercise session, and these blood lipids do not return to baseline values by 48 hours after the exercise session (Wallace et al. 1991). This effect needs to be accounted for in studies. These as well as other limitations indicate that the results of previous studies as well as the meta-analysis discussed earlier need to be viewed with caution, and that when changes in the blood lipid profile are a major training goal, aerobic training should be performed (Kelley and Kelley 2009a, 2009b). It is also important to note that nutritional counseling in conjunction with resistance training further contributes to positive changes in the blood lipid profile (Sallinen et al. 2005).

How resistance training might positively affect the lipid profile has not been completely elucidated. Decreased percent body fat has been reported to positively influence the lipid profile (Twisk, Kemper, and van Mechelen 2000; Williams et al. 1994), and resistance training can decrease percent body fat. Additionally, the meta-analysis indicates that decreases in body mass index are associated with greater improvements in TC, HDL-C, and TC/HDL-C ratio and that greater increases in fat-free mass are associated with greater increases in HDL-C. Thus, changes in body mass or body composition as a result of weight training may affect the lipid profile. Resistance training may improve the oxidative capacity of skeletal muscle because of an increase in the activity of specific aerobic-oxidative enzymes (Wang et al. 1993), which could positively affect the blood lipid profile. Such a change might occur as a result of fiber-type conversion from type IIx to type IIa (Staron et al. 1994) and an increase in capillaries per muscle fiber (McCall et al. 1996). Weight training could also negatively affect the lipid profile. People with a higher percentage of type I muscle fibers tend to have a higher HDL-C concentration (Tikkanen, Naveri, and Harkonen 1996). Some resistance training programs have the greatest hypertrophic effect on type II fibers (see Hypertrophy earlier in this chapter). The resulting decrease in the percentage area of type I fibers may negatively affect the lipid profile.

The meta-analysis also indicates some other interesting associations. Those with a lower initial HDL-C level show greater increases in HDL-C with training. Greater decreases in LDL-C are associated with a higher compliance rate to training, which may reflect greater benefits when there is a greater commitment to the training program. Although not explained, an association does exist between upper-body strength changes and changes in TC as a result of resistance training.

Further research is needed before a conclusion can be reached concerning the effect of resistance training on the lipid profile and what type of resistance training program is optimal when positive effects of the blood lipid profile are desired. However, an aptitude for power or speed athletic events, including weightlifting, does not offer protection from cardiovascular risk in former athletes. On the other hand, an aptitude for endurance athletic events and continuing vigorous physical activity after retirement from competitive sport do offer protection against cardiovascular risk (Kujala et al. 2000). Therefore, a prudent conclusion might be to encourage strength and power athletes to perform some aerobic training and follow dietary practices appropriate to bring about positive changes in the lipid profile. This may be especially important for long-term health after retirement from competition.

Cardiac Wall Thickness

Increased cardiac wall thicknesses are an adaptation to the intermittent elevated blood pressures during resistance training (Naylor, George et al. 2008; Rowland and Fernhall 2007). Both echocardiographic and magnetic resonance imaging (MRI) techniques (see figure 3.29) have been used to investigate changes in cardiac morphology as a result of weight training. Several literature reviews have concluded that highly strength-trained people can have greater-than-average absolute diastolic posterior left ventricular wall thickness (PWTd) (Fleck 1988, 2002; Naylor, George et al. 2008;

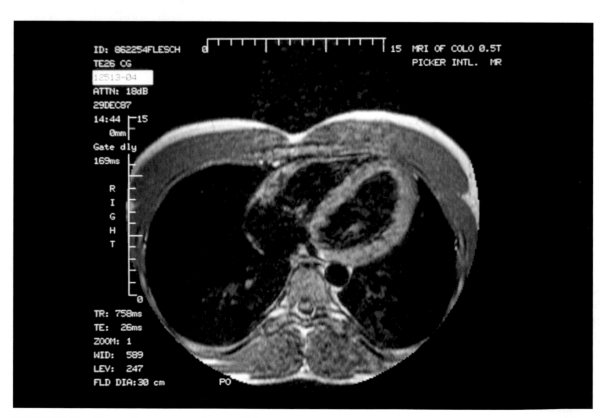

FIGURE 3.29 Magnetic resonance image (MRI) of the left ventricle (circular chamber with thick walls) and right ventricle (triangular chamber).

Courtesy of Dr. Steven Fleck's laboratory.

Urhausen and Kindermann 1992) and diastolic intraventricular septum wall thickness (IVSd) (Fleck 1988, 2002; Naylor, George et al. 2008; Perrault and Turcotte 1994; Urhausen and Kindermann 1992; Wolfe, Cunningham, and Boughner 1986). Similarly, a meta-analysis indicates IVSd to be significantly greater than normal in strength-trained athletes (normal: 10.5 mm vs. strength-trained: 11.8 mm), and that PWTd was greater in strength-trained athletes (normal: 10.3 mm vs. strength-trained: 11.0 mm), but not significantly so (Pluim et al. 1999). In general, absolute wall thickness in highly strength-trained people rarely exceeds the upper limits of normal (Urhausen and Kindermann 1992; Wolfe, Cunningham, and Boughner 1986) and is normally significantly lower than in those with diseases such as aortic stenosis, obstructive cardiomyopathy, and extreme hypertension (Wolfe, Cunningham, and Boughner 1986). Increased ventricular wall thicknesses are also apparent in many other types of athletes (Naylor, George et al. 2008). A ranking of 27 sports places weightlifting at number 8 in terms of left ventricular wall thickness (Spataro et al. 1994).

When cardiac wall thicknesses (PWTd and IVSd) of highly strength-trained people are expressed relative to body surface area or to fat-free mass, generally there is no difference from normal (Fleck 1988, 2002; Fleck, Bennett et al. 1989; Naylor, George et al. 2008; Perrault and Turcotte 1994; Urhausen and Kindermann 1992). This is important because it indicates a physiological adaptation rather than an adaptation to a pathological disease state. The caliber of athletes may have some correlation with ventricular wall thicknesses. A meta-analysis indicates IVSd thickness, but not PWTd, to be affected by the caliber of the athlete, and that national-, international-, and regional-caliber athletes have a greater IVSd thickness than recreational strength trainers do (Fleck 1988). However, this is not supported by all studies examining wall thickness changes in weight-trained athletes (Naylor, George et al. 2008).

Short-term longitudinal training studies also indicate that strength training can increase PWTd and IVSd; however, it is not a necessary outcome of all weight training programs (Fleck 1988, 2002; Naylor, George et al. 2008; Perrault and Turcotte 1994). The conclusion that not all resistance training programs result in an increase in ventricular wall thickness is supported by cross-sectional studies showing no significant difference from controls in ventricular wall thickness in female collegiate strength- and power-trained athletes (George et al. 1995) and junior and master national-caliber powerlifters (Haykowsky et al. 2000).

Whether an increase in left ventricular wall thickness occurs probably depends on differences in the training performed. The highest blood pressures during a set to concentric failure occur during the last few repetitions of a set (Fleck and Dean 1987; MacDougall et al. 1985; Sale et al. 1994). Exercises involving large-muscle mass, such as leg presses, result in higher blood pressures than small-muscle-mass exercises (MacDougall et al. 1985). Therefore, whether sets are carried to concentric failure and the exercises performed may affect the occurrence of increases in ventricular wall thickness. Other factors that may affect whether changes in ventricular wall thickness occur include training intensity, training volume, the duration of training, and the rest periods between sets.

The effect of weight training on other cardiac chamber wall thicknesses has received considerably less attention than the effect on left ventricular wall thickness. However, a magnetic resonance imaging study reports no difference in systolic and diastolic right ventricular wall thickness between male junior elite Olympic weightlifters and age- and weight-matched controls (Fleck, Henke, and Wilson 1989), which indicates that the right ventricle is not exposed to sufficiently elevated blood pressures to cause hypertrophy. However, it has also been reported that six months of weight training produces small but significant increases in right ventricular mass (Spence et al. 2013) indicating that the right ventricle does increase in size with weight training.

Resistance training can result in increased left ventricular wall thickness, but it is not a necessary consequence of all resistance training programs. Increased left ventricular wall thickness, when apparent, is caused by the intermittent elevated blood pressures encountered during strength training. When expressed relative to body surface area or fat-free mass, generally no increase in left ventricular wall thickness is demonstrated. Additionally, increased left ventricular wall thickness rarely exceeds the upper limits of normalcy and is significantly below wall thickness increases resulting from pathological conditions.

Heart Chamber Size

An increase in ventricular chamber size or volume is an indication of volume overload on the heart (i.e., the need to pump a large volume of blood).

The majority of cross-sectional data on highly strength-trained athletes and longitudinal short-term training studies show resistance training to have little or no effect on absolute left ventricular internal dimensions, an indicator of chamber size (Adler et al. 2008; Fleck 1988, 2002; Fleck, Henke, and Wilson 1989; George et al. 1995; Naylor, George et al. 2008; Perrault and Turcotte 1994; Urhausen and Kindermann 1992). This is true whether systolic or diastolic chamber dimensions are examined. However, a meta-analysis indicates that strength-trained athletes have a significantly greater-than-normal left ventricle internal diameter in diastole (LVIDd) (52.1 vs. 49.6 mm) (Pluim et al. 1999). It has also been reported that right ventricular end diastolic volume increases slightly, but significantly, with six months of weight training (Spence et al. 2013). Similar to left ventricular wall thickness, the left ventricular internal dimensions in highly strength-trained people normally do not exceed the upper limits of normal (Fleck 1988, 2002; Perrault and Turcotte 1994; Urhausen and Kindermann 1992; Wolfe, Cunningham, and Boughner 1986) and in most cases are not significantly different from normal when expressed relative to body surface area or fat-free mass (Fleck 1988, 2002; Urhausen and Kindermann 1992; Wolfe, Cunningham, and Boughner 1986).

Increases in cardiac chamber size do occur as a result of endurance training and participation in many other sports (D'Andrea, Cocchia et al. 2010; Naylor, George et al. 2008; Pluim et al. 1999). A comparison of nationally ranked athletes in 27 sports ranked weightlifters number 22 in terms of left ventricular internal dimensions (Spataro et al. 1994). The slight increase or no change in left ventricular internal dimensions coupled with no change or an increase in left ventricular wall thickness is an important difference between weight training and pathological cardiac hypertrophy, in which a large increase in wall thickness is not accompanied by an increase in left ventricular internal dimensions (Urhausen and Kindermann 1992). A meta-analysis of PWTd + IVSd / LVIDd, or mean relative wall thickness, indicates that strength-trained athletes had a mean wall-to-wall thickness that was greater than normal (Pluim et al. 1999). This indicates that wall thickness increases to a greater extent than left ventricular volume in strength-trained athletes.

Meta-analysis indicates that the caliber of the athlete does not influence whether the left ventricular internal dimension is significantly different from normal (Fleck 1988). Reports of nationally ranked junior and senior powerlifters having normal left ventricular internal dimensions (Haykowsky et al. 2000) and of national-caliber strength-trained athletes having a left ventricular internal dimension not significantly different from normal (Adler et al. 2008; Dickhuth et al. 1979; Fleck, Bennett et al. 1989) also indicate that the caliber of the athlete has little effect on left ventricular chamber size. Because changes in ventricular volume are normally associated with a volume overload, it might be hypothesized that the type of weight training program would have an effect on left ventricular chamber size.

A comparison of bodybuilders and weightlifters shows no significant difference between the two groups in left and right ventricular internal dimension, although the bodybuilders had slightly greater values. However, the bodybuilders, but not the weightlifters, had a greater absolute left and right ventricular internal dimension at rest (Deligiannis, Zahopoulou, and Mandroukas 1988) compared to normal. If expressed relative to body surface area or fat-free mass, the left ventricular internal dimension of neither the bodybuilders nor the weightlifters was significantly different from normal. However, the right ventricular internal dimension of the bodybuilders was significantly different from normal when expressed relative to body surface area and fat-free mass. This same study also reported the left atrial internal dimension of both bodybuilders and weightlifters to be greater than normal in absolute terms and relative to body surface area and fat-free mass terms; the bodybuilders had a significantly greater left atrial internal dimension than the weightlifters (Deligiannis, Zahopoulo, and Mandroukas 1988). In support of the preceding, increased left atrial volume relative to body surface area was associated with endurance, but not strength training, and with an increase in left ventricular volume, which typically does not occur with resistance training (D'Andrea, Cocchia et al. 2010). This information indicates that the type of weight training program may affect cardiac chamber size, but the effect is small.

Resistance training appears to result in a slight increase in cardiac chamber size as indicated by a meta-analysis showing a small significant (2.5%) increase in strength-trained athletes compared to normal (Fagard 1996). However, no difference from normal is generally apparent when examined relative to body surface area or fat-free mass. High-volume training programs may have the greatest potential to affect cardiac chamber sizes.

Left Ventricular Mass

An increase in left ventricular mass (LVM) can be brought about by an increase in either wall thickness or chamber size. Estimates of LVM have been obtained using echocardiographic and magnetic resonance imaging (MRI). The majority of cross-sectional studies on highly resistance-trained athletes (Fleck 1988, 2002; George et al. 1995; Haykowsky et al. 2000; Naylor, George et al. 2008) and of longitudinal short-term training studies (Fleck 1988, 2002; Naylor, George et al. 2008; Wolfe, Cunningham, and Boughner 1986) demonstrate absolute LVM to be greater than normal in resistance-trained athletes or increased as a result of weight training. This conclusion is supported by a meta-analysis indicating that LVM is greater than normal in strength-trained athletes (normal 174 g vs. strength-trained 267 g) (Pluim et al. 1999). However, increased LVM is not a necessary outcome of all resistance training programs, and the difference is greatly reduced or nonexistent relative to body surface area or fat-free mass. Some data indicate that national- and international-caliber weight-trained athletes have a greater LVM than lesser-caliber athletes (Effron 1989; Fleck 1988).

The type of weight training program may influence how LVM is increased. Both bodybuilders and weightlifters have a significantly greater-than-normal absolute LVM; however, they are not significantly different from each other (Deligiannis, Zahopoulou, and Mandroukas 1988). Bodybuilders and weightlifters both also have significantly greater-than-normal left ventricular wall thicknesses. However, only bodybuilders have a significantly greater-than-normal left ventricular end-diastolic dimension (Deligiannis, Zahopoulou, and Mandroukas 1988). Thus, in bodybuilders the increased LVM is caused by both greater left ventricular wall thickness and greater chamber size, whereas in weightlifters the increase is caused for the most part only by greater-than-normal wall thickness. It could be hypothesized that a weight training program that increases both left ventricular wall thickness and left ventricular internal dimensions would result in the greatest increase in estimated LVM. However, it has also been concluded that weight training volume does not affect the increase in LVM (Naylor, George et al 2008).

Resistance training can increase absolute LVM; however, such an increase does not occur with all weight training programs. The increased LVM can be caused by an increase in either wall thickness or chamber size, or a combination of both.

Cardiac Function

Abnormalities in systolic and diastolic function are associated with cardiac hypertrophy caused by pathological conditions, such as hypertension and valvular heart disease. This has raised concern that cardiac hypertrophy caused by resistance training may impair cardiac function. However, the majority of cross-sectional studies demonstrate that common measures of left ventricular systolic function—for example, percentage of fractional shortening, ejection fraction, and velocity of circumferential shortening—are unaffected by resistance training (Adler et al. 2008; Ellias et al. 1991; Fleck 1988, 2002; George et al. 1995; Haykowsky et al. 2000; Urhausen and Kindermann 1992). However, it has also been reported that the percentage of fractional shortening is significantly greater in strength-trained athletes than in normal subjects (Colan, Sanders, and Borrow 1987), indicating enhanced systolic function. Short-term longitudinal training studies also show no change (Lusiani et al. 1986) or a significant increase in the percentage of fractional shortening (Kanakis and Hickson 1980). The majority of studies indicate that weight training has no effect on systolic function, and minimal data indicate enhanced systolic function.

Left ventricular diastolic function has received less attention than systolic function. Cross-sectional data on highly weight-trained athletes indicate no significant change from normal (Urhausen and Kindermann 1992) or an increase in left ventricular diastolic function (Adler et al. 2008). Powerlifters competing at the national level, who have significantly greater absolute and relative-to-body-surface-area left ventricular mass, have been reported to have normal and even enhanced measures of diastolic function (peak rate of chamber enlargement and atrial peak filling rate) (Colan, Sanders, and Borrow 1985; Pearson et al. 1986).

A meta-analysis indicates that systolic and diastolic function are not significantly different from normal in strength-trained athletes (Pluim et al. 1999). Overall, both cross-sectional and longitudinal studies indicate that resistance training has no significant effect on either systolic or diastolic function.

Acute Cardiovascular Responses

The acute response to resistance training refers to physiological responses during one set of an exercise, several sets of an exercise(s), or one training session. Determining acute responses accurately can be difficult. Intra-arterial lines are necessary to accurately determine blood pressure because it is impossible with auscultatory sphygmomanometry to determine such things as blood pressure during the concentric and eccentric phases of repetitions. Finger plesmography has also been used to determine blood pressure continuously during resistance training. Cardiac impedance and echocardiographic techniques have been used to determine cardiac output, stroke volume, and left ventricular volume, but these techniques have limitations during physical activity. Thus, in some instances, conclusions drawn concerning the acute response to resistance training must be viewed with caution (see table 3.9).

Heart Rate and Blood Pressure

Heart rate and both systolic and diastolic blood pressure increase substantially during the performance of dynamic heavy resistance exercise (Fleck 1988; Hill and Butler 1991). This is true for machine, free weight, and isokinetic exercise (Fleck and Dean 1987; Gomides et al. 2010; Iellamo et al. 1997; Kleiner et al. 1996; MacDougall et al. 1985; Sale et al. 1993, 1994; Scharf et al. 1994). Mean peak systolic and diastolic blood pressures as high as 320/250 mmHg and a peak heart rate of 170 beats per minute occur during the performance of a two-legged leg press set to failure at 95% of 1RM, in which a Valsalva maneuver was allowed (MacDougall et al. 1985). However, heart rate and blood pressure responses are also substantial even when an attempt is made to limit the performance of a Valsalva maneuver. For example, mean peak blood pressures of 198/160 mmHg and a heart rate of 135 beats per minute occur during a single-legged knee extension set performed to concentric failure at 80% of 1RM when a Valsalva maneuver is discouraged (Fleck and Dean 1987).

Both blood pressure (see figure 3.30) and heart rate increase as the set progresses, so the highest values occur during the last several repetitions of a set to volitional fatigue whether or not a Valsalva maneuver is allowed (Fleck and Dean 1987; Gomides et al. 2010; MacDougall et al. 1985; Sale et al. 1994). When a Valsalva maneuver is allowed, the blood pressure and heart rate response are significantly higher during sets performed to volitional fatigue with submaximal resistances (50-95% of 1RM) than when a resistance of 100% of 1RM is used (MacDougall et al. 1985; Sale et al. 1994). When a Valsalva maneuver is discouraged, the blood pressure response is higher, but not significantly so, during sets at 90, 80, and 70% of 1RM compared to sets at 100 and 50% of 1RM to volitional fatigue (Fleck and Dean 1987). Although it is not clear whether a Valsalva maneuver was discouraged in people with hypertension, the blood pressure response is higher during sets of knee extension exercise at 80 and 40% of 1RM to

TABLE 3.9 Acute Response During Resistance Exercise Relative to Rest

Response	Portion of repetition	
	Concentric	Eccentric
Heart rate (no difference between concentric and eccentric)	Increase	Increase
Stroke volume (?) (eccentric value higher than concentric)	No difference or decrease	No difference or increase
Cardiac output (?) (eccentric value higher than concentric)	No difference or increase	Increase
Blood pressure (highest at exercise sticking point) Systolic increase Diastolic increase	Increase Increase	Increase Increase
Intrathoracic pressure (highest when a Valsalva maneuver is performed)	Increase	Increase

? = minimal data.

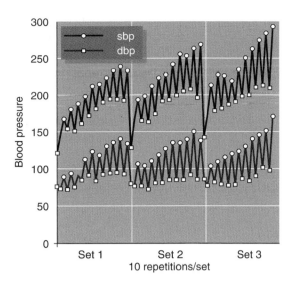

FIGURE 3.30 Blood pressure response increases during a two-legged leg press set to volitional fatigue as well as during three successive sets of 10 repetitions at a 10RM resistance. sbp = systolic blood pressure; dbp = diastolic blood pressure.

Reprinted, by permission, from R.W. Gotshall et al., 1999, "Noninvasive characterization of the blood pressure response to the double-leg press exercise" *Journal of Exercise Physiology 2(4): 1-6.*

failure compared to a set to failure with 100% of 1RM (Gomides et al. 2010).

The blood pressure and heart rate responses during dynamic weight training appear to be similar to the responses during isometric actions in that, as the duration of the activity increases, so does the heart rate and blood pressure response (Kahn, Kapitaniak, and Monod 1985; Ludbrook et al. 1978). Thus, both the heart rate and blood pressure responses are lower in a set to failure using 100% of 1RM (one repetition) compared to sets to failure at lower percentages (90% through 40%) of 1RM (Fleck and Dean 1987; Gomides et al. 2010). However, the pattern of peak blood pressure and heart rate response in sets to failure at 90 to 40% of 1RM are inconsistent. Both the peak heart rate and blood pressure responses have been shown to increase during submaximal sets to failure (50, 70, 80, 85, and 87.5% of 1RM) as the percentage of 1RM increases (Sale et al. 1994). Conversely, no significant difference in the peak blood pressure and heart rate response during sets to failure with 90, 80, 70 or 50% of 1RM during one-legged knee extension and one-armed overhead press have been shown (Fleck and Dean 1987). Similarly, no significant difference in knee extension sets to failure using 80 and 40% of 1RM in the peak blood pressure and heart rate response of people

with hypertension has been shown (Gomides et al. 2010).

The heart rate and blood pressure responses during successive sets to failure are also inconsistent. During three successive sets (see figure 3.30) to failure of the leg press exercise with three minutes of rest between sets, blood pressure increases with successive sets (Gotshall et al. 1999). However, in hypertensive people peak blood pressure in three successive sets of knee extension exercise at either 80% (8 to 10 repetitions per set) or 40% (14 to 20 repetitions per set) of 1RM with 90 seconds between sets does not significantly increase in successive sets (Gomides et al. 2010). Heart rate does not increase in three to five successive sets (bench press, knee extension, elbow flexion) with rest periods between sets of three to five minutes (Alcaraz, Sanchez-Lorente, and Blazevich 2008; Wickwire et al. 2009) or in hypertensive people in three successive sets of the knee extension as described earlier (Gomides et al. 2010).

Shorter rest period lengths (35 seconds) between sets of exercises for different muscle groups (alternating exercise order) can be used with no peak heart rate increase in successive sets (Alcaraz, Sanchez-Lorente, and Blazevich 2008). Between sets both the blood pressure and heart rate return toward resting values, but with rest periods between sets (one and a half to three minutes), they are still above resting values when the next set begins. Additionally, both heart rate and blood pressure responses increase with increased active muscle mass, but the response is not linear (Falkel, Fleck, and Murray 1992; Fleck 1988; MacDougall et al. 1985).

During dynamic resistance exercise, higher systolic and diastolic blood pressures, but not heart rates, have been reported during the concentric compared to the eccentric portion of repetitions (Falkel, Fleck, and Murray 1992; MacDougall et al. 1985; Miles et al. 1987). Therefore, the point in the range of motion during the eccentric or concentric portion of a repetition at which blood pressure is determined affects the value. The highest systolic and diastolic blood pressures (finger plesmography) occur at the start of the concentric portion of the leg press (see figure 3.31); blood pressure decreases as the concentric portion of the repetition progresses, reaching its lowest point when the legs are extended (Gotshall et al. 1999). Blood pressure then increases as the legs bend during the eccentric portion of a repetition and again reaches

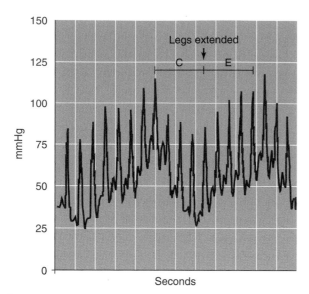

FIGURE 3.31 Blood pressure response during one complete repetition of a two-legged leg press exercise.

Reprinted, by permission, from R.W. Gotshall et al., 1999, "Noninvasive characterization of the blood pressure response to the double-leg press exercise" *Journal of Exercise Physiology* 2(4): 1-6.

its highest point when the legs are bent as far as possible. This indicates that the blood pressure response is highest at the sticking point of an exercise, when the muscular contraction is nearest its maximal force.

Investigations with isokinetic exercise give further insight into the acute blood pressure and heart rate responses. The velocity of isokinetic contraction (30 to 200 degrees per second) has little effect on the blood pressure and heart rate response (Haennel et al. 1989; Kleiner et al. 1999), whereas isokinetic exercise performed with both a concentric and eccentric phase results in a higher peak blood pressure than concentric exercise only (Sale et al. 1993). Thus, many factors, including active muscle mass, whether sets are carried to volitional fatigue, the number of sets performed, the rest periods between sets, the resistance used, where in the range of motion a measurement is obtained, and whether both concentric and eccentric muscular actions are performed, affect the blood pressure and heart rate responses during dynamic resistance training.

Stroke Volume and Cardiac Output

Estimates of stroke volume and cardiac output during resistance exercise are potentially affected by blood pressure during exercise, which, as discussed earlier, varies during the concentric and eccentric phases of the repetition and increases as a set progresses toward concentric failure. Thus, stroke volume and cardiac output may change depending on where during a repetition they are estimated and as a set continues toward concentric failure. Responses determined by electrical impedance techniques during knee extension exercise are shown to vary slightly depending on whether a Valsalva maneuver is performed. When attempts are made to limit the performance of a Valsalva maneuver, stroke volume and cardiac output during the concentric phase of the knee extension exercise (12 repetitions with a 12RM resistance) are not elevated significantly above resting values (Miles et al. 1987). During the concentric phase of the knee extension exercise, when a Valsalva maneuver is allowed (sets at 50, 80, and 100% of 1RM to fatigue), peak stroke volume is either significantly below resting values or not significantly different from resting values, and peak cardiac output is above resting values, but not always significantly so (Falkel, Fleck, and Murray 1992). During the eccentric repetition phase when a Valsalva maneuver is not allowed, peak stroke volume and cardiac output are significantly increased above resting values. When a Valsalva maneuver is allowed, peak stroke volume during the eccentric phase is significantly above or not significantly different from resting values, and peak cardiac output is always significantly greater than resting values. Thus, generally, with or without a Valsalva maneuver, peak stroke volume and cardiac output during the eccentric phase of knee extension exercise are generally higher compared to the concentric phase.

During a squat exercise at 50, 80, and 100% of 1RM to failure, the peak stroke volume and cardiac output response are also different between the eccentric and concentric repetition phases (Falkel, Fleck, and Murray 1992). During the eccentric phase, peak stroke volume is above resting values (sets at 50 and 100% of 1RM), but not always significantly so, or it is significantly below resting values (sets at 80% of 1RM). Peak stroke volume during the concentric phase of all sets is significantly below resting values. Peak cardiac output during the eccentric phase during all sets is significantly above resting values, and during the concentric phase of all sets it is always above resting values, but not always significantly so. Thus, as with the knee extension exercise, generally, peak stroke volume and cardiac output are higher in the eccentric phase of the squat exercise than in the concentric phase.

Heart rate is not significantly different between the concentric and eccentric phases of a repetition (Falkel, Fleck, and Murray 1992; MacDougall et al. 1985; Miles et al. 1987). As discussed earlier, stroke volume is significantly greater during the eccentric phase than during the concentric phase of a repetition. Thus, the greater cardiac output during the eccentric phase is due largely to a greater stroke volume during that phase.

A general pattern for both large-muscle-mass exercises (e.g., squat) and small-muscle-mass exercises (e.g., knee extension) for both peak stroke volume and cardiac output is that greater values occur during the eccentric phase than during the concentric phase. Stroke volume is generally below resting values during the concentric phase and generally above resting values during the eccentric phase. Cardiac output during the eccentric phase of both large- and small-muscle-mass exercises is generally above resting values. However, cardiac output during the concentric phase of large-muscle-group exercises may also be above resting values, but during small-muscle-group exercises can be either above or below the values.

Mechanisms of the Pressor Response

Several factors may influence the increase in blood pressure, or pressor response, during resistance training. Cardiac output can be increased above resting values during both the eccentric and concentric phases of resistance training exercise (Falkel, Fleck, and Murray 1992), which may contribute to the increase in blood pressure during weight training.

Increased intrathoracic or intra-abdominal pressures may have an effect on the blood pressure response during resistance training (Fleck 1988). Intrathoracic pressure increases during resistance training exercise (Falkel, Fleck, and Murray 1992; MacDougall et al. 1985; Sale et al. 1994) especially if a Valsalva maneuver is performed. Increased intrathoracic pressure may eventually decrease venous return to the heart and so decrease cardiac output. During resistance exercise an indirect measure (mouth pressure) of a Valsalva maneuver and intrathoracic pressure indicates a reduced cardiac output and stroke volume in people showing greater intrathoracic pressure than in those showing indications of less intrathoracic pressure (Falkel, Fleck, and Murray 1992). The increase in

intrathoracic pressure may limit venous return and thus cardiac output, but at the same time it may cause a buildup of blood in the systemic circulation, causing an increase in blood pressure. Cardiac output and stroke volume can be above resting values during resistance training exercise. For an increase in cardiac output and stroke volume to occur during resistance training, it can be speculated that the increase in blood pressure and the powerful muscle pump overcome the decrease in venous return because of an increase in intrathoracic pressure.

Increased intrathoracic pressure may have a protective function for the cerebral blood vessels similar to that thought to be active during a cough or strain (Hamilton, Woodbury, and Harper 1943). Any increase in intrathoracic pressure is transmitted to the cerebral spinal fluid because of its bearing on the intervertebral foramina. This reduces the transmural pressure of the cerebral blood vessels, protecting them from damage caused by the increase in blood pressure (MacDougall et al. 1985).

Increased intramuscular pressure during weight training exercise increases total peripheral resistance and occludes blood flow. Quite high intramuscular pressures (92 kPa) have been measured during static human muscular actions (Edwards, Hill, and McDonnell 1972). Although there is considerable intramuscular variability, static actions of 40 to 60% of maximum can occlude blood flow (Bonde-Peterson, Mork, and Nielsen 1975; Sadamoto, Bonde-Peterson, and Suzuki 1983). Increased intramuscular pressure during muscular actions is the most probable reason for blood pressures being reportedly higher during the concentric phase than during the eccentric phase (Miles et al. 1987) and is probably responsible for blood pressure being the highest at the sticking point of a repetition (Gotshall et al. 1999).

Increased blood pressure during weight training may help maintain perfusion pressure and so help maintain blood flow despite an increased intramuscular pressure (MacDougall et al. 1985). This appears to be true at least for small human muscles (Wright, McCloskey, and Fitzpatrick 2000). After fatiguing a thumb muscle (adductor pollicis) by performing rhythmic isometric actions, blood pressure was increased by contracting the knee extensors. Eighteen percent of the isometric force lost as a result of the fatigue of the small muscle was recovered for each 10% increase in blood pressure. The recovery of contractile force is probably related to an increase in perfusion pressure to the muscle. However, the applicability or magnitude of this mechanism to larger muscle groups is unclear.

During isometric exercise blood pressure continuously increases as the isometric action increases in duration and progresses toward fatigue. Although isometric exercise lacks a concentric and eccentric phase, examining the cardiovascular response to isometric exercise does offer some insight into the response during traditional resistance training. During knee extension isometric exercise (30% of maximal force), mean heart rate increases significantly and mean stroke volume decreases significantly (Rowland and Fernhall 2007). This results in a small increase in cardiac output even though mean arterial resistance has increased. This indicates that increased cardiac output was not the major cause of an increase in blood pressure and that blood pressure increases due to an increase in vascular resistance probably caused by an increase in intramuscular pressure occluding blood flow in the active muscle tissue. The resulting increase in blood pressure should have resulted in a greater decrease in stroke volume than shown. A decrease in stroke volume less than expected because of the increase in blood pressure is probably related to an increase in myocardial contractility resulting in a maintenance of or increase in ejection fraction.

During upper-body isometric action heart rate, systolic blood pressure, ejection fraction, and stroke volume all increase (Adler et al. 2008). The increase in stroke volume despite an increase in systolic blood pressure indicates an increase in myocardial contractility as evidenced by the increase in ejection fraction. The increase in stroke volume is also due to an increase in end diastolic volume and a decrease in end systolic volume (Adler et al. 2008). Even though isometric exercise lacks a concentric and eccentric phase, these results indicate that an increase in myocardial contractility helps to maintain or even increase stroke volume and thus cardiac output during traditional resistance training.

During isometric exercise no increase in blood flow to inactive muscle tissue occurs (Rowland and Fernhall 2007). This indicates that vasoconstriction occurs in inactive muscle tissue, which would limit blood flow to inactive tissue and possibly further increase blood pressure, and not vasodilation, which would tend to decrease blood pressure. So even though vasodilation in inactive muscle tissue would tend to decrease blood pressure, it does not appear to occur during isometric exercise. This indicates that the vasodilation of inactive tissue during traditional resistance training does not occur even though it would tend to decrease blood pressure. The applicability of vasodilation of inactive tissue to decrease blood pressure is especially questionable for large-muscle-group exercises (squat, deadlift), during which very little of the total muscle mass is inactive.

In summary, the pressor response during traditional resistance training is due predominantly to an increase in vascular resistance because of an increase in intramuscular pressure compressing blood vessels. If stroke volume and cardiac output increase during resistance training, the pressor response would also increase. Maintenance or an increase in stroke volume during resistance training is due to an increase in myocardial contractility.

Hypotensive Response

Following a bout of physical activity a significant decrease in systolic or diastolic blood pressure (or both) compared to resting values can take place; this is termed **postexercise hypotension**. This acute response may be important to consider if a chronic reduction in resting blood pressure is a training goal. A resistance training session can result in a postexercise hypotensive response that can last from 60 minutes (de Salles et al. 2010; Ruiz, Simão et al. 2011; Scher et al. 2011; Simão et al. 2005) to 24 hours (Queiroz et al. 2009). Resistance training sessions can also result in no significant change or even a slight increase in blood pressure during the immediate postexercise period (De Van et al. 2005; Focht and Koltyn 1999; O'Connor et al. 1993; Roltsch et al. 2001). It is also important to note that a hypotensive response can also occur in hypertensive people and that the response may be greater in people with this condition (Hardy and Tucker 1998; Melo et al. 2006). When apparent, the postexercise hypotensive response is related to the interaction among cardiac output, vascular resistance, and parasympathetic activity.

The effect of various resistance training variables on the postexercise hypotensive response has been investigated; however, more research is needed in this area. A postexercise hypotensive response does occur after a training session performed in a circuit or a set repetition format (Simão et al. 2005). Resistance training intensity can increase the duration, but not the magnitude, of the postexercise hypotensive response (Simão et al. 2005). However, no postexercise hypotensive response and no difference at various percentages of 1RM have been shown (Focht and Koltyn 1998). Training volume (increased number of sets of an exercise) has little or no effect on the postexercise hypotensive response (Simão et al. 2005), although the difference in volume was small (five vs. six sets of each exercise). However, the optimal value for acute training variables to bring about a postexercise hypotensive response remains to be elucidated.

The mechanism(s) responsible for a postexercise hypotensive response after resistance training are unclear. As with aerobic exercise, a postexercise hypotensive response is related to a decrease in vascular resistance, but the cause of this decrease is not clear. It is unlikely that the postexercise hypotensive response after aerobic training is due to thermoregulatory or blood volume changes; a decrease as well as no change in sympathetic nerve activity has been shown after aerobic training (MacDonald 2002). The cause of the postexercise hypotensive response after resistance raining requires further study.

Chronic Cardiovascular Adaptations During Exercise

Traditional cardiovascular training results in adaptations (e.g., reduced heart rate and blood pressure during activity) that allow the performance of physical activity with less cardiovascular stress. Resistance training can result in a similar response (see table 3.10).

Heart Rate and Blood Pressure

Cross-sectional data demonstrate that resistance training can reduce cardiovascular stress during weight training and other exercise tasks. Male bodybuilders have lower maximal intra-arterial systolic and diastolic blood pressures and maximal heart rates during sets to voluntary concentric failure at 50, 70, 80, 90, and 100% of 1RM than sedentary subjects and novice (six to nine months of training) resistance-trained males do (Fleck and Dean 1987). The bodybuilders were stronger than the other subjects, so they had a lower pressor response not only at the same relative workload, but also at greater absolute weight training workloads. Bodybuilders also had lower heart rates, but not blood pressures, than medical students during arm ergometry at the same absolute exercise intensity (Colliander and Tesch 1988). In addition, bodybuilders had lower heart rates at the same relative workloads (percentage of 1RM) than powerlifters during resistance training exercises (Falkel, Fleck, and Murray 1992). This indicates that high-volume programs may have the greatest effect on the pressor response during resistance training as well as other physical tasks. The lower pressor response shown by bodybuilders may be due in part to a smaller-magnitude Valsalva maneuver during resistance exercise compared to that of powerlifters (Falkel, Fleck, and Murray 1992). During upper-body isometric activity (50% of maximal force) national team weightlifters had significantly lower heart rates, but similar systolic and diastolic blood pressures compared to sedentary people (Adler et al. 2008).

Short-term training (12 to 16 weeks) also causes cardiovascular adaptations during the performance of exercise tasks. Heart rate and blood pressure do decrease as a result of weight training during bicycle ergometry, treadmill walking, and treadmill walking holding hand weights (Blessing et al. 1987; Goldberg, Elliot, and Kuehl 1988, 1994).

TABLE 3.10 Chronic Cardiovascular Adaptations During Exercise

Adaptation	Absolute workload*	Relative workload*
Heart rate	Decrease	No change
Blood pressure Systolic Diastolic	 Decrease Decrease	 No change or decrease or increase No change or decrease or increase
Stroke volume	Increase	?
Cardiac output	Increase	?
$\dot{V}O_2$peak	Increase	?

* = minimal data and contradictory data; ? = unknown.

Short-term training studies also demonstrate significant decreases in blood pressure and heart rate response during isometric actions (Goldberg, Elliot, and Kuehl 1994) and in both young adults (Sale et al. 1994) and 66-year-old adults (McCartney et al. 1993) during dynamic resistance training at the same absolute resistance. However, after 19 weeks of training, the systolic and diastolic blood pressure response at the same relative resistance may be unchanged or even increased (Sale et al. 1994). It is important to note that the same relative resistance (percentage of 1RM) after training is a greater absolute resistance. After the 19 weeks of training, maximal heart rate during all sets at the same relative resistance tended to be higher; at the same absolute resistance they tended to be lower, but not significantly so. Longitudinal information demonstrates that weight training can reduce the pressor response during a variety of physical activities. Both cross-sectional and longitudinal information indicate that weight training can reduce the heart rate and blood pressure response during various physical activities.

Stroke Volume and Cardiac Output

Weightlifters' cardiac output has been observed to increase to 30 L · min^{-1}—stroke volume increases up to 200 ml immediately after resistance training exercise—untrained people show no significant change (Vorobyev 1988). During upper-body isometric activity (50% of maximal force) national team weightlifters demonstrate a significantly higher stroke volume than sedentary people (Adler et al. 2008). The weightlifters' increased stroke volume was due to a significantly greater end-diastolic volume and significantly lower end-systolic volume resulting in a significantly greater ejection fraction compared to that of the sedentary subjects.

There may be a difference in the response of various types of resistance-trained athletes. Bodybuilders' peak stroke volume and cardiac output were significantly greater than those of powerlifters during sets to voluntary concentric failure at various percentages (50, 80, and 100%) of 1RM during both the knee extension and squat exercises (Falkel, Fleck, and Murray 1992). The bodybuilders' greater cardiac output and stroke volume were evident during both the concentric and eccentric phases of both exercises and may have been caused by the performance of a more limited Valsalva maneuver, which resulted in a smaller elevation of intrathoracic pressure. During most of the squat and knee extension exercise sets, the bodybuilders demonstrated a higher maximal heart rate than the powerlifters did. This indicates that cardiac output increased in the bodybuilders as the result of an increase in both stroke volume and heart rate. Thus, the type of resistance training program may affect the magnitude of any adaptation that results in the ability to maintain cardiac output during activity.

Short-term training may have an effect on the magnitude of the Valsalva maneuver (Sale et al. 1994). After 19 weeks of weight training, subjects' esophageal pressures during sets at the same relative resistance (percentage of 1RM) were unchanged. However, at the same absolute resistance, which is now a lower percentage of 1RM after training, esophageal pressures during the first several repetitions of a set were reduced. This indicates a less forceful Valsalva maneuver during the first several repetitions of a set at the same absolute resistance after weight training. A reduction in the forcefulness of the Valsalva maneuver may allow stroke volume and cardiac output to increase compared to pretraining. Esophageal pressure during the last repetitions of the set was unaffected by training and therefore did not alter stroke volume or cardiac output compared to pretraining values. This indicates a differential effect on the forcefulness of a Valsalva maneuver during different repetitions of a set and therefore differing effects on intrathoracic pressure, venous return, and cardiac output during different repetitions of a set.

Both cross-sectional and longitudinal information indicate that stroke volume and cardiac output may increase during weight training in strength-trained people compared to untrained people. Any changes in stroke volume and cardiac output brought about by chronic weight training may be related to a reduction in the forcefulness of a Valsalva maneuver after training and the type of training performed.

Peak Oxygen Consumption

Peak oxygen consumption ($\dot{V}O_2$peak) on a treadmill or bicycle ergometer is considered a marker of cardiorespiratory fitness. Relative $\dot{V}O_2$peak (ml · kg^{-1} · min^{-1}) of competitive Olympic weightlifters, powerlifters, and bodybuilders ranges from 41 to 55 ml · kg^{-1} · min^{-1} (Fleck 2003; George et al.

1995; Kraemer, Deschenes, and Fleck 1988; Saltin and Astrand 1967). These are average to moderately above average relative $\dot{V}O_2$peak values. This wide range indicates that resistance training may increase relative $\dot{V}O_2$peak, but that not all programs may bring about such an increase.

Insight into the type of programs that result in the greatest increase in $\dot{V}O_2$peak can be gained by examining short-term training studies. Traditional heavy resistance training using heavy resistances for a few number of repetitions per set and long rest periods result in small increases or no change in $\dot{V}O_2$peak (Fahey and Brown 1973; Gettman and Pollock 1981; Keeler et al. 2001; Lee et al. 1990). A seven-week Olympic-style weightlifting program can result in moderate gains in absolute $(L \cdot min^{-1})$ $\dot{V}O_2$peak (9%) and $\dot{V}O_2$peak relative to body weight (8%) (Stone et al. 1983). The first five weeks of training consisted of three to five sets of 10 repetitions for each exercise, rest periods between sets and exercises of three and a half to four minutes, and two training sessions per day, three days per week. Vertical jumps were performed two days per week for five sets of 10 repetitions. The majority of the increase in $\dot{V}O_2$peak occurred during the first five weeks of the program. Training during the next two weeks was identical to that of the first five weeks, except that three sets of five repetitions of each exercise were performed. This two-week training period resulted in no further gains in $\dot{V}O_2$peak. The results indicate that higher-volume weight training may be necessary to bring about significant gains in $\dot{V}O_2$peak. However, this conclusion must be viewed with caution because of the inclusion of vertical jump training in the total training program and the fact that the lower-volume program occurred after the higher-volume program, when adaptations are more likely to take place.

Circuit weight training generally consists of 12 to 15 repetitions per set using 40 to 60% of 1RM with short rest periods of 15 to 30 seconds between sets and exercises. This type of training results in increases in $\dot{V}O_2$peak of approximately 10 to 18% (see chapter 6, Circuit System).

For physical conditioning to elicit changes in $\dot{V}O_2$peak, heart rate must be maintained at a minimum of 60% of maximum for a minimum of 20 minutes. Exercising heart rate and total metabolic cost during a circuit weight training session is significantly higher than during a more traditional heavy weight training session (Pichon et al. 1996). This may explain in part why circuit weight training elicits a significant increase in $\dot{V}O_2$peak and a more traditional heavy weight training program elicits little or no change. Additionally, the relatively long rest periods taken in a traditional heavy weight training program allow the heart rate to decrease below the recommended 60% of maximum level needed to bring about a significant increase in $\dot{V}O_2$peak. Weight training programs intended to increase $\dot{V}O_2$ peak should consist of higher training volumes and use short rest periods between sets and exercises.

The increase in $\dot{V}O_2$peak caused by resistance training can be substantially less than the 15 to 20% increases associated with traditional endurance-oriented running, cycling, and swimming programs. If a major goal of a training program is to significantly increase $\dot{V}O_2$peak, some form of aerobic training needs to be included. The volume of aerobic training necessary to maintain or significantly increase $\dot{V}O_2$peak when performing weight training is minimal (Nakao, Inoue, and Murakami 1995). Moderately trained subjects minimally, but significantly, increased relative $\dot{V}O_2$peak (3 to 4 $ml \cdot kg^{-1} \cdot min^{-1}$) over one to two years of weight training when performing only one aerobic training session per week of running 2 miles (3.2 km) per session. Those who performed only weight training during the same training period demonstrated a small but significant decrease in relative $\dot{V}O_2$peak. No difference in maximal strength gains was demonstrated between the weight trainers who ran and those who did not.

In conclusion, resistance training exercise results in a pressor response that affects the cardiovascular system. Chronic performance of resistance training can result in positive adaptations to the cardiovascular system at rest and during physical activity.

Summary

Resistance training results in a multitude of physiological adaptations specifically related to the program design. The amount of muscle mass activated is both a local and general key to determining how many physiological systems will be involved in the maintenance of homeostasis and the support of muscular activity. In turn, those systems that are used in the performance of a resistance exercise and training protocol will adapt to reduce the physiological stress and improve performance. Exercise prescription factors, such as the volume and intensity of training, will influence to what extent any adaptation occurs. Chapter 4 examines how to integrate the various components of a total conditioning program.

SELECTED READINGS

Carroll, T.J., Selvanayagam, V.S., Riek, S., and Semmler, J.G. 2011. Neural adaptations to strength training: Moving beyond transcranial magnetic stimulation and reflex studies. *Acta Physiologica* (Oxford) 202: 119-140.

Fleck, S.J. 1988. Cardiovascular adaptations to resistance training. *Medicine & Science in Sports & Exercise* 20: S146-S151.

Fleck, S.J. 2002. Cardiovascular responses to strength training. In *Strength & power in sport*, edited by P.V. Komi. Oxford: Blackwell Science.

Hodson-Tole, E.F., and Wakeling, J.M. 2009. Motor unit recruitment for dynamic tasks: Current understanding and future directions. *Journal of Comparative Physiology B: Biochemical, Systemic, and Environmental Physiology* 179: 57-66.

Kraemer, W.J., Nindl, B.C., Volek, J.S., Marx, J.O., Gotshalk, L.A., Bush, J.A., Welsch, J.R., Vingren, J.L., Spiering, B.A., Fragala, M.S., Hatfield, D.L., Ho, J.Y., Maresh, C.M., Mastro, A.M., and Hymer, W.C. 2008. Influence of oral contraceptive use on growth hormone in vivo bioactivity following resistance exercise: Responses of molecular mass variants. *Growth Hormone and IGF Research* 18: 238-244.

Kraemer, W.J., and Ratamess, N.A. 2005. Hormonal responses and adaptations to resistance exercise and training. *Sports Medicine* 35: 339-361.

Kraemer, W.J., and Rogol, A.D. (eds.). 2005. *The endocrine system in sports and exercise*. Blackwell Publishing Ltd, Malden, MA.

Pette, D., and Staron, R.S. 2001. Transitions of muscle fiber phenotypic profiles. *Histochemistry and Cell Biology* 115: 359-372.

Rennie, M.J. 2001. How muscles know how to adapt. *Journal of Physiology* 535: 1.

Russel, B., Motlagh, D., and Ashley, W.W. 2000. Form follows function: How muscle shape is regulated by work. *Journal of Applied Physiology* 88: 1127-1132.

Schoenfeld, B.J. 2010. The mechanisms of muscle hypertrophy and their application to resistance training. *Journal of Strength and Conditioning Research* 24: 2857-2872.

Spence, A.L., Carter, H.H., Murray, C.P., Oxborough, D., Naylor, L.H., George, K.P., and Green, D.J. 2013. Magnetic resonance imaging–derived right ventricular adaptations to endurance versus resistance training. *Medicine & Science in Sports & Exercise* 45: 534-541.

Staron, R.S., and Hikida, R.S. 2001. Muscular responses to exercise and training. In *Exercise and sport science*, edited by W. E. Garrett Jr. and D.T. Kirkendall. Philadelphia: Lippincott Williams & Wilkins.

Sueck, G.C., and Regnier, M. 2001. Plasticity in skeletal, cardiac, and smooth muscle. Invited review: Plasticity and energetic demands of contraction in skeletal and cardiac muscle. *Journal of Applied Physiology* 90: 1158-1164.

Timmons, J.A. 2011. Variability in training-induced skeletal muscle adaptation. *Journal of Applied Physiology* 110: 846-853.

Toigo, M., and Boutellier, U. 2006. New fundamental resistance exercise determinants of molecular and cellular muscle adaptations. *European Journal of Applied Physiology* 97: 643-663.

Integrating Other Fitness Components

After reading this chapter, you should be able to

1. discuss the advantages and disadvantages of concurrent training, as well as how these concerns affect specific populations differently,

2. explain the physiological mechanisms behind adaptations to concurrent training,

3. explain the various forms of cardiovascular endurance training,

4. discuss the methods used to determine intensity in cardiovascular endurance training and how they relate to program prescription,

5. demonstrate the various forms of stretching, and

6. understand how flexibility and stretching impact sports performance.

Integrating a variety of components of physical activity into a **total conditioning program** requires a careful examination of training priorities. The compatibility of various modes of exercise must also be considered in relationship to fitness or performance goals. The timing, sequencing, and emphasis of the program will also affect the body's ability to adapt and achieve program goals. Therefore, an individualized exercise prescription is vital for creating a successful total conditioning program. Additionally, in today's world of fitness and sport conditioning, participant safety must be of paramount importance (Casa et al. 2012).

Resistance training is only one form of conditioning and must be integrated into a total conditioning program. A host of conditioning programs can be customized to meet the training goals of the individual. In addition, sport practices need to be accounted for in the total program, thus creating another component of the total conditioning program. A total conditioning program may consist of any or all of the following components:

- Flexibility
- Cardiorespiratory endurance
- Plyometrics
- Strength and power
- Anaerobic endurance and speed training
- Local muscular endurance

A resistance training program can be periodized in a variety of ways to integrate the aspects of the total program over a yearly training cycle.

This chapter presents the concepts that are important to consider when designing resistance training programs that can be integrated into total conditioning programs. Vital to this process is an understanding of the **compatibility of exercise,** which refers to whether two types of exercise positively or negatively affect adaptations to either type. Training goals can change over a yearly training cycle as a result of different physical demands (e.g., in-season, off-season) or where the person is in their athletic career. Changes in training goals will require changes in the periodization model being used at specific times in the year or athletic career.

Compatibility of Exercise Programs

Few resistance training programs are performed without the simultaneous use of other conditioning types. Our current understanding of the concurrent use of multiple conditioning types has been primarily based on the simultaneous use of resistance training and cardiorespiratory endurance training programs. Physiologically, this appears to be the most dramatic antagonistic combination because of the very different natures of the two training outcomes: high force versus high endurance. Yet, as we will see in this chapter, compatibility depends on many factors.

The compatibility of concurrent types of exercise is related to the physiological mechanisms causing adaptations to each type of exercise and whether they are pushing these adaptations in the same direction of change. For example, the physiological mechanisms to improve the oxidative endurance capabilities of muscle fibers are related to improving oxygen transport, delivery, and use. In this process, muscle fiber size may not increase or may even decrease to optimize transit distances for oxygen delivery. Conversely, with heavy resistance training, anabolic signaling causes muscle fibers to increase in size, the opposite of what happens with intense endurance training. This is one example of two physiological stimuli trying to drive muscle fiber size in opposite directions for different reasons. This incompatibility occurs in the motor units that are asked to perform both forms of exercise.

Many questions might be asked related to what makes exercise programs incompatible. What are the effects on strength, power, or cardiorespiratory endurance performances when these are all included in a total training program? Or, how can a trainee use both strength and endurance exercise without limiting adaptations to each? What about using different intensities of training over a particular cycle and prioritizing one training mode over another? What about eliminating one type of exercise during a training cycle? Understanding the compatibility of exercise is vital for designing programs that achieve training goals for strength and power as well as cardiorespiratory endurance.

Training adaptations are specific to the imposed training stimulus, and this appears to be an important factor when examining concurrent exercise program compatibilities. Compatibility studies typically have three training groups. For example, to study the compatibility of strength and endurance training, researchers separate subjects into three groups: one for strength training, one for endurance training, and one for both. Our understanding of exercise training compatibility primarily relates to the concurrent use of aerobic endurance and strength training programs, which is explored in the next section.

Concurrent Strength and Endurance Training

Studies examining concurrent strength and endurance training provide the following general conclusions (Aagaard and Andersen 2010; Chromiak and Mulvaney 1990; Dudley and Fleck 1987; García-Pallarés and Izquierdo 2011; Kraemer, Patton et al. 1995; Nader 2006; Wilson et al. 2012):

- High-intensity endurance training may compromise strength, especially at high velocities of muscle action.
- Power capabilities may be most affected by the performance of both strength and endurance training.
- High-intensity endurance training may negatively affect short-term anaerobic performance.
- The development of peak oxygen consumption is not compromised by heavy resistance training.
- Strength training does not negatively affect endurance capabilities.
- Strength and power training programs may benefit endurance performances by preventing injuries, increasing lactic acid threshold, and reducing the ground contact time during running.

However, whether incompatibility occurs may depend on training status; the intensity, volume, and frequency of both types of training; and whether both types are performed on alternate days or on the same training day. These factors are explored in the following sections.

In 1980, the compatibility of **concurrent training** programs directed at both cardiorespiratory endurance and maximal muscle strength became a major topic. During 10 weeks of concurrent training, a decreased capacity to continue to improve maximal strength was observed during the 9th and 10th weeks of training (Hickson 1980). The result was a realization that intense aerobic training may be detrimental to the development of strength. This started a line of research into exercise program compatibility that has continued to this day.

Given that the loss in strength or power was seen only after several weeks of concurrent training, many scientists thought that this might be due to overtraining. Although strength gains were compromised, aerobic capacity was not affected by concurrent training when strength and endurance exercise were performed on alternate days (Hickson 1980). This lack of an effect on oxygen consumption with concurrent training was again observed with the use of very high-intensity interval training performed along with intense isokinetic training. But isokinetic torque trainees at the faster velocities of movement (160-278 degrees per second) did not show the same gains as that of a strength-training-only group (Dudley and Djamil 1985). Note that isokinetic torque increases at the slower velocities of movement were affected by concurrent training to a lesser degree.

It was thought that lowering the number of training days per week as well as the intensity might limit the problems with compatibility (Hunter, Demment, and Miller 1987). However, for those just beginning to train, despite a training program with only three sets of 10RM four days a week for 12 weeks, strength in both bench press and squat 1RM was compromised by adding a 40-minute endurance running program four days a week at 75% of heart rate reserve. Again, maximal oxygen consumption was not negatively affected by the concurrent training programs. Interestingly, previously endurance-trained subjects did not show the negative effect on strength with concurrent training that beginners did. This suggests that the ability to tolerate aerobic conditioning may play a role in strength losses (Hunter, Demment, and Miller 1987) and if the frequency of training were reduced even further, maybe this would help reduce the incompatibility of training programs. In younger women exercising only two days a week for 11 weeks, no incompatibility of training programs for strength or endurance was seen (Silva

et al. 2012). Whether a continuous endurance training program or an interval training program was used, no interference in strength gains was observed. Thus, very low frequencies of training, which allow for more recovery, might minimize incompatibility for beginning trainees.

Unlike shorter programs, longer concurrent training programs (four days a week for 20 weeks) have shown that the rate of gain in maximal oxygen consumption significantly levels off later in the training program compared to endurance training only in trained people (Nelson et al. 1990). This indicates that endurance capacity may not be completely free of incompatibility problems. With 21 weeks of concurrent training, the use of lower frequency (two times per week for each modality) produced improvements in both maximal isometric strength and maximal oxygen consumption in untrained men (Mikkola et al. 2012). However, the rate of force development, or explosive power, was compromised with concurrent training.

Beginners using alternate days of training three days per week for each modality (which results in six days of training a week) may be exposed to too much total training volume, too few recovery days, or both. Training both modalities on the same day would provide more rest days over the week. Yet it has been proposed that training both modalities on the same day may still compromise strength (Sale et al. 1990). However, the combination of a less intense exercise program and a lower training frequency might be more effective when performing both programs on the same day. This was demonstrated with a comparison of a combined training group (training three-days-a-week with 5- to 7RM for eight resistance exercises along with 50 minutes of aerobic cycling at 70% of heart rate reserve for 10 weeks) with a resistance-training-only group and an aerobic-training-only group performing identical programs as the combined group (McCarthy et al. 1995). Similar gains were made in 1RM strength and aerobic capacity in the combined group when compared to the single training groups' improvements.

Training background and the frequency of training remain potential factors in determining the compatibility of concurrent training programs. It appears that high-intensity alternate-day training in relatively untrained men and women can produce decrements in maximal force production but not in peak oxygen consumption. This may be different in people with an endurance training background; they may not experience compromised maximal strength, but their endurance gains may plateau. Training both strength and endurance in the same workout three days per week using realistic training intensities may be optimal for beginners, who may need more rest days during the week. However, power development may take longer to improve under concurrent training conditions.

Concurrent Training in Trained Athletes

Compared to untrained or moderately trained people, far less is known about the impact of concurrent training with highly trained athletes. Most athletes use both strength and power and cardiorespiratory endurance programs to meet the demands of their sports (see figure 4.1). Early work did show an advantage to being in better aerobic condition at the start of concurrent training, because those with aerobic training backgrounds had greater strength gains from training concurrently (Hunter, Demment, and Miller 1987). However, in highly aerobically trained soldiers using both training modalities on the same day four days per week, power development in the Wingate test was compromised (Kraemer, Patton et al. 1995).

In elite Gaelic Athletic Association and rugby team members, the question of concurrent training was examined over eight weeks of training (Hennessy and Watson 1994). The combined group exercising five days per week saw improvements in endurance capacities, but no changes in lower-body strength, power, or speed. The endurance training group showed increases in endurance with no changes in strength, power, or speed. Finally, the strength training group maintained endurance and, as might be expected, increased strength and power. Thus, over short-term training cycles in athletes, care must be taken to prioritize training goals because interference in strength and power can occur and a degree of specificity exists. Concurrent training of athletes in various sports can be affected by sport conditioning drills and practice (see box 4.1).

In elite soccer players not familiar with strength training, a program consisting of aerobic interval training at 90 to 95% of maximal heart rate and half squat strength training with maximum resistances for four sets of four repetitions was performed twice a week over an eight-week training

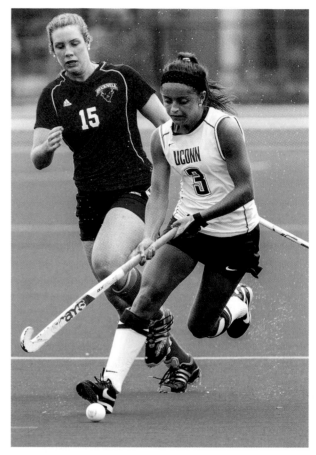

FIGURE 4.1 The effects of concurrent training in athletes who need high levels of strength, power, and cardiorespiratory endurance is a less-studied phenomenon, and careful attention to training and testing results are needed for determining whether performance decrements are reflective of exercise compatibility.

Photo courtesy of UConn Athletics.

cycle (Helgerud et al. 2011). Strength, power, 10 m sprint time, and maximal oxygen consumption all improved over the training cycle. The use of a lower training frequency (two days per week) along with typical sport training may have eliminated any type of incompatibility over the training cycle.

Using lighter resistances and lower-intensity aerobic conditioning may not present much of a compatibility problem in athletes. Well-conditioned female university soccer and volleyball players training three days per week over an 11-week training program demonstrated no incompatibility for strength and endurance gains (Davis et al. 2008). Two conditioning formats were used in this study, a serial and an integrated approach. Each used the same exercise intensities. The serial approach used a warm-up, a resistance training workout, and

Can Compatibility Issues Exist With Normal Sport Practice and Conditioning?

Yes they can, especially when the exercise volume increases dramatically to the point at which performance gains due to an off-season training program are lost. This is what happened to a group of National Collegiate Athletic Association Division I American football players in the off-season and spring practice program (Moore and Fry 2007).

For football players, year-round training is broken up into training phases (e.g., fall in-season, winter off-season, spring football, and summer preseason). Starting with the winter off-season program, players performed only a linear periodized heavy resistance training program during the first month of winter conditioning. In the following month a high-volume sport conditioning program (e.g., sprints, agility drills) was added to the strength training program. This was followed over the next month by the typical 15 spring football practices. After the first month, all of the 1RM strength tests showed improvement. Then, after the second month of performing heavy resistance training and conditioning drills, maximal squat and power clean 1RMs decreased, returning players to pre-first-month levels. By the end of the 15 football practice sessions, even upper-body bench press 1RMs had returned to pre-first-month levels. Speed and agility along with vertical jump improved after the first month and then remained unchanged for the rest of the winter program.

One might speculate that dramatically reducing the volume of resistance training while focusing on maintaining intensity might be a plausible approach for eliminating the loss of strength and power when conditioning and sport practices occur concurrently. Additionally, as pointed out in the study, more communication is needed between the strength and conditioning and sport coaches. Program modifications and careful monitoring are necessary when total exercise volume is dramatically increased in a training cycle.

Moore, C.A., and Fry, A.C. 2007. Nonfunctional overreaching during off-season training for skill position players in collegiate American football. *Journal of Strength and Conditioning Research* 21: 793-800.

then a 30-minute endurance training workout at 60 to 84% (average 65%) of the heart rate reserve (HRR) in sequence. The integrated approach used a warm-up, and then subjects performed the same nine resistance exercises for three sets of 8 to 12 repetitions at 50% of 1RM. However, before every resistance exercise, each subject did 30 to 60 seconds of vigorous aerobic treadmill exercise again at 60 to 84% (average 65%) of HRR. Both forms of training increased both strength and endurance, but the use of the integrated workout did show significantly greater percentage gains in strength and endurance and reductions in fat mass compared to the serial approach. Thus, incompatibility may be minimized with the use of lighter and lower-intensity circuit-type programs. This study suggests that incompatibility issues with concurrent training may depend on many factors such as training status, intensity, and volume (see table 4.1).

A variety of workout protocols have been used when examining the question of incompatibility. Depending on the design of the resistance and endurance training workouts, training adaptations for strength and power can be compromised (Hennessy and Watson 1994; Kraemer, Patton et al. 1995; Nelson et al. 1990) or unaffected (Bell et al. 1991b; Hortobagyi, Katch, and LaChance 1991; McCarthy et al. 1995; Sale et al. 1990), whereas endurance capabilities are typically not affected in untrained people. In athletes, whether incompatibility occurs is less clear and may be affected by the smaller increases in fitness expected in strength, power, speed, and aerobic capacity in athletes such as elite rugby athletes (Hennessy and Watson 1994). While lower-intensity training programs in women have shown no incompatibility, higher intensities may be needed over an entire training cycle to cause increases in specific training outcomes (Davis et al. 2008).

A meta-analysis has been used to study the concept of compatibility of exercise programs (Wilson et al. 2012). From this analysis, running appears to be more detrimental to strength and hypertrophy than cycling is. It was also determined

TABLE 4.1 Representative Studies on Concurrent Training Effects in Various Populations

Study	Subjects	Training protocol	Findings
Hickson 1980	17 M, 6 W RT: 22 y (7 M , 1 W) ET: 25 y (5 M, 3 W) ER: 26 y (5 M, 2 W) Some subjects were active but no regular training (~3 months prior to start of protocol)	10 weeks of training RT: 3 d/wk @ 80% of 1RM; 3 min rest (squat 5 × 5, knee flexion 3 × 5, knee extension 3 × 5); 2 d/wk (leg press 3 × 5, calf raise 3 × 20) ET: 6 d/wk Interval: 3 d/wk; six 5 min intervals on cycle ergometer @ $\dot{V}O_2$max; 2 min rest Continuous: treadmill, performed on alternate days (1st wk: 30 min/d, 2nd wk: 35 min/d, 3rd week and beyond: 40 min/d) ER: Same as RT and ET (2 hr rest between training sessions; RT before ET)	STR: RT (+44%); ET (no change); ER (+25%) $\dot{V}O_2$max: Bike —RT (+4); ET (+23%); ER (18%) Treadmill—RT (no change); ET (+17%); ER (+17%) BF%: RT (−0.8%); ET (−3.6%); ER (−2.3%)
Kraemer, Patton, et al. 1995	35 M soldiers RT: 24.3 ± 5.1 y (n = 9) ET: 21.4 ± 4.1 y (n = 8) ER: 18 total U/L: 23.3 ± 3.6 y (n = 9) U only: 22.9 ± 5.0 y (n = 9) Control: 22.4 ± 4.2 y (n = 5) Standard military training program 3×/wk for ~2 y	12 weeks of training RT: hypertrophy (2 d/wk; 1 min rest): Upper (U): BP and fly (3 × 10), military press and upright row (2 × 10), lat pull-down and seated row (3 × 10), curl (3 × 10), sit-up (2 × 25) Lower (L): split squat (3 × 10), one-legged knee extension (3 × 10), leg curl (3 × 10), calf raise (3 × 15) Strength (2 d/wk; 2-3 min rest): U: BP (5 × 5), Military press (5 × 5), curl (5 × 5), lat pull-down (5 × 5), oblique (5 × 5), sit-up (5 × 5) L: deadlift (4 × 6), leg press (5 × 5), double knee extension (5 × 5), calf raise (3 × 10) ET: Continuous: 2 d/wk; max distance 40 min @ 80-85% of $\dot{V}O_2$max Interval: 2 d/wk: 200-800 m interval @ 95-100+% $\dot{V}O_2$max (1:4 to 1:0.5 work:rest) ER: ET followed by RT (5-6 hr rest) U/L: Same as RT and ET U only: Same ET and U as RT	STR: Peak power LB: RT (+17.2%); ET (−1.2%); U/L (+2.7%); U only (+7.2%) Mean power LB: RT (+20.3%); ET (−3.2%); U/L (+4.6%); U only (+3.4%) Peak power UB: RT (+10.3%); ET (−0.5%); U/L (+5.1%); U only (+6.5%) Mean power UB: RT (+12.5%); ET (+4.55%); U/L (+8.4%); U only (+7.9%) Military press 1RM: RT(+30.0%); ET (+1.7%); U/L (+19.6%); U only (+9.6%) Double leg extension 1RM: RT (+34.4%); ET (+3.1%); U/L (+34.4%); U only (+10.9%) $\dot{V}O_2$max: RT (−0.99%); ET (+11.8%); U/L (+7.7%); U only (+9.62 ± 3.2%)
McCarthy et al. 1995	30 M RT: 27.9 ± 1.2 y (n = 10) ET: 26.6 ± 1.6 y (n = 10) ER: 27.3 ± 1.7 y (n = 10) No regular training (~3 months prior to start of protocol)	10 wk of training RT: 3 d/wk; training to failure (~6 reps/set); wk 1: 2 sets, 75 s rest; wk 2-10: 3 sets, 75 s rest; barbell squat, BP, curl, knee extension, leg curl, lat pull-down, overhead press, heel raise ET: 3 d/wk; wk 1: 30 min @ 70% of HRR; wk 2-10: 45 min @ 70% of HRR ER: Same exercise as ET and RT (~10-20 min rest between RT and ET). Order alternated each time (i.e., ET 1st, RT 2nd; then RT 1st, ET 2nd)	CMVJ: RT (+6%); ET (+2%); ER (+9%) STR: squat 1RM: RT (+23%); ET (−1%); ER (+22%) BP 1RM: RT (+18%); ET (+1%); ER (+18%) $\dot{V}O_2$max: RT (+9%); ET (+18%); ER(+16%) BF%: RT (−12%); ET (−9%); ER (−11%) BM%: RT (+3.4%); ET (+0.4%); ER (+5.3%)
Bell et al. 2000	45 subjects (27 M, 18 W); 22.3 ± 3.3 y RT: 7 M, 4 W ET: 7 M, 4 W ER: 8 M, 5 W Control: 5 M, 5 W All were physically active and had some strength training experience but no regular training (for either strength or endurance) at start of protocol.	12 weeks of training RT: 3 d/wk, 2-6 sets × 4-12 reps @ 72-84% (average intensity; increased 4% every 3 wk) L: leg press, one-legged knee flexion and extension, calf raise U: BP, lat pull-down, shoulder press, curl ET: Monark cycle ergometer Continuous: 2 d/wk (30 min progressing to 42 min; increase 4 min every 4 wk) Interval: 1×/wk, 4 sets of 1:1 work: rest (3 min exercise; then 3 min rest) Resistance was increased at wk 6; 1 set added every 4 wk until 7 sets ER: Same exercise as RT and ET; alternating order each day	STR: 1RM leg press increase: RT: W (64.5%); M (51.1%) ET: W (41.8%); M (24.5%) ER: W (83.8%); M (37.1%) Control: W (8.5%); M (11.3%) $\dot{V}O_2$max: RT: W (−6.0%); M (−1.4%) ET: W (+12.6%); M (+4.9%) ER: W (+7.5%); M (+6.2%) Control: W (−3.4%); M (−2.3%)
Gravelle and Gravelle 2000	19 W, college-aged RT: n = 6 ER: 13 total LR: lift first (n = 6) RL: row first (n = 7) All exercised 2-3×/wk. No regular training (for strength or endurance) more than 1×/wk for 3 months prior to start of protocol.	11 weeks of training RT: 3 d/wk; 1 min rest; wk 1 and 2: 2 × 10; wk 3 and 4: 3 × 10; wk 5-5.5: 4 × 10; wk 5.5-9: 4 × 10; wk 10 and 11; 4 × 6-8; leg press, squat, knee extension and flexion, straight-leg deadlift, heel raise ER: 3 d/wk; continuous rowing @ 70% of $\dot{V}O_2$max (duration began for 25 min, progressed to 45 min/wk by wk 5.5; wk 6- 11: start @ 70% of $\dot{V}O_2$max for a wk, then increased by 1 stroke per min/wk)	STR: 1RM leg press increase: RT (25.9%); ER (RL) (14.6%); ER (LR) (11.3%) $\dot{V}O_2$max: RT (+9.2%); ER (RL) (+5.3%); ER (LR) (+8.0%)

Study	Subjects	Training protocol	Findings
Häkkinen et al. 2003	27 healthy men RT: 38 ± 5 y ($n = 16$) ER: 37 ± 5 y ($n = 11$) All were considered active, yet had no background in strength training or competitive sports of any kind.	21 weeks of training RT: 2 d/wk, 1st 7 wk @ 50-70%; 3 or 4 × 10-15; 2nd 7 wk L: 3-5 × 8-12 or 5 6 U: 3-5 × 10-12; Last 7 wk L: 4-6 × 3-6 reps @ 70-80% or 8-12 reps @ 50-60% of 1RM U: 3-5 × 8-12 L: 2 leg exercises each day (leg press and uni- or bilateral knee extension Other: 4 or 5 exercises each day stressing major muscle groups (i.e., BP, triceps push-down, lat pull-down, sit-up, trunk extensors, uni- or bilateral elbow and knee extension and/or leg adduction/abduction exercises) ER: 2 d/wk RT (same as RT group) and 2 d/wk ET 1st 7 wk: 30 min cycling or walking; 2nd 7 wks: day 1— 45 min (15 min below aerobic threshold, 10 min between aerobic and anaerobic thresholds, 5 min above anaerobic threshold, 15 min under aerobic threshold; day 2—60 min under aerobic threshold Last 7 wk: day 1—60 min (15 min under aerobic threshold 2 × 10 min between aerobic and anaerobic thresholds, 2 × 5 min above anaerobic threshold, 15 min under aerobic threshold); day 2—60-90 min under aerobic threshold	STR: 1RM bilateral leg extension increase: RT (21%); ER (22%) $\dot{V}O_2$max: ER (+18.5%) BF%: RT (+1.5%); ER (−10.22%) BM%: RT (+2.38%); ER (−1.47%)
Izquierdo et al. 2004	31 healthy men RT: 64.8 ± 2.6 y ($n = 11$) ET: 68.2 ± 1.7 y ($n = 10$) ER: 66.4 ± 4.5 y ($n = 10$) All were untrained with no training (strength or otherwise) for ~5 y prior to start of protocol.	16 weeks of training RT: 2×/wk; machines only; combination heavy and explosive RT; 1st 8 wk—50-70%, 3 or 4 × 10-15; last 8 wk—70-80%, 3-5 × 5 or 6. Each day consisted of 2 L exercises (leg press and bilateral knee extension), 1 arm extension exercise (BP), and 4 or 5 exercises for the main muscle groups (i.e., lat pull-down, shoulder press, ab crunch or rotation, leg curl). ET: 2×/wk; self-reported cycling; 30-40 min/session (rate of 60 rpm; HR between 70 and 90% of HRmax or between 55 and 85% maximum aerobic workload) ER: 1×/wk RT; 1×/wk ET; same protocols as RT and ET; alternating days	STR: 1RM half squat increases (wk 8; wk 16): RT: 27%; 41% ET: 8%; 11% ER: 22%; 38% 1RM BP increases (wk 16): RT (36%); ET (0%); ER (22%) Peak power during cycling test to exhaustion (wk 16): RT (+10%); ET (+16%); ER (+18%) BF% (pretraining vs. wk 16): RT (−7.5%); ET (0%); ER (−1.9%)
Izquierdo, Hakkinen et al. 2005	31 healthy men RT: 43.5 ± 2.8 y ($n = 11$) ET: 42.3 ± 2.6 y ($n = 10$) ER: 41.8 ± 3.7 y ($n = 10$) Training status not specified.	16 weeks of training RT, ET, and ER same as above (Izquierdo et al. 2004)	STR: 1RM half squat increases (wk 8; wk 16): RT: 22%; 45% ER: 24%; 37% 1RM BP increases (wk 16): RT (37%); ET (0%); ER (15%) BF% (pretraining vs. wk 16): RT (−7.7%); ET (0%); ER (−4.5%)
Gergley 2009	30 sedentary, healthy young men and women RT: 20.7 ± 1.5 y (8 M, 2 F) ER(2 groups): C: 20.3 ± 1.6 y (7 M, 3 F) T: 19.7 ± 1.6 y (7 M, 3 F) No prior experience with intense strength or endurance training.	9 weeks of training RT: 2 d/wk; wk 1-3: 3 × 12 (90 s rest); wk 4-6: 3 × 10 (120 s rest); wk 7-9: 3 × 8 (+150 s rest); leg extension, leg curl, leg press ER: C (cycle ergometer; same strength program as RT) T (incline treadmill; same strength program as RT) Both (wk 1-3: 20 min @ 65% HRmax; wk 4-6: 30 min @ 65% HRmax; wk 7-9: 40 min @ 65% HRmax); same strength program as RT	STR: leg press 1RM: RT (+38.5 ± 3.5%); ER-C (+27.5 ± 4.0%); ER-T (+23.5 ± 2.8%) BF%: postraining RT greater than ER-C and ER-T BM%: posttraining ER-C and ER-T more than RT

>continued

TABLE 4.1 >*continued*

Study	Subjects	Training protocol	Findings
Levin, McGuigan, and Laursen 2009	14 well-trained male cyclists/triathletes ET: 37 ± 7 y (n = 7) ER: 25 ± 4 y (n = 7) Involved in competition for a minimum of 12 months prior to start of protocol.	6 weeks of training ET: self-reported cycling training; distance (avg/wk): 278 ± 34 km (173 ± 21 miles); duration (avg/wk): 613 ± 78 min ER: self-reported cycling training; distance (avg/wk): 274 ± 56 km (170 ± 35 miles); duration (avg/wk): 526 ± 85 min 3×/wk RT: ~180 min/wk, nonlinear periodization strength: 4 × 5 (2 min rest); lunge, squat, straight-leg dead-lift, calf raises, crunches Power: 3 × 6 (2 min rest); jump squat, one-legged jump squat, deadlift, one-legged calf, back extension Hypertrophy: 3 × 12 (2 min rest); one-legged leg press, knee extension, knee flexion, calves, crunches ER Pre 279 ± 84 km (173 ± 52 miles) During 21 weeks of training	STR: 1RM squat: ET (6.6%); ER (25.7%) $\dot{V}O_2$max: graded exercise test: ET (−0.95%); ER (−0.16%)
Sillanpaa et al. 2009	62 healthy, middle-aged women RT: 50.8 ± 7.9 (n = 17) ET: 51.7 ± 6.9 (n = 15) ER 48.9 ± 6.8 (n = 18) Control: 51.4 ± 7.8 (n = 12) Training status not specified, although those with training experience of 1 y were excluded.	21 weeks of training RT: 2 d/wk; wk 1-7: 3 or 4 × 15- to 20RM; wk 8-14: 3 or 4 × 10- to 12RM; wk 15-21: 3 or 4 × 6- to 8RM 2 leg extension exercises, 1 knee flexion exercise, 4 or 5 exercises for the major muscle groups ET: 2 d/wk cycle training; wk 1-7 (day 1: 30 min continuous; day 2: few 10 min intervals); wk 8-14 (day 1: 45 min inter-vals; day 2: 60 min continuous); wk 15-21 (day 1: 90 min continuous; day 2: 60 min continuous) ER: RT 2 d/wk (same protocol as RT) and ET 2 d/wk (same protocol as ET)	STR: leg extension: RT (9 ± 8%); ET (3 ± 4%); ER (12 ± 8%); control (0%) $\dot{V}O_2$max: ET (23 ± 18%); ER (16 ± 12%); RT and control (0%) BF%: RT (−0.9 ± 1.8%); ET (−2.1 ± 2.2%); ER (−1.9 ± 1.7%); control (−0.6 ± 1.5%)
Aagaard et al. 2011	14 elite male cyclists; 19.5 ± 0.8 y ET: n = 7 ER: n = 7 U-23 National Team, non-professionals only	16 weeks of training ET: 10-18 hr cycling /wk intensity-matched with ER ER: same cycling as ET, also 2 or 3×/wk RT; wk 1: 4 × 10-12; wk 2 and 3: 4 × 8-10; wk 4 and 5: 4 × 6-8; wk 6-16: 4 × 5 or 6. All sessions rest periods: 1-2 min between sets, 2-3 min between exercises; 4 exercises (knee extension, leg press, leg curl, calf raise)	STR: ER (+12%); ET (−1.53%) $\dot{V}O_2$max: ER (+2.95%); ET (+0.97%) BF%: ER (−14.75%); ET (−9.02%) Lean body mass: ER (+3.29%); ET (0%)
Cadore et al. 2011	23 healthy elderly men RT: 64 ± 3.5 y (n = 8) ET: 64 ± 3.5 y (n = 7) ER: 66.8 ± 4.8 y (n = 8) No regular training (~12 months prior to start of protocol).	12 weeks of training RT: 3 d/wk; all 90-120 s rest periods; wk 1-7: 2 × 18- to 20RM progress to 2 × 12- to 14RM; wk 8-12: 3 × 12- to 14RM progress to 6- to 8RM; 9 exer-cises: leg press, knee extension, leg curl, BP, pull-down, seated row, triceps extension, curl, and ab exercise ET: 3 d/wk cycle ergometer; wk 1 and 2: 20 min @ 80% of HRVT; wk 5 and 6: 25 min @ 85-90% HRVT; wk 7-10: 30 min @ 95% HRVT; wk 11 and 12: 6 × 4 min at 100% HRVT; 1min rest ER: Same protocols as ET and RT; RT followed by ET	$\dot{V}O_2$max: RT (+5.7 ± 7%); ET (+20.4 ± 10.6%); ER (+22 ± 10%) BF%: RT (−2.20%); ET (−6.23%); ER (−9.92%) BM%: RT (no change); ET (−1.39%); ER (+5.16%)
Ronnestad et al. 2012b	18 healthy men RT: 26 ± 2 y (n = 7); rec-reationally active ER: 27 ± 2 y (n = 11) ; well-trained cyclists Neither group had prior experience with strength training.	12 weeks of training RT: 2×/wk; wk 1-3: 1st bout 3 × 10RM, 2nd bout 3 × 6RM; wk 4-6: 1st bout 3 × 8RM, 2nd bout 3 × 5RM; wk 7-12: 1st bout 3 × 6RM, 2nd bout 3 × 4RM; 4 exercises (half squat, one-legged press, one-legged hip extension, ankle flexion) ER: cycling 9.9 ± 1.1 (h/wk); same strength training as RT; RT followed by ET	CMJ: squat jump (cm): RT (+13%); ER (+6.2%) STR: 1RM half squat and leg press: RT (+35%); ER (+25%) BM%: RT (+1.6%); ER (no change)

See also Bell et al. 1997; Dudley and Djamil 1985; Glowacki et al. 2004; Mikkola et al. 2007; Nelson et al. 1990; Ronnestad et al. 2011; Sale et al. 1990; Shaw et al. 2009.

M = men, W = women, y = years, wk = week, d = day, hr = hour, RT = resistance training, ET = endurance training, ER = concurrent training (endurance and resistance), 1RM = 1-repetition maximum, RM = repetition maximum, CMJ = countermovement jump, STR= strength, BF% = body fat percentage, BM% = body mass percentage, BP = bench press; U = upper body, L = lower body, UB = upper body (findings), LB = lower body (findings), HR = heart rate, HRR = heart rate reserve, HRmax = maximal heart rate, CMVJ = Counter Movement Vertical Jump, HRVT = Heart Rate Ventilatory Threshold.

that the interference effects of endurance training on strength and power are related to the type, frequency, and duration of endurance training. To limit such negative effects of endurance training when performing concurrent training, careful attention to these factors is vital (see box 4.2)

Will Resistance Training Affect Aerobic Performance?

One of the most consistent findings of concurrent training studies has been that even heavy resistance training does not typically impair endurance performance. In fact, several studies indicated that strength training may actually increase markers of endurance ability (Bastiaans et al. 2001; Hickson, Rosenkoetter, and Brown 1980; Hickson et al. 1988; Marcinik et al. 1991). For example, after subjects performed 12 weeks of weight training three days per week, peak cycling oxygen consumption was unchanged, but cycling lactate threshold and time to exhaustion were elevated 12 and 33%, respectively (Marcinik et al. 1991). When a group of elite runners dedicating 32% of their total training volume to explosive strength training was compared to another group of elite runners who allocated only 3% to explosive strength training over a nine-week training cycle, 5K run times decreased only in the group that spent more time

in the weight room performing explosive power training (Paavolainen et al. 1999). This may well have been the result of improvements in strength and power, leg stiffness, and running economy despite no change in maximal oxygen consumption kinetics as shown after 14 weeks of adding strength training to the total conditioning program (Millet et al. 2002).

Strength training added to the training program of recreational runners and elite runners appears to augment short-term (15 minutes) and long-term (7 hours) endurance performances. Strength training also increases the transition of type IIx to type IIa muscle fibers, gains in maximal strength, and rapid force production while enhancing neuromuscular function. National-level cyclists in Denmark were placed into one of two training groups (endurance only or strength and endurance training) to determine the effects of the addition of a strength training program over 16 weeks (Aagaard et al. 2011). The strength training consisted of a periodized resistance training program progressing from 10- to 12RM to 8- to 10RM to 5- to 6RM over the first eight weeks and then 5- to 6RM over the last eight weeks using normal lower-body exercises (isolated knee extension, incline leg press, hamstring curl, calf raise) with one- to two-minute rest periods at a frequency of two or three times per week. The endurance training consisted of 10 to

 BOX 4.2 **PRACTICAL QUESTION**

What Can Be Done to Eliminate Compatibility Problems When Multiple Forms of Exercise Are Required?

Although each situation must be addressed individually, in general, here are some approaches to limit the problems of exercise incompatibility:

- Develop a testing program to determine whether, in fact, a problem exists for each athlete.
- Reduce the intensity and volume of exercise.
- Use nonrunning forms of aerobic conditioning.
- Allow more rest days during the week, especially for beginners and athletes returning from a detraining period.
- Reduce the resistance training volume when other exercise demands are mandatory or part of the sport practices.
- Perform lower-body resistance training on days when lower-body cardiorespiratory exercise is not being performed.
- Perform upper-body exercises on days when lower-body musculature is being used for conditioning drills or endurance exercise.
- Provide at least one day of complete rest per week to allow for recovery.

18 hours of endurance training each week using a progressive periodized program. Forty-five-minute endurance capacity increased significantly (8%) in the combined training group but did not improve significantly in the endurance only group. A greater transition to type IIa muscle fibers from type IIx also occurred with combined training. However, no changes in muscle fiber area or capillary density were observed, potentially indicating the already high level of aerobic capability in elite cyclists and the potential for oxidative stress to minimize muscle fiber size increases.

In elite Norwegian men and women cross-country skiers, the addition of a strength training program over three months on a two-days-a-week schedule improved upper- and lower-body strength (Losnegard et al. 2011). No significant changes were observed in the cross-sectional area of thigh musculature, which again may be due to a combination of the low strength training frequency and potential interference on hypertrophy caused by the demanding endurance ski training. Interestingly, significant improvements in maximal oxygen consumption in sport-specific skate-roller-skiing and double-poling performance were observed in the combined group only. However, no changes were demonstrated in treadmill maximal oxygen consumption in either group, which shows a great deal of specificity for the expression of the improved upper- and lower-body strength on sport-specific endurance performance.

More strength training time may be needed to improve cardiorespiratory function in younger runners. Eight weeks of an explosive strength training program in young (16 to 18 years) runners significantly increased lower-body strength (Mikkola et al. 2007). This short-term training effect seemed to translate to improvements in the maximal speed in an anaerobic running test and 30 m sprint speed in only the strength training group with no significant change shown by a group of runners who did not perform the explosive strength training program. However, neither group demonstrated any significant improvements in maximal oxygen uptake or running economy.

The preceding study indicates that endurance performance can be enhanced via neuromuscular mechanisms with lower training frequencies (e.g., enhanced stretch-shortening cycle ability and reduced contact time with the ground). A combination of factors is probably involved to various extents depending on the type of endur-ance sport, including greater **tendon stiffness**, enhanced transition of type IIx to type IIa muscle fibers, no impact on capillary density or mitochondrial function, greater rate of force development, and increases in upper- and lower-body strength even when no hypertrophy occurs (Aagaard and Andersen 2010).

Concurrent Training and Aging

The use of both cardiorespiratory endurance and strength training has been promoted for health and disease prevention (Garber et al. 2011). Concerns about the use of these two exercise modes interfering with the development of either fitness outcome have not been identified. Low training frequencies (two days a week) with reduced training volume for the combined training programs present no real problems with incompatibility for men and women in the 60- to 84-year age group over a 12-week training period (Wood et al. 2001). When middle-aged (approx 40 years of age) men trained concurrently for both strength and aerobic endurance over 21 weeks, improvements in strength, power, and muscle fiber size were demonstrated (Häkkinen et al. 2003). Such findings show that when lower frequencies of training (two days of strength or explosive power training and two days of endurance training on a cycle ergometer) are used over relatively long training periods, muscle hypertrophy (muscle fiber size and thigh cross-sectional area), strength (1RM and maximal isometric force), and maximal oxygen consumption are not compromised. However, exceptions have been noted; training for 16 weeks with a low-frequency concurrent training (two days of strength and two days of aerobic endurance training) showed smaller gains in leg strength and no difference in cardiorespiratory fitness gains (Izquierdo et al. 2005). Such findings indicate that age and the duration of training may both influence the ability to adapt to both training stimuli.

Interference may increase with more intense training programs. For example, a study of older men (65 years) performing a linear periodized model with intensity increasing for both strength (one week at 25RM followed by two weeks at 18- to 20RM, 15- to 17RM, 12- to 14RM, 8- to 10RM, and 6- to 8RM) and endurance training (20 to 30 minutes at 80% of ventilatory threshold for nine weeks followed by six 4-minute intervals with one-minute rests at 100% of ventilator threshold) over 11 weeks showed some interference (Cadore et al. 2010). The combined group showed less improvement in lower-body strength. Increases were observed in maximal muscle activation only in the strength training group, suggesting that endurance training may compromise the neural adaptations needed for strength development in older men. Interestingly, the endurance training group, although not showing any improvements in strength, did show increases in aerobic capacity and decreases in free testosterone concentrations at rest. As with younger people, the impact of higher-intensity aerobic stress may well have played a major role in the interference observed.

Underlying Mechanisms of Incompatibility

The underlying physiological mechanism(s) that might explain the interference of one training modality with another has been a point of speculation for many years. Obviously, the program design of each conditioning workout is the first place to look for reasons for incompatibility as discussed earlier. However, it is important to understand what might explain the inhibition of optimal adaptations for either maximal force production or endurance adaptations, such as maximal or peak oxygen consumption with concurrent training. Changes in muscle protein synthesis with each mode of training appear to be highly specific; however, the signaling pathways are too complex to explain incompatibility based on one factor or protein synthesis signaling pathway (Baar 2006; Wilkinson et al. 2008).

Any incompatibility involves several factors. First, there is an upper genetic limit for any fitness parameter. In other words, the gain for any performance or physiological adaptation can only increase to a maximal value that is limited by the person's genetic profile. Second, for skeletal muscle, incompatibility typically exists only for those motor units that are recruited to perform both types of exercise. Third, not all training effects are targeted at skeletal muscle; although a major focus of most exercise programs is skeletal muscle, other systems such as the cardiovascular, endocrine, and immune systems and the connective tissues that support skeletal muscle function are also undergoing adaptations in the process of exercise training. Finally, the extent and type of motor unit recruitment dictates how much involvement from the various systems is needed to support exercise performance and recovery processes. For example, lifting a light weight one time will not require as much physiological support as lifting a heavy weight multiple times. The type and extent of physiological support needed to maintain homeostasis during exercise and into recovery thus depends on specific exercise demands.

A muscle fiber that is recruited is affected by the demands of the activity performed. With heavy resistance training, type IIa fibers are the end point of the type II subtype transformation (see chapter 3). Type IIx fibers are not detected after heavy resistance training, and the few that remain have a high concentration of aerobic enzymes compared to typical type IIx fibers and therefore are starting a transition to the type IIa phenotype (Ploutz et al. 1994). When muscle fibers are recruited to perform a repetitive oxidative activity, as in high-intensity aerobic training, oxygen moves from the circulation into the muscle's metabolic machinery to help in the production of the ATP energy needed for many physiological functions, including muscle contraction. In this process many enzymatic and signaling events are increased to optimize this function. The following changes result to accomplish aerobic adaptations in the muscle: an increased number of mitochondria, increased myoglobin to increase oxygen transport capability within the muscle fiber, increased capillary density, increased energy stores, and minimally increased muscle fiber size. All of these factors increase the ability to transport oxygen, increase the use of oxygen to provide ATP, and minimize the diffusion distances for oxygen. Conversely, when a muscle fiber is recruited to produce high amounts of force, the motor unit is stimulated with a high Hz electrical depolarization, which produces many anabolic signals related to contractile and noncontractile protein synthesis. Other changes include an increase in anabolic receptors and changes in neurological structure and function. The result is an increase in force capability and, with much resistance training, an increase in muscle fiber size. Thus, a conflict in cellular adaptations provides the basis for cellular incompatibility with concurrent training that can theoretically result in a reduction in either strength or endurance capabilities.

The muscle fiber associated with the motor unit recruited to perform both types of exercise is faced with the dilemma of trying to adapt to the oxidative stimulus to improve its aerobic function and to the stimulus from the heavy resistance training program to improve its force production ability (Nelson et al. 1990; Sale et al. 1990). So what happens to the muscle fiber population?

In a study of concurrent training that included high-intensity resistance and endurance training using highly endurance-trained members of the U.S. Army's 101st and 82nd Airborne units, lower-body power was inhibited in the combined group, but maximal oxygen consumption and strength were not affected by a periodized four-days-a-week program (Monday, Tuesday, Thursday, and Friday) over three months (Kraemer, Patton et al. 1995). However, the changes at the muscle fiber level gave some insight into what was happening at the cellular level. Training consisted of performing endurance training in the morning and resistance training in the afternoon on the same day separated by six hours. The high-intensity endurance training program included both high-intensity continuous and interval track sprint workouts. Strength training included two heavy resistance days and two short-rest metabolic training days each week. Muscle biopsies were obtained from the vastus lateralis of the thigh musculature to determine muscle fiber changes. In an endurance-training-only group, the type I muscle fibers showed a decrease in cross-sectional area pre- to posttraining and no changes in the type II muscle fiber cross-sectional areas. This demonstrated a type of exercise-induced atrophy. In a group that performed only upper-body resistance training and endurance training, no changes were observed in type I or type II muscle fiber cross-sectional areas. This supported the concept of specificity of training yet showed that even isometric forces of the lower body used for upper-body stabilization during resistance training were sufficient to eliminate type I muscle fiber atrophy. A strength-training-only group showed an increase in both type I and type II muscle fiber cross-sectional areas. Of specific interest for the question of incompatibility, a combined group performing both endurance and strength training with the lower body showed no change in type I muscle fiber cross-sectional area yet increases in type II fiber areas (see table 4.2).

These results reflect the cellular dilemma for optimization of muscle fiber size adaptations to meet the demands of either strength or endur-

TABLE 4.2 Muscle Fiber Characteristics Pre- and Posttraining

Group	C Pre	C Post	S Pre	S Post	E Pre	E Post	UBC Pre	UBC Post	Control Pre	Control Post
% of different muscle fiber types										
I	55.6 (±11.1)	57.7 (±11.1)	55.21 (±11.7)	55.44 (±1.5)	54.1 (±5.9)	54.6 (±5.3)	50.6 (±8.0)	51.1 (±7.9)	52.0 (±11.5)	52.8 (±10.8)
IIc	1.9 (±2.2)	1.8 (±2.7)	2.4 (±1.6)	2.0 (±1.3)	0.9 (±0.6)	2.5* (±2.0)	1.3 (±1.0)	3.0* (±2.2)	1.6 (±0.9)	1.3 (±1.3)
IIa	28.4 (±15.4)	39.3* (±11.1)	23.3 (±11.5)	40.5* (±10.6)	25.75 (±4.8)	34.1 (±3.9)	25.5 (±4.2)	34.2* (±6.9)	25.6 (±1.6)	26.6 (±4.6)
IIx	14.11 (±7.2)	1.6* (±0.8)	19.1 (±7.9)	1.9* (±0.8)	19.2 (±3.6)	8.8* (±4.4)	22.6 (±4.9)	11.6* (±5.3)	20.8 (±7.6)	19.2 (±6.4)
Cross-sectional muscle fiber area (μm^2)										
I	5,008 (±874)	4,756 (±692)	4,883 (±1286)	5,460* (±1214)	5,437 (±970)	4,853* (±966)	5,680 (±535)	5,376 (±702)	4,946 (±1309)	5,177 (±1344)
IIc	4,157 (±983)	4,658 (±771)	3,981.2 (±1535)	5,301* (±1956)	2,741 (±482)	2,402* (±351)	3,050 (±930)	2,918 (±1086)	3,733 (±1285)	4,062 (±1094)
IIa	5,862 (±997)	7,039* (±1151)	6,084 (±1339)	7,527* (±1981)	6,782 (±1267)	6,287 (±385)	6,393 (±1109)	6,357 (±1140)	6,310 (±593)	6,407 (±423)
IIx	5,190 (±712)	4,886 (±1171)	5,795 (±1495)	6,078 (±2604)	6,325 (±1860)	4,953 (±1405)	6,052 (±1890)	5,855 (±867)	5,917 (±896)	6,120 (±1089)

C = combined; S = strength; E = endurance; UBC = upper body combined.

* $p < .05$ from corresponding pretraining value.

Means (±SD).

Adapted, by permission, from W.J. Kraemer et al., 1995, "Compatibility of high intensity strength and endurance training on hormonal and skeletal muscle adaptations," *Journal of Applied Physiology* 78(3): 976-989.

ance training. High-intensity endurance training stimulated a decrease in type I muscle fiber size most likely as the result of an increase in aerobic signaling to favor oxygen diffusion distances and mitochondrial biosynthesis. A reduction in fiber size most likely also contributes to a decrease in strength, power, and rate of force development from the affected motor units. The lack of significant aerobic signaling in the strength-training-only group allowed for anabolic signaling for protein synthesis and accretion in all muscle fiber types resulting in increased fiber size. The additional use of metabolic resistance training protocols (e.g., short rest, supersets) potentially allowed for the maintenance of aerobic function. The upper-body-only training group did not show the decreases in fiber size that were seen in the endurance-training-only group, most likely as a result of the isometric force required for stabilization of the lower body when performing upper-body resistance exercises, especially during the 5RM training days. The combined training group showed a type of averaging of the resulting stimulus from each training modality, resulting in no significant change in type I muscle fiber size and an increase in type II muscle fiber size. This reflects the specificity of motor unit recruitment and the associated adaptations of each pool of motor units.

Other studies support the dramatic influence of oxidative stress with high-intensity endurance training on fiber hypertrophy. Typically, no change in any muscle fiber type's cross-sectional area is shown with this type of training. However, a transition from type IIx to IIa as a result of strength training occurs indicating that high-threshold motor units are recruited (Aagaard et al. 2010; Aagaard and Andersen 2011).

In the 1970s, studies showing a reduction of mitochondrial density resulted in many runners avoiding resistance training programs (MacDougall et al. 1979). Because mitochondria are the site of aerobic energy production, any decrease in the volume or density of mitochondria could theoretically decrease the oxidative capacity of the muscle. Thus, based on these results, many distance runners did not perform resistance training fearing that it would compromise their endurance capabilities. A decrease in mitochondrial density after resistance training would appear to support this belief. What distance runners did not know at the time was that resistance training offers other benefits, such as increases in connective tissue strength,

improved running economy and efficiency, and the prevention or reduction of overuse injuries. As previously discussed, later research did not support the contention that resistance training would compromise aerobic performance. Additionally, in comparison to a nonexercising group, a group that performed 12 weeks of combined strength and endurance training showed mitochondrial number increases, but changes took place in different anatomical regions of the muscle (Chilibeck, Syrotuik, and Bell 2002). The intermyofibrillar region undergoes a linear increase with training, whereas the subsarcolemmal region undergoes a preferential increase late in the training program. Thus, mitochondrial number and density need to be examined in all regions of the muscle fiber to understand the cellular effect of performing concurrent training.

In summary, the physiological mechanisms that may mediate adaptational responses to concurrent training remain speculative but appear related to alterations in neural recruitment patterns, attenuation of muscle hypertrophy, or both (Chromiak and Mulvaney 1990; Dudley and Djamil 1985; Dudley and Fleck 1987; Wilson et al. 2012). Additionally, with longer training periods or very intense training, a decrease in some performance outcomes may be due to nonfunctional overreaching or overtraining (Hennessy and Watson 1994; Nelson et al. 1990). Conversely, concurrent exercise training, when properly designed, may just require a longer duration for the summation of physiological adaptations thereby resolving compatibility issues.

No doubt, many people do not appear to be able to adapt optimally to both modes of training when high training frequencies and intensities that limit recovery are used. Thus, the stimuli created by the program design, as noted earlier in this chapter, are vital considerations for optimizing the concurrent use of both modes of training (Wilson et al. 2012). Prioritization of training (i.e., emphasizing one training type and de-emphasizing others in a training cycle) along with periodization of volumes and intensities may be important when several fitness components must be trained at the same time.

Signaling From Exercise Programs

Signaling systems play a vital role in the adaptation of a muscle fiber (Baar 2006; Gundersen 2011). Because signaling mechanisms are complex and highly redundant, singular explanations of anabolic and catabolic effects are difficult to attribute to one causative factor. As discussed in chapter 3, endocrine signaling plays a major role in helping to determine the status of the cell. Hormone signals include anabolic hormones such as testosterone, insulin-like growth factors, insulin, and various types of growth hormones as well as catabolic hormones such as cortisol, which at very high concentrations can dramatically affect tissue breakdown and suppress immune function (Spiering et al. 2008a, 2008b). Data that purely attribute one factor to the increase or decrease in muscle fiber size are limited because a whole series of signaling events are going on at the same time to maintain cellular and whole-body homeostasis during exercise and to restore tissue to normal or cause adaptations after exercise disruption or damage (see figure 4.2).

Signaling systems are put into action by various stimuli, such as hormonal binding. This is demonstrated by IGF-I binding to its receptors in skeletal muscle fibers and the stimulation of the mTOR (mammalian target of rapamycin), a protein and part of a system of signals that regulates cell growth, proliferation transcription, and survival, as well as protein synthesis. The mTOR system can also be stimulated by muscular contraction as well as by the nutritional intake of the branched-chain amino acid leucine (Matsakas and Patel 2009; Spiering et al. 2008b; Walker et al. 2011). The protein kinase B (Akt) mammalian target of rapamycin (mTOR) signaling system is also capable of stimulating protein synthesis while decreasing protein breakdown, thus promoting muscle fiber hypertrophy (Baar 2006).

A major antagonist of the mTOR system is the adenosine monophosphate (AMP), 5' adenosine monophosphate-activated protein kinase (AMPK), or the AMP/AMPK system (Kimball 2006; Gordon et al. 2008). This system can block the positive anabolic effects stimulated by mTOR. It stimulates catabolic pathways that provide energy for muscle cell function (such as fatty acid oxidation or improvement in glucose transport by increasing cellular glucose transporters). Recent findings show that the addition of aerobic exercise to a resistance exercise workout negatively alters some of the many anabolic signaling systems (Lundberg et al. 2012). The concurrent use of both heavy resistance and intense aerobic exercise diminishes the quality of the signals being conveyed to the genetic machinery needed for anabolism. Thus, allowing for adequate recovery from exercise (i.e., rest days) and nutritionally replacing energy substrates (i.e., ingesting protein, carbohydrate, and fat) appear to be important considerations when performing both forms of exercise concurrently. This might explain the reductions in performance when high-intensity, high-volume, and high-frequency training programs are performed, including concurrent training.

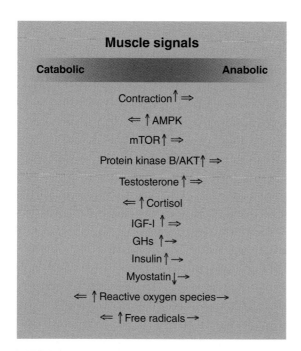

FIGURE 4.2 Signals to muscle originate from many cells, glands, and metabolic pathways. Some of the major signals that muscle responds to are shown here. The vertical arrows indicate increases or decreases in concentrations, and the horizontal arrows show the magnitude (single- or double-direction arrows) of its directional effect. The double arrow represents a higher magnitude of effect. The signals stimulate either anabolic or catabolic processes in the muscle.

Program Design Challenges

Exercise prescription must take into consideration the demands of the total program and ensure that the frequency, intensity, and volume of exercise do not become counterproductive to optimal physiological adaptations and performance (García-Pallarés and Izquierdo 2011). Those involved in exercise prescription should keep the following points in mind:

- Training program sequences should be prioritized according to how they relate to training program goals. Trainees should not attempt to perform high-intensity and high-volume strength and endurance training concurrently. The relative training volume for each mode of exercise needs to reflect the prioritization of each training cycle.
- Periodized training programs with planned rest phases should be used to allow for adequate recovery from sessions.
- Strength or power athletes should limit high-intensity aerobic training because the high oxidative stress accompanying high-volume or high-intensity endurance training appears to negatively affect power development.

Basics of Cardiorespiratory Training

As previously discussed, some degree of cardio-respiratory training is part of almost every total conditioning program. Continuous training and interval training are the primary program designs for cardiorespiratory training (Bishop, Girard, and Mendez-Villanueva 2011). Each can be prescribed from low intensity to high intensity. In many programs continuous aerobic training is used for low-intensity training and for recovery workouts.

The aerobic program design should be carefully examined so as not to create an interference with desired training adaptations from a resistance training program. Yet, there is a need to train at higher intensities if maximal aerobic capacity is a primary outcome. In such situations, prioritization of training and periodization of both the aerobic and resistance training programs is vital to training success. The modality used for aerobic training also needs to be considered. Running may be inherently more likely to cause incompatibility than cycling; running is more stressful at the same training intensity because of the ground impact forces and includes a full stretch-shortening cycle, including eccentric loading (Wilson et al. 2012).

The prescription of aerobic exercise should be individualized. Those who need more specific exercise prescriptions may benefit from a stress test to document their exact **functional capacity**

and to suggest heart rate zones. The results of treadmill or cycle ergometry testing can be very helpful for individualizing exercise prescription for endurance training (Garber et al. 2011). This is especially important for older adults or people whose functional capacity is in doubt (e.g., those with cardiovascular pathologies). However, testing can also provide very highly specific training data for elite athletes. The test modality should be specific to the exercise training or competition, even when cross-training is used. For example, the importance of a sport-specific assessment has been demonstrated with cross-country skiers, for whom strength training improved maximal oxygen consumption during skate-rollerskiing and double-poling performance, but not in a typical treadmill-running maximal oxygen consumption test (Losnegard et al. 2011).

Continuous Aerobic Training Program

Many programs use continuous exercise to train the aerobic ability. The typical goal of **aerobic conditioning** is to improve maximal or peak oxygen consumption and associated cardiorespiratory functions to support endurance performance (Garber et al. 2011). However, beyond training for caloric expenditure, blood pressure control, and health reasons, improving maximal oxygen consumption from a relatively trained state requires higher training intensities ($\geq 85\%$ of $\dot{V}O_2max$). This causes many athletes to use interval training to achieve higher exercise intensities. The use of higher aerobic training intensities along with strength training helps to enhance endurance capability by improving running economy and efficiency of movement (Guglielmo, Greco, and Denadai 2009; Millet et al. 2002).

The myth that people need extended, slow, long-distance running to provide an "aerobic base" before participating in other, more intense conditioning modalities most likely arises from the perceived need to use lower-intensity training during a "general conditioning phase," especially when untrained people begin training. However, the relationship between aerobic and anaerobic performances is limited and demonstrates that those who perform well in anaerobic tests do not necessarily perform well in aerobic tests (Koziris et al. 1996). This is most likely due to differences in body mass, the energy source predominantly used to perform a particular task, muscle fiber type, training background, or any combination of these. Nevertheless, whether using continuous or interval aerobic training methods, proper progression in the frequency, intensity, and duration is needed.

Aerobic training intensity is a key factor in optimizing compatibility with other training types, especially strength and power resistance training. One of the easiest ways to monitor aerobic intensity is with heart rate monitoring. A **heart rate training zone** is typically prescribed to control the intensity of the aerobic exercise stimulus. The person then performs steady-state exercise within the training zone. Generally, lower-intensity heart rate training zones are between 55 and 65% of maximal heart rate. Lower intensities are typically used by untrained or aerobically unfit people or as recovery exercise by highly trained athletes.

Despite the importance of individual exercise prescription, many people (most notably, coaches who are prescribing exercise for hundreds of athletes) do not have the resources available to obtain laboratory stress tests. Coaches and trainees must realize that for basic aerobic fitness, endurance training doesn't have to be overly stressful to be effective. This is not the case for competitive endurance athletes, who must use higher training intensities to prepare for competition. In addition, some athletes should not train at high aerobic intensities because such training may inhibit the strength and power adaptations important for performance in many activities (García-Pallarés and Izquierdo 2011).

The duration and frequency of aerobic exercise also needs to increase progressively as the person becomes more tolerant of exercise stress. For basic **cardiorespiratory endurance fitness,** exercise should be performed for 20 to 60 minutes three to five days per week (Garber et al. 2011). Running, bicycling, cross-country skiing, stair climbing, ellipse training, aerobics (e.g., bench-step aerobics), and swimming are some of the most popular and effective cardiorespiratory conditioning modalities (Kraemer, Keuning et al. 2001). However, a degree of specificity is necessary if the conditioning modality is vital to sport skills (e.g., run training if conditioning for soccer).

An endurance exercise training session consists of a warm-up, a training period, and a cool-down. The heart rate is checked and the pace of the exercise adjusted so that the trainee is exercising within his or her training zone. Heart rate watches are often used to monitor heart rate. However, a 10-second pulse rate can be obtained after a steady-state exercise duration is achieved (usually three to five minutes).

A pace test to assist with determining and monitoring training at the training heart rate over a specified distance can be conducted over a number of training sessions. Pace tests for running or cycling should be performed on flat terrain. Also, as fitness levels improve, it is important to check the pace against the heart rate response relationship. A less-conditioned person usually requires shorter pace distances to evaluate a training pace. It is important to ensure that steady-state exercise is achieved at the selected distance (exercise duration of three to five minutes after the warm-up).

Heart rate intensity can be determined using a percentage of maximal heart rate or the Karvonen formula, also termed the heart rate reserve method. To determine a 70 and 90% heart rate intensity for a 20-year-old using the Karvonen formula would require the following calculations in which HRmax= maximal heart rate, HRrest = heart rate at rest, HRR = heart rate reserve, THR = target heart rate, and bpm = beats per minute. Several equations can be used to estimate HRmax, but the following is very accurate (Gellish et al. 2007):

$$HRmax = 207 - (0.7 \times age\ in\ years)$$
$$HRmax = 207 - (0.7 \times 20\ years)$$
$$HRmax = 193\ bpm$$

HRR is the difference between resting heart rate and HRmax and is calculated as follows assuming a HRrest of 73 bpm:

$$HRR = (HRmax - HRrest)$$
$$HRR = (193\ bpm - 73\ bpm)$$
$$HRR = 120\ bpm$$

THR is then calculated as follows for 70 and 90% heart rate intensity:

$$THR = HRrest + (HRR \times desired\ intensity)$$
$$THR\ 70\% = 73\ bpm + (120\ bpm \times 0.70)$$
$$THR\ 70\% = 157\ bpm$$
$$THR\ 90\% = 73\ bpm + (120\ bpm \times 0.90)$$
$$THR\ 90\% = 181\ bpm$$

So a training intensity between 70% and 90% using the Karvonen method is a heart rate between 157 bpm and 181 bpm.

After HRmax has been estimated, the desired heart rate training zones can be calculated:

70% HRmax = 0.7 × 193 = 135 bpm
90% HRmax = 0.9 × 193 = 174 bpm
70-90% HRmax training zone =135 to 174 bpm

As previously discussed, the impact of exercise compatibility on strength and power development might be less if intensities and durations are carefully prescribed (McCarthy et al. 1995; Wilson et al. 2012). Thus, in the preceding example, on a light training day a heart rate of 135 bpm would be used if training at 70% of the heart rate target training zone. Other target heart rate training zones can easily be determined. Use of such zones is a quantitative method to prescribe intensity that takes into account many factors including the environment, psychological stress, arousal, and previous training.

Interval Training

Conditioning is necessary to enhance speed or anaerobic endurance. **Interval training** is one major cardiorespiratory training paradigm. Sprint activities of a few seconds require a higher power output than longer-duration sprints of one to two minutes (Kraemer, Fleck, and Deschenes 2012). Training needs to be related to both the distance and the duration of the activity performed in the particular sport. As an example, for an American football lineman, 5 to 20 yd sprints (one to three seconds) are appropriate, whereas a receiver may need to train using sprint distances ranging from 10 to 60 yd. An 800 m runner would need to train at distances and paces equivalent to the distance and pace needed in a race. Programs that require longer durations of high-intensity exercise (e.g., 800 and 1,500 m) also involve interval-type training.

It is important to differentiate between "quality" sprint training for maximal speed and "quantity" sprint conditioning used to enhance speed endurance, improve buffering capacity, and improve repeat sprint ability. Classic interval training has consisted of modulating the exercise work-to-rest ratios for years (Ben Sira et al. 2010). This ratio describes the relationship between the lengths of an interval to the rest allowed between intervals. For example, if an interval is 10 seconds in duration and 30-second rests are allowed between intervals, the work-to-rest ratio would be 1:3. In sprint speed training, rest periods are longer to ensure recovery prior to another sprint effort so it is performed at close to maximal velocity. Sprint interval training designed to improve buffering capacity, anaerobic

capacity, aerobic function, and repeat sprint ability require shorter rest periods. Higher and longer intensities of interval training must be carefully prioritized and periodized because such programs can detract from strength, power, and muscle size increases when performed concurrently, especially in untrained subjects (Aagaard and Andersen 2010; García-Pallarés and Izquierdo 2011).

The difference between the quantity and quality of interval training is shown by the following. Sprint training performed three days per week consisting of three 100 yd sprints followed by three 50 yd sprints with rest intervals of 3 minutes and 90 seconds, respectively, between each sprint and 5 minutes between sets resulted in increases in sprint speed, but no increases in peak oxygen consumption, over an eight-week training program (Callister et al. 1988). Conversely, when two sets of four sprint intervals of 20 seconds are separated by only one minute of rest, significant increases in the peak oxygen consumption can be attained by the eighth week of a 10-week training program (Kraemer et al. 1989). Thus, the exercise-to-rest ratio and the length of sprints are vital factors in determining the effects of sprint intervals on increases in peak oxygen consumption or sprint speed.

The preceding results are in part explained by shorter sprint training involving maximal or close-to-maximal exercise intensity. This results in the use of predominantly anaerobic energy sources and practicing maximal sprinting technique. As the exercise duration increases with the use of shorter rest periods, there is a shift toward more use of aerobic energy, which results in an increase of aerobic ability. Interval training programs using various interval durations and rest periods can be designed to address the anaerobic and aerobic metabolic needs of a wide variety of sports and activities.

Another important consideration in designing interval programs is the need to tolerate high acidity levels in certain sport activities (e.g., longer-duration sprinting, boxing, mixed martial arts, and wrestling), which necessitate training that increases lactate production and enhances lactate removal (Brooks and Fahey 1984). To train short sprint ability, typically 5- to 10-second intervals with exercise-to-rest ratios of 1:3 to 1:6 are used; to train the anaerobic glycolytic system, longer intervals of 30 seconds to 2 minutes with work-to-rest ratios of 1:3 are used (Karp 2000). The number of repetitions per training session varies with the training goals, interval duration, and fitness level of the trainee, but typically somewhere between 3 to 12 intervals are performed per session.

Inclined surfaces have also been used to improve power and to train the muscles associated with sprinting. During inclined run-sprint training, the average power and energy generated during hip flexion and extension in the swing phase are greater than during sprinting with no incline. Thus, incline sprint training provides for enhanced muscular loading of the hip musculature during both the swing and stance phases (Swanson and Caldwell 2000), which may be useful for enhancing sprint ability. In addition, the use of resistive devices (e.g., sled-towing devices) also has potential for enhancing sprint performance (West et al. 2013).

It must be kept in mind that sprint speed is different from speed during agility runs with two or more direction changes (Young, McDowell, and Scarlett 2001). The training effect for unidirectional speed development does not transfer highly to the multiple direction changes typical in many sports. Thus, training programs need to be designed to target specific goals. A typical interval workout could include the following:

- Warm-up consisting of low-intensity exercise and dynamic stretching
- Technique drills
- Start drills
- Conditioning phase or intervals
- Cool-down, which may include dynamic or static stretching (see Stretching and Flexibility)

In summary, typically, interval training to increase sprint speed uses longer rest periods and maximal or near-maximal short intervals, whereas interval training to increase maximal aerobic ability uses longer intervals with short rest periods. Additionally, interval training for some activities can include a sport-specific attribute, such as controlling a soccer ball, basketball, or water polo ball. This type of training enhances both the motor skill and the conditioning component needed for performance in a particular sport.

Stretching and Flexibility

As with most areas of fitness, the needs for flexibility and stretching must be determined accord-ing to the trainees' sports, goals, ability to safely perform movements with their current range of motion (ROM), and posture. Flexibility is affected by numerous internal and external influences or factors, such as the type of joint, the internal resistance within the joint, the temperature of the joint, and the elasticity of muscle tissue. The role of stretching in helping to develop flexibility or improve the absolute range of movement of a joint or series of joints has been well established (figure 4.3). Less clear is the type of stretching that should be used as part of a warm-up given the potential for a negative impact on performance. Additionally, the impact of flexibility or stretching on injury prevention has been a topic of interest.

Techniques for several methods of **flexibility training** are well documented (Anderson 2010). As with all training programs, stretching programs should be designed to meet the needs of the person and the activity or sport.

There are four basic types of stretching (Moore and Hutton 1980). Although the techniques of these types differ, a meta-analysis concludes that no significant difference in flexibility increases of the hamstring musculature exist among them (Decoster et al. 2005).

- Slow-movement stretching
- Static stretching
- Dynamic and ballistic stretching
- Proprioceptive neuromuscular facilitation (PNF)

Slow Movements

Slow-movement stretching is often done before any other types of stretching. Continuous slow movements such as neck rotations, arm rotations, and trunk rotations are also included in dynamic stretching. Slow-movement stretching may be more beneficial to warming up than to increasing flexibility. Use of slow movements prior to the faster dynamic movements of ballistic stretching may be a good progression in a warm-up.

Static Stretching

The most common type of stretching is **static stretching**, in which the person voluntarily relaxes the muscle while elongating it, and then holds the muscle in a stretched position. A simple example is the toe touch, in which one bends over and tries to touch one's toes while keeping the knees straight.

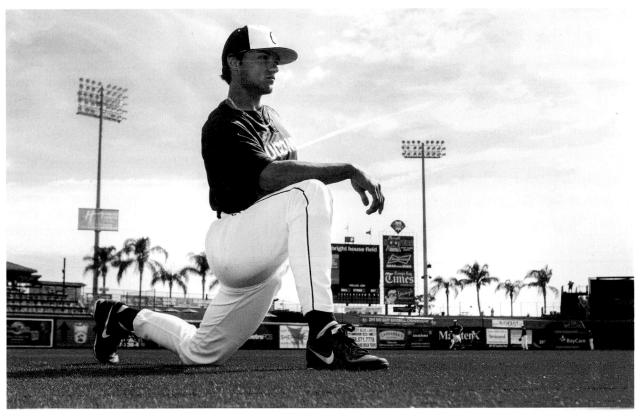

FIGURE 4.3 Stretching can be an important part of a total conditioning program, but the type of stretching performed, the timing of the stretching within a program, and the recovery from stretching are all important factors that must be considered.

Photo courtesy of UConn Athletics.

The stretching movement is typically held at the point of minimal discomfort. Stretching is typically performed progressively, meaning that the person tries to increase the range of movement slightly farther each time the stretch is performed to extend the range of motion. Subsequent stretching continues to improve the range of motion.

Static stretching is one of the most effective and desirable techniques when comfort and limited training time are major factors (Moore and Hutton 1980). After a stretching bout, there is an increase in a joint's range of motion, less EMG activity in the muscle stretched, and a decrease in resting muscle tension. This indicates a lower resting tension in the muscle is related to a person's ability to tolerate higher stretching strain and is associated with the increases in range of motion after a stretching bout (Wiemann and Hahn 1997). In addition, during static stretching, EMG activity is low in some muscles being stretched, indicating a partial neural mediation with stretching (Mohr et al. 1998). Interestingly, static stretching may be more

than twice as effective as dynamic range of motion flexibility exercises for increasing hamstring flexibility (11- vs. 4-degree increase) (Brandy, Irion, and Briggler 1998). In this study, dynamic range of motion training consisted of achieving a stretched position in five seconds, holding the stretch for five seconds, and then returning to an unstretched position in five seconds. Static stretching consisted of one 30-second static stretch. The use of stretching to improve flexibility is a widespread practice, but the effectiveness of various programs may be related to the change in stretch tolerance rather than to the passive properties of muscle (Magnusson 1998). In partial support of this theory, static stretching for 90 seconds was shown not to alter the viscoelastic properties of muscle (Magnusson, Aagaard, and Nielson 2000).

Many variations of this technique have been proposed, with stretch time ranging up to 60 seconds. Static stretch times beyond 30 seconds are not more effective when stretching is done each day (Brandy, Irion, and Briggler 1997). Holding stretches for 15 seconds was more effective than holding them for 5 seconds for improving active ROM, but not for increasing passive ROM (Roberts and Wilson 1999). Thus, performing 15- to 30-second stretches three to five times appears to be optimal. It has been demonstrated that the greatest decreases in tension occurs in the first 20 seconds of a held static stretch of the ankle joint (McNair et al. 2001).

Dynamic and Ballistic Stretching

Recent concerns about the use of static stretching in warm-ups prior to workouts or competition (see the section Typical Warm-Up Prior to Workouts or Competition later in this chapter) has increased the popularity of **dynamic stretching**. This type of stretching involves a dynamic movement during the stretch that results in movement through the entire range of motion of the joint(s) involved. **Ballistic stretching** involves a fast, dynamic movement through the entire range of motion and ends in a stretch. An example of dynamic stretching is walking lunges at a controlled velocity; an example of ballistic stretching is mimicking the punting action in American football.

Proprioceptive Neuromuscular Facilitation (PNF)

A more complex set of stretching techniques using various stretch-contract-relax protocols is termed **proprioceptive neuromuscular facilitation (PNF)** stretching. There are several variations of this technique, but the three major types are as follows (Shellock and Prentice 1985):

- Slow-reversal-hold
- Contract-relax/agonist
- Hold-relax

Using the hamstring stretch as an example, the slow-reversal-hold technique is as follows: The trainee lies on the back, with one knee extended and the ankle flexed to 90 degrees. A partner pushes on the leg, passively flexing the hip joint until the trainee feels slight discomfort in the hamstring. The trainee then pushes for 10 seconds against the resistance applied by the partner by activating the hamstring muscle. The hamstring muscles are then relaxed, and the antagonist quadriceps muscles are activated, while the partner applies force for 10 seconds to further stretch the hamstrings. The

leg should move so there is increased hip joint flexion. All muscles are then relaxed for 10 seconds, after which the stretch is repeated beginning at the increased hip flexion joint angle. This push–relax sequence is typically repeated at least three times.

The other two PNF techniques commonly used are similar to the slow-reversal-hold method. The contract-relax/agonist technique involves a dynamic concentric action before the relaxation/stretch phase. In the earlier example, the hamstrings are contracted so the leg moves toward the floor. The hold-relax technique uses an isometric action before the relaxation/stretch phase. These types of PNF techniques typically take longer to perform than other stretching techniques and also often require a partner.

Some argue that because PNF training is associated with greater discomfort, static stretching is more appropriate (Moore and Hutton 1980). In addition, in some movements the position may be more important than using a static or PNF technique (Sullivan, Dejulia, and Worrell 1992). It has been demonstrated that the position of the pelvic tilt used in a hamstring flexibility program plays a greater role in determining the improvement in the ranges of motion than the specific technique itself (Dejulia, Dejulia, and Worrell 1992). This emphasizes the concept that most flexibility techniques are effective, but other factors may influence their appropriateness in a given program design.

Development of Flexibility

Flexibility training can be performed in either the warm-up or cool-down portion of a workout or as a separate training session. Many programs recommend holding each static stretch for 6 to 12 seconds; holding for 10 to 30 seconds is also commonly recommended. The problem with holding static stretches for longer than 30 seconds is that the stretching program might last longer than the workouts (Alter 1998). All of the stretching techniques result in improvement in the absolute range of movement in a joint or series of joints. However, over the past 10 years using static and PNF stretching techniques as part of warm-ups immediately prior to workouts or competitions has been questioned. It appears that when high force, velocity, or power is needed within the first few minutes after a warm-up, dynamic stretching should be performed (Behm and Chaouachi 2011). Because the need for flexibility can vary among people and sports, assessing movement ranges can help in the design of a flexibility program. Many people have various areas in need of increased flexibility and a general level of inflexibility, which can be addressed by proper screening and stretching movements (Cook, Burton, and Hoogenboom 2006a, 2006b).

Typical Warm-Up Prior to Workouts or Competition

Warm-ups can improve performance by affecting the neuromuscular and viscoelastic properties of the connective tissues and joints. However, activities must be appropriate, such as light cardiorespiratory exercise and dynamic stretching. Other warm-up activities have to be used at specific times before workouts or competition or not used at all (e.g., long-duration static stretching) (Fradkin, Zazryn, and Smoliga 2010).

A warm-up should typically consist of submaximal aerobic activity followed by slow movements and large-muscle-group dynamic stretching complemented with sport-specific dynamic activities (Behm and Chaouachi 2011). A dynamic warm-up consisting of dynamic stretching and running improved hamstring flexibility, vertical jump power, and quadriceps strength in physically fit young men and women when compared to a static stretching warm-up even after five minutes of stationary cycling (Aguilar et al. 2012). Despite the overwhelming findings about the detrimental effects of static stretching on strength or power of the stretched muscle, a more directed static stretching of the hamstrings (the antagonist of the quadriceps) resulted in small but significant improvements in quadriceps strength and countermovement jump power in trained men compared to a no-stretching control condition (Sandberg et al. 2012). Using dynamic stretching in a warm-up may also enhance performance when environmental challenges such as cold exposure are present (see box 4.3).

The effects of static stretching on increases in the range of motion may well diminish with time after stretching. Performing three 45-second hamstring stretches separated by 30 seconds has been shown to produce a 20% viscoelastic stress relaxation. The investigators suggested that the static stretching protocol used in their study had no short-term effect on the viscoelastic properties of the human hamstring muscle group (Magnusson, Aagaard, and Nielson 2000). It has been suggested that poststretch force decrements appear to be more related to the inactivation of the muscles affected by the stretch than to the elasticity changes often thought to be the result of stretching the musculoconnective tissue components (Behm, Button, and Butt 2001). Using 30-second static stretches of the hamstrings has shown that increases in the range of motion resulting from static stretching appear to be transient, lasting for a short time after the stretch and then decreasing with time (Depino, Webright, and Arnold 2000). Thus, although acute static stretching does result in temporary ROM gains, it might not increase connective tissue extensibility for an extended period of time.

Likewise, the effects of static stretching on strength and power diminish with time after stretching. For example, 10 minutes after an upper-body static stretching protocol, no differences in upper-body power performances were seen in trained field event throwers (Torres et al. 2008). The duration of the rest period after a static stretch may be important to consider if such stretching is to be used in a warm-up protocol. Nevertheless, until more research is performed on the effects recovery duration after stretching has on performance, it may be prudent (see box 4.4) to use dynamic warm-ups prior to high-force, -power, or -speed workouts and competitions (Behm and Chaouachi 2011).

In addition to the studies presented in box 4.4, stretching has been found to negatively affect isokinetic knee extension torque production below 150 degrees per second (2.62 radians per second), but not at higher velocities of movement (Nelson, Allen et al. 2001). Static stretching may also affect the concentric isokinetic torque production more than the eccentric torque production (Cramer et al. 2006). Highly trained athletes such as National Collegiate Athletic Association Division I women's basketball players may be less susceptible to decrements in isolated, single-joint, isokinetic peak toque production with static stretching (Egan, Cramer et al. 2006). Therefore, differences may well exist between how recreationally active or highly trained athletes are affected by static stretching in closed and open kinetic chain movements. In addition, the inhibition of maximal isometric torque production with static stretching may be joint-angle specific to the stretch protocol used (Nelson, Guillory et al. 2001). Stretching types other than static stretching may also negatively

Does a Warm-Up Using Dynamic Stretching Provide a Performance Edge When Practicing or Competing in the Cold?

This was the question investigated in a research project aimed at understanding how important a warm-up routine of dynamic stretches and exercise was after subjects were exposed to a cold environment for 45 minutes (Dixon et al. 2010). In many sports (e.g., soccer, rugby), reserve players wait to get into the game; environmental conditions may affect the power performance of these players. In this investigation, nine collegiate athletes were tested with and without a warm-up protocol under both ambient (22 °C, or 71.6 °F) and cold (12 °C, or 53.6 °F) conditions. Power (W) in a countermovement vertical jump was used to determine the effects of the warm-up. Vertical jump power was assessed before, immediately after, and then again after two ambient (with and without warm-up) and two cold (with and without warm-up) conditions. The control condition was just standing and waiting for the testing for the same amount of time the warm-up took. The warm-up consisted of the following exercises:

Warm-Up
20 yd distance for each exercise

1. Arm circles forward: walking forward on the toes while circling the arms forward with the arms parallel to the ground

2. Backward heel walk with arm circles backward: walking backward on the heels while circling the arms backward with arms parallel to the ground

3. High-knee walk: walking forward and pulling the knee up to the chest with both arms, alternating legs while walking

4. High-knee skip: skipping forward and bringing the knee up so that the quadriceps are parallel to the ground

5. High-knee run: running while focusing on bringing the knees up so that the quadriceps are parallel to the ground

6. Butt kick: running while bringing the heels to the glutes

7. Tin soldiers: walking forward and kicking a single leg up in front while keeping the knee locked in extension (alternate)

8. One-legged slide walk forward: walking forward with straight legs and then leaning forward on one leg and reaching for the foot with the opposite hand

9. One-legged slide walk backward: walking backward with straight legs and then leaning forward on one leg and reaching for the foot with the opposite hand

10. Backward skip: skipping backward

11. Backward run: running backward and extending the rear foot behind

12. Back pedal: moving backward while shuffling the feet and keeping them low to the ground

13. Overhead lunge walk: doing walking lunges forward with hands on the head

14. Inchworm: starting in the push-up position, walking the feet to the hands; then walking the hands out to the push-up position

The primary finding of this study was that the warm-up used under cold conditions allowed for a greater power output (W) as measured on a force plate. Cold exposure without the warm-up resulted in a power output of 4,517 W, whereas cold exposure with the warm-up resulted in a power output of 5,190 W, which was significantly higher. The results of this study demonstrate that before practicing or playing in cold conditions, athletes should perform a dynamic warm-up to optimize performance.

Dixon, P.G., Kraemer, W.J., Volek, J.S., Howard, R.L., Gomez, A.L., Comstock, B.A., Dunn-Lewis, C., Fragala, M.S., Hooper, D.R., Häkkinen, K., and Maresh, C.M. 2010. The impact of cold-water immersion on power production in the vertical jump and the benefits of a dynamic exercise warm-up. *Journal of Strength and Conditioning Research* 24: 3313-3317.

BOX 4.4 RESEARCH

Static Stretching and Sprint Performance

Using static stretching in a warm-up immediately prior to sprinting might not be a good idea. A study involving nationally ranked track athletes showed that using static stretching slowed performance in a 40 m sprint; the second 20 m were most affected by using static stretching as a warm-up (Winchester et al. 2008). Subsequently, a study of the effects of static stretching on sprint speed in collegiate track and field athletes (sprinters and jumpers) showed that 100 m sprint time increased, but not significantly so (Kistler et al. 2010). A significant increase in time (0.03 seconds) occurred in the 20 to 40 m portion of the race. The 0 to 20, 40 to 60, and 60 to 100 m portions of the race were not significantly affected by static stretching. The total time of the 100 m sprint was not significantly affected by static stretching, but it was 0.06 seconds slower.

Both studies used a similar static stretch protocol of alternating the stretching of the legs using four passive static stretch sets that were intended to stretch the calf musculature, hamstrings, and thighs, in that order. Stretches were held for 30 seconds from the time of mild discomfort. Athletes rested for 20 seconds between stretches and 30 seconds between sets. In both of these studies, the static stretching was performed after a dynamic warm-up. This provides strong evidence that, even done after a dynamic warm-up, static stretching can be detrimental to sprint speed. Thus, static stretching should not be performed just prior to sprinting during a pre-event or preworkout warm-up.

Kistler, B.M., Walsh, M.S., Horn, T.S., and Cox, R.H. 2010. The acute effects of static stretching on the sprint performance of collegiate men in the 60- and 100-m dash after a dynamic warm-up. *Journal of Strength and Conditioning Research* 24: 2280-2284.

Winchester, J.B., Nelson, A.G., Landin, D., Young, M.A., and Schexnayder, I.C. 2008. Static stretching impairs sprint performance in collegiate track and field athletes. *Journal of Strength and Conditioning Research* 22: 13-19.

affect performance. For example, PNF stretching can negatively affect vertical jump performance in women (Church et al. 2001).

As previously discussed, small but significant decreases in sprint performances exist when static stretching is performed prior to the sprint (Kistler et al. 2010; Winchester et al. 2008). Additionally, static stretching produced significant decrements in drop jump performance and nonsignificant decreases in concentric explosive muscle performance, but PNF stretching had no significant effect on concentric stretch-shortening cycle muscle performance (Young and Elliott 2001). If the other proposed benefits of a warm-up can be achieved by using predominantly dynamic warm-up activities, then the possible negative acute effect of static stretching on force production can be eliminated (Behm and Chaouachi 2011).

Chronic Stretching

Whether chronic stretching over a longer period of time before workouts affects performance needs further study. How and if chronic stretch training affects performance may depend on the subject population, type of stretching, and other types of training being performed concurrently.

PNF stretching programs performed as separate workouts do not appear to hamper training-related strength, power, or speed performances (Higgs and Winter 2009). Six weeks of static stretching performed four days a week by highly trained female track and field athletes did not appear to improve power or speed performances, but no negative effects were noted (Bazett-Jones, Gibson, and McBride 2008). Nevertheless, the investigators suggested that static stretching should be performed postpractice to avoid any possible negative effects on workout performances.

Examining the effects of static stretching on strength and power without the performance of any other type of training over 10 weeks revealed improvements in flexibility (18.1%), standing long jump (2.3%), vertical jump (6.7%), 20 m sprint (1.3%), knee flexion 1RM (15.3%), knee extension 1RM (32.4%), knee flexion endurance (30.4%), and knee extension endurance (28.5%) (Kokkonen et al. 2007). A study of both static and ballistic stretching in a wide age spectrum (18 to 60 years) over a four-week period showed no effects on strength, power, or length–tension relationships and no differences between static and ballistic training groups (LaRoche, Lussier, and Roy

2008). In total, these results appear to show that the length of stretch training programs, concurrent training status, and when stretching is performed may play significant roles in the effects, if any, on force production. Each form of stretching seems to result in improvements in flexibility that are not detrimental to force or power production unless placed before a strength, power, or speed exercise test (Behm and Chaouachi 2011).

Chronic improvement in flexibility is an important component of physical fitness and needs to be addressed in the context of a resistance training program, especially given that range of movement incapabilities can hamper normal function or sport performance. Importantly, stretch training may have to be maintained because its effects on flexibility have been shown to be lost four weeks after the cessation of a six-week training protocol (i.e., back to pretraining levels) (Willy et al. 2001). In addition, the resumption of training for the same length of time after cessation did not result in any gains beyond the end point of the first six-week stretching program. This means that the participants essentially started over in terms of flexibility. The length and retention of flexibility training adaptations remain relatively unstudied at this point, but care should be taken to consider flexibility maintenance programs once flexibility goals have been met because of the potential loss of range of motion that may occur if flexibility training is discontinued.

Flexibility and Injury

Physical therapists and athletic trainers spend a great deal of time improving the flexibility of targeted areas related to an injury. However, the prevention of injury due to flexibility training before or around a workout or competition is not supported in the scientific literature (Thacker et al. 2004). In a study attempting to address the question of whether flexibility training can prevent injury, 1,538 men were randomized into two groups with a control group performing no stretching and the other group performing 20-second static stretches under supervision for six major muscle groups of the lower limbs (Pope et al. 2000). Ultimately, the inclusion of static stretching did not affect the exercise-related injury incidence, and the authors found that fitness levels may be more important in the prevention of injury than flexibility. The lack of clinical and scientific clarity

for any specific exercise prescription has made it difficult to make evidence-based prescriptions or programs for stretching, yet many warm-up procedures have been proposed (Herman et al. 2012; Stojanovic and Ostojic 2011).

Additionally, stretching immediately before or immediately after exercise does not appear to alleviate delayed-onset muscle soreness after a workout (Herbert, deNoronha, and Kamper 2011). In general, the use of stretching in a warm-up does not appear to influence overuse injury incidence. However, some evidence suggests that pre-event or preworkout stretching can reduce the incidence of muscle strains, but more controlled research is needed for verifying this (McHugh and Cosgrave 2010).

Resistance Training and Changes in Flexibility

It has been known for some time that heavy resistance training results in either an improvement or no change in flexibility (Massey and Chaudet 1956). More recent studies support this contention. An 11-week weight training program (three times per week, three sets of 8RM of exercises stressing all major muscle groups) demonstrated significant increases in ankle dorsiflexion and shoulder extension without any flexibility training (Thrash and Kelly 1987).

Flexibility improved in both young sedentary women (24 to 26 years old) who performed strength training (three sets of 10RM) for eight weeks (Santos et al. 2010) and adult sedentary women (37 years old) who performed strength training (three sets 8- to 12RM in a circuit) for 10 weeks (Monteiro et al. 2008). However, some movements, such as elbow and knee extension and flexion, did not show an increase in flexibility, which is probably related to the structure of these joints (elbow extension is limited by the olecranon contacting the humerus). A resistance training program can enhance flexibility when exercises are performed with a full range of motion (Morton et al. 2011). Even though resistance training can improve flexibility without concurrent flexibility exercises, the use of a stretching program concurrently has been recommended (Garber et al. 2011).

In untrained older people, only small increases in flexibility have been shown in response to a resistance training program (Barbosa et al. 2002;

Fatouros et al. 2002). If increased flexibility is a desired training outcome, flexibility training may need to be performed in addition to resistance training programs, especially in the elderly (Hurley et al. 1995). Older people (>50 years of age) may need an additional stretching program to gain further increases in range of motion (Girouard and Hurley 1995; Vandervoort 2009).

Competitive weightlifters possess average or above-average flexibility in most joints (Beedle, Jesse, and Stone 1991; Leighton 1955, 1957), although differences among athletes who resistance train have been observed (Beedle, Jesse, and Stone 1991). These differences were related to the type of training program performed (e.g., Olympic weightlifting vs. powerlifting). Olympic weightlifters and control subjects had greater flexibility on five flexibility measures, which indicates that powerlifting may require muscle size increases that can partially limit range of motion, or that those who are successful at powerlifting may be genetically or otherwise predisposed to decreased flexibility. In a descriptive study of several groups of athletes, Olympic weightlifters were second only to gymnasts in a composite flexibility score (Jensen and Fisher 1979). Furthermore, as muscle hypertrophy becomes extreme in competitive athletes such as bodybuilders and powerlifters, one might have to add joint-specific range of motion flexibility training and monitor needed ranges of motion. Thus, resistance training alone may not promote flexibility in some highly trained athletes. In some cases, limited range of motion may provide a competitive advantage for certain performances (Kraemer and Koziris 1994). Competitive powerlifters have limited flexibility, which may be due to the competitive task, especially in the upper body (i.e., bench press) (Beedle, Jesse, and Stone 1991; Chang, Buschbacker, and Edlich 1988).

In summary, resistance training alone can increase the flexibility of many joints; however, the resistance training program used and the person's initial level of flexibility affect the degree to which flexibility is increased by resistance training alone. To maintain or even increase flexibility, lifting techniques should stress the full range of motion of both the agonist and antagonist muscle groups, and exercises should be done that strengthen both the agonists and antagonists of a joint (see box 4.5).

BOX 4.5 PRACTICAL QUESTION

Is There Such a Thing as Being Muscle Bound?

The concept of being muscle bound is often associated with resistance training. Some people, including coaches, believe that resistance training results in a decrease in flexibility. Little scientific or empirical evidence supports this contention, provided that stretching is performed as part of a total conditioning program (Todd 1985).

One story is that the term *muscle bound* originated from the marketing wars of the early 1900s between Charles Atlas, who was selling mail order programs consisting of primarily body mass exercises, and Bob Hoffman of York Barbell, a company that sold barbells and weights. The story goes that, to diminish the sales of barbells, Charles Atlas hired a York Barbell lifter and paid him to say that lifting with barbells caused him to become "muscle bound."

Early in the 1950s it was demonstrated that heavy resistance training does not cause a decrease in joint flexibility when full range of motion resistance training was used and muscle groups on each side of the joint were trained (Massey and Chaudet 1956). However, if a movement around the joint is not trained (biceps but not triceps), some loss of flexibility can occur as a result of the overdevelopment of the muscle groups on one side of the joint (Massey and Chaudet 1956). Excessive hypertrophy may cause movement limitations, such as the powerlifter with short arms and very large chest musculature who cannot touch his elbows in front of his chest. Typically, going through the full range of motion with each exercise and performing supplemental stretching exercises limits inflexibility and makes the muscle-bound condition rare.

Massey, B.H., and Chaudet, N.L. 1956. Effects of heavy resistance exercise on range of joint movement in young male adults. *Research Quarterly* 27: 41-51.

Todd, T. 1985. The myth of the muscle-bound lifter *NSCA Journal* 7: 37-41.

Muscle–Tendon Complex

In addition to affecting muscle, training also affects tendons (Finni 2006; Fukashiro, Hay, and Nagano 2006; Nicol, Avela, and Komi 2006). This is in part because, when force is produced, a muscle's contractile forces are transmitted by the tendon to the bone, which results in movement about a joint (except with isometric muscle actions). This interaction of muscle and its tendon is termed the **muscle–tendon complex** (MTC). The study of the MTC has been aided by advances in ultrasound technology (Fath et al. 2010; Magnusson et al. 2008).

Much of the sports medicine literature focuses on MTC **stiffness.** However, it is important to understand that MTC stiffness should not be thought of in the same way that we typically think of the term *stiffness*. In this case, the term is defined as the relationship between the force applied to the MTC and the resultant change in the length of the unit. Thus, if a greater degree of force is needed to produce a given amount of stretch, or change in length, this is termed a stiffer MTC. If less force is needed to produce the same amount of stretch, then the MTC is thought to be more compliant. Short, thick tendons require more force to stretch, whereas long, thin tendons can be readily stretched and absorb more energy, but only a small amount of mechanical energy is recovered when the tendon returns to its original length. Interestingly, passive stretching and increases in ROM may not always reflect decreases in MTC stiffness (Hoge et al. 2010). New approaches to measuring MTC stiffness may well be important markers for tracking the adaptive changes of various conditioning programs (Joseph et al. 2012).

Another property of the MTC is **hysteresis**, or the amount of heat energy lost by the MTC during the recoil from a stretch. When less heat is lost in the recoil from the stretch, the movement is more efficient. With increasing temperature, the viscosity of the tendon lessens, which improves the tendon's response to its stretch and recoil. In part, effective warm-ups attempt to minimize heat loss by decreasing the tendon's viscosity and thereby reducing hysteresis, which can help improve performance (see box 4.3).

The analogy of a rubber band is helpful for understanding stiffness and hysteresis. The more force that is applied, the longer a rubber band or muscle will be stretched; when the rubber band is released, the recoil produces predominantly mechanical energy, although some energy is lost as heat. The mechanical energy contributes to the elastic component of the muscle that is a well-known part of stretch-shortening cycle movements (e.g., the countermovement vertical jump).

Muscle tendon stiffness can be advantageous to certain strength, power, and speed movements (Kubo, Kanehisa, and Fukunaga 2002; Mahieu, et al. 2007), depending on the movement. For example, in running or sprinting, a stiff MTC is beneficial to the ankle and knee, which use very short ranges of motion and have thick tendons. Conversely, joints in the shoulder and hip typically have longer ranges of motion and thinner tendons. Movements such as a serve in tennis may be optimized by an MTC that is more pliant, or less stiff. Thus, MTC stiffness is neither good nor bad; rather, in different movements a stiff tendon may be advantageous and in other movements a compliant tendon is advantageous. Field assessments of MTC status are being developed and will be needed for better prescribing sport-specific exercise protocols.

Training programs can affect the MTC. Resistance training can increase MTC stiffness, and detraining can return it to its pretraining condition (Kubo et al. 2012). Meanwhile, stretching has been shown to decrease MTC stiffness and hysteresis. Although all people can benefit from a decrease in hysteresis, a decrease in MTC stiffness may not be beneficial in some cases, especially just prior to a strength, power, or speed event (Ryan et al. 2008). This reflects the current practice of refraining from performing static stretches immediately prior to strength and power events or training exercises.

Summary

Designing each component of a total conditioning program requires thought and must be put into the context of the physiological demands or performance goals to be addressed. This overview of some of the major factors related to training for increased strength, power, local muscular endurance, cardiorespiratory function, and flexibility reveals that programs must be carefully integrated so they do not interfere with each other. Program designers must address the specific training of each component and also the timing, sequence, and prioritization of the exercise workouts in relation to the goals for each training cycle.

The compatibility of exercise programs is related to the specific demands placed on the neuromuscular unit. High-intensity aerobic training, in the form of longer-duration interval training or high-intensity continuous training, causes some inhibition of the muscle fiber hypertrophy needed for significant increases in muscle strength and power. Exercise training program incompatibility is typically observed in the areas of muscle fiber size increases, power improvements, and strength gains over time. This is most prominent in untrained people beginning a combined program of strength and aerobic training. In athletes, incompatibility might be due to short-term overreaching. The use of more rest days during the week or lower exercise intensities appears to be one way to minimize incompatibility.

Flexibility training can increase the ranges of motion used in sports. Resistance training increases MTC stiffness, whereas stretching typically decreases it. Program design should be based on the trainee's fitness level and the specific demands of the activity or sport to minimize compatibility problems.

SELECTED READINGS

Aagaard, P., and Andersen, J.L. 2010. Effects of strength training on endurance capacity in top-level endurance athletes. *Scandinavian Journal of Medicine and Science in Sports* 20 (Suppl. 2): 39-47.

Anderson, B. 2010. *Stretching*. Bolinas, CA: Shelter Publications.

Baar, K. 2006. Training for endurance and strength: Lessons from cell signaling. *Medicine & Science in Sports & Exercise* 38: 1939-1944.

Behm, D.G., and Chaouachi, A. 2011. A review of the acute effects of static and dynamic stretching on performance. *European Journal of Applied Physiology* 111: 2633-2651.

Bishop, D., Girard, O., and Mendez-Villanueva, A. 2011. Repeated-sprint ability—part II: Recommendations for training. *Sports Medicine* 41: 741-756.

Casa, D.J., Guskiewicz, K.M., Anderson,. S.A., Courson, R.W., Heck, J.F., Jimenez, C.C., McDermott, B.P., Miller, M.G., Stearns, R.L., Swartz, E.E., and Walsh, K.M. 2012. National Athletic Trainers' Association position statement: Preventing sudden death in sports. *Journal of Athletic Training* 47: 96-118.

Cook, G., Burton, L., and Hoogenboom, B. 2006a. The use of fundamental movements as an assessment of function—part 1. *North American Journal of Physical Therapy* 1: 62-72.

Cook, G., Burton, L., and Hoogenboom, B. 2006b. The use of fundamental movements as an assessment of function—part 2. *North American Journal of Physical Therapy* 1: 132-139.

García-Pallarés, J., and Izquierdo, M. 2011. Strategies to optimize concurrent training of strength and aerobic fitness for rowing and canoeing. *Sports Medicine* 41: 329-343.

Hennessy, L.C., and Watson, A.W.S. 1994. The interference effects of training for strength and endurance simultaneously. *Journal of Strength and Conditioning Research* 8: 12-19.

Laursen, P.B., and Jenkins, D.G. 2002. The scientific basis for high-intensity interval training: Optimizing training programs and maximizing performance in highly trained endurance athletes. *Sports Medicine* 32: 53-73.

Nader, G.A. 2006. Concurrent strength and endurance training: From molecules to man. *Medicine & Science in Sports & Exercise* 38: 1965-1970.

Wilson, J.M., Marin, P.J., Rhea, M.R., Wilson, S.M., Loenneke, J.P., and Anderson, J.C. 2012. Concurrent training: A meta-analysis examining interference of aerobic and resistance exercise. *Journal of Strength and Conditioning Research* 26: 2293-2307.

5

Developing the Individualized Resistance Training Workout

After studying this chapter, you should be able to

1. apply the principles of sound program design in order to develop an effective, individualized exercise stimulus,

2. ask the appropriate question that comprise the needs analysis, concerning biomechanical analysis, energy sources and injury prevention,

3. identify and understand the importance of manipulating the acute program variables to effect the acute workout stimuli and program design,

4. understand the specific physiological responses of the acute program variance and their impact on workout and program design,

5. understand the concept of training potential and the different windows of adaptations for different fitness levels and measures, and

6. develop effective individualized training goals that are testable, maintainable, attainable and prioritized.

A resistance training approach that works for one person may not work as well for another. Evaluating training goals and objectives and individualizing workouts is necessary for optimizing any resistance training program. The optimal program is individualized to meet specific goals and then placed into an appropriate periodized training model to optimize adaptations and recovery. **Program design** is a systematic process that uses a sound understanding of the basic principles of resistance training to meet the needs of each trainee. Program variables should be modulated to create an effective individualized exercise stimulus. Thus, a more involved program design system offers a larger tool box to use to develop, prescribe, and then modify resistance training workouts over a training period. This chapter outlines the major variables used in designing a single resistance exercise protocol that will create the exercise stimuli for physiological and performance adaptations to training.

Program Choices

Over the ages, strength has been the subject of myth and legend. Today, intense marketing strategies are used to sell commercial exercise programs, training styles, and equipment to promote muscular fitness and changes in body image. In this time of commercialized gym chains and packaged programs on the Internet, along with infomercials promoting equipment, it is important that trainers be able to systematically analyze the training variables involved in these programs and their potential effects on training adaptations.

Without properly individualized programs, unrealistic training goals may lead to exercise nonadherence when improvements do not meet trainees' expectations. Substantial improvements are often evident in the early phases of training, but such changes cannot be expected to continue with long-term training. Additionally, and potentially more serious, is the fact that overuse syndromes leading to injury may result when the demands of the program are too much for the person to tolerate. Thus, the challenge is to design resistance training programs that are effective, safe, and realistic.

What constitutes the best resistance training program is not a simple question; a host of factors need to be considered, particularly the goals of the trainee. These goals relate to the types of adaptations desired and the genetic potential of the person to attain them. Finally, other factors such as age and sex also play a part in training outcome. Thus, the argument can be made that one best program of exercises, sets, repetitions, and load does not exist.

The next question is whether any given training program will still be effective at another time. Because training goals may change and trainees will become fitter, it is doubtful that a given program will result in the same magnitude of adaptations over time. Thus, **progression**, or making the program more stressful, is an important principle in resistance training. Program designers must use the major principles of resistance training, such as progressive overload, specificity, and variation, while also paying special attention to making changes that meet the changing training goals and fitness level of each trainee. Today individualized programs and progressions are still missing from many programs from commercial fitness to sports.

An almost infinite number of programs can be designed from the many variations in resistance training components. Programs based on sound scientific principles will have positive effects related to the program design. For example, if a trainee uses a light weight and performs a high number of repetitions, local muscular endurance will improve, but little improvement in muscular strength will occur (Anderson and Kearney 1982). Such changes are also reflected at the level of the muscle fiber because light loads produce limited gains in muscle fiber size with training (Campos et al. 2002). These are examples of a specific training adaptation. Adaptations in strength, power, and underlying muscle fibers are predictable from our understanding of the physiological adaptations related to training with light loads (see chapter 3).

The program designer, however, must also consider the differences in the magnitude of the adaptation to training among individuals. For example, a male collegiate cross country runner will not have the same training-related gains in strength or muscle size as a male North American collegiate football player because of dramatic physiological and genetic differences in factors such as muscle fiber number, type, and size. The initial exercise prescription should be based on a scientific understanding of the training goals and acute program variables such as sets, repetitions, rest periods, and exercise choice needed to stimulate a physiological change. However, the training responses of individuals will vary, and exercise protocol may need to be modified if the desired effects are not observed. Each adaptation takes place on a unique time line because neural adaptations happen rapidly and muscle protein accretion leading to muscle hypertrophy takes longer (see chapter 3). Thus, the expectations for change must be kept within the physiological context of each variable's adaptation time course. Furthermore, genetics may also dictate whether the trainee is a low, moderate, or high responder for a given physiological trait such as muscle size or strength (Marshall, McEwen, and Robbins 2011). Such variations have also been seen with maximal oxygen consumption improvements with aerobic training (Skinner et al. 2001).

Some people cannot attain a high degree of improvement for a particular adaptation, such as muscle hypertrophy, because of their inherent genetics. This means that some people will attain their genetic potential more quickly than others with training and can move into maintenance programs for specific variables (e.g., strength in the bench press). Nevertheless, the overall program design can be adjusted over time to optimize each person's physiological potential for a particular training goal. Although it may be possible to predict a certain type of adaptation from a specific program design variable, such as intensity, people vary in the magnitude of change over time. For example, a periodized program that includes three heavy sets of 3- to 5RM will result in increased muscular strength in anyone; however, the degree of increase will vary from person to person.

Several questions remain: In what is the person trying to excel? How are the changes related to the testing outcome? Is testing specific to the task being trained for, or is testing for general fitness? A testing program should be specific to the task in which improvements are desired and should interface with the program design; moreover, the desired training effects of the program must be evaluated individually (Kraemer and Spiering, 2006). Coaches and personal trainers who assert that they do not test because they do not want their trainees to train for the test miss the point of having a valid testing program that reflects the types of physical performance capabilities their trainees are trying to develop. Some may simply not want their programs evaluated, which keeps them from learning what modifications may be necessary.

The absolute magnitude of a training adaptation will vary among trainees in the same training program. Thus, a general program for fitness, a sport, or another activity should be viewed only as a starting point for a trainee, from which the program design is adjusted to match the training needs of that person. Resistance training programs do not have the same objectives: Some are used for maintenance, whereas others are used for long-term, continued physiological development and improved performance. Both maintenance and building programs can occur within the same training program because each addresses unique training goals.

The key to successful program design is effective supervision by qualified coaches and personal trainers. In fact, several studies show that supervision by trained strength conditioning professionals and progression in the intensity and volume of the exercise are needed to cause maximal fitness gains. In men and women, and even in younger athletes (approximately 16 years old), greater strength gains are observed with supervision (Coutts, Murphy, and Dascombe 2004; Mazzetti et al. 2000; Ratamess et al. 2008). Coaches who supervise more than one trainee should try to keep their numbers low. A 1:5 coach-to-athlete supervision ratio produced much better training results than a 1:25 ratio (Gentil and Bottaro 2010). Thus, optimal supervision is one key to program success.

Supervision should include watching the trainee to ensure proper exercise technique and tolerance of the stresses created by the acute program variable combination, as well as to determine the person's ability to perform the workout. Monitoring training logs and the results of each workout to determine the next workout in the overall plan is another important part of the individualization process.

The development of individual training goals for specific training phases or cycles also becomes paramount in long-term program design. Thus, program designers are faced with making appropriate changes in the resistance training program over time to meet the trainee's changing needs and goals. This necessitates making sound clinical or coaching decisions based on a valid initial program design, the ability to monitor and test for progress, and an understanding of the needs and training responses of the trainee. To do this requires a basic understanding of resistance training principles and the underlying theory of the program design process. Also needed is an understanding of the needs of the sport or activity and how to use testing data to monitor the training effects for each person. The process of planning and changing the exercise prescription over time is vital for the ultimate success of any resistance training program (see figure 5.1).

Understanding the factors that go into creating the exercise stimulus is crucial to the success of the program design process. Creating an effective exercise stimulus starts with the development of a single training session directed at specific trainable characteristics, such as force production, power, or hypertrophy (see table 7.2 in chapter 7). Over time changes made in the acute program variables create the progressions, variations, and overloads needed to achieve physiological adaptations and improved performances. The sequence of correctly designed individual workouts makes up a periodized program that produces the desired and expected training outcomes. Thus, the planning process always starts with the individual training session (workout) and the acute program variables chosen to address the goals of the overall training cycle and program.

This chapter addresses the following components of program design: the needs analysis and the acute program variables such as intensity, volume, rest periods between sets and exercises, exercise selection and order, repetition speed, and training frequency.

Needs Analysis

A **needs analysis** is a process that involves answering a series of questions that assist in the design of a resistance training program (see figure 5.2)

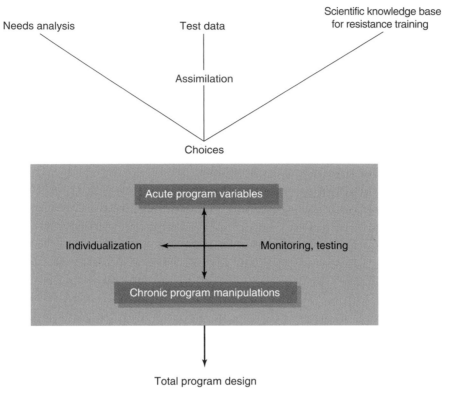

FIGURE 5.1 An exercise prescription model for resistance training.

Needs Analysis	**Acute Program Variables**
Exercise movements (biomechanics)	Choices of exercises
• Specific muscle used	• Structural, whole-body, multijoint
• Joint angles	• Body part, isolated joint
• Muscle action	Order of exercise
Metabolism	• Large-muscle groups first
• ATP-PC system	• Complex technique exercises first
• Anaerobic system	• Arm to leg or upper to lower body
• Aerobic system	• Arm to arm or leg to leg or upper to upper or lower to lower circuit formatting
Injury prevention	Number of sets
• Common sites of injury	Intensity of the dynamic constant external resistance
• Sites of prior injury	Rest period lengths
	• Short: <1 minute
	• Moderate: 2-3 minutes
	• Long: >3 minutes

FIGURE 5.2 A detailed component model for a needs analysis and the acute program variables.

(Kraemer 1983b). Program designers should take the time to examine each of these questions to give themselves a basic context in which to address each of the acute program variables.

The major questions in a needs analysis are as follows:

- What muscle groups should be trained?
- What basic energy sources (e.g., anaerobic, aerobic) should be trained?
- What type of muscle action(s) (e.g., isometric, eccentric) should be trained?
- What are the primary sites of injury for the particular sport or activity, and what is the prior injury history of the person?
- What are the specific needs for muscle strength, hypertrophy, endurance, power, speed, agility, flexibility, body composition, balance, and coordination?

Biomechanical Analysis to Determine Training Needs

What muscle groups should be trained? This first question requires an examination of the muscles and the joint angles that need to be trained. For any activity, including a sport, this involves a basic analysis of the movements performed. At the simplest level, the eyeball technique can be used to determine the movements and muscles activated in a sport or training activity. A fundamental understanding of biomechanics will be of help to further define this analysis.

With today's technology a variety of video analyses can be made, from the simplest (e.g., cell phone video camera, free video phone apps) to the more detailed (i.e., commercial image capture and analysis programs). Videos permit trainers to carefully examine specific aspects of movement patterns involved in activities and sports. Depending on the sophistication of the video capture equipment, they can evaluate the muscles, joint angles, movement velocities, and forces involved. With free video applications on phones, the ability to analyze sport and exercise techniques is now readily available. Video software applications also contain video libraries of proper sport and exercise techniques. In addition, two- and three-camera video biomechanical software for exercise and sport technique analyses is also available at a reasonable cost. These technologies give trainers the opportunity to examine the acute program variables, thereby ensuring that the movements being performed are specific to the task or sport for which the person is training.

The principle of **specificity**, a major tenet in resistance training, states that the exercise program must reflect, in part, the characteristics of the activity or sport for an adequate transfer to occur from the program to the activity. Biomechanical analyses permit the choice of specific exercises that use the muscles and types of muscular actions in a manner specific to the activity for which training is being performed (see box 5.1). Specificity assumes that the muscles used in the sport or activity must be trained in terms of the following:

- Joint around which movement occurs
- Joint range of motion
- Pattern of resistance throughout the range of motion
- Pattern of limb velocity throughout the range of motion
- Types of muscle actions that occur (concentric, eccentric, isometric)

Resistance training for any sport or activity should start with full range of motion exercises around all of the body's major joints. However, training for specific sports or activity movements, such as quarter squats for vertical jumping, should also be included in the workout to maximize the contribution of strength training to specific performance aspects. The best way to select such exercises is to analyze the sport or physical activity biomechanically and to match it to exercises according to the previously mentioned variables. Ideally, exercises are then chosen based on the analyses of the specific muscles used, the muscle action types, and the joint angles. For general fitness and muscular development, the large major muscle groups of the shoulders, chest, back, torso, thighs, and legs are always trained.

The principle of specificity is an overriding rule in the process of designing a resistance training program. Each exercise and resistance used in a program will have various amounts of transfer to the performance of an activity or sport. The amount of transfer will be related to the degree of specificity that can be achieved with the total program design and available equipment. When training for improved health and well-being, the specificity of the training will be related to choosing exercises that can affect a given physiological

❓ BOX 5.1 PRACTICAL QUESTION

Do I Need to Perform Both Flat and Incline Bench Presses?

Given that flat and incline bench presses train the same muscle groups, are both needed? Changing the biomechanics of an exercise does alter the recruitment pattern within the muscles that are involved in performing the exercise. For example, in the bench press the primary muscles involved are the pectoralis major and the anterior deltoid. Although a flat bench press and an incline bench press both use these muscles as primary movers, subtle differences have been seen when their electromyographic (EMG) patterns of activation have been compared (Trebs, Brandenburg, and Pitney 2010). An obvious change in the joint angles and motion between the two bench press exercises exists. But does this translate into different patterns of activation?

In a comparison of the flat bench press and the incline bench press, the activation of the two heads of the pectoralis major (clavicular head and the sternocostal head) and the anterior deltoid show EMG activation differences at different joint angles. Thus, using both exercises in a resistance training program ensures that all of the involved musculature is recruited and therefore trained. Changing the angles of an exercise creates different patterns of recruitment of the involved musculature. In this case, performing both exercises is important to provide for complete neuromuscular activation and fully train the involved musculature. As a resistance training program progresses, additional supplemental exercises should be chosen to stimulate all motor units within the involved musculature and fully train the targeted muscle.

Trebs, A.A., Brandenburg, J.P., and Pitney, W.A. 2010. An electromyography analysis of 3 muscles surrounding the shoulder joint during the performance of a chest press exercise at several angles. *Journal of Strength and Conditioning Research* 24: 1925-1930.

---

variable or desired adaptation. Other acute program variables, such as rest period length between sets and exercises, will also interact with acute and chronic responses of various physiological systems including the metabolic and hormonal systems needed for the support of the motor units recruited with training. Thus, one acute program variable will interact with others to create an integrated stimulus for the workout. The acute program variables are discussed in much greater detail later in this chapter.

The concept of **transfer specificity** refers to the fact that every training activity has a certain degree of carryover to other activities in terms of specificity. Except for practicing the specific task or sport itself, no conditioning activities will have 100% transfer. However, some exercise programs have a much higher degree of carryover to an activity or sport than others do because of greater specificity or similarities in biomechanical characteristics, neuromuscular recruitment patterns, and energy sources. Although specificity is vital for transferring training to performance, some exercise movements (e.g., squat, hang clean, seated row, bench press) and resistance loadings (i.e., from light to heavy) are used for general strength and power fitness. This provides a base for more advanced training techniques. Thus, each training cycle has clear objectives for each of the exercises and the resistance loading chosen.

Sometimes several exercises and loading schemes are required to completely train a movement. In essence, one must typically train the whole concentric force–velocity curve, from low-velocity, high-force to high-velocity, low-force movements, to fully develop the neuromuscular system for transfer to the activity or sport skill. For example, to enhance a vertical jump, power (defined as force × distance / time, or work / velocity) is vital. Heavy resistances are needed to improve the force component of the power equation, which develops maximal concentric and eccentric strength. However, to address the velocity factor in the power equation, one also needs to include high-velocity power movements by doing maximal vertical jumps (plyometrics) or squat jumps at various submaximal percentages of 1RM (e.g., 30 to 50%). This combination of training intensities enhances maximal strength, the rate of force production, and power (see figure 3.26), all of which are needed to enhance vertical jump capabilities (Kraemer and Newton 2000).

Most sport skills cannot be loaded without changing the movement pattern or technique.

For example, if a load is added to a baseball bat (e.g., a weighted ring), the movement pattern of the bat swing will be altered with a slower velocity requiring more force to move the bat. The optimal training program has a solid strength and power training base for all of the major muscle groups and then maximizes specificity to create the greatest carryover to the sport or activity targeted for improvement. Many factors contribute to performance development, including technique, coordination, force production, rate of force development, and the stretch-shortening cycle (Newton and Kraemer 1994). Resistance training addresses some of these factors and improves the physiological potential for performance.

Muscle Actions to Be Trained

Decisions regarding the use of isometric, dynamic concentric, dynamic eccentric, or isokinetic exercise modalities are important in the preliminary stages of planning a resistance training program for sport, fitness, or rehabilitation. The basic biomechanical analysis described previously is used to decide which muscles to train and to identify the type of muscle action(s) involved in the activity. Most activities and resistance training programs use several types of muscle actions, typically including concentric and eccentric along with some isometric.

When training for some tasks, one type of muscle action may receive emphasis to improve performance. For example, one factor that separates elite powerlifters from less competitive powerlifters is the rate at which the load is lowered in the squat and bench press (Madsen and McLaughlin 1984; McLaughlin, Dillman, and Lardner 1977). Elite powerlifters lower the weight at a slower rate than less competitive lifters do, even though the former use greater resistances. In this case, some heavy eccentric training may be advantageous for competitive powerlifters. In wrestling, on the other hand, many holds involve isometric muscle actions of various muscle groups. Therefore, some isometric training will help in the conditioning of wrestlers. It has been shown that isometric grip strength and "bear hug" isometric strength are both dramatically reduced over the course of a wrestling tournament (Kraemer, Fry et al. 2001). This is one example of how a specific movement in a sport can be assessed in the needs analysis and then placed into the program to provide for transfer specificity.

Energy Sources to Be Trained

The performance of every sport and activity derives a percentage of needed energy from all three energy sources (Fox 1979). However, many activities derive the majority of needed energy from one energy source (e.g., energy for the 50 m sprint comes predominantly from intramuscular ATP and PC). Therefore, the energy sources to be trained have a major impact on the program design (see box 5.2). Resistance training typically focuses on the improvement of energy use derived from the anaerobic energy sources (ATP-PC and anaerobic glycolytic energy systems). Improvement of whole-body aerobic metabolism has not been a traditional goal of classic resistance training. However, resistance training can contribute to an improvement in aerobic training as a result of its synergistic effects such as reductions in cardiovascular strain, more efficient recruitment patterns, increased fat-free mass, improved energy economy and efficiency, and improved blood flow dynamics under exercise stress. This is especially true in some populations, such as seniors.

Primary Sites of Injury

Determining the primary sites of injury in an activity, recreational sport, or competitive sport is crucial. This can be accomplished by a literature search or a conversation with an athletic trainer, sport physical therapist, or team physician. The best predictor of future injuries is prior injury, which is why the injury history of the person is important to know. The prescription of resistance training exercises can be directed at enhancing the strength and function of tissues so that they better resist injury or reinjury, recover faster when injured, and suffer less extensive tissue damage when injured. The classic term **prehabilitation** refers to preventing an injury by training the joints and muscles that are most susceptible to injury in an activity. Understanding the sport's or activity's typical injury profile, such as injury to the knee in soccer and wrestling, along with the person's prior history of injury, can help in properly designing a resistance training program.

The fundamental basis for a resistance exercise program designed to prevent injury is the strengthening of tissues so they can better tolerate physical stresses and the improvement of physiological capabilities to repair and remodel tissues. Resistance exercise stress does cause some muscle tissue

For Some Sports, Can an Athlete Use Short-Rest, High-Lactate-Producing Resistance Training All the Time?

A needs analysis of sports that produce high muscle and blood lactate concentrations, such as wrestling, boxing, and 800 m track, might suggest that athletes should perform short-rest, high-lactate-producing resistance exercise protocols all the time. However, every resistance exercise program should be individualized and periodized. The many popular high-intensity commercial programs do not address this issue. Using only one protocol is like using only one tool to build a house. Other protocols are needed to develop maximal strength and power, which provide the basis for both performance and injury prevention. No doubt athletes in such sports need short-rest protocols in their overall training program because this improves buffering capacities, which enhance performance and the tolerance of acidic conditions. Such programs are often used in the weeks leading up to the season because in-season sport practices adequately expose athletes to acidic conditions. Other strength and power capabilities need to be addressed to limit detraining during the season.

Optimal strength and power fitness components cannot be developed under the extreme conditions of fatigue produced with rest period lengths of one minute or less. In addition, the sole use of very low-rest protocols can create an accumulation of fatigue and diminished recovery when high training frequencies (e.g., six days a week) are used, as proposed by some commercial programs. Such workouts also are associated with high physiological stress (e.g., high adrenaline increases, high cortisol increases). Although this is important for stress adaptations, if rest and recovery are not provided in the training model (i.e., periodization), an overreaching or overtraining syndrome can result. More concerning is the potential for rhabdomyolysis if such protocols are used indiscriminately without proper progression and planning.

Many sport coaches do not understand the need for quality training and identify only with a misconceived concept of hard work. Today, too many sport coaches are turning to high-intensity commercial protocols as a result of marketing and the misperception that a real workout leaves the athlete drenched with sweat, exhausted, and maybe even a little sick. Some of the hallmark features of an inappropriate workout are nausea, dizziness, and mental fatigue as a result of inappropriate progressions or less-than-optimal training times, such as right after a holiday break. Although a proper progression of short-rest protocols can help athletes tolerate such physiological conditions, the steady use of *only* these types of very short-rest, high-intensity protocols limit the development of maximal strength and power. This is because trainees can express only a percentage of their maximal strength and power under low-rest conditions during training or competition.

damage. The response to normal breakdown and repair demands with resistance training is mediated in part by many of the inflammatory, immune, and endocrine processes that are involved in the repair of injured tissue. Resistance training can help condition and prepare these systems for the more extensive repair activities needed after injury and may result in faster injury recovery as well as help prevent injury as a result of stronger ligaments, tendons, and muscle tissues.

Other Training Outcomes

Determining the magnitude of improvement needed for variables such as muscle strength, power, hypertrophy, local muscular endurance, speed, balance, coordination, flexibility, and body composition is an important step in the overall process of designing a resistance training program. It may seem reasonable to assume that a resistance training program should improve all of these variables. To do so, various training phases may have to target specific fitness components at particular times over the course of a year. On the other hand, similar improvements in all of these variables may not be needed in all cases. For example, many sports, such as gymnastics, wrestling, and Olympic weightlifting, require a high strength-to-mass or a high power-to-mass ratio. In such cases resistance training programs are designed to maximize strength and power while minimizing increases in body mass. This is evident in sports that have weight classes such as weightlifting, powerlifting, and wrestling and for sports that require maximal sprinting speed or jumping ability (e.g., high jump, long jump), in which increasing body mass may be detrimental to sprint speed as well as maximal jump height or distance. In addition, some sports benefit from increasing body mass, such as North American football, a sport in which the force of impact is greater for a given body mass, assuming power is increased accordingly. Thus, the need for these components of muscular fitness must be evaluated to plan a proper resistance training program.

Program Design

After the needs analysis has been completed, an overall program must be designed. Training phases, or cycles, must be developed to provide variation in the exercise stimuli. Approaches to the "chronic program manipulations," or periodization of the various acute program variables, will be addressed in chapter 7. These workout sequences should address the specific goals and needs of the individual. Acute program variables serve as the framework of one specific resistance training session. Understanding the effects of acute program variables is very important because individual training sessions (workouts) make up all training programs.

Acute Program Variables

As early as 1983, Kraemer developed an approach to evaluating each workout for a specific set of training variables (Kraemer 1983b). Using statistical analyses, he determined that five acute program variable clusters exist, each of which contributes differently to making workouts unique. **The acute program variables** provide a general description of any workout protocol. By manipulating the variables in each cluster, as shown in figure 5.3, trainers can design single workouts. All training sessions result in specific physiological responses and eventually lead to the adaptations these stimuli produce. Therefore, the choices made regarding

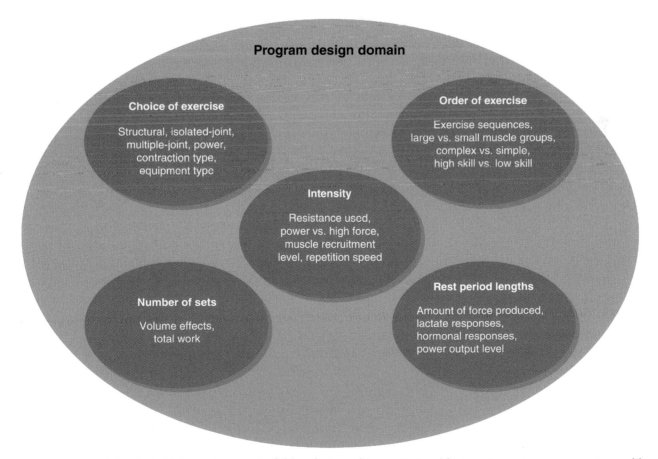

FIGURE 5.3 The clusters of acute program variables that can be manipulated in a resistance training program with example constituent factors to be addressed in each cluster.

acute program variables have an important impact on program design and effectiveness.

Choice of Exercise

As described in the needs analysis, the **choice of exercise** is related to the biomechanical characteristics of the activity. The number of joint angles and exercises is almost limitless. A change in joint angle affects the motor units in the muscle that are activated (e.g., toes pointing in, out, or straight forward during the standing calf raise) (Tesch and Dudley 1994). Motor units containing muscle fibers that are not activated do not benefit from resistance training. Exercises should be selected that stress the muscles and joint angles designated by the needs analysis.

Exercises can be arbitrarily designated as primary exercises or assistance exercises. **Primary exercises** train the prime movers in a particular movement and are typically major muscle group exercises, such as the squat, bench press, and power clean. **Assistance exercises** train predominantly one muscle or muscle group associated with the primary exercise. Exercises can also be classified as structural or body-part. **Structural exercises** include those whole-body lifts that require the coordinated action of more than one joint and several muscle groups. The power clean, power snatch, deadlift, and squat are good examples of structural whole-body exercises.

Exercises can also be classified as **multijoint** or **multi-muscle-group exercises,** which means that they require movement at more than one joint or the use of more than one muscle group. Exercises that attempt to isolate a particular muscle group are known as **body-part, single-joint,** or **single-muscle-group exercises**. The biceps curl, knee extension, and knee curl are examples of single-joint, single-muscle-group or body-part exercises. Many assistance exercises can be classified as body-part, single-muscle-group, or single-joint exercises.

Structural and multijoint exercises require neural coordination among muscles and joints. From an implementation perspective, we do know that multijoint exercises can require a longer initial period of learning, or neural adaptation phase, than single-joint exercises do (Chilibeck et al. 1998). Thus, teaching proper technique is vital during the early phases of training for those who are just being introduced to these types of exercises. However, even though more time may be needed for technique instruction, structural and multijoint exercises are crucial to include when training whole-body strength movements for particular activities. Most sports, military occupational tasks, and functional activities in everyday life (e.g., climbing stairs, getting out of a chair, shoveling snow, lifting grocery bags) depend on structural multijoint movements, which is why such movements are included in most resistance training programs.

In sports, whole-body strength and power movements are the basis for success. For example, running and jumping activities, tackling in North American football and rugby, wrestling skills, and hitting a baseball all require whole-body strength and power. Many times, structural exercises involve the need for advanced lifting techniques, such as power cleans and snatches, which require more technique coaching than simpler exercises do. Teachers and coaches should know how to teach such exercises or identify properly credentialed professionals who can teach and supervise them (e.g., certified United States Weightlifting coaches) before including them in training programs. Dropping them from a program because of a lack of qualified teachers can lower the effectiveness of the program; this is why qualified professionals are often needed for the optimal implementation of a program. For those interested in basic fitness, structural exercises are also advantageous when training time is limited because they allow the training of more than one muscle group with each exercise. The time economy achieved with structural and multijoint exercises is also an important consideration for an individual or team with a limited amount of time per training session.

Muscle Actions

Concentric, eccentric, and isometric muscle actions influence the adaptations to resistance exercise. Greater force is produced during eccentric muscle actions with the advantage of requiring less energy per unit of muscle force (Bonde-Peterson, Knuttgen, and Henriksson 1972; Eloranta and Komi 1980; Komi, Kaneko, and Aura 1987). It has been known for some time that an eccentric component of the repetition is needed to optimize muscle hypertrophy (Dudley et al. 1991; Hather, Mason, and Dudley 1991). Dynamic strength improvements and hypertrophy are greatest when eccentric actions are included in a repetition (Dudley et al. 1991). Thus, each repetition should contain a loaded concentric and eccentric muscle action for optimal results. Some equipment does not produce a loaded eccentric phase of the repetition (e.g., hydraulic and some isokinetic equipment).

Eccentric strength is greater than concentric strength (see figure 3.26) ranging from 105 to 120% of concentric 1RM depending on the exercise. Bodybuilders, powerlifters, long jumpers, figure skaters, and other types of athletes have used such techniques as accentuated negatives, heavy negatives, and "slow negatives" to maximize strength, power, or muscle hypertrophy or to help control deceleration forces with landings (see chapter 2). However, using resistances in excess of concentric 1RM in any exercise must be done with great care because the muscle tissue damage produced can be great. With heavy eccentric resistance exercise, especially in untrained people, delayed-onset muscle soreness can be more prominent than it is following heavy concentric-only actions, isometric training, and normal weight training including heavy concentric and eccentric action (see the discussion of postexercise soreness in chapter 2). In addition, performing a high-intensity training session or performing new exercises at novel joint angles can result in greater muscle soreness when an eccentric action is involved.

Isometric strength increases are specific to the joint angles trained (i.e., angular specificity), but have shown carryover to other joint angles (see the discussion of isometric training in chapter 2). Thus, isometric actions can be used to bring about strength gains at a certain point in the range of motion of an exercise or movement (see the discussion of functional isometrics in chapter 6). As noted previously, isometric training can be important for some sports such as wrestling or recreational activities such as rock climbing because of the importance of isometrics in a sport skill (e.g., grasping and holding in wrestling) or the physical demands of the activity (e.g., grasping a rock in rock climbing).

Order of Exercise

The order of exercise has recently received more attention in the development of a workout routine. Some have theorized that exercising the larger muscle groups first presents a superior training stimulus to all of the muscles involved. This is thought to be mediated by stimulating a greater neural, metabolic, endocrine, and circulatory response, which may augment the training with subsequent muscles or exercises later in the workout.

Exercise order is important in the sequencing of structural or multi- and single-joint exercises. Classically, multijoint exercises, such as the squat and power clean, are performed first followed by the single-joint exercises, such as the biceps curl and knee extension. The rationale for this order is that the exercises performed at the beginning of the workout require the greatest amount of muscle mass and energy for optimal performance. Trainees can develop greater neural stimulation with heavier weights because they are less fatigued at that time.

When structural exercises are performed early in the workout, more resistance can be used because fatigue is limited. To examine this concept, the authors examined the workout logs of 50 American football players performing squats at the beginning of the workout and then at the end of the workout. The players used significantly heavier resistances (195 ± 35 vs. 189 ± 31 kg [430 ± 77 vs. 417 ± 68 lb]) on heavy days (3- to 5RM) when they performed the squats first. Others have demonstrated that more total repetitions can be done if a large-muscle-group exercise, such as the squat, is performed at the beginning rather than at the end of the workout (Sforzo and Touey 1996; Spreuwenberg et al. 2006). Additionally, in an upper-body exercise sequence, more repetitions can be performed of both a large- and small-muscle-group exercise when the exercise is placed at the beginning rather than the end of a workout. The decrease in performance is even greater when only one-minute rest periods are used compared to three-minute rest periods (Miranda et al. 2010; Simão et al. 2007). Interestingly, ratings of perceived exertion (RPE) have not been found to be different with exercise orders, which is most likely due to high RPEs with any heavily loaded resistance exercise (Simão et al. 2007; Spreuwenberg et al. 2006). Thus, the quality of the exercise performance appears to be affected by prior fatigue both in the resistance that can be used and the number of repetitions that can be performed, which affects the total amount of work in the workout.

Order of exercise may also contribute to the concept of **postactivation potentiation** (PAP). Motor units may respond with greater force or power as a result of prior activity (Ebben 2006; Robbins 2005, 2010b). Thus, exercise order can be used to optimize the quality of subsequent force or power production. Complex training, or contrast loading, involves the performance of a strength exercise, such as the squat, and then after a short rest period a power-type exercise, such as the vertical jump. A wide variety of protocols that involve heavy loading before power-type training have been examined (Weber et al. 2008). Many factors are involved including the choice of the exercises, the amount of rest between the exercises, and the loads used in the complex training protocol (see box 5.3). Although complex training appears to increase power output, a general optimal model that works for everyone remains elusive. Thus, when using this training technique, an individualized approach is vital to determine whether an optimal PAP loading sequence exists. Not everyone will respond to this type of training sequence with improved power outputs in the second exercise performed.

Bodybuilders in the United States and weightlifters in the former Soviet Bloc countries have used various types of **pre-exhaustion** training methods that involve performing the small-muscle-group exercises before larger-muscle-group exercises. For example, a single-joint exercise, such as the triceps extension or dumbbell fly, is performed before a multijoint exercise, such as the bench press. The theory is that the fatigued smaller muscles will contribute less to the movement, thereby placing greater stress on other muscle groups. For example, muscular exhaustion during the bench press exercise is often related to fatigue of the triceps muscles. Many bodybuilders include the bench press to maximize hypertrophy of the chest muscles. Therefore, the rationale for performing a single-joint exercise such as the dumbbell fly is to pre-exhaust the chest muscles so that exhaustion during the bench press may be related to chest muscle fatigue

 BOX 5.3 RESEARCH

Choice of Exercise and Rest Period Lengths in Complex Training

Vertical jump performance is very important for many athletes, especially volleyball players. One approach to training is to use a complex training, or contrast loading, exercise order. This involves the performance of a strength exercise, such as the squat, and then, after a short rest period, a power-type exercise, such as the vertical jump (see Complex Training, or Contrast Loading in chapter 6). The mechanism that appears to mediate improvements in power production with prior exercise stress is postactivation potentiation (PAP). Although the theoretical concept has been around for many years, the characteristics of the program design for implementation have been elusive.

One research study gives some clarity to this training concept. NCAA Division I men and women volleyball players were studied to determine the efficacy of specific program characteristics to achieve PAP to enhance performance in the vertical jump (McCann and Flanagan 2010). Finding this optimal sequence would be important to optimize the quality of training for vertical jump performance. Athletes performed either a back squat or a hang clean from the mid-thigh with a resistance equal to 5RM followed by countermovement jumps with either four or five minutes of rest. The protocol that produced the greatest increase in vertical jump ability resulted in an increase of 5.7%. However, no one protocol produced the greatest vertical jump increase in every athlete. This indicates that the increase in power due to various complex training protocols is very individual. A lot of inter-individual variance was observed, indicating that there may be responders and nonresponders to each of the protocols. The conclusion is that complex training does increase power output, but the exact optimal protocol is not known and varies from person to person. Thus, coaches and trainers need to individualize program design when using complex training methods and directly evaluate the efficacy for each athlete. Additionally, complex training does appear to acutely increase power output, but no general prescription has yet been found that maximally increases power in all people (Robbins 2005).

McCann, M.R., and Flanagan, S.P. 2010. The effects of exercise selection and rest interval on postactivation potentiation of vertical jump performance. *Journal of Strength and Conditioning Research* 25: 1285-1291.

Robbins, D.W. 2005. Postactivation potentiation and its practical applicability: A brief review. *Journal of Strength and Conditioning Research* 19: 453–458.

as opposed to fatigue of the triceps. Pre-exhaustion of the chest musculature with flys did not significantly change electromyography (EMG) activity in the pectoralis major or anterior deltoid, but EMG activity in the triceps brachii did increase (Brennecke et al. 2009). Thus, the muscles that were pre-exhausted did not show increased EMG activity, but the muscle that was not pre-exhausted did. Practically, pre-exhaustion often results in a decrease in the amount of resistance used in the large-muscle-group exercise, which raises doubt as to its use in pure strength training.

Another method of pre-exhaustion involves fatiguing synergistic, or stabilizing, muscles before performing the primary exercise movement. An example is performing the lat pull-down or military press before the bench press. However, in one study this popular concept was brought into question because one set of a leg press exercise with and without a pre-exhaustion exercise consisting of one set of a knee extension, showed that muscle activation as measured by electromyography (EMG) of the quadriceps was less and fewer repetitions were performed when the antagonists were pre-exhausted (Augustsson et al. 2003). Thus muscles that are pre-exhausted may not experience increased activation.

The priority system, which involves focusing on the exercises performed first or early in the workout, has also been used extensively in resistance training (see Priority System in chapter 6). This system allows the trainee to use heavier resistances for the exercises performed early in the workout, thereby eliminating the issue of excessive fatigue. A corollary to the priority system is sequencing power exercises (e.g., power clean, plyometrics) so they are performed early in a session. This allows the lifter to develop and train maximal power before becoming fatigued, which hinders the training effects. However, in some instances, power-type exercises may be performed later in the session to improve anaerobic conditioning. For example, basketball players must not only have a high vertical jump, but also be able to jump during an overtime period when fatigued. In this instance, power exercises such as plyometrics may be performed later in the session to train the ability to develop maximal power of the lower limb under conditions of fatigue. However, some exercises, such as the Olympic lifts, may suffer severe technique degradation under extreme conditions of fatigue, heightening the potential for orthopedic

injury. Such a sequence should be used only as an adjunct to optimizing power development and care must be taken with regards to the choice of exercises used. Additionally, the fitness state of the athlete and program progression need to be carefully considered and planned for.

Another consideration in the exercise order is placing exercises that athletes are just learning, especially those with complex movements, near the beginning of the exercise order. For example, if an athlete is learning how to perform the power clean, this exercise would be placed in the beginning of the workout so that learning will not be inhibited by fatigue. During the learning phases of any lift, proper technique is important to master, and fatigue will have a negative effect on that learning.

The sequencing of exercises also applies to the order of exercises used in various types of circuit weight training protocols. The question of whether to follow a leg exercise with another leg exercise or to proceed to another muscle group has to be addressed (see the discussion of alternating muscle group order in chapter 6). The concept of pre-exhaustion discussed earlier can come into play here. Alternate muscle group ordering, such as arm-to-leg ordering, allows for some recovery of one muscle group while another is working. This is the most common order used in circuit weight training programs. Beginning lifters are less tolerant of arm-to-arm and leg-to-leg exercise orders or stacking exercises for a particular muscle group because of high blood lactate concentrations (10-14 mmol $\cdot$ L^{-1}), which is representative of high acidic conditions, lower buffering capacities, and high ATP turnover, especially when rest periods between exercises are short (60 seconds or less) (Kraemer et al. 1990, 1991; Roberts, Ghiasvand, and Parker 2004). However, stacking exercises is a common practice among elite bodybuilders in an attempt to increase muscular definition and reduce body fat during the "cut" phases of a training program leading to a competition. Normally, an alternating order of arm to leg or upper to lower body is used initially; then, if desired, stacked orders are gradually incorporated into the training program.

When functional strength (i.e., high transfer specificity) is the emphasis, basic strength and power exercises such as the squat, power clean, and bench press should be performed early in the workout. Training for enhanced speed and power typically necessitates the performance of total-body explosive lifts such as the power clean and jump squat near the beginning of a workout. Improper sequencing of exercises can compromise the lifter's ability to perform the desired number of repetitions with the desired resistance. Even more important, if fatigue is too great, alterations in exercise technique can lead to overuse syndromes or injury. Therefore, exercise order needs to correspond with specific training goals. A few general methods for sequencing exercises for both multi- and single-muscle-group training sessions are as follows:

- Large-muscle-group before small-muscle-group exercises
- Multijoint before single-joint exercises
- Alternating of push and pull exercises for total-body sessions
- Alternating of upper- and lower-body exercises for total-body sessions
- Exercises for weak points (priority) performed before exercises for strong points (of an individual)
- Olympic lifts before basic strength and single-joint exercises
- Power-type exercises before other exercise types

One final consideration about exercise order is to be aware of the fitness and training state of the trainee. The negative effect of fatigue on exercise technique can result in overuse or acute injury. As discussed earlier, training sessions should never be too stressful for the person, especially a beginning trainee or one who is coming off an extended break or an injury.

Number of Sets

All exercises in a training session need not be performed for the same number of sets. This concept was discussed in chapter 2. The number of sets is one of the factors affecting the volume of exercise (e.g., sets multiplied by repetitions multiplied by weight), or in other words, the total work (joules) performed. Typically, three to six sets are used to achieve optimal gains in strength, and the physiological responses appear to be different with three versus one set of exercises in a total-body workout (American College of Sports Medicine 2009; Gotshalk et al. 1997; Mulligan et al. 1996). It has been suggested that multiple-set systems work best for developing strength and local muscular endurance (American College of Sports Medicine 2009; Atha 1981; Kraemer 1997), and the gains will be made at a faster rate than those achieved through single-set systems (McDonagh and Davies 1984).

In many training studies, one set per exercise performed for 8- to 12RM at a slow velocity has been compared to both periodized and nonperiodized multiple-set programs. Figure 5.4 shows representative studies of a continuum of untrained to trained men and women that demonstrate the superiority of multiple-set programs for short-term and long-term strength improvement. The representative studies are listed in table 5.1.

Studies examining resistance-trained people have shown multiple-set programs to be superior for strength, power, hypertrophy, and high-

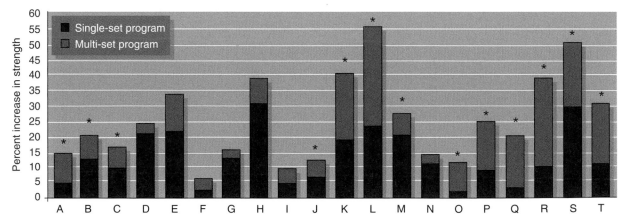

FIGURE 5.4 A comparison of muscle strength increases following single-set and multiple-set resistance training programs. Studies are arranged from short-term (six weeks) to long-term (nine months). Data presented are the mean percentage increases across all exercises used in testing for each study.

* = a difference between single-set and multiple-set programs.

TABLE 5.1 Comparative Examination of the Effects of Single- and Multiple-Set Programs on Strength Increase

Study	General protocol	Author	% increase (MS; SS)
A	1 × 6- to 9RM vs. 3 × 6- to 9RM in moderately trained (MT) women	Schlumberger, Stec, and Schmidtbleicher 2001	15%; 6%
B	1 × 7- to 7RM vs. 3 × 7- to 7RM of leg exercises In UT men	Paulsen et al. 2003	21%; 14%
C	1 × 10- to 12RM vs. 3 × 10- to 12RM and a periodized program in untrained (UT) men	Stowers et al. 1983	17.5%; 12.5%
D	1 × 10- to 12RM vs. 3 × 6RM in UT men	Silvester et al. 1984	25%; 24%
E	1 × 8- to 12RM vs. a periodized program in UT women	Sanborn et al. 2000	34.7%; 24.2%
F	1 × 7- to 12RM vs. 2 and 4 × 7- to 12RM in MT men	Ostrowski et al. 1997	7%; 4%
G	1 × 10- to 12RM vs. 2 × 8- to 10RM in UT men	Coleman 1977	15%; 16%
H	1× to failure (as many as possible) with 60-65% of 1RM vs. 3 × 6 (80-85% of 1RM) in UT men	Jacobson 1986	40%; 32%
I	1 × 8 to 20RM vs. 3 × 6 (75% of 1RM) in UT men	Messier and Dill 1985	10%; 6%
J	1 × 8- to 12RM vs. 3 × 8- to 12RM in resistance-trained (RT) men	Kraemer 1997	13%; 9%
K	1 × 10 (10RM) to 1 × 7 (7RM) vs. 3 × 10 (10RM) to 3 × 7 (7RM) of leg exercises in UT men	Ronnestad et al. 2007	41%; 21%
L	1 × 8- to 10RM, 6- to 8RM, 4- to 6RM vs. 3 × 8- to 10RM, 6- to 8RM, 4- to 6RM in MT men	Rhea et al. 2002	56%; 26%
M	1, 2, or 3 × 2-, 6-, or 10RM in UT men	Berger 1963d	28%; 23%
N	1 × 8- to 12RM vs. 3 × 8- to 12RM in MT men and women	Hass et al. 2000	13%;14%
O	1 × 8- to 12RM vs. a periodized program in RT men	Kraemer 1997	12%; 4%
P	1 × 8- to 12RM vs. 3 × 10RM and a periodized program in RT men	J.B. Kramer et al. 1997	25%; 12%
Q	1 × 8- to 12RM vs. a periodized program in RT men	Kraemer 1997	21%; 6%
R	1 × 8- to 12RM vs. a periodized program in UT women	Marx et al. 2001	40%; 13%
S	1 × 8- to 12RM vs. 3 × 8- to 12RM in UT men and women	Borst et al. 2001	51%; 31%
T	1 × 8- to 12RM vs. a periodized program in RT women	Kraemer et al. 2000	31%; 14%

MS = multiple set; SS = single set; RT = resistance trained; UT = untrained; MT = moderately trained.

intensity endurance improvements (e.g., Kraemer 1997; Kraemer et al. 2000; J.B. Kramer et al. 1997; Krieger 2010; Marx et al. 2001; McGee et al. 1992). These findings have prompted the American College of Sports Medicine (2009) to recommend periodized multiple-set programs when long-term progression (not maintenance) is the goal. With one exception, to date, the percentage gains in multiple-set programs are higher than those in single-set programs in short-term and long-term training studies in untrained and trained people.

Short-term and all long-term studies support the contention that training volume greater than one set is needed for improvement and progression in physical development and performance, especially after the initial training period starting from the untrained state. As noted in chapter 2, meta-analyses have demonstrated that for both trained and untrained people, multiple sets per muscle group elicit maximal strength gains. It must be kept in mind that these meta-analyses examined the number of sets per muscle group and not per exercise. Interestingly, one meta-analysis showed that untrained subjects experienced greater strength increases with increased volume (i.e., four sets vs. one set; Rhea et al. 2003). Two other meta-analyses demonstrated that about 40% greater hypertrophy and 46% greater strength gains occur with multiple-set training compared to single-set training in both trained and untrained subjects (Krieger 2009, 2010). Nevertheless, because the need for variation (including variation in volume during some training phases) is so critical for continued improvement, single-set or low-volume training might be useful during some workouts or training cycles over the course of an entire macrocycle. The key factor is periodization in training volume, rather than only increasing the number of sets, which represents only one factor in the volume and intensity equation in any periodization model.

Considering the number of variables involved in resistance training program design, comparing single- and multiple-set protocols may be an oversimplification. For example, several of the aforementioned studies compared programs that used different set numbers regardless of differences in intensity, exercise selection, and repetition speed. In addition, the use of untrained subjects during short-term training periods has also raised criticism (Stone et al. 1998), because untrained subjects have been reported to respond favorably to most programs (Häkkinen 1985).

In advanced lifters, further increases in volume may be counterproductive, but the correct manipulation of both volume and intensity seems to produce optimal performance gains and avoid overtraining (Häkkinen, Komi et al. 1987; Häkkinen, Pakarinen et al. 1988a). Yet one study showed that trained people may need in excess of four sets per exercise to see improvements in maximal squat strength (Marshall, McEwen, and Robbins 2011).

Multiple sets of an exercise present a training stimulus to the muscle during each set. Once initial fitness has been achieved, a multiple presentation of the stimulus (three or four sets) with specific rest periods between sets (to allow the use of the desired resistance) is superior to a single presentation of the training stimulus. Some advocates of single-set programs believe that a muscle or muscle group can perform maximal exercise only for a single set; however, this has not been demonstrated. In fact, highly trained bodybuilders (Kraemer, Noble et al. 1987) and athletes trained to tolerate short-rest-period protocols (Kraemer 1997) can repeat multiple sets at 10RM using the same resistance with as little as one minute of rest between sets.

Exercise volume is a vital concept of training progression. This is especially true in those who have already achieved a basic level of training or strength fitness. The interaction of the number of sets with the principle of variation in training, or more specifically, periodized training, may also augment training adaptations. The time course of volume changes is important to the change in the exercise stimulus in periodized training models. A constant-volume program may lead to staleness and lack of adherence to training. Ultimately, varying training volume by using both high- and low-volume protocols to provide different exercise stimuli over a long-term training period is important to provide rest and recovery periods. This is further discussed in chapter 7.

The number of sets performed per workout for multiple-set programs is highly variable and has not received much attention in the literature. In general, this number is affected by (1) the muscle groups trained and whether large- or small-muscle-mass exercises are performed; (2) the intensity of training; (3) the training phase (i.e., whether the goal is strength, power, hypertrophy, or endurance); (4) the training frequency and workout structure (e.g., total-body vs. upper- or lower-body splits vs. muscle group split workouts or two workouts in one day); (5) the level of conditioning; (6) the number of exercises in which a muscle group is involved; (7) the use of recovery strategies such as posttraining feedings; and (8) the use of anabolic drugs (which enable lifters to tolerate higher-than-normal training volumes). The number of sets is based on the individual lifter and depends on the needs analysis, phase of the training program, administrative factors, and other aforementioned factors.

Rest Periods Between Sets and Exercises

The effect of rest period length on bioenergetics, the acute hormonal response, and other physiological factors was discussed in detail in chapter 3. Rest period length between sets and exercises is an important acute program variable in workout design. It can affect the intensity used and the safety of lifters if it results in the degradation of exercise technique (for reviews, see de Salles et al. 2009; Willardson 2006).

Rest periods between sets and exercises determine the magnitude of ATP-PC energy source resynthesis and the concentrations of lactate in the muscle and blood. A short rest period between sets and exercises significantly increases the metabolic, hormonal, and cardiovascular responses to an acute bout of resistance exercise, as well as the performance of subsequent sets (Kraemer 1997; Kraemer, Dziados et al. 1993; Kraemer, Noble et al. 1987; Kraemer et al. 1990, 1991; Rahimi et al. 2010). Differences based on training background were noted in athletes who took three- versus one-minute rest periods between sets and exercises (Kraemer 1997). All of the athletes were able to perform 10 repetitions with 10RM loads for three sets with three-minute rest periods for the leg press and bench press. However, when rest periods were reduced to one minute, 10, 8, and 7 repetitions per set were performed in the first to third sets, respectively. When rest periods of one minute are compared to those of three minutes, fewer repetitions are performed by trained men in an upper-body workout (Miranda et al. 2007). Figure 5.5 shows

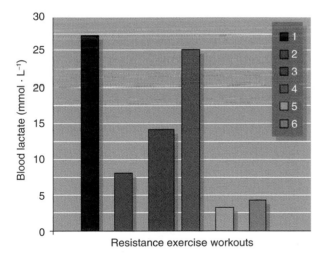

FIGURE 5.5 Average immediate postexercise lactate responses to various resistance exercise protocols with the first 4 workouts using short rest periods and the last 2 using long rest periods: (1) bodybuilding workout; (2) low-intensity circuit weight training; (3) high-intensity circuit weight training; (4) short-rest, high-intensity workout; (5) powerlifting; and (6) Olympic weightlifting.

Data from Kraemer et al., 1987; Gettman and Pollock 1981; and Keul et al. 1978.

the blood lactate response to exercise protocols using rest periods of various lengths. Thus, rest period length affects many physiological variables and fatigue level during a training session.

For advanced training emphasizing absolute strength or power, rest periods of at least two minutes are recommended for structural exercises such as squats, power cleans, and deadlifts, using maximal or near-maximal loads; less rest may be needed for smaller-muscle-mass exercises or single-joint movements (American College of Sports Medicine 2009; de Salles et al. 2009). Advanced lifters may require longer rest periods to accompany the heavy loads they need to cause strength gains. This is largely because these loads are near the lifter's genetic potential, and to attain these force levels, maximizing energy store recovery is crucial (de Salles et al. 2009).

When two- versus five-minute rest period lengths were used with recreationally weight-trained men, no differences were observed in hormonal responses to loading, gains related to muscle size and strength, or resting hormonal concentrations over six months of training (Ahtiainen et al. 2005). Three-minute rests resulted in a 7% increase in squat performance after five weeks of training, compared to a 2% increase as a result of 30-second rest periods (Robinson et al. 1995).

The role of rest period lengths has also been examined with isokinetic training. Quadriceps peak torque has been shown to significantly increase from 170 to ~198 Nm (14.1%) with 160 seconds of rest compared to a non-significant increase of 160 to 175 Nm (8.6%) with 40 seconds of rest. The amount of total work performed was greater with long rest periods than with short rest periods (13.2 vs. 7.2%, respectively), and power increased to a similar extent with both rest periods (Pincivero, Lephart, and Karunakara 1997). The role of short rest periods in an isokinetic training program was supported when it was again found that peak torque and average power of the quadriceps at 60 degrees per second increased only 0.7% using a short (40-second) rest period between sets but increased 5.9 and 8.1%, respectively, using a long (160-second) rest period (Pincivero et al. 2004). Rest periods of 60 seconds and less may have a dramatic impact on the intensity of the exercise and therefore will compromise the achievement of maximal strength and power development. Furthermore, very short rest periods may well compromise the technique of many lifts.

For novice to recreationally trained lifters, at least two minutes of rest may be needed to allow the recovery of force production necessary to optimize strength development.

Strength and power performance is highly dependent on anaerobic energy metabolism, primarily the ATP-PC (phosphagen energy) system. The majority of phosphagen repletion seems to occur within three minutes (Dawson et al. 1997; Fleck 1983; Volek and Kraemer 1996). In addition, removal of lactate and H^+ may require at least four minutes (Robinson et al. 1995). The performance of maximal lifts requires maximal energy substrate availability before sets, and this requires relatively long rest periods. Stressing the glycolytic and ATP-PC energy systems may enhance training for muscular endurance, and thus, less rest between sets appears to be effective (Kraemer 1997; Kraemer, Noble et al. 1987). Again, caution is needed regarding the choice of exercises and the intensity used to limit technique problems during the exercises.

Several studies (Kraemer et al. 1990, 1991; Kraemer, Fleck et al. 1993) have used various combinations of resistance and rest period lengths in a workout to investigate the acute blood lactate responses. These comparisons indicate that higher volumes of work result in higher blood lactate concentrations especially when short rest periods are used. These studies also indicate that a heavier resistance does not necessarily result in higher blood lactate concentrations. The effects of various rest period lengths between sets and exercises on blood lactate have been shown to be similar for both sexes. It appears that the amount of work performed and the duration of the force demands during a set influence the acute blood lactate concentrations. Therefore, when using a three-set format, a 10RM resistance allows for a relatively higher number of repetitions per set but still maintains the use of a relatively high percentage of the 1RM (75 to 85% of 1RM), which results in high blood lactate concentrations, especially when short rest period lengths are used. Thus, when two workouts use identical exercises, rest period lengths of two minutes, and equal total work, if heavier resistances are used, the acute blood lactate response is higher compared to when lighter resistances are used. This is true even though the lighter resistances result in greater power output. This indicates that force production has a more dominant influence than power on the glycolytic

demands of a workout (Bush et al. 1999).

From a practical standpoint it has been demonstrated that short-rest programs can cause greater psychological anxiety and fatigue (Tharion et al. 1991). This might be related to the greater discomfort, muscle fatigue, and high metabolic demands that occur when using very short rest period protocols (i.e., one minute and shorter). The psychological ramifications of using short-rest workouts must also be carefully considered when designing a training session. The increased anxiety appears to be due to the dramatic metabolic demands characterized by workouts using rest periods of one minute or less. Although the psychological stresses are higher, the changes in mood states do not constitute abnormal psychological changes and may be a part of the arousal process before a demanding workout.

Intense exercise results in high concentrations of hydrogen ions, decreases in pH, dramatic increases in the stress hormones epinephrine and cortisol, and increases in blood lactate (Gordon, Kraemer, and Pedro 1991; Kraemer, Noble et al. 1987). Such changes indicate severe metabolic stress, and performance depends on the body's buffering systems, such as bicarbonate buffering in the blood and phosphate and carnosine in the muscle, to tolerate such stress. Despite such physiological mechanisms, fatigue and performance decrements occur under such conditions. Workouts using rest periods of less than one minute and with a moderate to high volume of exercise result in metabolic and psychological stress as described earlier and possible severe health risks, especially when they are performed at the beginning of a training program or immediately after a break in training (see box 6.5 in chapter 6). The use of short-rest programs has become popular in many commercial programs and often for so-called work hardening in athletics and military training. However, nausea, dizziness, and vomiting are signs of being sick and overshooting one's physiological capabilities to cope with the stress, not of a good workout. Proper progression and appropriate frequency of such programs are needed. Otherwise, overuse, overreaching, or injury can occur.

Progressing from longer rest periods to shorter ones is important. Adverse symptoms, such as dizziness, light-headedness, nausea, vomiting, and fainting, need to be monitored during and after workouts (de Salles et al. 2009; Willardson 2006). Short-rest protocols must be carefully placed into an overall training program, and rest period length should be further decreased only when the symptoms mentioned earlier are not present. In sports in which athletes train and compete year-round, coaches should not add more of the same training stimuli. For example, wrestling practices and matches produce high glycolytic demands on the lactic acid system. Wrestlers who compete almost year-round do not also need short-rest protocols in the weight room. Recreating the same stimuli in the weight room is not beneficial or time effective; plus, it might lead to overreaching or overtraining. The time may be better spent working on basic strength and power attributes, the training for which requires long rest periods (e.g., three to five minutes) between sets and exercises. If short-rest workouts are desired, they should be performed within the larger context of a strength or power training program for sport (e.g., one or two short-rest workouts and two strength or power workouts in a week cycle) or as part of an 8- to 12-week preseason program. This is especially beneficial in sports in which athletes need to develop a tolerance of acidic conditions and their sport-specific training does not address this need in practices or competitions.

Short rest period length is also characteristic of circuit weight training (see Circuit System in chapter 6), but the resistances are typically lighter (i.e., 40-60% of 1RM) and sets may not be performed to concentric failure (Gettman and Pollock 1981). Such workouts do not result in as high a blood lactate concentration as do very short-rest, multiple-set 10RM workouts during which sets are carried to or close to failure. These circuit weight training workouts do not result in the fatigue caused by the short-rest, moderate- to high-volume programs discussed earlier.

Short rest periods affect the quality of a repetition or the power produced. See figure 5.6 for a comparison of repetition quality under various rest period conditions. The quality of a repetition is important, especially for maximal power development because submaximal power and velocities in the performance of a repetition do not enhance maximal power development. Fatigue affects the quality of the repetition. To develop maximal power and strength, trainees need to achieve optimal motor unit recruitment, or full recruitment, with the exercise stimuli. Such recruitment requires a longer rest period between sets (de Salles et al. 2009; Willardson 2006).

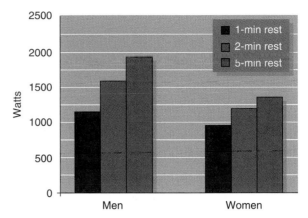

FIGURE 5.6 Average power per set in a squat jump using three sets at 60% of 1RM squat in trained men (*n* = 10) and women (*n* = 10) who were collegiate soccer athletes using various rest periods between sets. Significant (*p* ≤ .05) differences were observed between rest period lengths, and men demonstrated significantly higher power outputs at each rest period length than women did.

Courtesy of Dr. William J. Kraemer, Department of Kinesiology, University of Connecticut, Storrs, CT.

Rest period length influences many physiological and biomechanical factors of the workout. People use short rest periods primarily to enhance their buffering capacity to better tolerate activities and sports that place high demands on the anaerobic energy system. Today, many use this program design variable to enhance the perception of a hard workout or for metabolic caloric expenditure. However, short rest periods keep trainees from activating all of the motor units needed for strength and power development. Additionally, there is the increased potential for overuse or injury, or both, when short rest periods are used randomly or without an understanding of how to safely progress from longer periods to shorter ones.

Resistance Used (Intensity)

The amount of resistance used in any exercise is one of the most important variables in a resistance training program. It determines the number of motor units recruited, and only those motor units will benefit from the exercise performed (see the discussion of motor units in chapter 3). Historically, it has been one of the most examined acute program variables (Atha 1981; McDonagh and Davies 1984).

Designing a resistance training program includes choosing a resistance for each exercise. As discussed in chapter 2, one can use either repetition maximums (RMs) or the **repetition maximum (RM)**

target zone (e.g., 3 to 5RM).The goal of using RM target zones is to ensure staying within a repetition range while not necessarily going to failure in each set, and simultaneously making sure the resistance used does not result in performing fewer or more repetitions than prescribed. If fewer or more repetitions are performed, the resistance must be changed for the subsequent set or the next time the exercise is performed. One can also choose the resistance as a percentage of the 1RM and then perform a certain number of repetitions per set. Any of these methods allows for individual progression within a workout and between workouts and makes a training log an important evaluation tool in resistance load progressions.

In general, research has supported the basis for a repetitions-per-set continuum (see figure 5.7) (Anderson and Kearney 1982; Atha 1981; Clarke 1973; McDonagh and Davies 1984; Weiss, Coney, and Clark 1999). As heavier weights are used, more motor units are recruited in the muscle, resulting in more fibers undergoing training adaptations. Most of the studies historically examined nonvaried programs using the same resistance load over the entire training program. Advanced periodization models have used various training intensities spanning the entire force–velocity curve. Significant strength increases have been reported using a variety of resistance loads across the repetition continuum, but the magnitude of the increase is determined by the training level of the person (American College of Sports Medicine 2002; Delorme and Watkins 1948; Kraemer 1997; Kraemer, Fleck, and Evans 1996; Staron et al. 1994). Lighter loads (i.e., 12RM and lighter) have smaller effects on maximal strength in previously untrained people (Anderson and Kearney 1982; Weiss, Coney, and Clark 1999), but have proven to be very effective for increasing local muscular endurance (Campos et al. 2002; Stone and Coulter 1994). Using a variety of resistance loads appears to be more conducive to increasing muscular fitness than performing all exercises with the same load or constant resistance. No doubt, to optimize strength and muscular development, heavier sets are needed. Periodized training that includes resistance load variation appears most effective for long-term improvements in muscular fitness (see chapter 7). Nonvaried, or constant, load training over long periods of time is not consistent with training progression recommendations (American College of Sports Medicine 2009; Garber et al. 2011).

As lifters move away from six repetitions per set or fewer, with heavier weights, to lighter resistances and more repetitions, gains in strength diminish until they are negligible. The strength gains achieved above 25 repetitions per set are typically small to nonexistent in untrained people (Atha 1981; Anderson and Kearney 1982; Campos et al. 2002) and perhaps are related to enhanced motor performance or neural learning when they

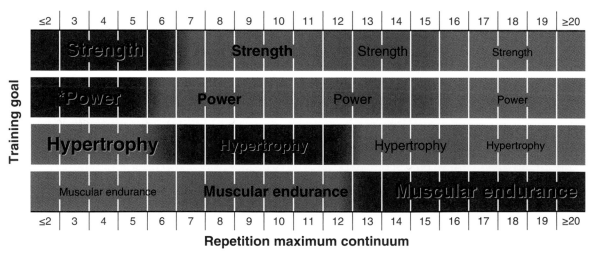

FIGURE 5.7 Theoretical repetitions-per-set continuum. Maximal power gains are made performing relatively few repetitions per set, and power improvements are specific to the resistance load on the force–velocity curve. See chapter 3 for further explanations on training goals.

do occur. A variety of individual responses due to genetic predisposition and pretraining status affect the training increases observed. After initial gains have been made as a result of neural or learning effects, primarily due to the eccentric phase of the repetition, heavier resistances are needed to optimize muscle strength and size gains. Historically, some have posited that going to failure with a lighter weight (e.g., 30-50%) will result in the further recruitment of the higher-threshold motor units used for heavier resistances. As discussed earlier, training study data are not consistent with such claims. This is further supported by electromyographic data (EMG). Even when one has been prefatigued prior to the performance of a lighter set of 50% of 1RM, the EMG does not reflect any higher motor unit recruitment. The same is also seen when performing the light resistance load to failure by itself (see figure 5.8).

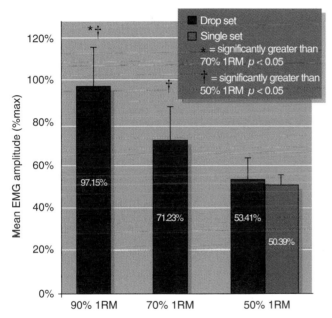

FIGURE 5.8 Electromyographic (EMG) data from the vastus lateralis muscle when performing a Smith machine squat using 90% of 1RM; then 70% of 1RM and then 50% of 1RM in a continuous drop set sequence. Increases are shown in each bar graph. Significance is also noted. The EMG amplitude is highest with the 90% of 1RM resistance, and even with prefatigue, the motor unit activation for the 50% of 1RM does not recruit more motor units. Percentages in the bars denote the percent of maximal motor unit recruitment for each intensity. Ratings of perceived exertion were similar when going to failure in this experiment showing that failure at any load gives the false perception of maximal recruitment.

Courtesy of Dr. William J. Kraemer, Department of Kinesiology, University of Connecticut, Storrs, CT.

Using percentages of 1RM is another common method of determining resistances for an exercise (e.g., 70 or 85%). If the trainee's 1RM for an exercise is 100 lb (45.4 kg), an 80% resistance would be 80 lb (36.3 kg). This method requires that maximal strength in lifts used within the training program be evaluated regularly. If 1RM is not tested regularly (weekly), the percentage of 1RM used in training will not be accurate. Thus, training intensity will be reduced and the lifter will be in danger of training with a less than optimal load. This is an especially important consideration at the beginning of a program. From a practical perspective, use of percentages of 1RM as the resistance for many commonly performed exercises (e.g., knee extension, upright row) may not be administratively effective because of the amount of testing time required. Use of an RM target or RM target zone allows the person to change resistances to stay at the RM target or within the RM target zone, thus developing the characteristics associated with that portion of the repetitions-per-set continuum.

The use of percentages of 1RM resistances is warranted for competitive Olympic lifts (i.e., clean and jerk, snatch, and variations), because these lifts require coordinated movements and optimal power development from many muscles to result in correct lifting technique. The movements cannot be performed at a true RM or complete momentary failure. Drastic reductions in velocity and power output experienced in the last repetition of a true RM set may not be conducive to correct technique in variations of the competitive Olympic lifts (e.g., power clean, hang clean, power snatch, hang snatch). Therefore, the percentage of 1RM is warranted to correctly calculate resistances for such lifts.

In two classic studies (see table 5.2), Hoeger and colleagues (1987, 1990) examined the use of appropriate exercises in the RM loading approach, the relationship between the percentage of 1RM, and the number of repetitions that both trained and untrained men and women could perform. This relationship varied with the amount of muscle mass needed for performing the exercise (i.e., leg presses require more muscle mass than knee extensions). When using machine resistances with 80% of 1RM, previously thought to be primarily a strength-related prescription, the number of repetitions the subjects could perform was typically greater than 10, especially for large-muscle-group exercises such as the leg press. The

TABLE 5.2 Number of Repetitions That Can Be Performed to Failure With a Set Percentage of 1RM

	40% x ± SD	60% x ± SD	80% x ± SD	1RM[b] x ± SD
Untrained males, n = 38				
LP	80.1 ± 7.9A[a]	33.9 ± 14.2A	15.2 ± 6.5A	137.9 ± 27.2
LD	41.5 ± 16.1B	19.7 ± 6.1B	9.8 ± 3.9B	59.9 ± 11.6
BP	34.9 ± 8.8B	19.7 ± 4.9B	9.8 ± 3.6B	63.9 ± 15.4
KE	23.4 ± 5.1C	15.4 ± 4.4C	9.3 ± 3.4BC	54.9 ± 13.3
SU	21.1 ± 7.5C	15.0 ± 5.6C	8.3 ± 4.1BCD	40.9 ± 12.6
AC	24.3 ± 7.0C	15.3 ± 4.9C	7.6 ± 3.5CD	33.2 ± 5.9
LC	18.6 ± 5.7C	11.2 ± 2.9D	6.3 ± 2.7D	33.0 ± 8.5
Trained males, n = 25				
LP	77.6 ± 34.2A	45.5 ± 23.5A	19.4 ± 9.0A	167.2 ± 43.2
LD	42.9 ± 16.0B	23.5 ± 5.5B	12.2 ± 3.72B	77.8 ± 15.7
BP	38.8 ± 8.2B	22.6 ± 4.4B	12.2 ± 2.87B	95.5 ± 24.8
KE	32.9 ± 8.8BCD	18.3 ± 5.6BC	11.6 ± 4.47B	72.5 ± 19.8
SU	27.1 ± 8.76CD	18.9 ± 6.8BC	12.2 ± 6.42B	59.9 ± 15.0
AC	35.3 ± 11.6BC	21.3 ± 6.2BC	11.4 ± 4.15B	41.2 ± 9.6
LC	24.3 ± 7.9D	15.4 ± 5.9C	7.2 ± 3.08C	38.8 ± 7.1
Untrained females, n = 40				
LP	83.6 ± 38.6A	38.0 ± 19.2A	11.9 ± 7.0A	85.3 ± 16.6
LD	45.9 ± 19.9B	23.7 ± 10.0B	10.0 ± 5.6AB	29.2 ± 5.6
BP	[c]	20.3 ± 8.2B	10.3 ± 4.2AB	27.7 ± 23.7
KE	19.2 ± 5.3C	13.4 ± 3.9C	7.9 ± 2.9BC	26.7 ± 7.8
SU	20.2 ± 11.6C	13.3 ± 8.2C	7.1 ± 5.2C	19.3 ± 8.3
AC	24.8 ± 11.0C	13.8 ± 5.3C	5.9 ± 3.6C	13.8 ± 2.7
LC	16.4 ± 4.4C	10.5 ± 3.4C	5.9 ± 2.6C	15.8 ± 3.7
Trained females, n = 26				
LP	146 ± 66.9A	57.3 ± 27.9A	22.4 ± 10.7A	107.5 ± 16.0
LD	81.3 ± 41.8B	25.2 ± 7.9CB	10.2 ± 3.9C	34.8 ± 6.0
BP	[c]	27.9 ± 7.9B	14.3 ± 4.4B	35.6 ± 4.9
KE	28.5 ± 10.9C	16.5 ± 5.3ED	9.4 ± 4.3CD	40.3 ± 10.2
SU	34.5 ± 16.8C	20.3 ± 8.1CD	12.0 ± 6.5CB	23.8 ± 6.4
AC	33.4 ± 10.4C	16.3 ± 5.0ED	6.9 ± 3.1ED	17.3 ± 3.8
LC	23.2 ± 7.7C	12.4 ± 5.1E	5.3 ± 2.6E	21.7 ± 5.0

LP = leg press (knees apart at a 100° angle for the starting position); LD = lateral pull-down (resistance pulled behind the head to the base of the neck); BP = bench press; KE = knee extension; SU = sit-up (horizontal board, feet held in place, knees at a 100° angle, and resistance held on chest); AC = arm curl (low pulley); LC = leg curl (to 90° of flexion).

[a]Letters indicate significantly different groupings: alpha level = 0.05; same letter = no difference.

[b]1RM expressed in kg.

[c]Data unobtainable because of resistance limitations on the Universal Gym equipment.

Adapted, by permission, from W.W.K. Hoeger, et al., 1990, "Relationship between repetitions and selected percentages of one repetition maximum: A comparison between untrained and trained males and females," *Journal of Applied Sport Science Research* 4: 47-54.

larger-muscle-group exercises appear to need much higher percentages of 1RM to stay within the strength repetitions-per-set zone, or any other zone, of the repetitions-per-set continuum.

It has been shown that powerlifters can lift 80% of their 1RM in the leg press for 22 repetitions, or a 22RM, and untrained controls can perform only 12 repetitions at 80% of their 1RM, or a 12RM (Kraemer et al. 1999). Such data, along with the data presented in the two previous studies (Hoeger et al. 1987, 1990), clearly indicate that if the percentage of 1RM method is used in determining the resistance for a specific number of repetitions, it must be carefully considered for each muscle group and for each type of lift and the exercise mode used (e.g., free weight squat vs. leg press machine). It is also important to note the great deal of variation in the number of repetitions possible at a specific percentage of 1RM, as shown by the large standard deviations in table 5.2. These results beg the question, Even though a high percentage of the 1RM was used, will performing 22 repetitions per set result in optimal strength increases? Although some have postulated that high-repetition training (e.g., 30RM) is useful for strength development, training data do not support this contention (Anderson and Kearney 1982; Campos et al. 2002).

Based on the repetitions-per-set continuum, 22 repetitions per set is primarily related to the development of local muscular endurance and not optimal for the development of maximal strength and power. In general, a certain percentage of 1RM with free weight exercises will allow fewer repetitions than the same percentage of 1RM on a similar exercise performed on a machine (see table 1.1). This is due, most likely, to the need for greater balance and control in three planes of movement with free weights. With machines, control of movement is generally needed in only one spatial plane. This relationship between the number of repetitions performed at a given percentage of 1RM is different when using free weights, as noted in chapter 1 (Shimano et al. 2006).

The U.S. National Football League's 225 lb (102 kg) test is popular for predicting the 1RM bench press score of North American football players based on the maximal number of repetitions performed with this weight (Hetzler et al. 2010). Also, charts or prediction equations are often used to predict the 1RM strength from the maximal number of repetitions performed with submaximal loads (Mayhew, Ball, and Bowen 1992; Shimano,

Kraemer et al. 2006; Morales and Sobonya 1996; Ware et al. 1995). One of the most popular prediction equations for many exercises is the Epley equation. Using the maximal number of repetitions performed using a given weight, it provides an estimate of 1RM strength (Epley 1985). The equation is as follows:

$$1RM = [(0.033 \times \# \text{ of reps}) \times (\text{weight})] + \text{weight}$$

Charts and equations provide only an estimate of 1RM, and some are closer than others for particular exercises (for a review, see Shimano et al. 2006). Any prediction of 1RM is more accurate the fewer the number of repetitions performed, which means lifting a heavier weight to failure. It appears that 1RM prediction is most accurate when three to five repetitions are performed and 80 to 85% of 1RM is used (Brechue and Mayhew 2009, 2012).

It is obvious that the amount of weight lifted in a set is highly dependent on other acute program variables such as exercise order, muscle action, repetition speed, and rest period length (Kraemer and Ratamess 2000). Thus, the repetitions-per-set zone, or number of repetitions possible at a specific percentage of 1RM, is affected by whether an exercise is performed early or late in a training session.

The resistance required to increase maximal strength may depend on training status. Beginning lifters with no prior resistance training experience need a minimal resistance of 40 to 50% of 1RM to increase dynamic muscular strength (American College of Sports Medicine 2009; Baechle, Earle, and Wathen 2000; Garber et al. 2011). However, experienced lifters need greater resistances to realize maximal strength gains (American College of Sports Medicine 2009). Häkkinen, Alen, and Komi (1985) reported that at least 80% of 1RM was needed to produce any further neural adaptations in experienced weight trainers. The need for increased intensity (percentage of 1RM) as training progresses is shown by the results of a meta-analysis (Rhea et al. 2003). A mean training resistance of 60% of 1RM resulted in maximal strength in untrained people, whereas a mean training resistance of 80% of 1RM produced maximal strength in trained people. Neural adaptations are crucial to resistance training, because they precede hypertrophy during intense training periods. Thus, a variety of resistances, and so percentages of 1RM, appear necessary to optimally increase both neural function (i.e., increased motor unit recruitment, firing rate, and synchronization) and hypertrophy. No matter how the training resistance is chosen, a proper training progression is needed for safe long-term fitness gains.

Repetition Speed

The speed used to perform dynamic muscle actions, or **repetition speed,** affects the adaptations to resistance training. Repetition speed is dependent on training resistance, fatigue, and goals and has been shown to significantly affect neural (Eloranta and Komi 1980; Häkkinen, Alen, and Komi 1985; Häkkinen, Komi, and Alen 1985), hypertrophy (Coyle et al. 1981; Housh et al. 1992), and metabolic (Ballor, Becque, and Katch 1987) adaptations to resistance training. Force production and repetition speed directly interact during exercise performance. Generally, concentric force production is higher at slower speeds and lower at higher speeds. This relationship is graphically represented as a force–velocity curve (see figure 3.26). The implications of the force–velocity curve demonstrate that training at slow velocities with maximal force is effective for strength training, and training at higher velocities is effective for power and speed enhancement. This generally is the case; however, training with a variety of velocities may be most effective for optimizing both strength and power development.

A distinction needs to be made between intentional and unintentional slow-speed repetitions. Unintentionally slow lifting speeds are dictated by the resistance used during heavy repetitions, such as 1- to 6RMs. In this case, resistance loading, fatigue, or both, are responsible for the longer repetition duration (i.e., slow speed). For example, the concentric phase of a 1RM bench press and the last repetition of a 5RM set may last three to five seconds (Mookerjee and Ratamess 1999). This may be considered slow; however, lifting the weight faster is not possible under these high-force requirement conditions. This type of unintentionally slow lifting speed in the concentric phase of the repetition is a function of the force–velocity curve and the fatigue pattern leading to failure in a heavy set of multiple repetitions. In other words, the force needed for a 5RM is high, and the velocity at which it can be moved is therefore slow. With each consecutive repetition to a point of failure, the velocity continues to decrease (Sanchez-Medina and Gonzalez-Badillo 2011). This is

typical of any set in which failure (i.e., RM) is the targeted end point: Repetition velocity slows down progressively.

The speed at which repetitions are performed does change the qualities of the repetitions, such as power output and maximal force. A comparison of Smith machine bench press repetitions using 55% of 1RM with both the eccentric and concentric phases lasting five seconds (slow training velocity), 30% of 1RM with the concentric phase performed in a ballistic manner so that the bar was thrown into the air and then caught before performing the eccentric phase of each repetition (power training), and six repetitions with a 6RM resistance (traditional heavy weight training) revealed differences in the qualities of repetitions (Keogh, Wilson, and Weatherby 1999). Both slow training velocity and power training resulted in significantly lower levels of force during both the eccentric and concentric phases of repetitions and lower levels of electromyographic (EMG) activity than traditional heavy weight training did. When compared to traditional heavy weight training, time under tension was longer during slow training and shorter during power training. Understanding that differences do occur in the force and power measures based on the way the repetition is performed, and the fact that this may well affect the specific training adaptation from a training program, is of vital importance when instructing and implementing a workout protocol.

Significantly reducing the resistance used is an inevitable result of intentionally performing repetitions slowly. It has been shown that intentionally slowing down a conventional load in an exercise results in significantly fewer repetitions (Hatfield et al. 2006). In a study in which subjects performed the squat and shoulder press at 60 and 80% of 1RM using volitional and an intentional very slow speed of 10 seconds for both the concentric and eccentric phases of the repetition, significantly fewer repetitions were completed with the intentional slow repetition speed (i.e., squat, 60% of 1RM; super slow, 5RM; volitional speed, 24RM, 80% of 1RM; super slow, 2RM; normal volitional speed, 12RM). In addition, power output was dramatically reduced for each set, and total work was reduced with the intentional slow training. Only one study has shown slow training to be superior (Westcott et al. 2001) to traditional training speeds in strength development. Most others have found slow velocity training to be less than optimal compared to traditional training for strength increases (Keeler et al. 2001; Rana et al. 2008).

Intentionally slow-speed repetitions must be performed with submaximal loads so the lifter has greater control of the repetition speed; such repetitions do result in longer time under tension. However, during this time under tension predominantly the lower-threshold motor units are recruited and trained. Thus, intentionally slow lifting may be most suitable for increasing local muscular endurance when using lighter resistances.

Both fast and moderate lifting speeds can increase local muscular endurance depending on the number of repetitions performed and the rest taken between sets and exercises. Interestingly, slow-speed training (6- to 10 RM, 10-second concentric, 4-second eccentric) has been shown to improve local muscular endurance but not more than traditional loading (6- to 10RM, one-second concentric, two-second eccentric) or traditional local muscular endurance (20- to 30RM) training protocols (Rana et al. 2008). Training with volitionally fast speeds is the most effective way to enhance muscular power and speed, and it is also effective for strength enhancement (Morrissey et al. 1998; Thomas et al. 2007). However, such training is not as effective for increasing hypertrophy as slow or moderate speeds are (Häkkinen, Komi, and Alen 1985), most likely because fewer high-threshold motor units are recruited because of lower force demands. High-speed repetitions impose fewer metabolic demands in exercises such as the leg extension, squat, row, and arm curl compared to slow- and moderate-speed repetitions (Ballor, Becque, and Katch 1987). In addition, when periodization is not used during short-term training programs, training for power is best accomplished by lifting lighter weight (30% of 1RM) with maximal speed (Wilson et al. 1993).

Self-paced pull-ups and push-ups result in more total work, more repetitions performed, and greater power output in less time than exercises performed at a pace of 2 seconds for both the concentric and eccentric phases (2/2 cadence) and 2 seconds and 4 seconds, respectively, for the concentric and eccentric (2/4 cadence) phases (LaChance and Hortobagyi 1994). The self-paced cadence was at a faster repetition velocity than the other two cadences. The number of repetitions, total work, and power output of the 2/2 cadence were midway between those of the self-paced and 2/4 cadence. Regardless of the format, artificial pacing (e.g., counting, using a metronome) always results in motor learning challenges as the person attempts to meet the external cues. With resistance exercise, it affects the characteristics of the set performed.

Historically, another technique that has been used for both strength and power training is **compensatory acceleration** (Hatfield 1989; Wilson 1994). This requires the lifter to accelerate the load maximally throughout the exercise's range of motion (regardless of momentum) during the concentric repetition phase, striving to increase velocity to maximal levels. However, care must be taken to avoid injury and joint stress. Heavier resistances are needed when using this technique so as not to create undue joint stress in exercises that end with the weight being held or still in contact with the limb and the joint being fully locked out (e.g., bench press, leg press, leg extension). A major advantage of this technique is that it can be used with heavy loads and is quite effective with multijoint exercises (Jones et al. 1999). Accordingly, Hunter and Culpepper (1995) and Jones and colleagues (1999) reported significant strength and power increases throughout the range of motion when lifters used compensatory acceleration; the increases were significantly greater than those achieved by training at a slower speed (Jones et al. 1999). Having the cognitive intention to attempt to maximally accelerate even the heaviest resistance loads may provide additional neurological stimulation.

Repetition speed affects training outcomes. Generally, faster concentric repetition speed should be used when training for power increases. The resistance used will affect how fast it can be moved (i.e., force–velocity curve). For general fitness, normal or volitional repetition velocities can be used. Super slow repetitions may be useful for local muscular endurance training but offer no advantage when training for strength or muscle hypertrophy (see Super Slow Systems in chapter 6).

Rest Periods Between Workouts (Training Frequency)

The number of training sessions performed during a time period, such as a week, may affect subsequent training adaptations (see the discussion of dynamic constant external resistance training in chapter 2). Frequency is best described as the number of times certain exercises or muscle groups are trained per week, and it is based on several factors such as volume, intensity, exercise selection, level of conditioning or training status, recovery ability, nutrition, and training goals. Typically, an exercise is used two days per week (Peterson 2004). Reduced frequency is adequate if the goal of training is to maintain adaptations (e.g., maintenance training). Training one or two days per week may be adequate for mass, power, and strength retention (Zatsiorsky 1995). However, this appears to be effective only for short-term periods, as long-term maintenance training (i.e., reduced frequency and volume) leads to detraining.

A frequency of two or three times per week has been shown to be very effective initially and has been recommended by the American College of Sports Medicine (American College of Sports Medicine 2009; Garber et al. 2011). This has been supported by many resistance training studies that have used frequencies of two or three alternating days per week with untrained subjects (Dudley et al. 1991; Hickson, Hidaka, and Foster 1994). Some studies have shown that training three days a week is superior to training two days a week (Graves et al. 1989), whereas training three to five days a week was superior in other studies (Gillam 1981; Hunter 1985). A meta-analysis indicates that for untrained subjects a training frequency of three times per week of a muscle group produces maximal strength gains (Rhea et al. 2003). The progression from beginning to intermediate lifting does not necessitate a change in frequency, but may be more dependent on alterations in other acute variables such as exercise choice, volume, and intensity. However, intermediate lifters commonly train three or four days a week. Increasing training frequency allows for greater volume and specialization or greater exercise choice per muscle group, greater volume in accordance with more specific goals, or both.

Many intermediate lifters use an upper/lower body split or muscle group split routine. Similar improvements in performance have been observed between an upper/lower split routine and a total-body workout in untrained women (Calder et al. 1994). In addition, similar muscle groups or selected exercises are not recommended to be performed on consecutive days during split routine programs to allow adequate recovery and minimize the risk of nonfunctional overreaching or overtraining. Furthermore, a recovery day is even more important when training involves intense, short-rest metabolic workouts (e.g., Monday, strength and power workout; Tuesday, short-rest metabolic workout; Wednesday, rest; Thursday, strength and power workout; Friday, short-rest metabolic workout; Saturday and Sunday, rest) (Kraemer, Patton et al. 1995).

Training frequency for advanced or elite athletes may vary considerably (depending on intensity, volume, and goals) and is typically greater than the training frequency of intermediate lifters. Frequencies as high as 18 sessions per week have been reported in Bulgarian weightlifters (Zatsiorsky 1995), but this is an extreme example.

One aspect of frequency that must always be kept in mind is how many times per week a muscle group is trained. In many situations, the higher total frequencies of advanced lifters are achieved by performing sessions dedicated to specific muscle groups (i.e., body-part programs). A meta-analysis showed that the optimal frequency for trained people was two days per week per muscle group and not three days per week, as shown for untrained people (Rhea et al. 2003). The lower frequency for the trained people was in part due to a higher training volume per session. One study demonstrated that American football players training four or five days a week achieved better results than those self-selecting frequencies of three and six days a week (Hoffman et al. 1990). However, each muscle group was trained only two or three days per week. Weightlifters and bodybuilders typically use high-frequency training (i.e., four to six sessions per week). Two training sessions per day have been used (Häkkinen, Pakarinen et al. 1988a; Zatsiorsky 1995) during preparatory training phases, which may result in 8 to 12 training sessions per week (see Two Training Sessions in One Day in chapter 7).

The rationale for high-frequency training is that frequent, short sessions followed by periods of recovery, supplementation, and food intake enhance the quality of high-intensity training as a result of maximal energy recovery and reduced fatigue during exercise (Baechle, Earle, and Wathen 2000). Greater increases in muscle size and strength have been shown when training volume was divided into two sessions per day as opposed to one in female athletes (Häkkinen and Kallinen

1994). In addition, exercises (i.e., total-body lifts) performed by Olympic weightlifters require technique mastery, which may increase total training volume and frequency. Elite powerlifters typically perform four to six sessions per week (Kraemer and Koziris 1992). It should be noted that training at such high frequencies would result in nonfunctional overreaching or eventually to overtraining in most people if high volumes are implemented without progression. The superior conditioning of elite athletes as a result of years of training progression and genetic predisposition may contribute to the successful use of very high-frequency programs.

Historically, anabolic drug use also may have aided recovery and the tolerance of extremely high volumes and frequencies of training. Without anabolic drug use, optimal nutritional strategies are crucial for supporting such training programs. Advanced periodized training cycles now use more variations in training volume and frequency to alter the exercise stimulus, enhance the exercise stimulus, and provide adequate natural recovery between sessions. Training with heavy loads necessitates increased recovery time before subsequent sessions, especially those that involve multijoint exercises. This may be primarily due to the greater resistance during the eccentric portion of the repetition. Studies show that eccentric exercise is more likely to cause delayed-onset muscle soreness (DOMS) than concentric-only training (Ebbling and Clarkson 1989; Fleck and Schutt 1985; Talag 1973). Eccentric training causes greater muscle fiber and connective tissue disruption, greater enzyme release, DOMS, and impaired neuromuscular function, which limits force production and range of motion (Saxton et al. 1995). Thus, recovery times of at least 72 hours may be required before initiating another session requiring several heavy sets or supramaximal eccentric lifts (Zatsiorsky 1995).

A study of untrained subjects compared frequencies of one day per week to two or three days per week (Sorichter et al. 1997). Each session consisted of seven sets of 10 one- to two-second eccentric-only muscle actions of the quadriceps. Both training groups showed strength improvement after training. However, the results showed that eccentric training once a week was effective for maintenance, whereas eccentric training twice a week was more effective for strength increases. Thus, the inclusion of heavy eccentric repetitions may necessitate a change in frequency (or the muscle groups trained per session) compared to normal concentric–eccentric resistance training or the use of periodized lighter loads that do not recruit the muscle fibers that are part of the high-threshold motor units involved with high force production but also more prone to tissue damage.

Training frequency may need to be adjusted based on the type of training program. Meta-analyses indicate that an optimal training frequency for highly resistance-trained people is two days per week per muscle group; this is likely due to the use of greater training volumes per session (Peterson et al. 2003; Rhea et al. 2003). Frequency may also need to be adjusted based on training experience. Higher frequencies of four to six sessions per week may be needed in highly resistance-trained people to cause further gains (American College of Sports Medicine 2009). Additionally, two sessions per day may also be useful as an advanced training strategy (see Two Training Sessions in One Day in chapter 7).

Training frequency should be carefully matched with the goals and targeted outcomes of the trainee. Using periodized training models, the person's needs and goals (e.g., for a particular physiological or performance variable) should determine the amount of exercise. Progression in frequency is a key component in successful resistance training programs. Frequency of training will vary depending on the phase of the training cycle, the fitness level of the person, the goals of the program, and the person's training history. Careful choices need to be made regarding rest days between training days to avoid overreaching or overtraining syndromes. These choices should be based on the progress toward specific training goals and the tolerance of the person of the changes made. Excessive soreness the morning after a workout may indicate that the exercise stress is too demanding. If this is the case, the workout loads, sets, rest periods between sets, and training frequency need to be evaluated and adjusted. Additionally, trainers should always remember that many younger people have a great potential to tolerate errors in training, but physiologically they may not be adapting positively to the program. Thus, monitoring progress and understanding the types of stresses associated with each workout design is vital to successful progressions.

Summary of Acute Program Variables

The following acute program variables are addressed in the design of a resistance training workout:

- Exercise and muscle groups trained
- Order of exercise
- Number of sets and set structure
- Rest periods
- Load or resistance used
- Repetition speed

The configuration of these variables determines the exercise stimulus for a particular workout. Since workouts should periodically be altered to meet changing training goals and to provide training variation, this paradigm is also used to describe, modify, and control resistance exercise programming. Finally, rest and recovery between workouts is important, and the implementation of planned rest and recovery periods may promote more effective periodization, and thus greater training adaptations.

Many workouts are possible with the manipulation of the preceding variables. Understanding the influence and importance of each is vital for optimizing specific training goals and for providing variation in workout design, which is important for periodization of training.

Using the acute program variables to develop workouts that enhance certain characteristics is vital to physical development. It is also possible to train different muscles or muscle groups in different ways resulting in programs for different muscle(s) with different training goals. For example, a person could train the chest muscles for maximal strength while training the leg muscles for power and the abdominal muscles for local muscular endurance. Proper manipulation of the acute program variables when developing a single workout, and changing the workout over time (i.e., periodization) are the basis of successful program design. No one should use the same resistance training program for long periods of time. Claims of a single program's superiority, often seen in magazines, on the Internet, and elsewhere, are simply marketing or self-promotion and should be viewed with caution.

The prescription of resistance training is both a science and an art. The key is to translate the science of resistance training into the practical implementation in the weight room, thereby bridging the gap between science and practice. Ultimately, individualized programs provide the best results and the best overall training responses. This chapter provides a paradigm for exercise prescription and a framework for the optimal design of resistance training programs.

This paradigm is a general-to-specific model of resistance training progression (American College of Sports Medicine 2009). Beginning programs should be simple until an adequate fitness and strength foundation is built. A simple program may improve all aspects of fitness, especially in untrained people. However, this is not the case with advanced training as more complex program designs are required to meet training or performance goals, or both. As programs progress, more variation should be introduced. With advanced levels of training, great variation is needed because the principle of specificity is an important determinant of further fitness gains. That is, it is virtually impossible to improve in multiple variables of fitness (i.e., strength, size, power, endurance, speed, body composition) at this stage at one time. Thus, specific training cycles need to be included to address each of these variables individually and to ensure progression.

Although guidelines can be given, the art of designing effective resistance training programs comes from logical exercise prescription followed by evaluation, testing, and interaction with the trainee. The prescription of resistance training is a dynamic process that requires the trainee and the strength and conditioning specialist or personal trainer to respond to the changing levels of adaptations and functional capacities of the trainee with altered program designs to meet changing training and performance goals.

Training Potential

The initial gains made during resistance training are large compared to those made after several months or years of training. As training proceeds, the size of gains decreases as the trainee approaches his or her genetic potential (see the top of the curve in figure 5.9). Understanding this concept is important to understanding the adaptations and changes that occur over time. Furthermore, one can see that almost any resistance training program might work for an untrained person in

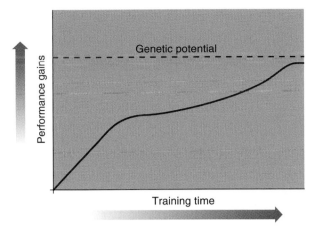

FIGURE 5.9 A theoretical training curve. Gains are made quickly on the lower portion of the curve as people start to train and become slower as they approach their genetic potential.

the early phases of training because the potential for increases in any fitness variable is significant. However, as fitness increases, the need for changes in the acute program variables and periodization becomes very important to bring about further increases in fitness. This is because the window of adaptations gets smaller as a result of training progression (see chapter 7, Advanced Training Strategies).

Window of Adaptation

The opportunity for improvement in a particular variable has been called the window of adaptation (Newton and Kraemer 1994). This means that the more untrained you are, the greater your potential for improvement and so the greater your relative gains will be. In addition, it could also mean that the greater your genetic potential is (e.g., the number of muscle fibers you have), the greater your absolute gains will be. The window of adaptation gets smaller as you train a specific variable and progress toward your theoretical genetic ceiling. Therefore, if at the start of a training program, you already have a high level of adaptation or fitness, the starting window for adaptation will be small. Training expectations must therefore be kept in perspective in terms of both the relative gains that can be made in a specific fitness variable and the absolute gains that can be made starting with a specific genetic predisposition. Furthermore, all training adaptations are specific to the program performed, and not all training improvements are made in the same time frame (e.g., neural versus

hypertrophy; see chapter 3) over the course of a training program.

The window of adaptation concept is exemplified in highly trained athletes, who sometimes experience miniscule gains in a performance variable over a long period of time. In fact, in elite North American college football players, many of the gains occur in the first year or so as a result of being highly trained in high school, which placed them closer to their genetic potential for strength and power (Miller et al. 2002).

The window of adaptation is also different for different fitness measures. College American football players had a choice among frequencies of training per week over a 10-week off-season conditioning program (Hoffman et al. 1990). The groups that chose three and six days a week made no gains in 1RM bench press (see table 5.3). The authors suggested that the three-days-a-week program was not a sufficient stimulus to elicit significant strength improvements in already conditioned athletes who had participated in an intensive in-season heavy resistance training program. The lack of changes in 1RM bench press for players using a six-days-a-week program was postulated to be the result of a short-term overreaching or overtraining syndrome. However, squat strength improved for all groups except the three-days-a-week group, indicating that not all muscle groups (i.e., bench press vs. squat) respond in the same manner to all training programs. Interestingly, none of the groups demonstrated an improvement in 40 yd sprint times, which demonstrates how difficult it is for athletes who already have achieved a high degree of fitness in a particular variable to make improvements consequent to short-term training. Nevertheless, although small changes (e.g., 0.1 second) in a 40 yd dash may not be statistically significant, the practitioner should not overlook the practical importance of such an effect.

Thus, the length of the training program, the fitness level of the athlete in a particular lift or performance task, genetic potential, and the training program design all influence the training adaptations. The expectation of continual large strength or performance gains in all aspects of an athlete's or fitness enthusiast's fitness profile is unrealistic.

Several studies have shown that differences in the rate of fitness improvement can be detected during short-term training. Some short-term training programs produce substantially greater changes in strength than others do (Keeler et al. 2001; Rana

TABLE 5.3 Results of Performance and Anthropometric Testing in College American Football Players Using a Selected Frequency of Training

Variable	Test	3 days	4 days	5 days	6 days
BW (kg)	Pre	80.3 ± 5.1	94.2 ± 12.7	99.2 ± 14.4	112.3 ± 12.4
	Post	79.6 ± 6.4	93.1 ± 12.0*	98.7 ± 13.7	111.0 ± 12.1
BP (kg)	Pre	107.2 ± 11.6	127.7 ± 13.9	131.1 ± 20.1	143.9 ± 12.0
	Post	109.1 ± 28.7	132.2 ± 14.5	135.3 ± 9.0*	149.7 ± 17.3
SQ (kg)	Pre	140.1 ± 18.6	173.6 ± 36.2	170.6 ± 19.4	191.6 ± 34.9
	Post	147.7 ± 38.9	186.3 ± 31.9*	183.4 ± 22.1*	204.1 ± 39.5*
40 (s)	Pre	4.83 ± 0.14	5.01 ± 0.22	4.97 ± 0.23	5.23 ± 0.20
	Post	4.82 ± 0.19	4.97 ± 0.18	4.93 ± 0.24	5.18 ± 0.20
VJ (cm)	Pre	70.2 ± 7.7	65.9 ± 8.4	64.5 ± 8.6	59.9 ± 6.7
	Post	71.7 ± 7.6	66.0 ± 8.8	66.0 ± 7.9	62.5 ± 7.1
2 MI (s)	Pre	933.1 ± 49.7	945.0 ± 61.3	960.8 ± 99.3	982.2 ± 65.0
	Post	811.1 ± 77.1*	830.7 ± 55.5*	834.2 ± 84.8*	879.8 ± 68.7*
SF (mm)	Pre	54.7 ± 12.2	79.7 ± 15.3	83.6 ± 20.0	100.3 ± 13.0
	Post	50.9 ± 10.5*	72.9 ± 12.7*	79.0 ± 19.7*	92.4 ± 15.2*
TH (cm)	Pre	56.0 ± 2.5	59.5 ± 4.6	59.8 ± 4.6	63.9 ± 3.4
	Post	56.7 ± 1.6	61.4 ± 3.5*	61.5 ± 4.2*	65.0 ± 3.2
CH (cm)	Pre	92.8 ± 3.9	103.3 ± 7.2	105.9 ± 8.4	111.9 ± 7.1
	Post	94.8 ± 3.1*	105.5 ± 6.9*	107.1 ± 8.2*	112.3 ± 6.1

* = $p \leq .05$

BW = body weight; BP = bench press; SQ = squat; 40 = 40 yd sprint; VJ = vertical jump; 2 MI = 2 mi run; SF = sum of skinfolds; TH = thigh circumference; CH = chest circumference.

Adapted, by permission, from J.R. Hoffman, et al. 1990, "The effects of self-selection for frequency of training in a winter conditioning program for football," *Journal of Applied Sport Science Research* 4: 76-82.

et al. 2008; Schlumberger, Stec, and Schmidtbleicher 2001; Staron et al. 1994). For example, over 10 weeks of training, a single-set program was superior to a super slow program in untrained women (Keeler et al. 2001). Over six weeks of training, a three-set program was superior to a one-set program in trained women (Schlumberger, Stec, and Schmidtbleicher 2001). This indicates that during the early phase of training the rate of improvement appears to be affected by the type and speed of the muscle action and the volume of training.

Nevertheless, an accumulation, or "banking," of training time is needed to see comprehensive and dramatic differences among various programs over longer training periods. Such long-term training adaptations are also more resistant to the effects of detraining. This concept has been demonstrated over six and nine months. In a nine-month study of collegiate women tennis players, a periodized training program was shown to be superior to a low-volume single-set training program in both the development of muscular strength and power

in addition to improvements in ball velocity in the tennis serve, and forehand and backhand strokes (Kraemer et al. 2000). In a six-month training program untrained women showed similar findings in the performance of a 40 yd sprint, body composition measures, and strength and power measures, demonstrating that a periodized multiple-set training program was superior to a low-volume single-set circuit-type program (Marx et al. 2001). Thus, certain training principles (e.g., specificity, periodization, volume of exercise) appear to affect the rate and magnitude of fitness gains observed over a given training period. However, in both studies it took two to three months before superiority of the periodized program was shown in some fitness measures, demonstrating that long training periods may be needed before training programs start to differentiate themselves and show differences in fitness gains. This is most likely because in the early phase of training almost any program will produce rapid gains, which may mask the differences among programs.

Setting Program Goals

An effective resistance training program requires specific goals. Factors such as age, physical maturity, training history, and psychological and physical tolerance need to be considered in any goal development process and individual program design. In addition, designers must prioritize goals so that training programs do not compete for adaptation priority (e.g., endurance training reduces power development). Among the many common program goals in resistance training that are related to improvements in function are increased muscular strength, increased power, increased local muscular endurance, and improvements in physiological training effects such as increased fat-free mass. Other functional gains such as increases in coordination, agility, balance, and speed are also common goals of conditioning programs, especially for athletes. In addition, it is becoming clear that fitness attributes such as balance may also have important implications for injury prevention, such as limiting falls in older people or preventing knee injury in athletes. Other physiological changes related to increased fat-free mass through muscle hypertrophy or the improvement of other physiological functions such as lower blood pressure, decreased body fat, and increased resting metabolic rate to help with long-term weight control are also goals of resistance training programs. Resistance training affects almost every physiological function and can enhance physical development and performance at all ages (Kraemer, Fleck, and Evans 1996; Kraemer and Ratamess 2004).

For the most part, training goals should be testable variables, such as 1RM strength, power, vertical jump height, and body composition, so trainers can judge objectively whether gains are made. The examination of a workout log can be invaluable in evaluating the effects of a resistance training program. Formal tests to determine functional changes in strength can be performed on a variety of equipment, including isokinetic dynamometers, free weights, and machines (Kraemer, Ratamess, Fry, and French 2006). Examining the results of specific tests can help both trainers and trainees modify the exercise program if improvements are not being made or decide whether to repeat a program in which the trainee was unsuccessful.

In some cases training for high-level sport performance does not coincide with improving health. Many elite athletes train excessively (e.g., lifting seven days a week or running 100 miles in a week or training four to six hours a day), more than what they need to optimize their health and general fitness. In fact, short-rest-period, high-volume (termed *extreme fitness*) programs performed without proper preparation and recovery can lead to acute overreaching if not serious muscle damage and injury. The goals in resistance training have to be put into the context of the desired outcome for the person. For example, trying to gain maximal amounts of body mass (including fat and muscle) to be a lineman in American football may not be healthy; however, large athletes are sought after at the college and professional levels (Kraemer and Gotshalk 2000). In this case, health and sport fitness goals may not be compatible. The competitive athlete must seriously consider whether training for a sport career will be detrimental to a healthy lifestyle after the career is completed. Not much is known about detraining "bulked-up" athletes except that they should reduce body mass and eliminate some of the major risk factors for cardiovascular disease and diabetes, which may lead to premature death, especially in professional North American football players (Helzberg et al. 2010; Kraemer 1983a; Mazzetti, Ratamess, and Kraemer 2000). Changing training goals after completion of a sport career is important to continued health and fitness.

Maintenance of Training Goals

The term capping is used to describe the decision to stop attempting to train certain characteristics when it is clear that small gains require large amounts of time and volume to achieve. This may be related to performance (e.g., bench press 1RM strength) or some form of physical development (e.g., calf girth). Capping is a difficult decision that comes only after an adequate period of training and observation of the person's potential for improvement. At some point, the trainer and trainee must make a value judgment as to how to best spend training time. When the decision is made not to devote further training time to developing a particular muscle characteristic (e.g., strength, size, power), the trainee enters into a maintenance training program. In maintenance programs all exercises need not be performed for the same number of sets, repetitions, and intensity despite the widespread use of such standardized programs. The time saved can be used to address other training goals. Such program design decisions allow trainees to prioritize other aspects of fitness over a given training period.

Many examples of training overkill can be found in sports. For example, although the continued development of whole-body power is advantageous to an American football player, an exercise such as the bench press may not be a good measure of playing ability (Fry and Kraemer 1991). The physical attributes needed for bench pressing a great amount of weight are a large, muscular torso, including large chest and back musculature, and short arms. Large upper-body musculature is a positive attribute for American football players because of the sport's dependence on body mass. However, because of the advantages of taller players in today's game, especially for linemen, few elite football players have the short arms needed for great success in the bench press (Kraemer and Gotshalk 2000).

Should the bench press lift be a part of the exercise prescription for American football players? It should, but the expectations of performance for each player must be kept in perspective. Furthermore, the potential for injuring the shoulders with this lift is a concern. Thus, each player's physical dimensions must be considered when developing short-term (e.g., bench press strength after a 10-week summer conditioning program) and long-term (e.g., bench press strength increase over the course of a college career) goals. Furthermore, the importance of a given lift to the performance of the sport should be evaluated. Spending extra time on the bench press to gain an extra 10 or 20 lb (4.5 or 9.1 kg) in the lift at the cost of not training, for example, hang cleans, which develop the structural power vital for performance in American football, would be an unwise use of training time (Barker et al. 1993; Fry and Kraemer 1991). For example, consider a player who has been training for over a year and has achieved a bench press 1RM of 355 lb (161 kg). The extra training time needed for achieving a 400 lb (181.4 kg) bench press may be better used to train another lift (e.g., hang clean), improve sprint speed or agility, or participate in more sport practice. Furthermore, elite players may not have the physical dimensions (e.g., short arms) needed for a 400 lb (181.4 kg) bench press (Kraemer and Gotshalk 2000). Maintenance or capping of the bench press may be called for in this case.

Such training decisions are among the many clinical and coaching decisions that must be made when monitoring the progression of resistance training. Are the training goals realistic in relationship to the sport or a health improvement goal? Is the attainment of a particular training goal vital to the person's success or health? These are difficult questions that need to be asked continually as training progresses.

Unrealistic Goals

Careful attention must be paid to the magnitude of the performance goal and how much training time will be needed for achieving it. Too often, goals are open ended or unrealistic. For many men the 23 in. (58.4 cm) upper arms, 36 in. (91.4 cm) thighs, 20 in. (50.8 cm) neck, 400 lb (181.4 kg) bench press, or 50 in. (127 cm) chest are unrealistic goals because of genetic limitations. Women, too, can develop unrealistic goals, although not the same kinds as men have. Their goals may include drastic decreases in limb or body size to reflect the media culture's ideals for women. Again, based on genetics, such changes may not be possible in many women. Many women mistakenly believe that large gains in strength, muscle definition, and body fat loss can be achieved using very light resistance training programs (e.g., 2 to 5 lb [0.9 to 2.3 kg] handheld weights) to "spot build" a particular body part or muscle. Although one may be able to successfully develop hypertrophy in a specific body part, it is not possible with excessively light resistances. Ultimately, for both men and women, the question is whether the resistance training program can stimulate the desired body changes. Those changes must be examined carefully and honestly.

Unrealistic expectations of equipment and programs develop when they are not evaluated based on sound scientific principles. In today's high-tech and big-hype culture of infomercial marketing of products, programs, and equipment, the average person can develop unrealistic training expectations. In addition, movie actors, models, and elite athletes project desired body images and performance levels, but for most people such levels of physical development, body types, and performances are unrealistic. Short-rest, high-intensity, extreme programs pay little attention to individualization or periodization. Too much too soon, as previously noted, is an invitation to overuse, overtraining, or injury.

Proper goal development is accomplished by starting out small and making gradual progress.

Goal setting is preceded by an evaluation of the person's current fitness level. Most people make the mistake of wanting too much too soon, with too little effort expended, and those marketing commercial programs take advantage of this psychological desire. Although initial gains may be made in using any fitness program, if it is not individualized and then periodized over time, acute overuse injuries can occur from doing too much too soon. Making progress in resistance training requires a long-term commitment to a total conditioning program. This means addressing more than one fitness goal, a principle commonly lacking in commercial programs (e.g., solely emphasizing local muscular endurance or body fat reduction). In addition, proper nutrition and lifestyle behaviors can support training goals and facilitate physical development. A careful evaluation of the training goals and the equipment needed for achieving them can avoid wasted time, money, and effort. Trainees must also remember that as they progress in a training program, their goals will change, and programming must be changed accordingly.

Prioritization of Training Goals

Although any strength training program will result in a host of concomitant adaptations in the body, prioritizing training goals helps the program designer create the optimal stimulus. For example, although performing four sets of 3RM in a particular exercise will enhance power by affecting the force component of the power equation, it does not address the velocity component of the power equation. Thus, a program that also has workouts (six sets of three repetitions at 30% of 1RM) or training cycles that address this goal will optimize power development. This becomes even more important as training progresses and the window of adaptation for performance decreases. Priorities for a specific goal can be set for a workout, a specific training phase or cycle, or a period of time. Many periodization models take this concept into consideration by manipulating the exercise stimuli used either over a training cycle (linear periodization) or weekly (daily nonlinear periodization).

Although different resistance training programs can produce different effects in the body related to the production of force and the development of muscle, the careful examination of a conditioning program is crucial when other forms of exercise are included. Program designers must carefully consider the compatibility of training types as they relate to a specific goal (see chapter 4). Placing too much emphasis on long-distance running to maintain a low body mass in sports such as gymnastics or wrestling, for instance, can be detrimental to the power development vital for these sports. Conversely, the typical fitness enthusiast may not be as concerned with any negative effects on power development if the primary goal is body mass control and cardiovascular health. In this case, power capabilities take second place in the goals of the conditioning program. However, athletes who are serious about recreational basketball league play and performance, for example, may want to consider training for vertical jump power and cardiorespiratory fitness by using an interval training program. Other types of conditioning elements must also be examined in the context of the resistance training program. These include plyometric training, sprint training, flexibility training, weight-gain and weight-loss programs, and sport practice and competitions.

Prioritization of training goals and the associated program designs must be considered in the more global context of the person's entire exercise exposure. The key is to detect any competing exercise stimuli that will compromise recovery or the achievement of a specific high-priority training goal. The simultaneous development of training goals often requires careful partitioning of the program's design over time either within a week or within a training cycle.

Individualization

Little individualization occurs in today's commercial, video, and Internet programs. Random workouts created by online programs cannot achieve the individualization needed for proper progression and safe participation. Each program must be designed to meet the individual's needs and training goals. The teacher, personal trainer, coach, and trainee must all evaluate and understand the trainee's fitness level. Keep in mind, however, that a person's fitness level should not be evaluated until it is determined that the person can tolerate the demands of the test (e.g., 1RM strength test) and that the data generated are reliable and meaningful (Kraemer, Fry, Ratamess, and French 2006). One of the most serious mistakes made in designing a workout is placing intolerable levels of stress on the trainee (i.e., "too much, too soon"). Insufficient rest between sets and exercises, excessive volume, excessive intensity, no individual progression beyond "do what you can," too many workouts in a row without rest days, and no formal programming variation are just a few of the many potential barriers to optimal progression in a resistance training program.

Progress in a resistance training program should follow the staircase principle (see figure 5.10). A person begins a training session at a particular strength level. During the training session, strength decreases as a result of fatigue; at the conclusion of the session, strength is at its lowest point. After recovering from the first session, the person should begin the next training session at a slightly higher strength level. This staircase effect should be observable as training sessions, weeks, months, and years progress and the person approaches his or her genetic potential. (This principle may be intentionally violated during a functional overreaching period, because training volume is subsequently decreased to allow the trainee to experience supercompensation (a dramatic improvement in the exercise goal).) Designing training programs that demonstrate this staircase effect is the biggest challenge in the field of resistance training.

Computerized training equipment as well as mobile and handheld devices have greatly enhanced our ability to monitor feedback and truly achieve individualized resistance training programs for large groups of people. Designers of training programs for athletic teams or large fitness facilities commonly distribute a generalized program for all to follow. Generalized programs do not produce the same results in each person, and in sports different positions can require very different training programs. Thus, general programs written for a particular group of people or sport should be viewed as a starting point for each person. Additions, deletions, changes, and progressions can then be applied to meet individuals' rates of progression and needs. This applies to athletes as well as to those training for general fitness.

Summary

The combination of program variables makes up the exercise stimuli configuration that is presented to the body in a resistance training program. The purpose of program design is to produce the most effective combination of training variables to create the desired stimuli so that adaptation will occur in the manner desired. In many ways the prescription of resistance exercise has for a long time been more of an art than a science, leading to many myths, fads, and commercial systems that are related more to philosophy than to fact. However, the growing number of scientific studies on resistance training continues to expand our understanding and can play a vital role in the exercise prescription process.

No matter how much science is available, the responsibility for making sound decisions concerning each program rests with the coach, the personal trainer, or the trainee. In each case a greater understanding of the knowledge base will help with training guidelines and offer initial answers to questions of program design. Program decisions should be based on a sound rationale and have some basis in scientific fact.

This chapter addressed the developmental process of program design. The next chapter offers descriptions of many systems of resistance training that have evolved over time. Chapter 7 covers long-term resistance exercise programming, with a particular emphasis on training periodization. The foundation presented in this chapter will help you understand the basis for both of these concepts.

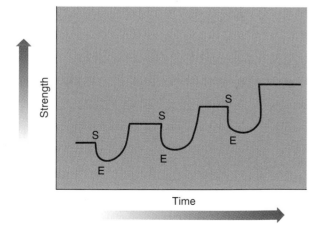

FIGURE 5.10 A resistance training program should produce a staircase effect. S and E designate the start and end of a workout, respectively.

SELECTED READINGS

American College of Sports Medicine. 2002. Position stand. Progression models in resistance training for healthy adults. *Medicine & Science in Sports & Exercise* 34: 364-380.

Calder, A.W., Chilibeck, P.D., Webber, C.E., and Sale, D.G. 1994. Comparison of whole and split weight training routines in young women. *Canadian Journal of Applied Physiology* 19: 185-199.

Cormie, P., McGuigan, M.R., and Newton, R.U. 2011. Developing maximal neuromuscular power: Part 1. Biological basis for maximal power. *Sports Medicine* 41: 17-38.

Cormie, P., McGuigan, M.R., and Newton, R.U. 2011. Developing maximal neuromuscular power: Part 2. Training considerations for improving maximal power production. *Sports Medicine* 41: 125-146.

Garber, C.E., Blissmer, B., Deschenes, M.R., Franklin, B.A., Lamonte, M.J., Lee, I.M., Nieman, D.C., and Swain, D.P. 2011. Quantity and quality of exercise for developing and maintaining cardiorespiratory, musculoskeletal, and neuromotor fitness in apparently healthy adults: Guidance for prescribing exercise. *Medicine & Science in Sports & Exercise* 43: 1334-1359.

Hoffman, J.R., Kraemer, W.J., Fry, A.C., Deschenes, M., and Kemp, M. 1990. The effects of self-selection for frequency of training in a winter conditioning program for football. *Journal of Applied Sport Science Research* 4: 76-82.

Jones, K., Hunter, G., Fleisig, G., Escamilla, R., and Lemak, L. 1999. The effects of compensatory acceleration on upper-body strength and power in collegiate football players. *Journal of Strength and Conditioning Research* 13: 99-105.

Keogh, J.W.L., Wilson, G.J., and Weatherby, R.P. 1999. A cross-sectional comparison of different resistance training techniques in the bench press. *Journal of Strength and Conditioning Research* 13: 247-258.

Kraemer, W.J. 1997. A series of studies: The physiological basis for strength training in American football: Fact over philosophy. *Journal of Strength and Conditioning Research* 11: 131-142.

Kraemer, W.J., Duncan, N.D., and Harman, F.S. 1998. Physiologic basis for strength training in the prevention of and rehabilitation from injury. In *Rehabilitation in sports medicine*, edited by P.K. Canavan, 49-59. Stamford, CT: Appleton and Lange.

Kraemer, W.J., and Fry, A.C. 1995. Strength testing: Development and evaluation of methodology. In *Physiological assessment of human fitness*, edited by P. Maud and C. Foster. Champaign, IL: Human Kinetics.

Kraemer, W.J., and Gómez, A.L. 2001. Establishing a solid fitness base. In *High-performance sports conditioning*, edited by B. Foran, 3-16. Champaign, IL: Human Kinetics.

Kraemer, W.J., and Gotshalk, L.A. 2000. Physiology of American football. In *Exercise and sport science*, edited by

W.E. Garrett and D.T. Kirkendall, 798-813. Philadelphia: Lippincott, Williams & Wilkins.

Kraemer, W.J., Mazzetti, S.A., Ratamess, N.A., and Fleck, S.J. 2000. Specificity of training modes. In *Isokinetics in human performance*, edited by L.E. Brown, 25-41. Champaign, IL: Human Kinetics.

Kraemer, W.J., and Newton, R.U. 2000. Training for muscular power. In *Clinics in sports medicine*, edited by J. Young, 341-368. Philadelphia: W.B. Saunders.

Kraemer, W.J., and Nindl, B.A. 1998. Factors involved with overtraining for strength and power. In *Overtraining in athletic conditioning*, edited by R.F. Kreider and A.M. O'Toole, 69-86. Champaign, IL: Human Kinetics.

Kraemer, W.J., and Ratamess, N.A. 2000. Physiology of resistance training: Current issues. In *Orthopaedic physical therapy clinics of North America*, edited by C. Hughes, 467-513. Philadelphia: W.B. Saunders.

Kraemer, W.J., and Ratamess, N.A. 2004. Fundamentals of resistance training: Progression and exercise prescription. *Medicine & Science in Sports & Exercise* 36: 674-678.

Kraemer, W.J., Ratamess, N.A., and Rubin, M.R. 2000. Basic principles of resistance training. In *Nutrition and the strength athlete*, 1-29. Boca Raton, FL: CRC Press.

Mazzetti, S.A., Kraemer, W.J., Volek, J.S., Duncan, N.D., Ratamess, N.A., Gómez, A.L., Newton, R.U., Häkkinen, K., and Fleck, S.J. 2000. The influence of direct supervision of resistance training on strength performance. *Medicine & Science in Sports & Exercise* 32: 1043-1050.

Mazzetti, S.A., Ratamess, N.A., and Kraemer, W.J. 2000. Pumping down: After years of bulking up, when they graduate, strength-trained athletes must be shown how to safely detrain. *Training and Conditioning* 10: 10-13.

Pearson, D., Faigenbaum, A., Conley, M., and Kraemer, W.J. 2000. The National Strength and Conditioning Association's basic guidelines for the resistance training of athletes. *Strength and Conditioning Journal* 22 (4): 14-30.

Robbins, D.W., Young, W.B., Behm, D.G., and Payne, W.R. 2010. Agonist–antagonist paired set resistance training: A brief review. *Journal of Strength and Conditioning Research* 24: 2873–2882.

Sforzo, G.A., and Touey, P.R. 1996. Manipulating exercise order affects muscular performance during a resistance exercise training session. *Journal of Strength and Conditioning Research* 10: 20-24.

6

Resistance Training Systems and Techniques

After studying this chapter, you should be able to

1. describe the acute training variables that must be known to perform a training system or training technique,

2. discuss the advantages of single-set and multiple set training programs,

3. describe different exercise order training systems,

4. describe training techniques, such as cheating, sets to failure, forced repetitions, partial repetitions, and vascular occlusion,

5. describe specialized training systems, such as functional isometrics, implement, vibration, negative, unstable surface, extreme, and chain training, and

6. discuss what is known from research concerning training techniques and specialized training systems.

Most resistance training systems and techniques were designed by strength coaches, powerlifters, Olympic weightlifters, bodybuilders, or personal trainers. Systems were, for the most part, originally designed to meet the needs and goals of specific groups, and the majority were designed for young, healthy adults or athletes. The needs and goals of a group include not only training outcomes, such as increased strength or changes in body composition, but also administrative concerns, such as the total training time available, the type of training traditionally performed, and equipment availability.

The fact that a system or technique has been used by enough people to have name recognition indicates that it has a good success rate in bringing about desired training adaptations for a particular group. However, virtually any weight training system or technique performed consistently will bring about training adaptations over short training periods, especially in untrained

people. Generally, specific systems and techniques are not popular because they have been scientifically shown to be superior to other systems or techniques in terms of bringing about changes in strength, power, or body composition. Rather, they are popular because they have been used and marketed by an individual, group, or company. A system or technique may also be popular with a specific group because of administrative considerations, such as taking less time to perform than another system or technique.

A great deal of speculation exists about why various systems and techniques are effective and how they physiologically cause training adaptations. Generally, more research is needed, especially in resistance-trained people, concerning the effectiveness of all training systems and techniques. In particular, long-term studies (i.e., six months or longer) are needed to demonstrate whether a particular system or technique brings about continued gains in fitness or results in a training plateau after several months. Knowledge of the various systems and techniques is of value when designing a training program to meet the goals and needs of, as well as to address the administrative concerns for, a particular individual or group. Such knowledge is also helpful when a training plateau is encountered, because a change in training is one way to move beyond a training plateau.

The variety of training systems and techniques demonstrates the vast array of acute training variable combinations that have been used and the almost limitless combinations that are possible (see box 6.1). Many practitioners adopt one training system or technique and then apply only that system to all trainees for long periods of time. Using nonvaried training over the course of months can lead to a training plateau in strength, power, and body composition (Kraemer et al. 2000; Kraemer, Häkkinen et al. 2003; Marx et al. 2001; Willoughby 1993). Additionally, the indefinite use of one system or technique can result in strength plateaus in certain exercises after months of training (Willoughby 1993). Thus, the indefinite use of a single system or technique can lead to less-than-optimal fitness gains. The use of different training systems or techniques is one way to bring training variation into a program thereby helping to avoid training plateaus.

One common mistake novice practitioners make is assuming that a system or technique used by a champion bodybuilder, powerlifter, Olympic weightlifter, or other type of athlete is the best system or technique for a novice lifter or recreational athlete. Programs used by elite athletes are often too intense or have a training volume that is too high for the novice lifter or recreational athlete. Elite athletes may have taken years of training to achieve the fitness levels necessary to tolerate and to make physiological adaptations with the programs they use. Elite strength and power athletes may also have a genetic potential to tolerate the high-intensity or high-volume programs they use and still achieve gains in strength, power, and hypertrophy.

A training record is invaluable for determining which training system or variation of a system or technique works best for an individual, group, or team. Without a detailed record of workouts, trainees will not remember the progression in enough detail to repeat it. Furthermore, the sets, repetitions, exercises, and resistances used in a program need to be documented to plan the next training session and training phase. Training records answer many questions about people's responses to particular programs, including which systems or techniques work best and how long they can continue with a particular training technique before reaching a plateau. Training logs are also motivational because trainees can see their progress over the course of weeks or months of training.

Single-Set Systems

The **single-set system,** the performance of each exercise in a program for one set, is one of the oldest resistance training systems. The effects of

BOX 6.1 PRACTICAL QUESTION

What Needs to Be Known to Use a System or Technique Correctly?

With any type of resistance training program, technique, or system, the traditional acute program variables need to be known. These include the number of repetitions per set, resistance used, exercises, exercise order, rest between sets and exercises, sets per exercise, and velocity of movement. A complete description might also include the training frequency per week, the total time under tension, the amount of rest between repetitions (if any), the time distribution of contraction types (concentric, eccentric, isometric) during repetitions, the range of motion of the exercise, whether sets are carried to failure, and the recovery between training sessions. Some systems or techniques describe additional variables, such as the rest between repetitions during the rest-pause technique. Many systems and techniques require descriptions of not only the traditional acute training variables, but also these additional variables. Before using a particular resistance training technique or system, a complete understanding of all of the acute program variables is necessary. However, many do not describe all of the acute training variables, making them difficult to follow.

single and multiple sets when performing various types of resistance training were discussed extensively in chapter 2. A single-set system described in 1925 (Liederman 1925) consisted of heavy resistances and a few repetitions per set with a five-minute rest between exercises. Single-set systems are still popular and have been recommended as a time-efficient way to develop and maintain muscular fitness in novice and older weight trainers (American College of Sports Medicine 2011).

Single-set systems do result in significant increases in strength and significant changes in body composition (American College of Sports Medicine 2009). Some studies report no significant difference in strength gains between nonvaried single- and multiple-set programs in untrained people, whereas other studies show a superiority of multiple-set programs (American College of Sports Medicine 2009). This discrepancy may be due in part to the length of the studies. Some comparisons of nonvaried multiple-set systems and nonvaried single-set systems report no significant difference in strength gains during the first 16 weeks of training; however, generally, studies lasting 17 to 40 weeks show that multiple-set programs result in greater strength gains than single-set programs (American College of Sports Medicine 2009; Wolfe, LeMura, and Cole 2004). Meta-analyses support that longer training durations with multiple sets do result in greater strength gains and that multiple-set programs are superior to single-set programs for strength gains in both untrained and trained people (Rhea et al. 2003; Rhea, Alvar, and Burkett 2002; Wolfe, LeMura, and Cole 2004). Interestingly, the difference in strength gains between single- and multiple-set programs may be greater in untrained people than in trained people (Rhea, Alvar, and Burkett 2002). Comparisons of various multiple-set periodized systems to nonvaried single-set systems show the periodized systems to result in greater increases (and in many cases, significantly greater increases) in strength and motor performance, as well as body composition changes (Fleck 1999; Kraemer et al. 1997, 2000; Marx et al. 2001).

A single-set system results in significant strength gains, especially during the initial weeks of training (6-16 weeks). However, over longer training periods, multiple-set programs produce greater strength gains and may be needed to increase training volume enough to cause continued strength gains (American College of Sports Medicine 2009).

Single-set systems are a reasonable choice for those with limited time for resistance training and for athletes during an in-season program or any other training phase when less time can be dedicated to resistance training.

Express Circuits

Personal trainers have developed express circuits for clients with minimal time available for resistance training, as well as any other type of fitness training. Express circuits are typically variations of a single-set system. Normally, the person performs one set of 6 to 12 repetitions of each exercise with 30 seconds to one minute of rest between exercises. Express circuits have been developed using both multijoint and single-joint exercises and typically involve at least one exercise for each major muscle group. Depending on the choice of exercise, this results in approximately 8 to 10 exercises per session. An express circuit has all the advantages and limitations of a single-set system.

Multiple-Set Systems

A **multiple-set system** can involve performing multiple sets with the same resistance or multiple sets with varying resistances (i.e., heavy to light, light to heavy), with varying numbers or the same number of repetitions per set and with all, some, or no sets carried to volitional fatigue. Virtually any training system that consists of more than one set of an exercise can be classified as a multiple-set system. One of the original multiple-set systems consisted of two or three warm-up sets of increasing resistance followed by several sets at the same resistance. This training system became popular in the 1940s (Darden 1973) and appears to be the forerunner of the vast array of the multiple-set systems of today.

Meta-analyses indicate that multiple-set programs result in greater strength (Peterson, Rhea, and Alvar 2004; Rhea et al. 2003; Rhea, Alvar, and Burkett 2002; Wolfe, LeMura, and Cole 2004) and hypertrophy (Krieger 2010) gains than single-set programs. When considering the number of sets, trainers need to distinguish between the number of sets per exercise and the number of sets per muscle group. For example, if two sets of two types of arm curl are performed, the biceps perform four sets. Meta-analyses indicate that four sets per muscle group for trained and nontrained people

(Rhea, Alvar, and Burkett 2002), and eight sets per muscle group for trained people (Peterson, Rhea, and Alvar 2004) produce near-maximal strength gains. As discussed earlier in the section on single-set systems, meta-analyses also indicate that strength gains may be more pronounced as a result of performing multiple sets and that greater strength gains with multiple-set programs may be more apparent with longer training durations (17-40 weeks) compared to shorter training durations (6-16 weeks). However, performance of a multiple-set system with no change in training variables for long periods of time can result in a plateau in strength (Willoughby 1993).

Although multiple-set programs generally produce significantly greater fitness gains than single-set programs, this is not always the case. For example, training three days per week with either a three- or one-set program with similar training intensity (percentage of 1RM) showed lower-body strength and muscle hypertrophy, but not upper-body strength and hypertrophy, to be greater with three sets (Ronnestad et al. 2007). Additionally, comparisons (see chapter 7) of periodized multiple-set systems and nonvaried multiple-set systems have generally shown the periodized systems to result in greater fitness gains.

Circuit System

Circuit systems consist of a series of resistance training exercises performed in succession with minimal rest (15 to 30 seconds) between exercises. Typically, approximately 10 to 15 repetitions of each exercise are performed per circuit with a resistance of 40 to 60% of 1RM. One to several circuits of the exercises can be performed. However, when one set of each exercise is performed, the training protocol would more likely be termed an express circuit. The exercises can be chosen to train any muscle group. This system is very time efficient when large numbers of people are trained, because each piece of equipment is in virtually constant use. It is also very time efficient for those with a limited amount of training time (see box 6.2).

The use of 40 to 60% of 1RM for 10 to 15 repetitions for some exercises will result in the set not being performed close to volitional fatigue and therefore may limit gains in maximal strength. In untrained and trained males and females, the number of repetitions in a set carried to volitional fatigue of the leg press ranges from 78 to 146 repetitions when 40% of 1RM is used and from 34 to 57 repetitions when 60% of 1RM is used (Hoeger et al. 1990). Substantially more than 15 repetitions per set of the lat pull-down can also be performed at these percentages of 1RM. Thus, if one goal of a circuit system is to increase maximal strength, it may be advisable to increase the percentage of 1RM used in many exercises or design the circuit using 10- to 15RM resistances or close to RM resistances for the exercises.

As expected, a circuit program (three sets × 10 repetitions per set at 12RM) using approximately 67% of 1RM does increase heart rate, blood pressure, and oxygen consumption (Ortego et al. 2009). However, there are some differences between the sexes. Men demonstrated a significantly greater oxygen consumption, total energy expenditure, and systolic, but not diastolic, blood pressure during the circuit than women did. Average heart rate increased for both men and women during the three circuits and reached approximately 86% of

---

 BOX 6.2 PRACTICAL QUESTION

What Are the Exercises in a Typical Circuit Weight Training Program?

The exercises included in a circuit weight training program can vary depending on the goals of the program. However, circuit weight training is often designed as a total-body program using an alternating exercise order (see the section Exercise Order Systems later in this chapter) with multijoint exercises used at the beginning of circuits. Many circuits are also performed using weight training machines because this allows quick changes in the resistance when several people (or more) are performing the same circuit at the same time. The number of circuits can be increased as the person adapts to the training. An example of a total-body circuit weight training program is as follows: leg press, chest press, leg curl, lat pull-down, leg extension, overhead press, calf raise, arm curl, back extension, triceps extension, and abdominal crunch.

maximal heart rate for both sexes during the third circuit (i.e., there was no significant difference between the sexes).

The preceding acute effects of circuit training support the proposed benefit of a circuit system on cardiorespiratory fitness. This benefit is in part related to the use of short rest periods between exercises, which results in the heart rate remaining elevated during the entire circuit compared to traditional longer rest periods (35 seconds vs. 3 minutes) during a training session (Alcaraz, Sanchez-Lorente, and Blazevich 2008). Circuit programs do increase maximal oxygen consumption, but the increase can vary substantially. Generally, short-duration (8-20 weeks) circuit systems increase peak oxygen consumption approximately 4 and 8% in healthy men and women, respectively (Gettman and Pollock 1981). However, the increase can vary substantially. For example, in college-aged women and men, circuit training results in an increase of approximately 10% and 0%, respectively (Wilmore et al. 1978). Formerly sedentary people show an increase of 12% (Camargo et al. 2008) in maximal oxygen consumption. Postmenopausal women with low pretraining (24 ml $\cdot$ kg^{-1} $\cdot$ min^{-1}) peak oxygen consumption performing circuit training in a periodized manner (progressing from 45-50% 1RM for two sets of 15-20 repetitions per set to 55-60% 1RM for three sets of 10-12 repetitions per set) during 24 weeks of training significantly increased peak oxygen consumption (18.6%; Brentano et al. 2008). One-repetition maximum strength in both the upper (26.4%) and lower (42.2%) body also increased significantly. Thus, the increase in peak oxygen consumption may vary substantially depending on the population performing circuit training, and when initial peak oxygen consumption is low, greater gains in peak oxygen consumption can be expected.

If one goal of a weight training system is to increase cardiorespiratory endurance, then a variation of a circuit is a good choice. However, to meet that goal, a traditional endurance training component, such as running, cycling, elliptical training, or swimming, needs to be included in the total training program.

There are many possible variations of a circuit program. One is the peripheral heart action system, in which the training session is divided into several sequences (Gaja 1965). A sequence is a group of four to six exercises, each for a different body part. The number of repetitions per set of each exercise in a sequence varies with the goals of the program, but normally 8 to 12 repetitions per set are performed. One training session consists of performing all of the exercises in the first sequence three times in a circuit fashion. The remaining sequences are then performed one after the other in the same fashion as the first sequence. An example of the exercises in a peripheral heart action training session is given in table 6.1.

The triset system is similar to the peripheral heart action system in that it incorporates groups or sequences of exercises. As the name implies, it consists of groups of three exercises. The exercises performed in a triset are for the same major body segment, such as the arms or the legs, but they can train different muscle groups as well. Little or no rest between exercises is allowed, and normally three sets of each exercise are performed. The exercises constituting a triset are, for example, the arm curl, triceps extension, and military press. Trisets are one of the dynamic types of resistance training compared in table 6.2 for isometric strength gains and were shown to be very effective for increasing isometric strength.

Both of these circuit system variations (peripheral heart action and triset) are fatiguing and result in maintenance of a relatively high heart

TABLE 6.1 Example of a Four-Sequence Peripheral Heart Action Training Session

Body part	Sequence			
	1	2	3	4
Chest	Bench press	Incline press	Decline bench	Chest fly
Back	Lat pull-down	Seated row	Bent-over row	T-bar row
Shoulders	Military press	Upright row	Lateral raise	Front shoulder raise
Legs	Squat	Knee extension	Back squat	Split squat
Abdomen	Sit-up	Crunch	Roman chair sit-up	V-up

TABLE 6.2   **Comparison of Isometric Strength Gains From Eight Resistance Training Systems**

	Cheat	Delorme	Descending half-triangle	Double progressive	Isometric[a]	Oxford	Superset	Triset
Elbow flexion	23*	9*	11*	7	0	7*	12*	25*
Elbow extension	66**	16	9**	25*	35*	28**	9	30**
Back and leg	27*	0	24*	13	–5	11	21*	17*

Strength values given are percentage changes from pre- to posttraining; **significant increase pre- to posttraining at 0.01 level of significance; *significant increase pre- to posttraining at 0.05 level of significance; [a] isometric training consisted of one maximal action 6 seconds in duration; Oxford is a heavy-to-light system; Delorme is a light-to-heavy system.

Adapted, by permission, from J.R. Leighton et al., 1967, "A study of the effectiveness of ten different methods of progressive resistance exercise on the development of strength, flexibility, girth and body weight," *Journal of the Association for Physical and Mental Rehabilitation* 21: 79.

rate during training. Therefore, both are probably reasonable choices, as are all types of circuit programs, when the training goal is to increase cardiorespiratory fitness as well as local muscular endurance.

Drop, or Strip, Sets

Drop, or strip, sets involve performing a set of an exercise to volitional fatigue, dropping, or stripping, some resistance, and then performing another set of the same exercise to volitional fatigue. Normally, little or no rest is used between sets, and although any number of repetitions per set could be performed, 8 to 12 are typical. Bodybuilders and some fitness enthusiasts use this type of training to increase muscle hypertrophy, but it may also result in gains in local muscular endurance. Decreasing the resistance and performing more sets can be repeated as often as desired, although two or three drop sets per exercise are usually performed.

Gains in 1RM over nine weeks of training were significantly greater for the biceps curl (13.2 vs. 8.2%) and bench press (16.5 vs. 10.6%) with three sets of 6 to 10 repetitions using drop sets compared to one set of 6 to 10 repetitions (Humburg et al. 2007). Although one-legged leg press ability showed greater 1RM gains (right and left leg, 13.3 vs. 9.7% and 15.5 vs. 9.4%) with the three-drop-set program, no significant difference was noted between the three-drop-set and the one-set programs. Both training programs used sets to failure (see the section Sets to Failure Technique later in this chapter). The results indicate that drop sets do result in increased strength but offer no information about how this technique compares with other techniques. The results do suggest that drop sets for multiple sets result in greater strength increases than a one-set program

and that this comparison is affected by differences in training volume.

One goal of this type of training is to maintain the total training volume by maintaining the number of repetitions per set, but it must be remembered that decreasing resistance will result in a decrease in total training volume. Performing successive sets using the same resistance and relatively short rest periods (e.g., one minute) does result in a decrease in the number of repetitions in successive sets. For example, back squats for four sets at an 8RM resistance results in 5.93, 4.47, and 4.20 repetitions per set in the second to fourth sets, respectively (Willardson and Burkett 2005). Similarly, back squats for five successive sets at 15RM result in 10.67, 8.40, 6.27, and 6.33 repetitions per set in the second to fifth sets, respectively (Willardson and Burkett 2006).

To maintain the number of repetitions per set at approximately 10 using a 10RM resistance with a one-minute rest between sets of each exercise and two minutes between exercises in three consecutive sets each of the back squat, knee curl, and knee extension requires a decrease in resistance per set of approximately 15% (Willardson et al. 2010). Decreases in resistance of 5 and 10% resulted in a decrease in the number of repetitions per set of the back squat and knee curl, the first two exercises performed. For example, with a 5% decrease in resistance, the mean number of repetitions for all three sets of the back squat was eight. Surprisingly, even though the knee extension was performed last in the exercise sequence, decreases in resistance were not necessary for maintaining approximately 10 repetitions per set. This indicates that the effect of decreasing resistance on the number of repetitions per set may vary depending on the exercise or be affected by where the exercise is in a sequence of exercises. Previous resistance training with the goal of increasing local muscular endurance (moderate resistance and short rest periods) may also affect the ability to maintain a certain number of repetitions per set with no change in resistance or result in smaller decreases in the resistance needed to maintain the same number of repetitions per set.

Other names, such as multi-poundage and breakdown training, are used to describe drop sets. To some, these other names are synonymous with drop sets; to others, they imply a variation of this type of training. The multi-poundage system uses drop sets with a 4- or 5RM resistance for four or five repetitions in the first set. After the first set the resistance is decreased and the trainee performs another set of four or five repetitions. This procedure continues for several sets (Poole 1964).

In breakdown training, after the trainee carries a set to voluntary muscular fatigue, the resistance is immediately reduced so that an additional two to four repetitions can be performed. A comparison of breakdown training to traditional training indicates greater strength increases with breakdown training (Westcott 1994). Both types of training were performed for one set of 10 to 12 repetitions at a 10- to 12RM resistance for one month. During the next month of training half of the subjects continued with this program while the other half performed breakdown training. After reaching volitional fatigue, the resistance used by subjects performing breakdown training was reduced by 10 lb (4.5 kg), and they performed an additional two to four repetitions. The average increase in resistance used for training was 7 lb (3.2 kg) more with breakdown training at the end of the two months of training. The study did not statistically analyze whether this difference between groups was significant. Because one group performed the same training program for the entire two months of training while the other group performed one type of training for one month and another type (breakdown training) for the second month, these results could be interpreted to mean that training variation and not breakdown training per se resulted in the additional strength gain. However, the project does indicate that breakdown training can increase strength in untrained people.

Safe performance of any drop set variation with free weights requires one or two spotters. If machines are used, spotters may not be needed. Additionally, this type of training is very fatiguing and will probably result in a significant amount of muscle soreness at first. Therefore, drop sets should be introduced into any training program slowly.

Triangle, or Pyramid, System

Many powerlifters and people interested in increasing 1RM lifting ability use triangle, or pyramid, systems. A complete **triangle,** or **pyramid, system** begins with a set of 10 to 12 repetitions with a light resistance. The resistance is then increased over several sets so that fewer and fewer repetitions are performed, until only a 1RM is performed. Then the same sets and resistances are repeated in reverse order, with the last set consisting of 10 to 12 repetitions (see figure 6.1). Generally, the resistance used and the number of repetitions performed are close to RMs. Any combination of repetition numbers per set can be termed a triangle system as long as the number of repetitions per set initially decreases and then increases.

Light-to-Heavy System

As the name implies, the light-to-heavy system involves progressing from light to heavy resistances. One type of light-to-heavy system is the ascending half triangle, or ascending half-pyramid (see figure 6.1). In this system the person performs only the first half of a triangle system by progressing from higher numbers of repetitions per set with light resistances to fewer numbers of repetitions per set with heavier resistances. A variation of an

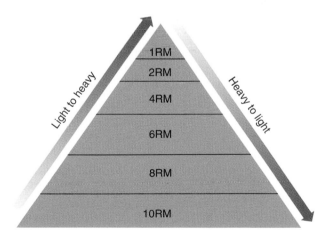

FIGURE 6.1 A system that consists of sets that progress from light to heavy resistances is called a light-to-heavy system (ascending half triangle). One that progress from heavy to light resistances is called a heavy-to-light system (descending half triangle). A full triangle, or pyramid, consists of both the ascending and descending portions of the triangle.

ascending half triangle system was one of the more effective systems for increasing isometric back and leg strength in the study results shown in table 6.2.

One variation of the light-to-heavy system became popular in the 1930s and 1940s among Olympic lifters (Hatfield and Krotee 1978). It consists of performing a set of three to five repetitions with a relatively light resistance. Five pounds (2.3 kg) are then added to the resistance, and another set of three to five repetitions is performed. This is continued until only one repetition can be performed. The Delorme regime, one of the earliest light-to-heavy systems scientifically examined, consists of three sets of 10 repetitions with the resistance progressing from 50 to 66 to 100% of 10RM in successive sets. This system causes significant increases in strength over short-term training periods (Delorme, Ferris, and Gallagher 1952; Delorme and Watkins 1948). The Delorme system was evaluated in the study results shown in table 6.2 and demonstrated a significant increase in isometric elbow flexion, but no significant increases in isometric elbow extension or back and leg strength.

Heavy-to-Light System

In a heavy-to-light system, after a few warm-up sets, the heaviest set is performed, and then the resistance is reduced for each succeeding set. Some heavy-to-light systems can also be termed descending half triangle, or descending half pyramid, systems (see figure 6.1). In this type of heavy-to-light system (a descending half triangle) the first set performed is the heaviest set with the fewest repetitions; the resistance is then decreased and the number of repetitions is increased.

The Oxford system, a relatively old training system, is a heavy-to-light system consisting of three sets of 10 repetitions progressing from 100 to 66 to 50% of 10RM in each successive set. Significant gains in strength have been demonstrated with this system (McMorris and Elkins 1954; Zinovieff 1951). The Oxford system was evaluated in the study depicted in table 6.2 and demonstrated significant increases in isometric elbow flexion and elbow extension, but a nonsignificant change in back and leg strength. Comparisons of the heavy-to-light Oxford system and light-to-heavy DeLorme systems are equivocal in terms of strength gain. One study found the heavy-to-light system to be superior to the light-

to-heavy system in strength gains, but indicated that further research is necessary (McMorris and Elkins 1954). The study results shown in table 6.2 found little difference between the Delorme and Oxford systems for increasing isometric elbow flexion strength, but found that the heavy-to-light Oxford system was superior to the light-to-heavy Delorme system for increasing isometric elbow extension and back and leg strength.

Double Progressive System

The double progressive system could be described as a descending half triangle followed by an ascending half triangle; however, during the first several sets, or the descending portion, the resistance is not changed. In the double progressive system both the number of repetitions per set and the resistance used are varied. During the first several sets the resistance is held constant while the number of repetitions per set is increased until a specified number of sets has been performed. The resistance is then increased and the number of repetitions per set decreased until the number of repetitions performed has returned to the number performed in the first set. This process is then repeated for each exercise performed. An example of this system is given in table 6.3. Of the systems compared in table 6.2 the double progressive system appears to be one of the least effective for increasing isometric strength. The double progressive system is very time-consuming. Additionally, the first sets appear to be warm-up sets, as they are not performed close to volitional fatigue and because more repetitions with the same resistance in the following sets can be performed. Although

TABLE 6.3 **Example of the Double Progressive System**

Set	Repetitions	Resistance (lb/kg)
1	4	120/54.4
2	6	120/54.4
3	8	120/54.4
4	10	120/54.4
5	12	120/54.4
6	10	140/63.5
7	8	160/72.6
8	6	175/79.4
9	4	185/83.9

minimal research is available, the research we do have indicates that the use of the double progressive system is unwarranted.

Exercise Order Systems

Exercise order systems dictate the order in which exercises are performed. There are two major types of exercise order. The first, which involves not performing exercises for a particular muscle group in succession, is called **alternating muscle group order**. The second involves performing exercises for the same muscle group in succession and is commonly termed **stacking exercise order**. All exercise order systems are some derivation of these two concepts.

A comparison of an alternating muscle group order of three sets of two exercises (bench press and bench pull) using 4RM and a traditional exercise order of performing all three sets of each exercise in succession offers some insight into the effect of an alternating exercise order (Robbins et al. 2010c; Robbins, Young, and Behm 2010). This type of alternating muscle group order (i.e., performing one set of an exercise and then performing one set of another exercise using muscle groups antagonistic to those used in the first exercise) has been termed **paired set training**, but could also be termed an agonist–antagonist superset (see the section Supersetting Systems later in this chapter). The rest periods between exercises in the alternating muscle group order were two minutes, which resulted in approximately four minutes between successive sets of an exercise. The rest period in the traditional exercise order was four minutes between sets. Although the total rest period between sets of the same exercise was four minutes in both exercise orders, the time to perform the alternating exercise order was half (10 vs. 20 minutes) of that to perform the traditional exercise order.

One advantage of an alternating muscle group order is that it provides some recovery for the muscle groups used in the other exercise. This advantage was not substantiated by EMG activity, which was the same with both exercise orders. However, it was substantiated by the total training volume, which showed a smaller decrease from the first to thirds sets with the alternating exercise order (bench press 36 vs. 51% and bench pull 17 vs. 35%).

Flushing

The flushing system was developed by bodybuilders to produce hypertrophy, definition, and vascularity. The number of exercises, sets, repetitions per set, and rest periods is not clearly defined. Flushing involves performing two or more exercises for the same muscle group, which is a stacking exercise order, or for two muscle groups in close proximity to each other. The hypothesis behind flushing is to keep blood in the muscle group or groups for a long period of time. Advocates for this system believe that this will develop muscle hypertrophy. Many bodybuilders do train a muscle group with several exercises in succession during the same training session, so practical experience indicates that this practice may result in hypertrophy. Because it is unknown how blood flow mediates changes in hypertrophy, such mechanisms are speculative. It could be hypothesized that higher blood flow allows more of the natural anabolic factors found in the blood, such as growth hormone or testosterone, to bind to receptors in muscle and connective tissue, or that increased blood flow increases the availability of necessary nutrients for protein synthesis.

Flushing does result in increased temporary hypertrophy, or the "pump" caused by weight training. Increased cell volume as a result of increased water content has been shown to be one of the regulating factors of protein synthesis (Waldegger et al. 1997). Over time, this could result in increased muscle hypertrophy. However, the effectiveness of the flushing system to increase hypertrophy is unknown because supporting scientific evidence is lacking.

Priority System

The priority system can be applied to virtually all resistance training systems. It involves performing the exercises that apply to the training program's major goal(s) early in a training session, so they can be performed with maximal intensity for the desired number of repetitions. For example, if single-joint exercises involving the muscles used in the squat or bench press are performed before the priority exercises, total force (repetitions × weight lifted) will be less and fatigue rate greater in the bench press and squat (Sforzo and Touey 1996; Simão et al. 2005, 2007). The same is true for the single-joint exercises if the exercise order is reversed. If exercises relating to the program's major goal(s) are performed late in the training session, fatigue may prevent the trainee from using maximal resistances for the desired number of repetitions, which may limit adaptation to the training.

Consider a bodybuilder whose weakest muscle group in terms of definition and hypertrophy is the quadriceps group. Using the priority concept, exercises for the quadriceps group would be performed at the beginning of the training session. A basketball coach may decide that a power forward's greatest weakness is lack of upper-body strength, which causes the player to be pushed around under the boards. Thus, major upper-body exercises would be placed at beginning of the training session for this player. Likewise, an American football or rugby player may want to promote strength and power development of the hips and low back, and therefore would perform exercises meant to develop this characteristic, such as hang cleans and squats, at the beginning of the training session.

Supersetting Systems

Supersetting has evolved into two distinct systems. One involves performing alternate sets of two exercises for agonist and antagonistic muscle groups of one body part. Examples of this type of supersetting are arm curls alternated with triceps extensions, or knee extensions alternated with knee curls. Significant increases in strength from this type of supersetting have been reported (see table 6.2). Of the eight systems compared in table 6.2, this type of supersetting is one of the most effective for increasing back and leg isometric strength. The earlier discussion of a superset using 4RM, which is higher than the normal intensity of 8 to -12RM typically used in a superset, indicates that supersets of agonist and antagonist muscle groups do allow greater training volume compared to a traditional exercise order.

Some evidence indicates that bench press power can be acutely increased (4.7%) by one set (eight repetitions) of an exercise involving the upper back musculature, the antagonists of the muscles involved in the bench press (Baker and Newton 2005). However, performing an isokinetic set of knee flexion (antagonist) followed by knee extension (agonist) for three sets in an alternating fashion results in decreased agonist force capabilities especially at slow velocities (60 degrees per second), increased agonist time to maximal force,

and decreased power (Maynard and Ebben 2003). This suggests a limitation of agonist–antagonist superset training in terms of force and power capabilities. Although no difference in measures of power changes during three sets between an agonist–antagonist exercise order (bench pull and bench press throw) and a traditional exercise order has been shown, the time to perform the agonist–antagonist exercise order was less (Robbins et al. 2010b). It is important to note that this exercise order involved a strength exercise (bench pull) and a power exercise (bench press throw). Thus, further research is needed concerning agonist–antagonist supersetting effects on power output with consideration given to the types of exercises included in the protocol.

As with all alternating exercise orders, one advantage of agonist–antagonist supersets is time efficiency. A comparison of agonist–antagonist supersetting of six exercises for four sets each using 10RM and one-minute rest periods between exercises, and the traditional exercise order of performing all sets of exercise prior to performing the next exercise, shows that this type of supersetting is time efficient for energy expenditure (Kelleher et al. 2010). Although total energy expenditure was not different between the two exercise orders, energy expenditure per minute of training time was 32% greater with supersetting. Additionally, blood lactate was also significantly higher with supersetting. The greater total energy expenditure per minute of training may be an advantage for someone with limited training time and a training goal of decreasing total body fat.

The second type of supersetting is similar to the triset system. It involves performing one set of two to three exercises in rapid succession for the same muscle group or body part. An example of this is lat pull-downs, seated rows, and bent-over rows. This type of supersetting has resulted in significant strength gains, changes in body composition, and increases in vertical jump performance when performed as part of a periodized weight training program (Kraemer 1997).

Both types of supersetting typically involve sets of 8 to 12 (or more) repetitions with little or no rest between sets and exercises. Supersetting is popular among bodybuilders and fitness enthusiasts, suggesting that these systems result in muscle hypertrophy. The fact that short rest periods between sets and exercises result in substantially increased blood acidity indicates that these systems are applicable when the training goal is to increase local muscular endurance.

Split-Body System

Some bodybuilders, athletes, and fitness enthusiasts use a split-body system in which, typically, the body is divided into two major portions, such as upper and lower. This system allows the performance of more exercises per body part or muscle group than would be possible in a training session of reasonable length if all muscle groups were trained in a single training session. Many variations of a split routine are possible. An example would be training the arms, legs, and abdomen on Mondays, Wednesdays, and Fridays, and the chest, shoulders, and back on Tuesdays, Thursdays, and Saturdays. The routine allows the performance of several exercises for a body part in a training session of reasonable length, but means that training is performed six days per week.

Variations of the split-body system can be developed so that training sessions take place four or five days per week. Even though training sessions are quite frequent, sufficient recovery of muscle groups between training sessions is possible because body parts are not necessarily trained on successive days. A split-body system allows the training intensity for a particular body part or group of exercises to be higher than would be possible if the four to six sessions were combined into two or three long sessions of equivalent training volume. It is also possible to develop split routines in which the total training volume per body part is higher than that of a typical total-body training session because in a split-body routine each training session is dedicated to a smaller number of body parts or muscle groups.

One possible advantage of a split-body system is allowing the performance of assistance exercises. In highly strength-trained athletes, such as college American football players, short-term (10-week) strength gains in the bench press and squat in part depend on the use of assistance exercises (Hoffman et al. 1990). Because split routines allow the performance of more assistance exercises, they may also be useful for enhancing strength development.

A split-body routine using linear periodization resulted in significant increases in strength and lean mass as well as decreased fat mass and percent body fat in both young (18- to 22-year-old) and middle-aged (35- to 50-year-old) men (Kerksick et al. 2009). In this split-body routine all upper-body and lower-body exercises were performed in two different training sessions; each session was performed two days per week resulting in a total of four sessions per week.

A comparison of a total-body training routine and a split-body routine in young women who were previously not weight trained demonstrated no significant differences between groups in 1RM ability, lean body mass, or percent body fat changes (Calder et al. 1994). The total-body group performed four upper-body exercises (five sets, 6- to 10RM) and three lower-body exercises (five sets, 10- to 12RM) per session twice a week for 20 weeks. The split-body group used the same exercises and set repetition scheme, but performed both the upper- and lower-body exercises two days per week for a total of four training sessions on four different days per week. The results indicate that total-body and split-body routines using the same total training volume produce similar results in healthy young women during the first 20 weeks of training.

Practically, split-body routines do offer some advantages, such as increased volume for a muscle group or body part; thus, they may be most applicable when increased volume is desired. However, if training volume is equal between a split-body and total-body program, training outcomes will be similar.

Body-Part System

Body-part systems are similar to a split-body system in that specific body parts or muscle groups are trained on specific days. However, with a body-part system typically only one or two body parts or major muscle groups are trained per training session. A typical body-part program would train the following muscle groups on specific days of the week: day 1, back; day 2, quadriceps, calves, and abdominals; day 3, chest and triceps; day 4, no training; day 5, back and biceps; day 6, hamstrings, gluteals, and biceps; and day 7, trapezius, deltoids, and abdominals.

Body-part systems are popular among bodybuilders and fitness enthusiasts. Typically, multiple exercises for each body part and multiple sets of each exercise are performed. This allows the performance of a high volume of training for a specific muscle group in one training session followed by several days of rest for that muscle group. Advocates of body-part systems believe that high-volume training followed by several days of rest for a specific muscle group is necessary to induce optimal gains in hypertrophy.

Blitz, or Isolated Split, System

The blitz, or isolated split, system is a variation of a body-part system. Rather than training several body parts during each training session, people train only one body part per session. The duration of the training session is not reduced. Thus, more sets and exercises per body part can be performed. An example of a blitz system is performing all arm, chest, leg, trunk, back, and shoulder exercises on Monday through Saturday, respectively. Some bodybuilders have performed this type of program in preparation for a contest. A short-duration blitz program may also be appropriate if an athlete's performance is limited by the strength of a particular muscle group or groups. A long jumper might perform a variation of a blitz program for the legs before the start of the season, which might involve training only the legs two days per week.

Training Techniques Applicable to Other Systems

Many training techniques can be used with virtually all training systems. For example, people can perform partial repetitions with any training system— single-set, multiple-set, or superset. The following training techniques are applicable to most types of training systems.

Cheating Technique

The cheating technique is popular among bodybuilders. As the name implies, it involves cheating, or breaking strict exercise form (Weider 1954). As an example, rather than maintaining an erect upper body when performing standing barbell arm curls, the lifter uses a slight torso swing to start the barbell moving from the elbow-extended position. The torso swing is not grossly exaggerated, but it is sufficient to allow the trainee to lift 10 to 20 lb (4.5 to 9.1 kg) more resistance than is possible with strict exercise form. The barbell curl has a bell-shaped strength curve, and having the arms fully extended is a weak position. The strongest position is when the elbow joint is at approximately a 90-degree angle. When barbell curls are performed with strict form, the maximum resistance that can be lifted depends on the resistance that can be moved from the weak, fully extended position.

With a constant resistance the muscles involved in flexing the elbow, therefore, are not maximally active during the stronger positions of the exercise's range of motion. The goal of cheating is to allow the use of a heavier resistance, which forces the muscle(s) to develop a force closer to maximal through a greater portion of the exercise's range of motion, thus enhancing strength and hypertrophy gains. Cheating can also be performed at the end of the set once volitional fatigue has occurred.

Lifters should be cautious when using the cheating technique. The heavier resistance and the cheating movement can increase the chance of injury. As an example, the torso-swinging movement when performing arm curls can place additional stress on the low back.

Comparisons of strength gains due to the cheating technique and those due to other training systems or techniques indicate that this technique is quite effective (see table 6.2). The cheating technique was one of the most effective systems or techniques for increasing elbow flexion, elbow extension, and back and leg isometric strength.

Sets to Failure Technique

A set to failure means that the set is performed until no further complete repetitions with good exercise technique can be performed. Synonymous with sets to failure are the terms *sets to volitional fatigue* and *sets to concentric failure*. Sets to failure can be incorporated into virtually any training system. Advocates of this technique believe that it promotes a greater recruitment of motor units and a greater secretion of growth-promoting hormones than when sets are not carried to failure, which results in a greater training stimulus. This, in turn, will lead to greater strength and hypertrophy gains. Many descriptions of training studies and programs use terms indicating that sets were performed to failure. The use of a repetition maximum (RM) or an **RM training zone** (e.g., 4-6 with RM) in a training program indicates that sets were carried to failure.

Fitness gains can be achieved when all sets in a training program are carried to failure. However, significant strength, motor performance, and body composition changes have also been shown when some, but not all, sets in a training program are carried to failure (Marx et al. 2001; Stone et al. 2000; Willardson et al. 2008). Significantly greater gains in strength have also been reported when no sets in multiple-set programs are carried to failure compared to a single-set program in which all sets were carried to momentary muscular failure (Kramer et al. 1997). It is important to note that in these studies, even though some sets were not carried to failure, the number of repetitions performed and the resistances used resulted in sets being performed close to failure.

Clearly, when sets are carried to failure, the velocity of the bar decreases as the set progresses and exercise technique changes (Duffy and Challis 2007; Izquierdo et al. 2006). In some exercises, such as the power clean and power snatch, even though a set may not be carried to failure (i.e., the lifter cannot complete the repetition), fatigue of some motor units has occurred. Even if another repetition can be performed with good exercise technique, the maximal velocity of the bar is decreased, indicating the fatigue of some motor units. A slowing of maximal velocity in these exercises may be indicated by a greater knee angle when the bar is caught. Thus, from the perspective of maximal achievable bar velocity, the set has been carried to a point of momentary failure of some motor units.

Studies have specifically examined the effect of sets to failure compared to not training to failure. One of the earlier studies (Rooney et al. 1994) reported that, in untrained subjects, training to failure resulted in greater isometric and dynamic strength increases of the elbow flexors compared to not training to failure. After six weeks of training using the back squat, knee curl, and knee extension, training to failure showed no advantage in lower-body muscular endurance (work in back squat, knee curl, and knee extension at 100, 90, and 80% of 15RM to failure) compared to not training to failure (Willardson et al. 2008). One aspect of this study was that total training volume was equal between training to failure (three sets 13-15 repetitions, 60-115% of 15RM) and not training to failure (four sets of 10-12 repetitions, 60-115% of 15RM). This indicates that when total training volume is equal, there is no advantage to local muscular endurance in training to failure.

A 16-week study demonstrated increased local muscular endurance when training to failure, but greater power gains with not training to failure (Izquierdo et al. 2006). This study used a periodized training program and a peaking phase. Training not to failure for the first 11 weeks consisted of performing half of the repetitions at the same intensity as training to failure (see box 6.3).

This 11-week training period was followed by 5 weeks of a peaking phase with both groups training with 85 to 90% 1RM for three sets of two to four repetitions per set. During the peaking phase both groups also performed a ballistic training program consisting of vertical jump and medicine ball drills. Both the training-to-failure and not-training-to-failure groups significantly increased 1RM bench press (20 and 20%, respectively) and squat (19 and 20%, respectively) ability after 11 weeks of training. Bench press 1RM did not change significantly after the peaking phase, whereas squat 1RM increased significantly in both groups (3% for both). No significant difference between the groups after 11 weeks of training was shown for arm power, leg power, or maximal number of repetitions performed to failure (75% of 1RM) in the squat. Training to failure resulted in a significantly greater number of repetitions to failure in the bench press (46 vs. 28%) after 11 weeks of training and after the peaking phase (85 vs. 69%). After the peaking phase not training to failure resulted in a significantly greater increase in leg power. Results indicate that training to failure offers an advantage when training for local muscular endurance especially of the upper body (bench press), whereas not training to failure offers an advantage in lower-body power after a peaking phase.

Contradicting the preceding conclusions, a study of trained rowers who performed eight weeks of periodized weight training not to failure in conjunction with endurance training revealed significantly greater gains in bench press 1RM. However, in agreement with the preceding study, bench press power and rowing performance improved significantly more with training not to failure compared to training to failure (Izquierdo-Gabarren et al. 2010). Both studies indicate that not training to failure may increase power or sport performance.

The effects on the hormonal response when training to failure is inconclusive. Sets to failure result in a significantly greater acute hormonal response (growth hormone, testosterone) compared to sets not to failure (Linnamo et al. 2005). However, 16 weeks of training with sets not to failure resulted in a lower resting blood cortisol and higher testosterone concentration compared to training to failure; this indicates a more positive anabolic environment when training not to failure (Izquierdo et al. 2006).

More information concerning the effect of performing sets to failure is needed. It is clear

BOX 6.3 **RESEARCH**

The Effectiveness of Sets to Failure

Determining what is meant by a set not to failure can be difficult. In one of the studies discussed previously (Izquierdo et al. 2006), athletes experienced in weight training performed their normal periodized training for 16 weeks. For the first six weeks "not failure" was defined as performing six sets of five repetitions at a 10RM resistance in the bench press and the same number of sets and repetitions in the squat using 80% of 10RM. In weeks 7 to 11 it was defined as performing six sets of three repetitions at 6RM in the bench press and the same number of sets and repetitions at 80% of 6RM in the squat. During weeks 12 to 16, both "to failure" and "not to failure" training consisted of a peaking phase consisting of using 85 to 90% of 1RM or approximately 5RM and performing three sets of two to four repetitions per set.

In another study (Izquierdo-Gabarren et al. 2010) in which rowers were trained for eight weeks, "sets to failure" consisted of performing four sets at initially 10 repetitions per set at 75% of 1RM and progressing to four repetitions per set at 92% of 1RM. "Sets not to failure" was defined in two different ways: initially performing four sets of five repetitions per set and progressing toward two repetitions per set at the same intensities as the "to failure" training, or performing only two sets for the same number of repetitions at the same intensities as the "to failure" training.

The first study resulted in similar gains in strength using both "to failure" and "not to failure" training, but greater gains in local muscular endurance with training to failure and greater gains in power with training not to failure. The second study showed greater increases in maximal strength and power when four sets were performed not to failure compared to two sets not to failure. Interestingly, both the four-set and two-set "not to failure" training resulted in significantly greater increases in rowing power in 10 maximal strokes or over 20 minutes of rowing than training to failure did.

In both of these studies, "not to failure" training generally consisted of performing half of the repetitions per set as the "to failure" training. Yet in both studies "not to failure" training resulted in greater increases in some measure of power, and similar or greater increases in strength. This indicates that athletes performing other types of training may not need to carry sets to failure to bring about increases in performance.

Izquierdo, M., Ibanez, J., Gonzalez-Badillo, J.J., Häkkinen, K., Ratamess, N.A., Kraemer, W.J., French, D.N., Eslava, J., Altadill, A., Asiain, X., and Gorostiaga, E.M. 2006. Different effects of strength training leading to failure versus not to failure of hormonal responses, strength, and muscle power games. *Journal of Applied Physiology* 100: 1647-1656.

Izquierdo-Gabarren, M., Gonzalez De Txabarri Exposito, R., Gracia-Pallares, J., Sanchez-Medina, L., De Villarreal, G., and Izquierdo, M. 2010. Concurrent endurance and strength training not to failure optimizes performance gains. *Medicine & Science in Sports & Exercise* 42: 1191-1199.

that performing sets to failure is not necessary for increasing maximal strength, local muscular endurance, or hypertrophy. Additionally, the decision of whether to carry sets to failure may in part depend on whether the major training goal is an increase in local muscular endurance or an increase in some other factor, such as power. One inherent difficulty in such comparisons is defining what constitutes "not to failure." It could be defined as the point at which one or two more repetitions could be performed, or the point at which any other number of additional repetitions could be performed. Short periods of sets to failure may be helpful for advanced lifters who want to break through a training plateau (Willardson 2007a). However, training to failure repeatedly over long training periods is not recommended because of the increased risk of overtraining and overuse injuries (Willardson 2007a).

Burn Technique

The burn technique is an extension of the sets to failure technique. After a set has been performed to momentary concentric failure, the lifter performs half or partial repetitions. Normally, five or six partial repetitions are performed, which cause an aching or burning sensation, giving this system its name (Richford 1966). The burning sensation is in part probably due to an increase in intramuscular acidity. Advocates of the burn technique believe that performing partial repetitions in a fatigued state fatigues more motor units resulting in greater gains in strength and hypertrophy. This technique is claimed to be especially effective in training the calves and arms.

Forced Repetition, or Assisted Repetition, Technique

One form of the forced repetition technique is an extension of the sets to failure technique. After a set to failure has been completed, training partner(s) assist the trainee by lifting the resistance just enough to allow completion of two to four more repetitions. Assistance is only provided during the concentric, or lifting, phase of repetitions; the lifter performs the eccentric, or lowering, phase without assistance. Assistance can also be provided on some machines by performing the concentric phase of a repetition with two limbs and the eccentric phase with only one limb. Forced repetition has also come to mean to some weight trainers a type of heavy negative training. With this forced repetition technique two or three repetitions are performed with a resistance close to 1RM for the exercise. Similar to the first forced repetition technique described, assistance is provided during the concentric, but not the eccentric, phase of repetitions.

Advocates of forced repetitions believe that because the muscle is forced to continue to produce force after concentric failure or with a resistance greater than can be lifted during the concentric phase, more motor units are fatigued resulting in greater gains in strength, hypertrophy, and local muscular endurance. Increased fatigue as a result of forced repetitions is indicated by EMG data in experienced strength-trained athletes (powerlifters and Olympic weightlifters), but not people with no weight training experience (Ahtiainen and Häkkinen 2009). EMG activity decreased in the quadriceps of the strength-trained athletes but not in experienced weight trainers during four forced repetitions. This indicates increased fatigue and increased motor unit activation in the strength-trained athletes during forced repetitions. It also indicates that the response to forced repetitions may be different between trained and untrained people.

Lifters who can lift greater weights in the bench press and squat lower the resistance more slowly compared to lifters who lift a lighter resistance (Madsen and McLaughlin 1984; McLaughlin, Dillman, and Lardner 1977). Because the eccentric phase of a repetition is performed without assistance during forced repetitions, it can be hypothesized that this system helps develop the neural adaptations necessary for lowering a heavy resistance with good exercise technique. Therefore, this technique may be of value when attempting to increase the 1RM of exercises, such as the bench press, in which performing the eccentric portion of a repetition at a slow velocity of movement is advantageous because the resistance develops little momentum that needs to be overcome when beginning the concentric repetition phase.

Gains in 1RM over nine weeks of training were significantly greater for the biceps curl (13.2 vs. 8.2%) and bench press (16.5 vs. 10.6%) with three sets of 6 to 10 repetitions performed to failure followed by two assisted repetitions compared to one set of 6 to 10 repetitions performed to failure followed by two assisted repetitions (Humburg et al. 2007). However, although the one-legged leg press showed greater 1RM gains (right and left leg, 13.3 vs. 9.7% and 15.5 vs. 9.4%) with the three-set program, no significant difference was noted between the three-set and one-set programs. This study also used drop sets with the three-set program, which may compromise conclusions concerning assisted repetitions. However, results indicate that assisted repetitions may bring about greater increases in strength when used in conjunction with multiple-set programs compared to single-set programs.

A study comparing a single-set circuit system (8- to 12RM) with forced repetitions compared to a three-set circuit system without forced repetitions showed that the three-set circuit system resulted in significantly greater gains in bench press and leg press 1RM and in the number of repetitions possible at 80 and 85% of 1RM in the bench press and leg press, respectively (Kraemer 1997). Although confounded by the difference in the number of sets performed, the results do demonstrate that a three-set circuit system results in significantly greater gains in strength and local muscular endurance than a single-set circuit system with forced repetitions does. Forced repetitions with multiple-set training of the bench press showed that three or four forced repetitions compared to one forced repetition per training session resulted in no significant difference in 3RM ability, bench press throw, peak power, or mean power (Drinkwater et al. 2007). Thus, one forced repetition of an exercise per training session may be all that is necessary for achieving the benefits of this technique.

Forced, or assisted, repetitions must be used with caution because muscle soreness may easily develop, especially in lifters not accustomed to this technique. Additionally, because the forced repetitions are performed under conditions of fatigue (after a set has been carried to failure or with a weight too heavy to complete the concentric of phase of all repetitions in the set), the lifter will encounter acute discomfort and must attempt to complete the forced repetitions despite discomfort. The spotters need to be extremely attentive and capable of lifting all of the resistance being used if the lifter loses proper exercise technique or is fatigued to the point of being unable to complete a repetition.

Partial Repetition Technique

A partial repetition is a repetition performed within a restricted range of motion of an exercise. Normally, partial repetitions are performed for both the concentric and eccentric phases of a repetition for one to five repetitions per set with approximately 100% of 1RM. The amount of weight possible to use for a partial repetition depends on the strength curve of the exercise (i.e., ascending, descending, or bell shaped) and the range of motion in which the partial repetition is performed. For example, performance of the upper portion of the range of motion in a squat with greater resistance than possible for a complete repetition is due to the squat having an ascending strength curve. Advocates of the partial repetition technique believe that by using very heavy weights within a restricted range of motion, trainees increase their maximal strength.

Partial repetitions have been used successfully to increase isometric strength within the partial repetition range of motion and the full range of motion of an exercise in subjects with limited range of motion (Graves et al. 1989, 1992). In healthy weight-trained males, one bench press training session including both full range of motion and partial range of motion repetitions results in a significant increase in the partial repetition 1RM (4.8%) and 5RM (4.1%) weights, but no significant change in the full range of motion 1RM and 5RM weights (Mookerjee and Ratamess 1999). The partial repetition range of motion used for the bench press was from an elbow angle of 90 degrees to completion of a repetition.

Increases in strength or power with partial repetition training are probably due to neural adaptations, such as more muscle fiber recruitment within the partial repetition range of motion. Functional isometric training has been shown to increase full range of motion 1RM strength only when the training is performed at the sticking point of an exercise (see Functional Isometrics later in this chapter). This is related to the joint-angle specificity of isometric training. The lack of improvement in the bench press full range of motion repetition maximum weight with only one training session in the study described earlier, in which partial range of motion training did not include the sticking point in the bench press, may be related to the neural joint-angle specificity of the partial repetition technique.

Two studies following identical training programs indicate that full range of motion repetitions of the bench press increase strength significantly more than partial repetitions in untrained females but not untrained males (Massey et al. 2004, 2005). Normal full range of motion training, partial range of motion training at 100% 1RM, and a mixed training program with two sets of partial range of motion and one set of normal range of motion for five weeks followed by one set of partial range of motion and two sets of full range of motion for the last five weeks of training were compared. The partial range of motion repetitions were performed in the top portion (elbows extended) of the bench press's range of motion when muscles involved are at a relatively short length. All groups significantly improved bench press 1RM. Training with a full range of motion (35%) increased 1RM in women significantly more than training with partial repetitions (22%) and the mixed training protocol (23%). No significant difference in bench press 1RM between training programs was shown for men.

Dynamic constant external resistance (DCER) training of the knee extensors and flexors from a knee angle of 80 to 115 degrees and 170 to 135 degrees, respectively, increased power significantly (Ullrich, Kleinder, and Bruggemann 2010). During both of these ranges of motion the muscles are at relatively long lengths, which indicates that partial repetitions with the muscle at long lengths do significantly increase power. The previously described studies of the bench press indicate that strength may be increased when the partial repetition is performed with the muscle in a relatively shortened length. Thus, strength or power may be increased with partial repetitions with either the muscle in a shortened or lengthened position; however, whether a shortened or lengthened muscle length is more advantageous is unclear.

Partial range of motion squats (knee angle to 120 degrees) compared to full range of motion squats (thighs parallel to floor) can result in greater force and power (Drinkwater, Moore, and Bird 2012). Both types of squats were performed for 10 or 5 repetitions using 67 and 83% of 1RM, respectively. Velocity of movement was not controlled, and the velocity used was at the discretion of the lifters. Power and maximal force during the partial range of motion squat with 87% of 1RM were greater than they were during the other three sets of squats. The maximal velocity was greater during the full range of motion squats with 63% of 1RM compared to the other squat sets. The results indicate that partial range of motion squats can result in greater power and force output than full range of motion squats when lifters choose the velocity of movement, but this is only true with heavier resistances.

Partial range of motion repetitions do significantly increase maximal range of motion strength and may be a useful adjunct to full range of motion training in some situations. Additionally, in healthy people partial repetitions do appear to increase maximal strength very quickly (one training session) within the range of motion of the partial repetition. Thus, partial repetitions may be appropriate for those who want to quickly increase maximal strength within a certain range of motion of an exercise.

Super Slow Systems

Super slow systems involve performing repetitions at a slow velocity. Although any slow velocity can be used, typically with super slow training only one or two sets of an exercise are performed with 10-second concentric and 4- or 5-second eccentric repetition phases. Proponents of super slow systems believe that the increased amount of time that a muscle is under tension enhances strength development, hypertrophy, and aerobic capabilities more than the use of traditional repetition velocities does.

Bench press super slow training at 55% of 1RM with both concentric and eccentric repetition phases lasting five seconds were compared to traditional heavy weight training (six repetitions at 6RM); EMG activity of the pectoralis major and triceps brachii, during both the eccentric and con-

centric phases, was significantly greater with the traditional heavy weight training (Keogh, Wilson, and Weatherby 1999). This was true during the first, middle, and last repetitions of the set. This indicates less muscle fiber recruitment with the super slow system.

Early studies demonstrate that super slow training can increase maximal strength. Super slow training with one set of four to six repetitions with a 10-second concentric and a 4-second eccentric repetition phase resulted in similar strength gains as a typical one-set program of 8 to 12 repetitions using a 2-second concentric and a 4-second eccentric repetition phase (Westcott 1994). In a similar study, subjects performed both eccentric-emphasized training (10-second eccentric and 4-second concentric repetition phases) and concentric-emphasized training (4-second eccentric and 10-second concentric repetition phases) for one set of four to six repetitions (Westcott 1995). Strength increases were similar between the concentric- and eccentric-emphasized training. Neither of these studies statistically analyzed the results, but both indicate that super slow training can increase strength. Training with either eccentric-emphasized (6-second eccentric, 2-second concentric) or concentric-emphasized (6-second eccentric, 2-second concentric) training does significantly increase strength (Gillies, Putman, and Bell 2006). Although both programs resulted in significant increases in concentric (21%), eccentric (44%), and normal (25%) repetition 1RM, no significant difference in strength gains was shown.

Several studies have compared super slow and traditional resistance training. A study in which untrained women performed either super slow training (50% of 1RM, 10-second concentric and 5-second eccentric phases) or traditional weight training (2-second concentric and 4-second eccentric phases) for one set showed that traditional weight training resulted in significantly greater strength improvement in five of eight exercises (Keeler et al. 2001). For example, 1RM for the bench press (34 vs. 11%), leg press (33 vs. 7%), and knee curl (40 vs. 15%) were all significantly greater with traditional training. Additionally, neither training group significantly changed body composition (BOD POD) or maximal oxygen consumption.

A four-week comparison of super slow training for one set (10-second concentric and eccentric repetition phases at 50% of 1RM) and traditional training for three sets of eight repetitions (2-second concentric and eccentric repetition phases at 80% of 1RM) showed no significant difference in strength gains between the two types of training, but only the traditional training showed significantly greater strength gains than a control group (Kim et al. 2011). A comparison of super slow (50% of 1RM, 10-second concentric and 5-second eccentric phases) and traditional training (80% of 1RM, 2-second concentric and 4-second eccentric phases) showed no significant difference in strength gains in untrained men (Neils et al. 2005). Both groups performed seven exercises for six to eight repetitions per set. Both groups did significantly increase 1RM squat (traditional 6.8% vs. super slow 3.6%) and bench press (traditional 8.6% vs. super slow 9.1%) ability, but no significant difference between groups was demonstrated. Additionally, body composition (dual-energy X-ray absorptiometry) did not change significantly in either group. However, peak power and counter-movement jump ability significantly increased with the traditional training, but not with the super slow training. The results indicate that strength and power gains may be greater with traditional training velocities, but body composition changes are similar with both types of training.

Middle-aged men and women trained either with a super slow program (10-second concentric and 4-second eccentric phases) or a traditional training program; both showed significant increases in strength (Wescott et al. 2001). Training consisted of one set of 13 different exercises. Those in the super slow group did show significantly greater strength gains than those who undertook traditional training. However, a limitation of the study was that 5RM and 10RM strength was tested in the super slow and traditional training groups, respectively.

Traditional training (80-85% of 1RM, 1- to 2-second concentric and eccentric phases) does result in different muscle fiber adaptations compared to super slow (40-60% of 1RM, 10-second concentric and 4-second eccentric phases) training (Herman 2009). Both groups trained the legs with three sets of three exercises (leg press, squat, and knee extension). Muscle fiber–type changes were examined in the vastus lateralis. The cross-sectional area of all major fiber types (type I, IIa, and IIx) significantly increased with traditional training, whereas with super slow training only two major fiber types significantly increased in cross-sectional area (IIa and IIx). Additionally, only traditional training showed an increase in the percentage of IIa fibers, and traditional training showed an increase in satellite cell content in more fiber types (I, IIa, IIax, IIx vs. IIax, IIx) than super slow training did. The results indicate that traditional training results in a greater overall muscle fiber response than super slow training does.

Collectively, the studies indicate that super slow training can increase maximal strength. However, it may not result in greater 1RM strength gains, greater increases in power, or greater overall muscle fiber type response. It is interesting to note that total energy expenditure resulting from performing 10 exercises with traditional training may be as high as 48% greater (172 vs. 116 kcal) than that of super slow training (Hunter, Seelhorst, and Snyder 2003). Both training sessions lasted 29 minutes; however, during traditional training two sets of each exercise were performed, whereas with super slow training one set was performed. Even though those in the traditional training group performed more sets of each exercise, because total training time was equal, traditional training results in a greater caloric expenditure per unit of time, which suggests that a greater decrease in body fat may occur with traditional training.

Vascular Occlusion

Vascular occlusion is a relatively new resistance training technique. It involves using a narrow cuff to compress the major artery supplying the muscle or muscles to be trained, which decreases blood flow to the muscle(s). The cuff is normally inflated to approximately diastolic blood pressure (Manni and Clark 2009). Normally, low resistance training intensities (20-50% of 1RM) are used in conjunction with vascular occlusion. This type of training was used as early as the 1980s in Japan and is known as Kaatsu training. Kaatsu walk training compared to walk training without occlusion increases muscle cross-sectional area (4-7%) and isometric strength (8-10%), whereas normal walk training has no significant effect on these measures (Abe, Kearns, and Sato 2005).

Vascular occlusion training received a major impetus in 2000 when a 16-week low-intensity (30-50% of 1RM) with occlusion training program in older women was reported to result in similar strength and muscle cross-sectional area increases as a high-intensity (50-80% of 1RM) without occlusion training program (Takarada, Nakamura, et al. 2000). Other training studies have concluded that vascular occlusion training at 50% of 1RM results in significantly greater increases in muscle cross-sectional area and strength gains in untrained athletes (Moore et al. 2004) as well as trained athletes (Takarada, Sato, and Ishii 2002) compared to training at the same intensity without vascular occlusion.

Although some advantage with vascular occlusion training at approximately 20% of 1RM is shown for strength (isokinetic peak torque had a significantly greater increase at 60 degrees per second, but not at 180 degrees per second), no significant difference in muscle cross-sectional area compared to the same training program without occlusion is shown (Sumide et al. 2009). However, other studies show that vascular occlusion training at 50% of 1RM (Baurgomaster et al. 2003) or 60% of 1RM (approximately 12RM) and 80% of 1RM (approximately 6RM) resulted in no greater strength or muscle size gains than performing the same training program without occlusion (Laurentino et al. 2008). Similarly, training with occlusion at 20% of 1RM (40%) shows no significant difference in 1RM increases compared to training without occlusion at 20% (21%) or 80% (36%) of 1RM (Laurentino et al. 2012). However, only the training with occlusion at 20% of 1RM and 80% of 1RM without occlusion significantly increased muscle cross-sectional area (6%) and decreased myostatin gene expression, which may be related to these two types of training showing increased muscle cross-sectional area. Thus, not all studies show a clear advantage in strength or muscle size increases with vascular occlusion training.

Why vascular occlusion training would result in greater strength and muscle size gains is unclear. It is clear that using vascular occlusion while performing weight training results in a greater reliance on anaerobic metabolism, an increase in some hormones (the growth hormone norepinephrine), increased acidity within the muscle being trained, and increased free radicals or reactive oxygen molecules compared to the same training without occlusion (Abe, Kearns, and Sato 2006; Manni and Clark 2009; Takarada, Nakamura et al. 2000; Takarada Takazawa et al. 2000). Whether these factors directly or indirectly affect maximal strength gains or increase muscle protein synthesis resulting in increased muscle hypertrophy remains to be elucidated. Thus, the effectiveness of vascular occlusion in conjunction with low-intensity resistance training is unclear.

Small Increment Technique

The resistance used for an exercise is traditionally increased when a certain number of repetitions per set can be performed. With free weights and plate-loaded machines, normally the smallest resistance increase is 2.5 lb (1.1 kg). With selectorized resistance training machines, the smallest resistance increase can be quite large (10 lb [4.5 kg] or more) if lighter weights that attach in some manner to the weight stack are not available. The small increment technique uses smaller increases in resistance than are typically used.

A short-duration (eight-week) training study demonstrated that the small increment technique resulted in 1RM gains in the bench press and triceps press equivalent to those of a more traditional increase in resistance technique (Hostler, Crill et al. 2001). With the small increment technique the resistance was increased 0.5 lb (0.23 kg) when seven or eight repetitions could be performed per set and 1 lb (0.45 kg) when nine or more repetitions could be performed per set. During training the resistance was increased approximately four times as often for the bench press and two times as often for the triceps press as with a traditional technique. The use of a small increment technique may improve the satisfaction of novice lifters and increase the likelihood of their continuing a program as a result of the positive feedback of increasing resistance at a rapid rate. This system may also be of use with experienced lifters who are experiencing a training plateau (Hostler, Crill et al. 2001).

Specialized Systems and Techniques

Specialized systems and techniques are designed to produce particular training goals in advanced lifters. Typically, goals of advanced lifters include increasing 1RM, motor performance, or muscle hypertrophy. Specialized systems and techniques are normally recommended only for advanced lifters who have already mastered exercise technique and have made substantial physiological adaptations to weight training.

Functional Isometrics

Functional isometrics attempts to take advantage of the joint-angle-specific strength gains caused by isometric training (see Isometric Training in chapter 2). Functional isometrics entails performing a dynamic concentric action for a portion of the concentric phase of a repetition until the resistance hits the pins of a power rack (see figure 6.2). The trainee then continues to attempt to lift the resistance with a maximal effort performing an isometric action for five to seven seconds. Note that in figure 6.2 pins in the power rack are also set at the lowest point of the range of motion for the safety of the lifter.

The objective of this system is to use joint-angle specificity to cause increases in strength at the joint angle at which the isometric action is performed. The joint angle chosen to perform the isometric action is normally the sticking point (i.e., the weakest point in the concentric range of motion) for the exercise. The maximal amount of resistance that can be lifted concentrically in any exercise is determined by the amount of resistance that can be moved through the sticking point. It is thought that increasing strength at the sticking point results in increases in 1RM.

The need to perform the isometric action at the sticking point of an exercise is supported by research. Short-term training studies comparing the use of functional isometrics in a training program to a normal DCER program indicate that significantly greater increases in 1RM bench press (19 vs. 11%, Jackson et al. 1985) and squat (26 vs. 10%, O'Shea and O'Shea 1989) occur when functional isometrics are performed at or near the exercise's sticking point. However, in both the bench press and the squat, when functional isometrics are performed at an elbow or knee angle of 170 degrees, which is not near the sticking point for either of these exercises, there is no significant difference in 1RM increases compared to a normal DCER training program (Giorgi et al. 1998).

Adding a three-second functional isometric squat after a five-minute low-intensity cycling warm-up may significantly increase countermovement vertical jump ability compared to the low-intensity warm-up alone (Berning et al. 2010). An increase of approximately 5% at four and five minutes after the functional isometric squat compared to the warm-up alone was shown in men with resistance training experience, but not in men with no resistance training experience. This indicates that functional isometrics may increase performance after a warm-up in experienced weight trainers.

Many powerlifters use functional isometrics without a power rack during the last repetition of a heavy set (e.g., 1- to 6RM). They attempt to perform the greatest range of motion as possible in the concentric phase of the last repetition, and when they cannot lift the weight any farther, they continue to produce force isometrically at the exact angle at which the sticking point occurs. This type of training requires very attentive spotters. It appears that, to use this system optimally, lifters

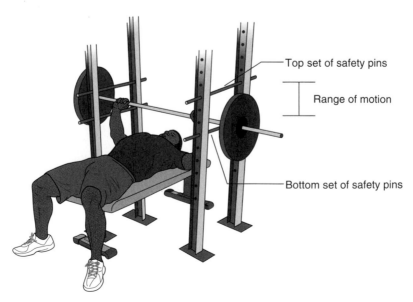

Top set of safety pins

Range of motion

Bottom set of safety pins

FIGURE 6.2 Functional isometrics used at the sticking point in the bench press. The top pin is placed at the exact point in the range of motion desired to be trained. The bottom pin is placed at the lowest point in the range of motion.

must know the sticking point in their range of motion to optimize training. This system is appropriate when the major goal of the program is to increase the 1RM capability of a particular exercise.

Implement Training

Implement training uses a variety of objects as the resistance to be lifted or moved (see figure 6.3). It can involve lifting water-filled dumbbells, water-filled barrels, kettlebells, or a tire (Bennett 2008; Hedrick 2003). Some forms of implement training are termed strongman training because of their resemblance to tasks in strongman contests. Advocates of implement training believe that lifting an unstable object, such as a water-filled barrel in which the water moves while the barrel is lifted, simulates lifting or moving unstable objects encountered in daily life activities or sports. Some types of implements, such as kettlebells, allow rotational and other movements that are difficult to perform with traditional dumbbells or barbells; these movements also resemble movements or tasks in various sporting events. These types of exercises are incorporated into some strength and conditioning programs; however, little research is available on most types of implement training.

Success in the tire flip, in which a large tire is flipped end over end, depends in large part on the duration of time from when the tire is just past the knees until the hands leave the tire to be repositioned on the tire as it nears an upright position (figure 6.4). The tire flip also results in significant elevations in heart rate and blood lactate indicating its benefit as an anaerobic conditioning exercise (Keogh et al. 2010). However, similar to most implement training methods, evidence of carryover to sport performance is lacking.

Kettlebell training and normal weight training for six weeks both significantly increase vertical jump, 1RM squat, and power clean ability (Otto et al. 2012). In this study, normal weight training included the squat, power clean, and other exercises. Kettlebell training included a variety of exercises. Vertical jump (approximately 2%) and 1RM power clean ability increased significantly with both types of training, but the percentage of increase in the power clean was greater with normal weight training (9 vs. 4%). Squat 1RM increased with both types of training, but the increase with normal weight training was significantly greater (13.5 vs. 4.5%). Kettlebell swing training with ten 35-second intervals separated by 25-second rest intervals does increase heart rate sufficiently to cause increases in aerobic ability (Hulsey et al. 2012). Thus, kettlebell training can be used to increase strength, power, and aerobic ability.

Perhaps the implement training that is most researched is the use of under- and overweight

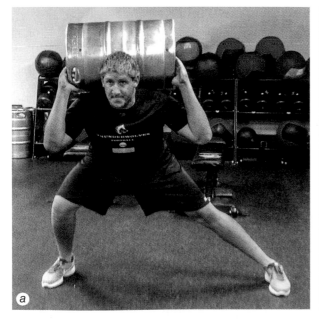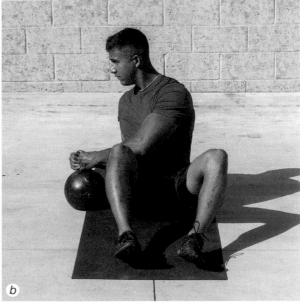

FIGURE 6.3 Implement training uses implements as the resistance to be lifted or moved: *(a)* a water-filled barrel being used in a side lunge–type movement, *(b)* a kettlebell being lifted in a torso rotation movement.

Photo 6.3a courtesy of Allen Hedrick, Colorado State University-Pueblo.

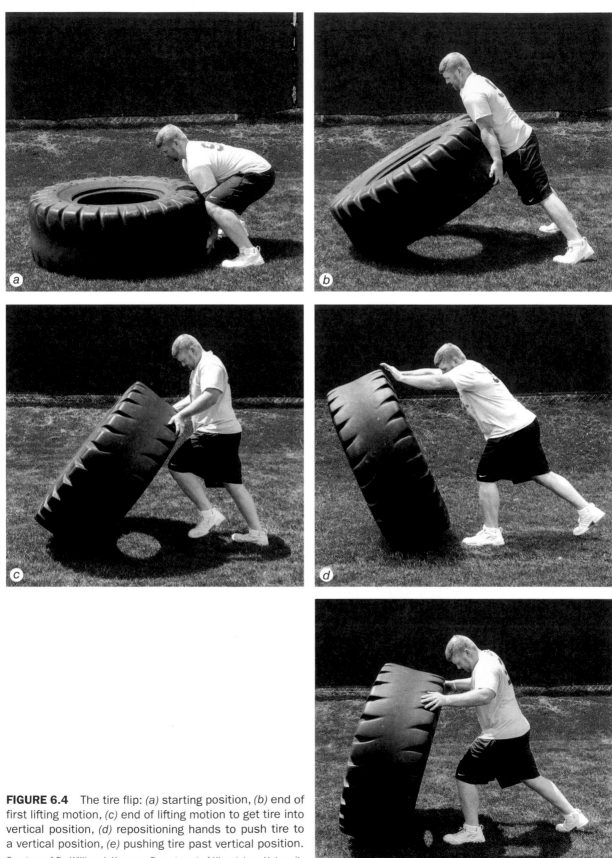

FIGURE 6.4 The tire flip: *(a)* starting position, *(b)* end of first lifting motion, *(c)* end of lifting motion to get tire into vertical position, *(d)* repositioning hands to push tire to a vertical position, *(e)* pushing tire past vertical position.

balls and bats to increase throwing and bat velocity, respectively, in baseball and softball players. Training by throwing both under- and overweight baseballs does increase maximal throwing velocity, and the use of a slightly under- or overweight ball (+ 20% of a normal baseball of 5 oz, or 142 grams) does not significantly affect throwing movement patterns (Szymanski, DeRenne, and Spaniol 2009). Similarly, training using under- and overweight bats (–12 to +100% of a normal bat) can significantly increase bat velocity (Szymanski, DeRenne, and Spaniol 2009). However, the increase in bat velocity due to the use of under- and overweight bats in training varies from no significant change to as much as a 10% increase (Szymanski, DeRenne, and Spaniol 2009). It is important to note that bat velocity increases can also occur as a result of swing training with a standard bat. Under- and overweight bats are also used as a warm-up prior to hitting to increase bat velocity significantly. The acute effects of using under- and overweight bats in a warm-up to increase bat velocity are contradictory; increases of approximately 6% (Reyes and Doly 2009) and no significant change have been shown (Szymamski e al. 2011).

Thus, under- and overweight balls and bats may increase performance in sport-related tasks of baseball and softball players. Similarly, kicking weighted soccer balls may be useful for increasing ball-kicking velocity (Young et al. 2011). However, the majority of implement training methods lack supporting research.

Vibration Training

Vibration training is quite popular. Vibration can be used acutely, such as in a warm-up to increase physical performance in an upcoming activity, or during long-term training to enhance strength and power gains. The most popular type is whole-body vibration, in which a person stands on a vibrating platform. Other types of vibration training include using vibrating dumbbells and equipment that applies vibration directly to a tendon or other body part.

Several physiological mechanisms have been suggested to explain how vibration training increases physical performance (Rehn et al. 2007). It may happen as a result of increased sensitivity of the stretch reflex or muscle spindles, which initiate muscle contraction, or by increased muscle fiber recruitment. Both of these neural mechanisms may increase the force or power of a muscle. Specific hormonal responses, such as increased testosterone or growth hormone, as well as increased hypertrophy may also increase performance. However, there is no clear consensus on how vibration may enhance neuromuscular performance.

Many factors may affect whether a significant change in strength and power takes place as a result of vibration. The frequency or number of vibrations per second (Hz) and amplitude (displacement), or how far the vibrating platform or vibrating implement travels during each vibration, are the most frequently described variables.

The two major types of whole-body vibration platforms (the most popular type of vibration used in training) are vertical and oscillating. Vertical vibration platforms, as the name implies, vibrate predominantly vertically; oscillating platforms vibrate through rotation about a horizontal axis. Table 6.4 lists other factors that could affect whether changes in strength, power, or

TABLE 6.4 Factors Affecting Vibration Training

Factor	Explanation
Frequency of vibration	Number of vibrations per second (Hz)
Amplitude of vibration	Displacement of the vibration
Damping	Use of footwear or padded handles may affect the frequency or magnitude of the vibration
Direction of vibration	Direction in which the vibration occurs; vertical and oscillating whole-body vibrating platforms are the most common
Duration	How long vibration takes place during each session, the number of vibration sessions, and the number of exercises performed with vibration
Timing of performance measurement	Acutely, the time between the vibration and the performance measurement; in long-term training, the time between the last vibration training session and the performance measurement
Posture	Body position in which vibration takes place
Rest periods	Length of rest periods between vibration sessions or exercises performed with vibration

performance occur as a result of vibration training. Any or all of these factors may determine whether vibration affects performance acutely or during long-term training.

Whole-body vibration is most commonly used in training and in research in part because whole-body vibration platforms are commercially available. Normally, vibration training involves performing an exercise movement, such as a squat or maintaining a partial squat position (quarter or half squat), which results in an isometric action of the leg musculature, while standing on a whole-body vibration platform. Measures of force and power are made shortly after the vibration training bout to determine the acute effects. Acute exposure to whole-body oscillating vibration does increase countermovement jump ability in female field hockey athletes (Cochrane and Stannard 2005) and recreationally active males (Turner, Sanderson, and Attwood 2011). Similarly, maximal isometric force is also increased significantly immediately after (9.4%) and eight minutes after (10.4%) performing squat-type exercises with vertical whole-body vibration (McBride, Nuzzo et al. 2010). Thus, whole-body vibration can acutely increase strength and power.

However, a critical review of the acute effects of whole-body vibration concludes that there is no clear evidence that vibration acutely affects muscular performance (Rehn et al. 2007). A meta-analysis concludes that there is no acute effect on strength using either vertical or oscillating whole-body vibration platforms (Marin and Rhea 2010).

Inconsistent changes in strength, power, or jumping ability due to acute vibration exposure are apparent. However, just as important, and perhaps more important, are the effects of vibration on other measures of performance, such as sprint ability. Sprint performance (5, 10, and 40 m) after whole-body vibration (30, 40, and 50 Hz) is not significantly affected; however, a trend toward a decrease in sprint time with the frequency of 30 Hz was shown (Guggenheimer et al. 2009). When vertical whole-body vibration is used between two bouts of countermovement jumps and short sprints, smaller decreases in performance are apparent compared to no vibration between the two bouts of exercise (Bullock et al. 2008). This suggests that acute vibration may have small positive effects on sprint performance.

Whole-body vibration can be added to a long-term training program by performing it in addition to the normal training program (e.g., prior to normal training sessions) or by performing it between sets of a resistance training program. In either case, similar to examining the acute effects of vibration, long-term vibration training typically involves performing a movement, such as a squat movement, or an isometric action, such as holding a quarter squat position while standing on a whole-body vibration platform. All of the factors previously discussed could determine whether vibration training positively affects strength, power, or another measure of performance.

Adding vertical whole-body vibration training to the program of ballerinas did significantly increase countermovement jump performance (6.3%) and average power against various resistances (50, 70, and 100 kg, or 110, 154, and 220 lb) in a press-type movement (Annino et al. 2007). Note that no comparison to another type of training in the ballerinas' total training program was made. A nine-week comparison of normal squat training and squat training with added resistance on an oscillating whole-body vibration platform resulted in both groups significantly increasing maximal isometric force in a one-legged leg press; no significant difference was seen between the training programs (Kvorning et al. 2006). However, countermovement jump height and power increased significantly only with the normal squat training program. One possible explanation for this result is changes in the hormonal response to training. Although both the vibration and no-vibration training programs resulted in a significant increase in testosterone and growth hormone during training sessions, the vibration training resulted in a significantly greater increase in growth hormone.

Adding vertical whole-body vibration training to the training program of women basketball players, which included resistance training, showed no significant advantage in various measures of strength and power compared to the normal training program (Fernandez-Rio et al. 2010). The added whole-body vibration training consisted of performing isometric actions for the leg musculature (half squat and standing on the toes) while standing on the vibrating platform. A series of studies adding vertical whole-body vibration training (isometric quarter squat) between sets during a six-week periodized squat training program demonstrated some small significant advantages in the initial rate of force development (up to 150 ms) during countermovement jumps and weighted squat jumps compared to the same training program without vibration training (Lamont et al. 2008, 2009, 2010).

The preceding discussion makes it clear that responses to whole-body vibration training can be varied, probably due to the frequency, duration, and other factors related to vibration training. A systematic review concludes that long-term whole-body vibration can have positive effects on leg musculature performance in untrained people and elderly women (Rehn et al. 2007). A meta-analysis also noted positive effects on performance as a result of long-term whole-body vibration training (Marin and Rhea 2010). However, these effects depend in part on the characteristics of the training. Vertical whole-body vibration causes a significantly greater long-term effect on strength than oscillating vibration does. Low vibration frequencies (<35 Hz) and high frequencies (>40 Hz) are less effective than moderate frequencies (35-40 Hz), which indicates that moderate frequencies are most appropriate for whole-body vibration.

The conclusion that moderate vibration frequencies are best for increasing strength is in agreement with an acute study indicating that a frequency of 40 Hz increases countermovement jump ability significantly (6%), but that other frequencies have no significant effect (Turner, Sanderson, and Attwood 2011). Vibration amplitudes of less than 6 mm are effective; an amplitude of 8 to 10 mm is the most effective for power increases. The total training time ranged from 360 to 720 seconds per training session; however, it is unclear whether short sets (15 to 30 seconds) or longer sets (several minutes) are optimal for increasing power.

Although whole-body vibration is the most common type of vibration training, vibration can also be applied directly to a tendon or a specific muscle group using specialized or custom-built equipment. Several acute studies show inconsistent effects of this type of vibration. One bout of vibration applied to the knee extensors while performing knee extension exercise at 35 or 70% of 1RM did increase strength and power during exercise as well as 1RM after exercise (Mileva et al. 2006). Vibration applied using a vibrating barbell between successive sets of the bench press does increase average power with a trend ($p = .06$) toward increased peak power during a bench press with 70% of 1RM (Poston et al. 2007). However, upper-body vibration using a vibrating dumbbell does not affect measures of upper-body power

(medicine ball throw), grip strength, or climbing-specific performance in experienced rock climbers (Cochrane and Hawke 2007).

Similar to whole-body vibration, whether an acute change in strength or power occurs as a result of the vibration of a tendon or a specific muscle group may depend on the characteristics of the vibration used. For example, vibration applied to the biceps musculature at frequencies of 6, 12, and 24 Hz all result in increased maximal isometric force, whereas a higher frequency of 48 Hz decreased maximal isometric force (Kin-Isler, Acikada, and Artian 2006). However, vibration applied directly to the biceps tendon at 65 Hz does not affect power output during successive sets of bicep curls using 70% of 1RM or at one and a half and eight minutes after the last set of biceps curls (Moran, McNamara, and Luo 2007). These results indicate that acute exposure to lower-frequency vibration may increase strength and power, whereas exposure to higher frequencies does not.

Studies of the long-term effects of training with vibrating dumbbells, or some other device that applies vibration directly to a tendon or muscle, are inconclusive. A few have examined the long-term effects of such devices and show small effects (effect size 0.02), but an insufficient number of studies are available to come to conclusions concerning these type of devices (Marin and Rhea 2010). However, a four-week isometric training study demonstrated that adding vibration while performing an arm curl exercise increased maximal isometric strength significantly more (26 vs. 10%) than the same training program without vibration (Silva et al. 2008).

Clearly, frequency, amplitude, and other characteristics of vibration can determine whether vibration training results in an acute or chronic effect. The rest period length between vibration bouts in a training session does affect the response. When vertical whole-body vibration is used for multiple stimulation bouts (six bouts of one minute, 30 Hz, 4 mm amplitude) in one training session, rest periods between successive bouts of two and one minute both significantly increase squat jump ability, countermovement jump ability, and leg musculature power; bouts using three-minute rest periods have no significant effect on these measures (DaSilva-Grigoletto et al. 2009). However, bouts with two-minute rest periods resulted in significantly greater increases in these measures than did bouts using the other two rest period lengths. When one- or two-minute rest periods are used in a similar training program for four weeks, both conditions produced significant increases in measures of strength and power (DaSilva-Grigoletto et al. 2009). However, the increases in squat jump (9 vs. 4%), countermovement jump (7 vs. 4%), and 4RM squat (13 vs. 11%) ability were significantly greater with the one-minute rest periods. Thus, the optimal length of rest period may depend on whether an acute or long-term training effect is desired.

Neural changes or adaptations are one possible explanation for vibration training effects on performance. However, the study results on the acute effects of vibration on EMG measures are inconsistent. Leg musculature EMG activity can increase during exercise performed during vertical whole-body vibration (Roelants et al. 2006), and whole-body oscillating vibration increases muscle spindle sensitivity (Hopkins et al. 2008). Similarly, vibration applied to the knee extensors during knee extensor exercise increases EMG measures (firing frequency, conduction velocity) of motor unit excitability (Mileva et al. 2006). However, EMG measures of motor neuron excitability have also been shown not to be affected by vertical whole-body vibration (McBride, Nuzzo et al. 2010), and biceps EMG activity is not affected by vibration applied directly to the biceps tendon (Moran, McNamara, and Luo 2007).

Dampening of vibration may also affect whether a change in strength, power, or performance occurs. Wearing shoes, or the type of shoe worn, may affect the EMG response of muscles to whole-body vibration. For example, with or without shoes the EMG response of the vastus lateralis and medial gastrocnemius are both greater during vertical whole-body vibration with an amplitude of 4 mm compared to 2 mm. However, vastus lateralis EMG activity is greatest without shoes, and medial gastrocnemius EMG activity is greatest with shoes at an amplitude of 4 mm (Narin et al. 2009). Thus, the response of different muscles may be affected differently by the dampening effect of wearing shoes during whole-body vibration.

Frequency, amplitude, duration, and the timing of a performance measure all affect whether a change in strength or power occurs. Increases in countermovement jump one minute after vertical whole-body vibration with various combinations of frequency, amplitude, and duration indicate

that as little as 30 seconds of whole-body vibration can increase countermovement jump ability immediately after and five minutes after, but not 10 minutes after, whole-body vibration (Adams et al. 2009). However, it has also been shown that countermovement jump ability immediately after vertical whole-body vibration is significantly increased, whereas 5, 15, and 30 minutes after whole-body vibration no significant effect on countermovement jump ability is found (Cormie et al. 2006). Thus, the acute effect of any performance increase due to whole-body vibration may be relatively short-lived. Additionally, high frequencies (40 and 50 Hz) coupled with large amplitude (4-6 mm) and low frequencies (30 and 35 Hz) coupled with small amplitude (2-4 mm) may provide the optimal stimulus for acutely increasing countermovement vertical jump ability (Adams et al. 2009).

Another factor that may affect whether a change in performance occurs is the muscle length at which force or power is measured. Several lengths (various joint angles) of the elbow flexors show significant increases in maximal isometric force when force is measured during vibration, but no difference in the increase is shown among various muscle lengths (Kin-Isler, Acikada, and Artian 2006). However, plantar flexion isokinetic peak torque occurs at a longer muscle length after a bout of whole-body vibration while dorsiflexion peak torque is not affected significantly by a bout of whole-body vibration and so shows no effect of muscle length at which peak torque occurs after whole-body vibration (Kemertzis et al. 2008). Thus, the effects of muscle length on increases in force or power are unclear.

Perhaps one of the more consistent findings is an increase in flexibility shortly after exposure to vibration. Increased flexibility has been shown in athletes (women field hockey and young male and female gymnasts) after whole-body vibration, vibration of specific muscle groups, and stretching while vibration is applied to specific muscle groups (Cochrane and Stannard 2005; Kinser et al. 2008; Sands et al. 2006, 2008). The effect of long-term flexibility training with vibration has received little study, but it appears to increase flexibility during four weeks of training and appears to be promising as a way to increase flexibility during long-term training (Sands et al. 2006). Vibration may also decrease delayed-onset muscle soreness (DOMS) after eccentric (downhill walking) exercise, which could be important as a recovery method between training sessions (Bakhitary et al. 2006). This suggests that vibration training may offer other benefits in addition to increases in strength or power.

This discussion makes it clear that the effects of acute exposure to vibration and long-term vibration training depend on the frequency and amplitude as well as other characteristics of the vibration used. As with many types of training, large differences in the individual response to a specific vibration stimulus are also apparent. Another factor complicating the possible effect of vibration training is the consistency of the vibration produced by the equipment, such as any changes in the displacement of a vibration platform with increased body mass. There do appear to be positive effects of both acute and long-term vibration training, but further study is warranted.

Negative Training

During most resistance exercises the negative, or eccentric, portion of the repetition is the lowering of the resistance. During this phase the muscles are actively lengthening to lower the resistance in a controlled manner. Conversely, in most exercises the lifting of the resistance is termed the positive, or concentric, portion of a repetition. The effects of isokinetic eccentric, DCER eccentric only, and accentuated eccentric training as well as comparisons of eccentric and concentric training were discussed in chapter 2. Here the discussion will be limited to the use of negative, or eccentric, training as an adjunct to traditional resistance training.

It is possible to lower more weight in the negative phase of a repetition than is lifted in the positive phase. Thus, it is possible to use more than the 1RM for a complete repetition when performing negative training. **Negative training** involves lowering, or performing the eccentric portion of repetitions, with more than the 1RM for a complete repetition. Accentuated eccentric training refers to training in which a complete repetition is performed but more resistance is used in the eccentric phase than in the concentric phase. This type of training was discussed in chapter 2 and will not be discussed here.

Negative training can be done by having spotters help the lifter raise the weight, which the lifter then lowers unassisted. It can also be performed on some resistance training machines by lifting the weight with both arms or legs and then lowering the resistance with only one arm or leg. Some machines are specifically built to allow the use of more resistance in the eccentric phase of a repetition. Proper exercise technique and safe spotting techniques must be used for all exercises performed in a heavy negative fashion.

Ranges of 105 to 140% of the concentric 1RM have been proposed for use during negative training. Seniors (mean age 68 years) safely used a range of 115 to 140% of the concentric 1RM during the eccentric phase of repetitions of six machine exercises during training (Nichols, Hitzelberger et al. 1995); during negative-only knee extension, 11.7 repetitions can be performed with 120% of a normal (concentric–eccentric repetition) 1RM (Carpinelli and Gutin 1991). Thus, using greater than the concentric 1RM during eccentric training appears to be safe. However, the amount of resistance that can be used during eccentric training may vary substantially from one exercise to another and by sex (table 6.5).

Men's eccentric-only 1RMs determined on machines were between 27 and 49% greater than the machines' concentric-only 1RM (see table 6.5), whereas women's eccentric-only 1RMs on machines varied between 66 and 161% greater than the concentric-only 1RM. Note that the men's eccentric-only 1RM is generally within the proposed percentages of concentric 1RM for use during eccentric training. However, women's eccentric-only 1RM for some exercises is substantially greater than the proposed limits of concentric 1RM for use during eccentric training. Additionally, the resistance used for negative training may depend on whether a machine or free weights are used. Heavier negative resistances may be possible with machines because they reduce the need for balancing the resistance in all three planes of movement.

Advocates of negative training believe that the use of more resistance during the negative portion of the exercise results in greater increases in strength. Neural adaptations may contribute to the benefit of heavy negative training. In a comparison of maximal eccentric-only and maximal concentric-only training, EMG activity during maximal eccentric actions was enhanced 86% after maximal eccentric training, but only 11% after maximal concentric training (Hortobagyi et al. 1996). During maximal concentric actions, EMG

TABLE 6.5 Percentage of Eccentric 1RM Greater Than Concentric 1RM of Machine Exercises

Exercise	Men (% eccentric greater than concentric 1RM)	Women (% eccentric greater than concentric 1RM)
Lat pull-down	32	29
Leg press	44	66
Bench press	40	146
Leg extension	35	55
Military press	49	161
Leg curl	27	82

Data from Hollander et al. 2007.

activity was increased 8 and 12% as a result of eccentric and concentric training, respectively. An increase in EMG activity during maximal eccentric actions may be advantageous (as discussed in the section Forced Repetition, or Assisted Repetition, Technique later in this chapter) for increasing 1RM strength. Performing a heavy eccentric repetition (105% of concentric 1RM) immediately prior to performing a concentric action results in a significantly increased concentric 1RM (Doan et al. 2002). This indicates that the eccentric action may enhance neural facilitation during the concentric movement. Thus, there is some evidence that heavy eccentric training may result in neural adaptations that may enhance strength.

Some studies previously discussed concerning accentuated eccentric (negative) training (see chapter 2) indicate that greater than the concentric 1RM must be used with accentuated eccentric training to achieve greater strength gains than occur with normal resistance training. These same studies also indicate that accentuated eccentric training can be safely performed with up to 125% of normal 1RM in the eccentric repetition phase. All of these previous studies examined the effects of accentuated eccentric, or negative-only, training on moderately resistance-trained or untrained people.

The effect of accentuated eccentric training in competitive Olympic weightlifters does indicate that it is advantageous for maximal strength gains over 12 weeks of training (Häkkinen and Komi 1981). Lifters performing 25% of the eccentric actions in their training with 100 to 130% of the 1RM concentric action significantly increased 10% in the snatch and 13% in the clean and jerk. Lifters performing their normal training over this same time frame improved 7% in the snatch and 6% in the clean and jerk. The improvement in the clean and jerk shown by lifters performing accentuated eccentric training was significantly greater than that of the group performing normal training. Both groups also improved significantly in various measures of isometric, concentric, and eccentric force during a leg press–type movement and a knee extension, but there was no significant difference between the groups. For these competitive athletes, their performance is measured by 1RM in the snatch and clean and jerk. Thus, accentuated eccentric training did offer the Olympic weightlifters some competitive advantage.

Super-Overload System

The super-overload system is a type of negative weight training. Partial repetitions are performed using 125% of the 1RM resistance. For example, if a person's 1RM in the bench press is 200 lb (90.7 kg), 250 lb (113.4 kg) is used (200 lb [90.7 kg] × 1.25 = 250 lb [113.4 kg]) for the partial repetitions. For example, in the bench press spotters help the lifter get the weight in the extended-elbow position. The lifter lowers the weight as far as possible before lifting the weight back to the extended-elbow position without assistance from the spotters. The lifter performs 7 to 10 such partial repetitions per set. After the partial repetitions the resistance is lowered slowly to the chest-touch position, and the spotters help lift the weight back to the extended-elbow position. Normally, three such sets per exercise are performed in a training session.

After eight weeks of training three days per week with at least one day of rest between training sessions, the super-overload system results in 1RM bench and leg press increases equal to those achieved with conventional weight training (Powers, Browning, and Groves 1978). This indicates that the super-overload system is as effective as conventional weight training in developing 1RM strength. Because resistances greater than 1RM are used in this type of training, spotters are mandatory when using free weights. It is also possible to use some machines with this system. As with other negative systems, on some machines the resistance may be lifted with both arms or legs and the partial repetitions performed with only one arm or leg.

Unstable Surface Training

Unstable surface training involves performing exercises on a Swiss ball, inflatable disc, wobble board, or other unstable surface (see figure 6.5). The exercises can be performed with body mass only or with additional resistance. Proponents of this type of training assert that it enhances athletic

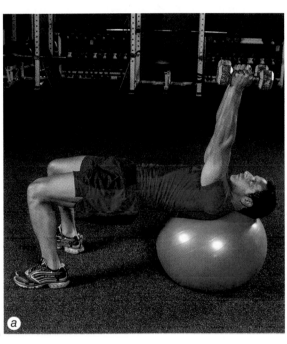
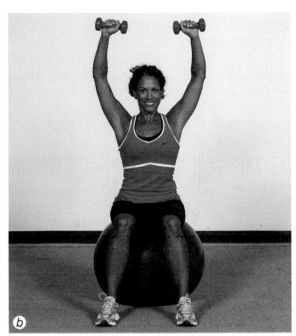
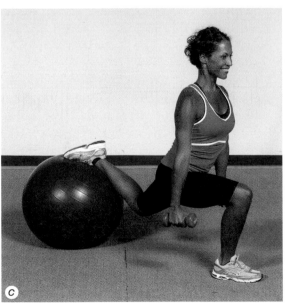
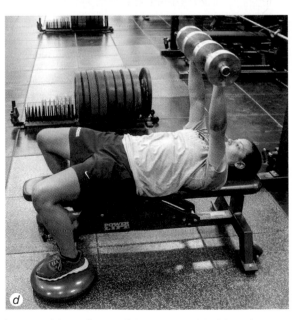

FIGURE 6.5   Many types of equipment can be used during unstable surface training: *(a)* dumbbell bench press on a Swiss ball, *(b)* seated overhead press on a Swiss ball, *(c)* lunge with one foot on a Swiss ball, *(d)* bench press with feet on inflatable discs.

Figure 6.5d Courtesy of Dr. William J. Kraemer, Department of Kinesiology, University of Connecticut, Storrs, CT.

performance as a result of improvements in balance, kinesthetic sense, proprioception, and core stability. They assert that because all movements require stability and mobility, training both of these qualities simultaneously and increasing core stability results in greater transfer of force production by the musculature of the upper and lower limbs during daily life and sport-specific actions.

The **core musculature** can be defined as the axial skeleton and all muscles, ligaments, and other soft tissues with attachments originating on the axial skeleton whether this tissue terminates on the axial or appendicular (arm or leg) skeleton. Increasing core stability may help to control the position and motion of the trunk over the pelvis to allow optimum force production, transfer and control of force, and the motion of the limbs during athletic activities. Unstable surface training was originally developed to be used in rehabilitation settings. This type of training does appear to increase balance, especially in those with impaired balance ability, such as seniors, and seems to prevent some types of injuries, such as low back injuries (DiStefano, Clark, and Padua 2009; Hibbs et al. 2008; Schilling et al. 2009; Willardson 2007b). However, many factors can affect whether unstable surface training increases core stability or performance in daily life or athletic activities.

Many types of unstable surface equipment and training programs have been used to determine whether unstable surface training increases the ability to perform athletic activities (DiStefano, Clark, and Padua 2009; Hibbs et al. 2008; Willardson 2007b). Additionally, the type of balance test used may also determine whether balance improves. Static balance (standing stationary) on a firm surface or on an unstable surface, and dynamic balance, or the ability to stabilize oneself in a static stance after or while moving, could all be used to evaluate whether an increase in balance took place as a result of training.

Generally, balance training, including unstable surface training, appears to improve static balance ability on stable and unstable surfaces as well as dynamic balance. Thus, elite athletes may improve static balance on an unstable surface and dynamic balance, but stable balance on a stable surface appears to have a ceiling (DiStefano, Clark, and Padua 2009). This indicates that if stable balance on a stable surface is already good, training may not improve it substantially. This is an important

consideration because most athletic activities are performed on stable surfaces (gym floors, solid playing surfaces). Athletes in sports performed on unstable surfaces, such as surfing, wind surfing, swimming, and snowboarding, however, may benefit from unstable surface training more than athletes in other types of sports.

Generally, a decrease in maximal force capabilities and an increase in EMG activity are demonstrated when an exercise is performed on an unstable surface (Behm et al. 2010; Norwood et al. 2007; Willardson 2007b). However, EMG activity may depend on whether the comparison is made between the same absolute resistance or a percentage of 1RM specific to the stable or unstable condition (McBride, Larkin et al. 2010). Generally, EMG activity is greater in muscles used in squatting in a stable condition when 70, 80, or 90% of stable 1RM is lifted compared to lifting unstable 1RM in an unstable condition. However, when lifting an absolute resistance (59, 67, or 75 kg, or 130, 148, or 165 lb), although EMG activity is greater in the stable condition, it is not generally significantly so. Increased EMG activity represents an increase in muscle activation and rate coding of motor units.

EMG activity may also depend on the unstable surface used and the muscle in question. For example, when performing a seated overhead press using either a barbell or a dumbbell while seated on a Swiss ball or on a normal bench, the 10RM is significantly (10-23%) less when seated on the Swiss ball (Kohler, Flanagan, and Whitting 2010). However, the EMG of the triceps was greater in the stable bench press, probably due to the increased resistance used, and the upper erector spinae showed the greatest EMG activity when subjects performed the exercises seated on the Swiss ball. During a dumbbell bench press on a Swiss ball using 60% of 1RM determined for a normal stable bench press, EMG activity of various muscles, including the abdominal muscles, is greater than during a normal stable bench press at the same resistance (Marshall and Murphy 2006). However, the resistance used was probably a greater percentage of 1RM in the unstable bench press performed on a Swiss ball, which may have resulted in the greater EMG activity.

In contradiction to both of the preceding studies, 1RM barbell bench press and EMG activity in various muscles was shown not to be significantly different between a bench press performed on a

Swiss ball and one performed on a stable normal bench (Goodman et al. 2008). So whether the resistance used is an absolute resistance (certain weight) or the same percentage of 1RM in the stable and unstable exercise, and the muscle in question, may affect EMG activity when performing exercises in unstable situations.

Similarly, the type of unstable equipment used will also affect EMG activity. Squatting while standing on a Swiss ball or on a wobble board generally shows increased muscle activation compared to the same exercise in a stable condition in highly experienced weight-trained people (Wahl and Behm 2008). However, squatting with both feet on one inflatable disc or with each foot on a separate inflatable disc did not demonstrate significant increases in muscle activation. This indicates that moderately unstable equipment, such as inflatable discs, do not produce enough instability to increase muscle activation in highly weight-trained people.

Many exercises using unstable surfaces have the goal of increasing core stability by increasing the activity of the core musculature, including the abdominal and low back muscles. Several advanced Swiss ball exercises have been shown not to activate the majority of muscles sufficiently to increase strength (Marshall and Desai 2010). Only one of six of the advanced exercises (prone hold and praying mantis, single-leg squat, hold and crunch, bridge, hip extension, and roll) showed sufficient EMG activity to indicate that the rectus abdominis, external obliques, or lumbar erector spinae were activated sufficiently to increase maximal strength. The bridge activated the rectus abdominis sufficiently to indicate that maximal strength would increase. Thus, the use of unstable surface exercises to increase maximal strength may be limited; however, when performed with a sufficient number of repetitions, muscular endurance could increase.

Whether unstable surface training increases performance in a specific activity could depend on whether the activity is performed in an unstable environment. For some activities played in unstable environments, such as ice hockey, no significant correlation between wobble board ability and skating speed in highly skilled players is apparent (Behm et al. 2005). This indicates that unstable surface training may not improve performance in these sports.

Including wobble board training in the training program for women Division I athletes does improve performance in a one-minute sit-up test indicating increased strength and endurance of the abdominal musculature and single-leg squat ability (Oliver and Di Brezzo 2009). However, athletes performing their normal training program showed a similar increase in one-minute sit-up ability.

A 10-week study in which some male Division I athletes performed exercises on inflatable discs and others performed them without the discs did not show any advantage with the discs (Cressey et al. 2007). The normal training resulted in a significant increase in drop jump (3.2%) and countermovement jump (2.4%) ability, whereas the unstable surface training resulted in no change in these same measures. Both the unstable surface training and the normal training resulted in a significant decrease (40 yd, –1.8 and –3.9%, 10 yd, –4.0 and –7.6%, respectively) in 40 yd and 10 yd sprint ability. The decrease in 40 yd sprint ability with the normal training was significantly greater than that shown with unstable surface training. Both groups also significantly improved in an agility test (T-test), but no significant difference between training modes was demonstrated.

Adding six weeks of Swiss ball training to the regimes of aerobically conditioned athletes (maximal oxygen consumption 55 ml · kg^{-1} · min^{-1}) does significantly increase core stability; however, maximal oxygen consumption and running economy were not significantly affected (Stanton, Reaburn, and Humphries 2004). Team handball throwing velocity is significantly increased (4.9%) after six weeks of core stability training using a variety of unstable surface devices (slings, discs; Saeterbakken, van den Tillaar, and Seiler 2011). Collectively, these studies indicate that not all types of unstable surface training or programs will produce significant improvements in measures of athletic performance.

Unstable surface training performed for at least 10 minutes per session for three sessions per week for at least four weeks improves balance in healthy people (DiStefano, Clark, and Padua 2009). Although clear evidence that unstable surface training will improve athletic performance is lacking, this type of training does appear to reduce the risk of some types of injuries. Guidelines for using unstable surface training in yearly training programs for athletes have been developed (see box 6.4).

? BOX 6.4 PRACTICAL QUESTION

What Are Guidelines for Unstable Surface Training?

As with all types of resistance training, no one training technique should be used exclusively in a training program. Unstable surface training does have some advantages and disadvantages compared to normal resistance training. One goal of developing a yearlong or long-term training program for athletes or fitness enthusiasts is to use a variety of training techniques to bring about desired adaptations. Thus, for fitness- and health-conscious people and athletes at all levels, ground-based free weight lifts, such as back squats, deadlifts, Olympic lifts, and lifts that involve trunk rotation, should form the foundation of their programs to train the core musculature. However, those who are training for health-related fitness who do not want to experience the training stresses associated with ground-based free weight lifts or do not have access to facilities to perform such exercises can achieve resistance training adaptations and functional health benefits with unstable training devices and exercises.

Guidelines for unstable surface training during a yearly training cycle have been proposed. During the preseason and in-season training, performing traditional exercises while standing on a stable surface is recommended for increases in core strength and power (DiStefano, Clark, and Padua 2009). During the postseason and off-season, unstable surface training (Swiss ball) exercises involving isometric actions, low resistances, and long tension times are recommended for increasing core endurance (DiStefano, Clark, and Padua 2009). Additionally, unstable surface training equipment (inflatable discs and balance boards) should be used in conjunction with plyometric exercises to improve proprioception, which may reduce the likelihood of lower-extremity injuries (DiStefano, Clark, and Padua 2009). In summary, training programs may include both traditional and unstable surface training exercises.

DiStefano, L.J., Clark, M.A., and Padua, D.A. 2009. Evidence supporting balance training in healthy individuals: A systematic review. *Journal of Strength and Conditioning Research* 23: 2718- 2731.

Sling Training

Sling training involves grasping a sling or placing another body part, such as a foot, in a sling and then performing exercises (figure 6.6). Because the sling is free to move, this type of exercise can be viewed as an unstable surface exercise. A wide variety of sling exercises can be performed, including push-ups, variations of rowing exercises, and abdominal or core stability exercises. Because of the unstable nature of the sling, this type of exercise results in many of the characteristics of other unstable training techniques, such as increased balance ability and core stability.

Sling training is effective for increasing strength. For example, female college students training with either sling exercises or traditional weight training exercises show significant increases in isokinetic torque in a variety of movements as well as 1RM bench press and leg press ability with no significant difference shown between training programs (Dannelly et al. 2011). However, the sling training resulted in a significantly greater increase in sling push-up ability than the traditional weight train-

ing program did. Both groups also significantly improved balance ability with no significant difference shown between groups. The results indicate that sling training is as effective as normal weight training in the initial training period of previously untrained people.

Sling training also improves motor performance. Combining it with other unstable surface training (discs) for six weeks significantly improves the throwing velocity (4.9%) of high school female handball players (Saeterbakken, van den Tillaar, and Seiler 2011). This type of training also improves throwing velocity in female college softball players (Prokopy et al. 2008). Sling training can also be used as a warm-up. Performing a sling-based warm-up increases throwing velocity and accuracy in collegiate baseball players to the same extent that a more traditional warm-up does (Huang et al. 2011). The preceding indicates that sling-based exercise is an efficient means of increasing strength and motor performance. One limitation of many sling-based exercises is that the resistance is limited by body mass. However,

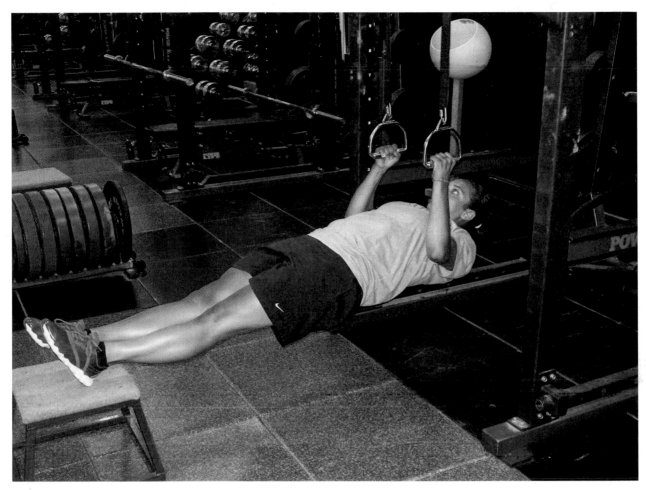

FIGURE 6.6 Many different sling exercises can be performed, including inverted rowing, shown here.

Courtesy of Dr. William J. Kraemer, Department of Kinesiology, University of Connecticut, Storrs, CT.

this limitation could be overcome by the use of additional resistance, such as weighted vests.

Functional Training

A term associated with unstable surface training and core stability is *functional training*, which has come to mean different things to different groups. The general definition of **functional training** is training that is meant to increase performance in some type of functional task, such as activities of daily living or tests related to athletic performance. Thus, functional training could refer to virtually any type of training meant to increase motor performance. To some, functional training refers to various forms of unstable surface training, the goal of which is to increase balance and core strength. Unstable surface training was originally developed for use in rehabilitative settings to increase balance (especially in those with impaired balance abil-

ity, such as seniors), and to prevent some types of injuries. Functional training also addresses task performance, such as rising from a chair or climbing stairs. This type of training is frequently included in programs to improve activities of daily living in seniors.

To others, functional training refers to various types of exercises, including unstable surface training, meant to increase performance in not only activities of daily living, but also athletic endeavors. Functional exercises of this type typically include various forms of plyometrics, rotational-type exercises for the core musculature, as well as other types of training such as kettlebell training, which includes ballistic and rotational movements.

Thus, functional training is defined differently by different people. The information presented in this chapter as well as other chapters suggests that no matter how functional training is defined, it can increase strength and motor performance.

Extreme Conditioning Programs

Extreme conditioning programs are high-volume, short-rest-period, multi-exercise programs, many of which have become very popular (e.g., CrossFit, Insanity, Gym Jones). Additionally, these programs typically have a high training frequency; some are performed five or six days per week. Some include a large number of multijoint exercises, variations of the Olympic lifts, as well as interval training and plyometrics. Because of the variety of extreme conditioning programs, there is no representative training session. However, a typical session consists of 10 repetitions of squat, bench press, and deadlift performed in a circuit fashion followed by successive sets in which the number of repetitions

per set decreases by one until only one repetition per set is performed. The resistance used is 80% of 1RM. Although lifters can rest between exercises, the goal is to perform the circuits with as little rest as possible between exercises.

Positive aspects of these types of programs are that they reduce body fat and increase local muscular endurance as a result of high volume (Bergeron et al. 2011). Negative aspects, also due to high volume, include deterioration of exercise technique resulting in fatigue, possible overuse injuries, and acute injuries. Exertional rhabdomyolysis (see box 6.5) and overreaching and overtraining are also concerns (Bergeron et al. 2011). To avoid these potential problems, trainers should individualize strength conditioning programs and increase volume, intensity, and frequency slowly to allow physiological adaptations to take place. Programs should also be periodized and sufficient

---

 BOX 6.5 RESEARCH

Exertional Rhabdomyolysis

Research has shown that any exercise causes muscle tissue damage and breakdown, which are essential for muscle growth. However, exercise that is too extreme, either in one exercise session or successive sessions, can lead to serious complications. Of great concern is the development of exertional rhabdomyolysis (called "rhabdo" for short), which is a dangerous condition in which excessive muscle tissue breakdown results in large amounts of muscle constituents, such as myoglobin, potassium ions, phosphate ions, creatine kinase [CK], uric acid, and other breakdown products, being released into the interstitial fluid and bloodstream. Inflammation occurs with the invasion of white blood cells into the injured tissue area, further complicating the process. The high levels of myoglobin and uric acid in the blood can then collect in kidney tubules, which can lead to renal failure. Additionally, the release of potassium ions can cause high levels in the blood and disrupt normal ionic balances. This can lead to a disruption of the heart's normal rhythm and is potentially fatal.

Rhabdomyolysis is a medical emergency that, if left untreated, can cause death. Even competitive American football players are not immune to this problem, as noted in news stories over the past few years about football players performing high-volume, short-rest protocols or high-volume, heavy-eccentric-load training and developing rhabdo. Rhabdo can also occur in untrained people wanting to get into shape who take on extreme fitness programs (e.g., high-volume, short-rest protocols) and do too much too soon. Performing such extreme programs after a break or a detraining period, not individualizing a program, using too much volume and too little rest during and between workouts, and not progressing training are factors that have led to incidents of rhabdo.

In one case study, rhabdo was observed in an 18-year-old college NCAA Division 1 American football player who was involved in a late summer conditioning session after four weeks of an intensive team training camp (Moeckel-Cole and Clarkson 2009). The authors reported that rhabdo occurred in the absence of dehydration, which many have erroneously thought was necessary for its development. The authors reported the following:

> The players were instructed by the strength and conditioning coach to perform 10 sets of 30 repetitions of squat exercises (300 total) using resistance bands attached to a platform beneath the feet and stretched over the shoulders. There was a 1-minute break

between each set. The patient recalled that this was the most painful exercise he had ever performed. After the 10 sets of squats, the players were next instructed to perform 30 Romanian dead lifts using 40-lb dumbbells. Finally, they all performed 30 shoulder shrug bicep curls using 80-lb dumbbells. The training session was held in the late afternoon and the room was not air-conditioned. At the time of the training session, the patient reported that the temperature of the room was very warm but not hot, somewhere in the range of 78-84 °F. The patient reported that during the incidental training session he consumed water (6-8 oz each time) between each set of exercises. Following the exercise session, the patient reported that he felt dizzy and was experiencing pain in the quadriceps group. The patient also reported that several other players were stressed by the session and were vomiting during the training. (p. 1056)

The player then had problems with movement and severe pain in his thighs after returning to his dorm room and this continued the next day. After consultation with the athletic trainer and no changes in the pain and movement problems he checked into the emergency room and was found to be fully hydrated but upon examination he had a CK value of 84,629 $IU \cdot L^{-1}$ (normal resting values range from about 25 to 100 $IU \cdot L^{-1}$ and after typical resistance exercises increase to about 250-350 $IU \cdot L^{-1}$). After 8 days in the hospital, it took one month for this athlete to recover and be ready to resume normal activities. This study showed that severe and extreme exercise protocols, even in fit athletes who are hydrated, can lead to the medical emergency of rhabdo. Hydration alone is not sufficient to prevent rhabdo, and important monitoring of symptoms such as severe muscular pain and dark brown urine in trainees is vital so that immediate medical care can be given. When designing and implementing a conditioning program it is vital that athletes have had a proper progression for intensity, volume, and rest period length and are ready for the workout that is designed. Too often workouts are mistakenly used for punishment or work hardening. However, it is becoming more apparent that no matter how fit an individual is, if excessive exercise prescriptions are used, the potential for rhabdo and its complications exist.

Moeckel-Cole, S.A., and Clarkson, P.M. 2009. Rhabdomyolysis in a collegiate football player. *Journal of Strength and Conditioning Research* 23: 1055-1059.

rest allowed between sessions so that recovery takes place.

Rest-Pause, or Interrepetition Rest, Technique

The rest-pause, or interrepetition rest, technique involves performing one or several repetitions with a relatively heavy resistance and then resting for a short period of time before performing one or several more repetitions. This type of training has also been termed cluster training because sets are broken into clusters of repetitions separated by short rest periods. Between repetitions or sets the lifter puts the weight down and rests for short periods of time. As an example, the lifter performs one repetition of an exercise with 250 lb (113.4 kg), which is near the 1RM for the exercise. The lifter then puts the weight down, rests 10 to 15 seconds, and then performs another repetition (or several) with the same resistance. This is repeated for four or five times. If the lifter cannot perform a

complete repetition, spotters assist just enough to allow the completion of the four or five repetitions. One or several sets of an exercise can be performed. Proponents of this technique believe that using a heavy resistance for several repetitions and then resting briefly before performing several more enables the lifter to use a heavier resistance or to maintain power (or both) in successive repetitions. Either of these results may cause greater strength or power increases with training.

Resting between repetitions for several repetitions does increase power output compared to no rest between repetitions (Lawton, Cronin, and Lindsell 2006). Athletes who performed the concentric repetition phase as fast as possible in a normal set of six repetitions at 6RM compared to using the same resistance for six sets of one repetition and resting 20 seconds between sets, three sets of two repetitions and resting for 50 seconds between sets, and two sets of three repetitions and resting 100 seconds between sets showed significantly greater power output in repetitions 4 through 6 (25-49%) when rest was allowed. Total power output during all sets with a rest between repetitions was also greater (21.6-25.1%) compared to the traditional 6RM set. No significant difference in power output was shown among the three protocols.

Subjects who performed power cleans for three sets of six repetitions with no rest between repetitions or 20 and 40 seconds of rest between repetitions showed a similar maintenance of power with rest between repetitions (Hardee et al. 2012). Peak power and force decreased significantly less during the three sets when 20 seconds of rest (6 and 2.7%, respectively) and 40 seconds of rest (3 and 0.4%, respectively) were allowed compared to when no rest was allowed (16 and 7%, respectively). Similarly, power is better maintained during four sets of six repetitions of squat jumps when 12 seconds of rest is allowed between repetitions, 30 seconds is allowed between groups of two repetitions, and 60 seconds is allowed between groups of three repetitions (Hansen, Cronin, and Newton 2011). Because of the greater power and force outputs when using rest intervals between repetitions, this type of training may be of value when the training goal is to increase power or strength.

Although rest between repetitions or groups of repetitions may allow greater power and force output while training, when applied to training over six weeks, no difference in power output is shown (Lawton et al. 2004). Athletes performed the concentric repetition phase of repetitions of the bench press as fast as possible for either four sets of six repetitions with approximately four minutes of rest between sets or eight sets of three repetitions with approximately 1.7 minutes of rest between sets. The total training volume and percentage of 6RM used by both groups was identical. Both groups improved power output in a bench press throw (20, 30, and 40 kg [44, 66, and 88 lb] resistance) ranging from 5.8 to 10.9%; however, no significant difference was shown between the groups. The four-set, six-repetition training did show a significantly greater increase in bench press 6RM strength (9.7 vs. 4.0%). A limitation of this study is that even though the concentric repetition phase was performed as fast as possible with both types of training, the eight-set, three-repetition program trained using percentages of 6RM as opposed to percentages of 3RM. Thus, the three-repetition sets were not performed with a resistance close to 3RM, which could limit maximal strength gains.

Another training study eight weeks in duration trained highly trained rugby athletes with either a traditional program or rest between groups of repetitions or clusters of an exercise (Hansen et al. 2011). Both training programs followed a periodized program. The cluster training technique was used only for the multijoint strength and power exercises, such as the squat, power clean, clean pull, and jump squat. Both training programs significantly increased 1RM squat ability, but the increase was significantly greater with the traditional training (18 vs. 15%). Neither training program significantly increased measures of power. However, cluster training may have had a greater effect on some measures of power than the traditional training did. For example, peak power during a jump squat carrying 40 kg (88 lb) favored the cluster training (4.7 vs. 0% increase), and peak velocity during a body weight jump squat favored the cluster training (3.8 vs. 0.5%). Thus, the effects of chronic use of the rest-pause technique, or cluster training, is not clear, but this type of training may offer a small advantage in power development.

A variation of the rest-pause technique has been shown to result in significant strength gains, but the strength gains were not as a large as those that occurred with a more conventional program (Rooney, Herbert, and Balwave 1994). The rest-pause technique consisted of performing one set of 6 to 10 repetitions at a 6RM weight with 30 seconds of rest between repetitions. Strength gains from the rest-pause technique were compared to one set of six repetitions using a resistance of 6RM. Both groups experienced significantly greater increases in 1RM than a control group did. However, the 1RM increase shown by the normal, or no-rest-between-repetitions, group (56%) was significantly greater than the increase shown by the rest-between-repetitions group (41%). Increases in maximal isometric strength of both groups were significantly greater than those of the control group. However, the difference between the rest and no-rest groups was not significant. The results indicate that this variation of the rest-pause technique compared to a no-rest-between-repetitions system was not as effective in increasing dynamic strength and resulted in equivalent isometric strength gains.

Neither of the training studies discussed earlier used the RM resistance for the number of repetitions performed with the rest-pause training.

However, as discussed in the earlier section Sets to Failure Technique, not training to failure may result in greater power increases than training to failure. These studies could be interpreted to mean that if a rest-pause technique is to result in greater strength increase than more traditional training, trainees would need to use close to the RM resistance for the number of repetitions performed. Rest-pause training does not appear to offer any advantage for increasing maximal strength, but it may be useful when training for power output.

Chain or Elastic Band Technique for Added Resistance

The chain training technique involves using hooks to hang chains from both ends of a barbell. When the barbell is in the lowest position of an exercise, such as the chest-touch position in the bench press, a relatively small section of chain is added to the mass of the barbell; the rest of the chain lies on the floor. As the barbell is lifted during the concentric repetition phase, more and more chain is picked up off the floor adding additional mass to the resistance being lifted. Attaching elastic bands to the ends of a barbell works in a similar manner because the elastic bands are stretched during the concentric repetition phase as resistance increases. This results in ever-increasing resistance as the barbell is lifted from the chest-touch to the elbow-straight position. Conversely, as the barbell is lowered from the elbow-straight position to the chest-touch position, the resistance decreases.

Chain and elastic band training are popular adjuncts to normal training among elite lifters. Fifty-seven percent and 39% of powerlifters (Swinton et al. 2011) and 56 and 38% of strongman competitors (Winwood, Keogh, and Harris 2011) incorporate chain or elastic band training, respectively, into their total training programs. Anecdotally, these techniques appear to be most prevalent in multijoint exercises, such as the bench press, squat, and deadlift, which have an ascending strength curve, or Olympic lifts in which the acceleration of the barbell and power are necessary for completing a repetition.

Several methods of hanging chain from a barbell have been developed. With the linear technique, one or more chains are hung from each side of the barbell (see figure 6.7). With the double-loop technique, one end of a smaller chain is attached to the barbell and the other end is attached to a larger chain (see figure 6.7). This results in a large increase in resistance when the larger chain begins to be lifted off of the floor. With both techniques the chain can be looped several times to increase the resistance, and chains of different sizes can be used to vary the resistance. With the double-loop technique the change in resistance can be substantially more than with the linear technique (Neely, Terry, and Morris 2010). For example, in a back squat the double-loop technique provides nearly twice the increase in resistance as the linear technique.

Test–retest reliability of a chain 1RM bench press (McCurdy et al. 2008) is high in both men ($r = .99$) and women ($r = .93$). More important from a training perspective, chain 1RM bench press ability significantly correlates with normal bench press 1RM in both men and women ($r = .95$ and .80, respectively). This indicates that if chain 1RM bench press is increased, normal bench press 1RM will also increase (McCurdy et al. 2008). During a normal back squat and squat performed with chains, EMG activity of the quadriceps and hamstring muscle groups and vertical ground reaction forces are not significantly different between the last repetition of five repetitions performed with a 5RM resistance, which indicates no advantage to chain training (Ebben and Jensen 2002). During performance of the chain squat, approximately 10% of the mass on the barbell was removed and replaced by the chains.

As might be expected, using chains does change the velocity of movement during an exercise. For example, in a comparison of a bench press performed using 75% of 1RM and one using 60% of 1RM with chains increasing resistance to a maximal resistance of approximately 75% of 1RM, concentric lifting velocity increased approximately 10% with the use of chains (Baker and Newton 2009). Likewise, eccentric lifting velocity was also increased with the use of chains.

In deadlifts at 30, 50, and 70% of 1RM with chains adding 20 or 40% of 1RM, velocity of movement and other measures were also affected (Swinton et al. 2011). The deadlifts were performed at as fast a velocity as possible. With the use of chains, peak velocity (–17 to 30%), peak power (–5 to 25%), and rate of force development (–3 to 11%) were significantly decreased; peak force (+2 to 10%) increased significantly; and greater force was maintained at the end of the concentric repetition phase.

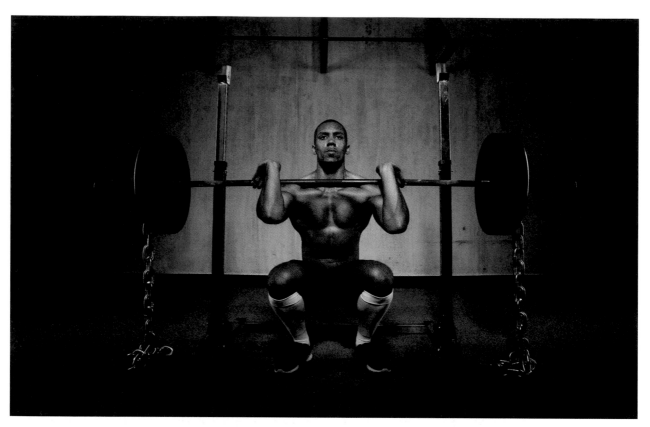

FIGURE 6.7 With the linear technique of using chains, one chain is hung from each side of a barbell.

© matthiasdrobeck/iStockphoto

The difference in velocity between the preceding two studies is probably due to how the resistance with chains was added. In the bench press chains were used to add resistance so that the same percentage of 1RM was used with and without chains, whereas in the deadlift chains were used to add resistance to a certain percentage of 1RM. In both cases, changes in velocity were likely due to the changing resistance during the concentric and eccentric repetition phases. How chains are used to change the resistance in an exercise may affect whether their use increases or decreases velocity, power, and force relative to a no-chain repetition. Additionally, if eccentric velocity is increased with the use of chains, unloading due to the use of chains in the eccentric repetition phase may result in a more rapid stretch-shortening cycle.

Training studies favor the use of chains and elastic bands. A seven-week training study using elastic bands demonstrated a significantly greater increase in 1RM back squat (16 vs. 6%) and bench press (8 vs. 4%) compared to normal training (Anderson, Sforzo, and Sigg 2008). Normal and elastic band training resistances were equated: During elastic band training, 80% of the resistance was supplied by free weights and 20% was supplied by elastic bands. Bench press training of untrained males for three weeks with 15% of the resistance supplied by elastic bands compared to normal free weight training showed the elastic band training to increase 1RM, significantly more than normal training did (10 vs. 7%) (Bellar et al. 2011). During a seven-week training period increases in predicted 1RM bench press were not significantly different with chain and elastic band training compared to normal training (Ghigiarelli et al. 2009), although increases in 5RM peak power showed a trend ($p = .11$) favoring the elastic band (4%) and chain (2.5%) compared to the normal training (1%).

Use of chains during the Olympic lifts appears to offer little or no advantage (Berning, Coker, and Briggs 2008; Coker, Berning, and Briggs 2006). Vertical ground reaction forces, vertical bar displacement, bar velocity, and rate of force production are not different when using chains in the clean and snatch lifts. These variables were examined when experienced Olympic weightlifters used 80 and 85% of 1RM and then had 5% of these resistances removed from the barbell and replaced with chains (75% of 1RM + 5% of 1RM from chains, 80% of 1RM + 5% of 1RM from chains). However, the lifters reported that greater effort was required throughout the entire lift when using chains and that greater effort was required to stabilize the bar because of the oscillation of the chains, especially during the catch phrase of the snatch. This suggests a possible psychological or physiological advantage to using chains in training.

Use of chains and elastic bands in training is quite popular among some groups of athletes. Many variations in changing the resistance are possible. However, further research is needed to determine the efficacy of this training practice.

Complex Training, or Contrast Loading

Complex training, or **contrast loading,** involves performing a strength exercise, such as a squat, and then after a short rest period performing a power-type exercise, such as a vertical jump (Fleck and Kontor 1986). The exercise sequence may consist of one or multiple sets of both the strength and power-type exercise. In a training session the exercise sequence may consist of several types of strength and power exercises. For example, complex training could consist of alternating sets of the bench press or squat with a resistance greater than 80% of 1RM, followed by bench press throws or vertical jumps using a resistance of 30 to 45% of 1RM or some other type of plyometric or stretch-shortening cycle exercise. The goal of this type of training is to acutely or over long-term training enhance power output in tasks such as jumping, sprinting, and throwing a ball.

The term *postactivation potentiation* is used to describe the increased performance or power output after performing a strength exercise. The postactivation potentiation may be due to some type of short-term neural accommodation resulting in an increased ability to recruit muscle fibers or the inhibition of neural protective mechanisms (Golgi tendon organs), although this explanation lacks a clear physiological mechanism. Another explanation of postactivation potentiation is increased phosphorylation of the myosin light-chain molecules in muscle resulting in increased calcium sensitivity of the muscle contractile pro-

teins (Babault, Maffiuletti, and Pousson 2008; J.C. Smith and Fry 2007; Tillin and Bishop 2009).

Some studies have shown that complex training acutely increases power output and velocity of movement (Babault, Maffiuletti, and Pousson 2008; Baker 2001a, 2001b; Paasuke et al. 2007; Rixon, Lamont, and Bemben 2007; Robbins 2005; Stone et al. 2008). However, many factors could affect whether power or strength are acutely affected by complex training. Whether an increase in power occurs depends on a balance of the fatigue caused by the strength exercise, recovery from the strength exercise, and the time frame of any postactivation potentiation (Tillin and Bishop 2009). Thus, the time between the performance of the strength exercise and when power output is determined could affect whether an increase in power is demonstrated.

Postactivation potentiation, when present, may be most apparent between 4 and 12 minutes (Batista et al. 2007) and 8 and 12 minutes (Kilduff et al. 2007) after completion of the strength exercise. Postactivation potentiation may also last as long as six hours (Saez Saez de Villarreal Gonzalez-Badillo, and Izquierdo 2007). However, not all information agrees with the preceding time frames. Postactivation potentiation was most apparent one to three minutes after a maximal isometric action and then decreased four to five minutes after the isometric action; it was not apparent at 10 minutes (Miyamoto et al. 2011).

Postactivation potentiation may also be most apparent in muscles with a high proportion of type II fibers (Hamada et al. 2000). Muscle contraction type also affects postactivation potentiation. Increased force or power capabilities are more apparent after isometric actions compared to dynamic actions; during fast concentric actions compared to slow ones (30 vs. 150 degrees per second); after isometric compared to concentric, eccentric, and concentric–eccentric actions (Esformes et al. 2011); and during concentric compared to eccentric actions (Babault, Maffiuletti, and Pousson 2008; Rixon, Lamont, and Bemben 2007). Training status or maximal strength may also affect postactivation potentiation: Trained athletes and resistance-trained athletes show a greater response than untrained people (Rixon, Lamont, and Bemben 2007; Robbins 2005), and power-trained athletes show a greater response than endurance-trained athletes (Paasuke et al.

2007). Likewise, maximal strength may also affect postactivation potentiation: Stronger people have a greater response than weaker ones (Tillin and Bishop 2009).

Given that all of the preceding factors may affect whether postactivation potentiation occurs, it is not surprising that a great deal of variation in the postactivation potentiation response has been shown (Comyns et al. 2006; Mangus et al. 2006). Research to date is equivocal concerning whether a complex training results in a postactivation response (Tillin and Bishop 2009).

Typically, a resistance of 3- to 5RM is used to elicit a postactivation potentiation, although as discussed earlier, isometric actions may be more effective in producing a postactivation potentiation response. The following examples demonstrate some of the difficulties in determining whether postactivation potentiation occurs. Following three sets of a 3RM bench press exercise, throwing velocity (seated medicine ball throw) was significantly improved when throwing a 4 kg (8.8 lb) medicine ball (8.3%), but not when throwing a 0.55 kg (1.2 lb) ball (Markovic, Simek, and Bradic 2008). No significant change in power in a bench press throw using a resistance of 45% of 1RM occurred after performing bench press repetitions at 100, 75, or 50% of 1RM (Brandenburg 2005). The results of these two studies indicate that the resistance used when determining whether a postactivation potentiation occurs may affect the results.

After track and field athletes performed five back squat repetitions at 85% of 1RM, vertical jump peak height (4.7%), and peak ground reaction force (4.6%) during a squat jump significantly increased (Weber et al. 2008). Recreationally resistance-trained people after performing one set of eight repetitions using 40% of 1RM or one set of four repetitions using 80% of 1RM in the back squat showed no significant change in counter-movement vertical jump peak ground reaction force or ground contact time (Hanson, Leigh, and Mynark 2007). Although the training histories of the subjects in these two studies differed, using a similar resistance (80 or 85% of 1RM) in the back squat showed a significant increase in and no significant postactivation potentiation.

Although, typically, one set of a strength exercise is used to try to bring about postactivation potentiation, multiple sets and other types of exercises may also cause postactivation potentiation (Saez Villarreal, Gonzalez-Badillo, and Izquierdo 2007). Three sets of five jumps with an added resistance that brings about maximal power output in a jump; two sets of four repetitions at 80% of 1RM and two sets of two repetitions at 85% of 1RM in the back squat; two sets of four repetitions at 80%; two sets of two repetitions at 90%; and two sets of one repetition at 95% of 1RM in the back squat all bring about a significant increase in drop jump height (3 to 5.5%) and countermovement jump height with an added resistance that causes maximal power (2.5 to 11.4%). Performing one set of three vertical jumps significantly increases (5.4%) power output in a set of six vertical jumps with an added resistance of 88 lb (40 kg) (Baker 2001a). These two studies indicate that multiple sets of an activity and power-type activities may also cause postactivation potentiation.

Little information concerning the long-term effects of complex training is available. Six weeks of plyometric-only, resistance-only, or complex training all increased 1RM squat, calf raise, and Romanian deadlift ability, but no significant difference was shown among training types (MacDonald, Lamont, and Garner 2012). Four weeks of complex, plyometric-only, and weight training all showed significant improvements in some motor performance tasks. However, the complex training showed the greatest overall improvements and improvement in more motor performance tasks (Dodd and Alvar 2007). Complex training significantly improved sprint ability (20 yd, 0.55%; 40 yd, 0.26%; 60 yd, 0.27%), vertical jump ability (0.98%), standing long jump ability (1.8%), and T-agility time (2.33%). Resistance training significantly improved only sprint ability (60 yd, 0.15%), vertical jump ability (0.36%), standing long jump ability (0.67%), and T-agility time (1.24%). Plyometric training improved only vertical jump ability (1.91%) and standing long jump ability (1.1%).

In 10 weeks complex training (resistance exercise followed by a series of plyometric exercises) significantly increased squat jump and countermovement jump ability in young (14- and 15-year-old) basketball players (Santos and Janeira 2008). Although no comparison to another type of training was included in this study, it does indicate that complex training can be effective. Three weeks of complex training or compound training result in similar increases (5 vs. 9%) in vertical jump height (Mihalik et al. 2008). Compound training consisted of performing the same exercises as in complex training, but on different days of the week (weight training and plyometric training were not performed in the same session). Complex training does appear to result in postactivation potentiation in some situations. However, the effect of long-term complex training needs further research.

Summary

The possibilities for creating new resistance training systems and techniques appears almost infinite. All of the systems and techniques discussed in this chapter were designed to address specific training goals. They evolved from a variety of sources, including bodybuilding, powerlifting, Olympic weightlifting, and personal trainers. When groups realize their desired adaptations using certain systems and techniques, they continue to use them. Some equipment companies promote resistance training systems and techniques that suit their equipment characteristics or fit into their marketing strategies. Thus, many factors other than a sound scientific basis affect whether a training system or technique becomes popular.

It should be possible to describe each system and technique in terms of its acute program variables. However, for most systems and techniques the acute program variables were never completely defined. The choice of a training system or technique depends on the goals of the program, time constraints, equipment availability, and how the goals of the resistance training program relate to the goals of the total fitness program. Different training systems and techniques can be incorporated into advanced training strategies (see chapter 7).

SELECTED READINGS

Ahtiainen, J.P., and Häkkinen, K. 2009. Strength athletes are capable to produce greater muscle activation and neural fatigue during high-intensity resistance exercise than nonathletes. *Journal of Strength and Conditioning Research* 23: 1129 1134.

Behm, D.G., Drinkwater, E.J., Willardson, J.M., and Cowley, P.M. 2010. Canadian Society for Exercise Physiology positions stand: The use of instability to train the core in athletic and nonathletic conditioning. *Applied Physiology, Nutrition and Metabolism* 35: 109-112.

Giorgi, A., Wilson, G.J., Weatherby, R.P., and Murphy, A. 1998. Functional isometric weight training: Its effects on the development of muscular function and the endocrine system over an 8-week training period. *Journal of Strength and Conditioning Research* 12: 18-25.

Izquierdo, M., Ibanez, J., Gonzalez-Badillo, J.J., Häkkinen, K., Ratamess, N.A., Kraemer, W.J., French, D.N., Eslava, J., Altadill, A., Asiain, X., and Gorostiaga, E.M. 2006. Different effects of strength training leading to failure versus not to failure of hormonal responses, strength, and muscle power games. *Journal of Applied Physiology* 100: 1647-1656.

Keogh, J.W.L., Wilson, G.J., and Weatherby, R.P. 1999. A cross-sectional comparison of different resistance training techniques in the bench press. *Journal of Strength and Conditioning Research* 13: 247-258.

Krieger, J.W. 2010. Single vs. multiple sets of resistance exercise for muscle hypertrophy: A meta-analysis. *Journal of Strength Conditioning Research* 24: 1150-1159.

Lawton, T.W., Cronin, J.B., Drinkwater, E., Lindsell, R., and Pyne, D. 2004. The effect of continuous repetition training and intra-set rest training on bench press strength and power. *Journal of Sports Medicine and Physical Fitness* 44: 361-367.

Marin, P.J., and Rhea, M.R. 2010. Effects of vibration training on muscle strength: A meta-analysis. *Journal of Strength and Conditioning Research* 24: 548-556.

Mookerjee, S., and Ratamess, N. 1999. Comparison of strength differences and joint action durations between full and partial range-of-motion bench press exercise. *Journal of Strength and Conditioning Research* 13: 76-81.

Tillin, N.A., and Bishop, D. 2009. Factors modulating post-activation potentiation and its effect on performance of subsequent explosive activities. *Sports Medicine* 39: 147-166.

Waller, M., Miller, J., and Hannon, J. 2011. Resistance circuit training: Its application for the adult population. *Strength and Conditioning Journal* 33: 16-22.

Willardson, J.M. 2007. Application of training to failure in periodized multiple-set resistance exercise programs. *Journal of Strength and Conditioning Research* 21: 628-631.

7

Advanced Training Strategies

---

1. describe the typical pattern of training intensity and volume used for linear and nonlinear periodization,

2. describe what is known from research concerning changes in strength, motor performance, and body composition due to linear and nonlinear periodization,

3. define power training and discuss how rate of force development, weight lifted, velocity of movement and the deceleration phase affect power output in an exercise,

4. describe what is known from research concerning designing the optimal plyometric training program, and

5. discuss why two weight training sessions per day might be advantageous to athletes.

The search for advanced training strategies probably began shortly after the development of the first resistance training programs. After performing a resistance training program for a short period of time and making substantial gains in strength and hypertrophy, someone probably wondered, What can I do to improve my current weight training program? The search for advanced training strategies that began at that point continues today. The popularity of advanced training strategies is demonstrated by surveys indicating that 95% of American high school coaches, 69% of American National Football League coaches, 80% of strongman competitors, 85% of American National Basketball Association coaches, 86% of American Major League Baseball strength and conditioning coaches, and 96% of elite British powerlifters use some type of periodized training (Duehring, Feldman, and Ebben 2009; Ebben and Blackard 2001; Ebben, Hintz, and Simenz 2005; Simenz, Dugan, and Ebben 2005; Swinton et al. 2009; Winwood, Keogh, and Harris 2011). Similarly, in the United States, 100% of high school, 100% of National Basketball Association, 95% of

Major League Baseball, and 94% of National Football League strength and conditioning coaches use plyometric training in their total training programs (Duehring, Feldman, and Ebben 2009; Ebben and Blackard 2001; Ebben, Hintz, and Simenz 2005; Simenz, Dugan, and Ebben 2005).

Advanced training strategies are necessary in part because as people become physically fitter, gains in fitness slow and training plateaus occur. Advanced training strategies are also necessary to optimally develop some fitness variables, such as power and muscular rate of force development, in highly fit people. Although new training strategies are developed frequently by coaches, personal trainers, and strength conditioning specialists, many are not studied scientifically. The advanced training strategies discussed in this chapter are periodization of resistance training, power training, plyometric or stretch-shortening cycle training, and multiple training sessions on the same day. All of these strategies have received a significant amount of attention from the sport science community. Therefore, there is sufficient research from which to draw conclusions and develop training guidelines.

Periodization of Resistance Training

Periodization of training refers to planned changes in any of the acute training program variables, such as exercise order, exercise choice, number of sets, number of repetitions per set, rest periods between sets and exercises, exercise intensity, and number of training sessions per day, to bring about continued and optimal fitness gains. Sport scientists, coaches, and athletes of the former Eastern Bloc countries of the Soviet Union and East Germany are credited with developing and researching the concept of periodization. However, anecdotal evidence also indicates that athletes were performing periodized programs in the United States, Europe, and other Western countries as early as the 1950s.

The main goals of periodized training are optimizing training adaptations during both short periods of time, such as weeks and months, and long periods of time, such as years or an entire athletic career. Some periodized plans also have as a goal to peak physical performance at a particular point in time, such as a major competition. Another goal of periodized training is to avoid training plateaus. During long-term training any program can result in a training plateau in part because people are approaching their genetic maximal capabilities for a specific characteristic, such as strength. However, comparative studies of nonvaried programs and periodized programs in which serial testing was performed demonstrate that nonvaried programs can result in training plateaus (see table 7.1), whereas periodized programs result in more consistent fitness gains.

TABLE 7.1   **Percentage Changes During Various Training Periods Demonstrating Training Plateaus With Nonperiodized Training**

Bench press 1RM			
	Pretraining to 12 weeks	Pretraining to 24 weeks	12 to 24 weeks
Nonlinear periodization	23[a, c]	47[a, c]	19[b]
1 set × 8-12 reps	12[a]	12[a]	0
Leg press 1RM			
Nonlinear periodization	21[a, c]	32[a, c]	9[c]
1 set × 8-12 reps	8[a]	11[a]	3
Bench press reps at 80% of 1RM			
Nonlinear periodization	14[a, c]	24[a, c]	9[b]
1 set × 8-12 reps	2	10[a]	8
Leg press reps at 80% of 1RM			
Nonlinear periodization	35[a, c]	65[a, c]	22[b]
1 set × 8-12 reps	16[a]	19[a]	2
Wingate peak power			
Nonlinear periodization	14[a, c]	27[a, c]	12[b]
1 set × 8-12 reps	1	4	4
Sit-ups in 1 min			
Nonlinear periodization	26[a, c]	42[a, c]	13[b]
1 set × 8-12 reps	8[a]	13[a]	2
Vertical jump power			
Nonlinear periodization	24[a, c]	40[a, c]	13[b]
1 set × 8-12 reps	9[a]	10[a]	1
40 yd sprint			
Nonlinear periodization	−3[a, c]	−6[a, c]	−3[b]
1 set × 8-12 reps	+1	−1	−1

a = significant difference from pretest; b = significant difference from 12 weeks; c = significant difference from one-set group.

Data from Marx et al. 2001.

Bench press 1RM

	Pretraining to 4 weeks	Pretraining to 16 weeks	4 to 8 weeks	8 to 12 weeks	12 to 16 weeks
Linear periodization	7[a]	24[a, b]	4	8	5
5 × 10RM	5[a]	8[a]	0	1	2
6 × 8RM	7[a]	10[a]	−2	2	3

Squat 1RM

	Pretraining to 4 weeks	Pretraining to 16 weeks	4 to 8 weeks	8 to 12 weeks	12 to 16 weeks
Linear periodization	9[a, c]	33[a, b]	3	9	12
5 × 10RM	4[a]	15[a]	3	3	5
6 × 8RM	10[a, c]	22[a, c]	2	7	3

a = significant increase from control group; b = significant difference from other two groups; c = significant difference from 5 × 10RM group.

Data from Willoughby 1993.

Bench press 1RM

	Pretraining to 16 weeks	Pretraining to 36 weeks	16 to 24 weeks	24 to 36 weeks
Nonlinear periodization	22[a]	25[a]	0[a]	4[a, c]
1 set × 8-12 reps	10[a]	10[a]	0[a]	0[a]

Leg press 1RM

	Pretraining to 16 weeks	Pretraining to 36 weeks	16 to 24 weeks	24 to 36 weeks
Nonlinear periodization	11[a]	18[a]	5[a, b]	3[a, c]
1 set × 8-12 reps	6[a]	7[a]	0[a]	0[a]

Shoulder press 1RM

	Pretraining to 16 weeks	Pretraining to 36 weeks	16 to 24 weeks	24 to 36 weeks
Nonlinear periodization	19[a]	28[a]	7[a, b]	2[a, c]
1 set × 8-12 reps	14[a]	14[a]	3[a]	−3[a]

Vertical jump

	Pretraining to 16 weeks	Pretraining to 36 weeks	16 to 24 weeks	24 to 36 weeks
Nonlinear periodization	26[a]	48[a]	6[a]	17[a, c]
1 set × 8-12 reps	5	5	0	0

Wingate power

	Pretraining to 16 weeks	Pretraining to 36 weeks	16 to 24 weeks	24 to 36 weeks
Nonlinear periodization	8	14[a]	4	3
1 set × 8-12 reps	0	0	0	0

Serve velocity

	Pretraining to 16 weeks	Pretraining to 36 weeks	16 to 24 weeks	24 to 36 weeks
Nonlinear periodization	21[a]	23[a]	2[a, b]	0[a]
1 set × 8-12 reps	4	4	3	−3

a = significant difference from pretest; b = significant difference from 16 weeks; c = significant difference from 24 weeks.

Data from Kraemer et al. 2000.

Bench press 1RM

	Pretraining to 4 weeks	Pretraining to 12 weeks	4 to 8 weeks	8 to 12 weeks
Nonlinear periodization	15[a]	28[a, c]	6[b]	5[b]
Linear periodization	4	9	1	5
3 × 8- to 10RM	3	9	2	3

Leg press 1 RM

	Pretraining to 4 weeks	Pretraining to 12 weeks	4 to 8 weeks	8 to 12 weeks
Nonlinear periodization	15[a, c]	39[a, c]	11[b]	8[b]
Linear periodization	5	16[a]	5	5
3 × 8- to 10RM	4	8	1	3

a = significant difference from pretest; b = significant difference from previous time point; c = significant difference from linear periodization and control group.

Data from Monteior et al. 2009.

A meta-analysis indicates that periodized resistance training programs result in greater strength increases in both sexes, untrained people, and trained people than nonvaried programs do (Rhea and Alderman 2004). Although periodized programs result in strength gains in both sexes performing the same periodized training program, relative strength gains may be greater in females than in males (Kell 2011). Perhaps surprisingly, untrained people experience greater strength gains (effect size = 1.59) compared to trained people (effect size = 0.78) and athletes (effect size = 0.84) with periodized programs.

Periodized programs also result in greater strength gains than nonvaried programs do whether the training program is 1 to 8, 9 to 20, or 20 to 40 weeks long; however, the greatest difference between periodized programs and nonvaried programs is shown with a training duration of 9 to 20 weeks. Periodized programs may not result in greater strength gains in some populations, such as seniors with a mean age of 71 years (DeBeliso et al. 2005). This is partially supported by the preceding meta-analysis, which indicated that people 55 years and younger (effect size = 1.34) experience greater strength gains with periodized programs compared to nonperiodized programs than those 55 years and older (effect size = 0.85).

Periodized training programs use different combinations of acute training program variables to emphasize different training outcomes, such as hypertrophy, maximal strength, local muscular endurance, and maximal power. This does not mean that a training session emphasizing one training outcome over time will not result in increases in other training outcomes; rather, it means that the training session is meant to develop one training outcome to a greater extent than others. As an example, a training session emphasizing maximal strength will result in muscle hypertrophy over time; however, the session is meant to develop maximal strength to a greater extent than hypertrophy. Guidelines have been developed (see table 7.2) to emphasize various training outcomes for novice, intermediate, and advanced weight-trained people (American College of Sports Medicine 2009). These guidelines can be used to develop periodized resistance training sessions.

The manipulation of resistance training's acute training program variables results in a virtually limitless number of possibilities and so a limitless number of both short- and long-term training strategies. To date, the sport science community has investigated two major types of periodized resistance training: linear periodization and nonlinear periodization.

Linear Periodization

Linear periodization is the older of the two major types of periodized resistance training. Also termed **classic strength and power periodization** and **stepwise periodization**, this type follows a general trend of decreasing training volume and increasing training intensity as training progresses (see figure 7.1). For weight training this means that a relatively high number of repetitions is performed at a low intensity when training is initiated, and as training progresses, the number of repetitions decreases and training intensity increases.

When linear periodization was first developed, only one or two major sport competitions took place per year (e.g., national and world championships). Thus, the training plan followed a yearly or six-month cycle to peak physical performance at the time of major competitions. This resulted in training volume reaching its lowest point and training intensity its highest point once or twice a year corresponding with major competitions. However, to allow for some physical and psychological recovery before the major competition, the highest training intensity occurred a short time before the major competition. Skill training for a particular sport or activity followed a very similar trend as training intensity, except that it normally reached its highest intensity slightly closer to a major competition.

Training phases emphasize particular training outcomes within the linear periodized plan. When used to prepare athletes for yearly or twice-yearly competitions, each of the major training phases lasted approximately three to four months. Anecdotal evidence and research indicate that substantial strength and performance gains are possible with shorter training phases. Thus, the training plan time frame has evolved so that that phases now last anywhere from two to six weeks. Thus, the time needed for one complete training cycle, or the performance of all training phases, is approximately 8 to 24 weeks. Studies examining linear periodization use these shorter training phases.

Terminology describing various time periods developed along with periodized training concepts. A macrocycle typically refers to one year of training, and a mesocycle refers to three to four

TABLE 7.2 **American College of Sports Medicine Guidelines to Emphasize Various Training Outcomes**

Type of trainee	Frequency per week	Number of sets per exercise	Number of repetitions per set	Intensity (% 1RM)	Rest between sets (min)
Emphasize strength					
Novice trainee	2 or 3 total-body sessions	1-3	8-12	60-70	2-3 major exercises, 1-2 assistance exercises
Intermediate trainee	3 for total-body sessions, 4 for split routines	Multiple	8-12	60-70	2-3 major exercises, 1-2 assistance exercises
Advanced trainee	4-6 split routines	Multiple	1-12	Up to 100 in a periodized manner	2-3 major exercises, 1-2 assistance exercises
Emphasize hypertrophy					
Novice trainee	2 or 3 total-body sessions	1-3	8-12	70-85	1-2
Intermediate trainee	3 for total-body sessions, 4 for split routines	1-3	8-12	70-85	1-2
Advanced trainee	4-6 split routines	3-6	1-12 (mostly 6-12)	70-100 in a periodized manner	2-3 major exercises, 1-2 assistance exercises
Emphasize local muscular endurance					
Novice trainee	2 or 3 total-body sessions	Multiple	10-15	Low	1 or less
Intermediate trainee	3 for total-body sessions, 4 for split routines	Multiple	10-15	Low	1 or less
Advanced trainee	4-6 split routines	Multiple	10-25	Various percentages	1 or less for 10-15 reps; 1-2 for 15-25 reps
Emphasize power					
Novice trainee	2 or 3 total-body sessions	Maximal strength training + 1-3 power-type exercises	3-6 not to failure	Upper body: 30-60 Lower body: 0-60	2-3 major exercises with high intensity, 1-2 assistance and major exercises with low intensity
Intermediate trainee	3 or 4 for total-body or split routines	Novice + 3-6 power-type exercises	Novice + 1-6	Novice + 85-100	2-3 for major exercises with high intensity, 1-2 assistance and major exercises with low intensity
Advanced trainee	4 or 5 for total-body or split routines	Novice + 3-6 power-type exercises	Novice + 1-6	Novice + 85-100	2-3 for major exercises with high intensity, 1-2 assistance and major exercises with low intensity

Based on American College of Sports Medicine, 2009.

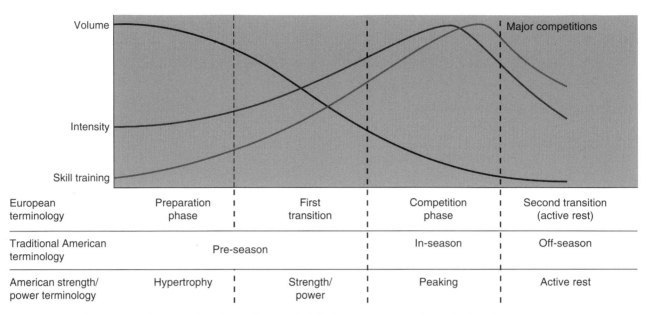

FIGURE 7.1 Linear periodization strength and power training pattern of volume and intensity.

months of a macrocycle. A microcycle typically refers to one to four weeks within a mesocycle. Several terminologies describing specific training phases also developed (see figure 7.1). For example, a mesocycle using classic European terminology is the preparation phase. The training terminology most frequently used in sport science studies examining linear periodization is the American strength and power terminology. Typically, regardless of the terminology used, training phases have specific goals normally in large part described by their names. For example, in the American strength and power terminology the peaking phase's major goal is to maximize, or peak, the expression of strength or power.

Active recovery phases are incorporated into the linear periodization model. However, active recovery does not mean complete cessation of physical activity or training, nor is this phase typically very long. This would result in substantial deconditioning, and trainees would then have to spend training time regaining their former physical condition, rather than improving it. Active recovery phases often consist of a reduction in total training volume and intensity rather than cessation of training. So within an active recovery phase not only are the volume and intensity of weight training decreased, but also other forms of training, such as interval training, aerobic training, and skill training, are decreased. It is also possible that within an active recovery phase the performance of one

type of training ceases completely while other types are continued at a low volume and intensity. Long active recovery phases are incorporated into some programs according to the sport's and athlete's requirements; they may also relate to the level of training and experience of the athlete. For example, the active recovery phase of an experienced and successful athlete immediately after a major competition or competitive season may be longer than that of a less experienced athlete.

Because the American strength and power periodization terminology and model are used most frequently in studies examining linear periodization, a detailed description of each training phase in this model is warranted (see table 7.3). Note that training volume decreases and intensity increases from the hypertrophy to peaking training phases. Additionally, note that a range of sets and repetitions per set exists for each exercise in a particular training phase. So, although training volume and intensity do follow a general trend of decreasing and increasing as training progresses, variations in volume and intensity can and do occur on a daily or weekly basis in most training plans.

The variation in the number of sets and repetitions also allows for variation in volume and intensity in specific exercises. For example, a person may have different intensities and volumes for specific muscle groups or exercises based on his needs and goals. Training volume and intensity are also affected by the number of exercises performed

TABLE 7.3 **Linear Periodization Model**

	Training phase				
	Hypertrophy	**Strength**	**Power**	**Peaking**	**Active rest**
Sets/exercise	3-5	3-5	3-5	1-3	Light physical activity
Reps/set	8-12	2-6	2 or 3	1-3	
Intensity	Low	Moderate	High	Very high	
Volume	Very high	High	Moderate	Low	

Based on Stone, O'Bryant, and Garhammer, 1981.

per session. In many training plans, as the training progresses, especially in the power and peaking phases, the number of exercises performed per session is decreased. This results in a decrease in training volume and allows for an increase in intensity as less fatigue occurs during a session allowing the lifting of a higher percentage of 1RM in the exercises performed. Additionally, as the training progresses, the choice of exercises performed may also change depending on the goals and needs of the trainee. Typically, for many athletes the number of single-joint exercises performed decreases as the training progresses and multijoint exercises are emphasized. Moreover, a greater emphasis, especially in the power and peaking phases, is placed on power-type exercises, such as variations of the Olympic lifts, lower-body plyometrics, and plyometric medicine ball upper-body exercises. In many programs only multijoint exercises are periodized. Although the general pattern of the American strength and power periodized plan is used by sport science studies, a wide variation in training phase length, number of sets, and number of repetitions per set has been used in training studies (see table 7.4).

Nonlinear Periodization

Nonlinear periodization is a more recent type of periodization than the linear model. A major goal in many linear training models is to peak strength and power immediately at the end of the peaking phase. However, for sports or activities with long seasons, in which competitive success depends on performance throughout the entire season, developing and maintaining physical fitness during the entire season is important. Peaking strength and power for major competitions normally occurring at the end of the season is also important. However, without success during the season, qualification for major tournaments and competitions does not occur. Therefore, goals of a training model

for sports or activities with long seasons, such as volleyball, basketball, baseball, and soccer, should be to develop physical fitness to ensure success during the season and yet continue to increase fitness throughout the season.

Nonlinear models are gaining popularity in sports and activities with long seasons for several reasons. A typical strength and power training program sometimes results in strength and power peaking immediately before the season, yet the major competitions occur at the end of the season. On the other hand, performing high-volume training during the initial portion of the season to attain peak strength and power at the end of the season might result in residual fatigue and thus poor performance at the start of the season. This could result in the athlete or team not qualifying for a major competition or tournament at the end of the season.

Nonlinear periodization varies training volume and intensity so that fitness gains occur over long training periods, such as long seasons; peaking of physical fitness at a certain point in time is a minor training goal. With **nonlinear periodization**, training intensity and volume are varied by using different RM or near-RM training zones. Typically, three training zones are used, such as 4- to 6RM, 8- to 10RM, and 12- to 15RM zones or close to RM zones. Other training zones could also be incorporated into a nonlinear model. For example, a very heavy resistance training zone such as 1- to 3RM or a very low intensity, such as 20- to 25RM, could also be included in a nonlinear model. The training zones are most often varied on a training session basis, which is termed **daily nonlinear periodization**. However, training zones can also be varied in a weekly, or biweekly manner (see box 7.1). Because training zones are not necessarily performed in a certain order, intensity or volume does not follow a pattern of consistently increasing or decreasing over time.

TABLE 7.4 Representative Linear Periodization Versus Nonvaried Training Studies

Reference	Mean age (yr) and sex	Training length (wk)	Frequency per week	Sets × reps	Intensity	Exercises trained	Test	Percentage increase
Stone et al. 1981	High school M	6	4	Multiple sets 3 × 6	Progressed at own rate	SQ and 5 others	SQ VJ	?* ?*
				Linear periodization wk 1-3: 5 × 10 wk 4: 5 × 5 wk 5: 3 × 3 wk 6: 3 × 2	Progressed at own rate	SQ and 5 others	SQ VJ	?*[a] ?*[a]
Stowers et al. 1983	College M	7	3	1 × 10	10RM	Combination of 8	BP SQ VJ	7* 14* 0
				3 × 10	10RM	Combination of 8	BP SQ VJ	9* 20* 1
				Linear periodization wk 1 and 2: 5 × 10 wk 3-5: 3 × 5 wk 6 and 7: 2 × 3	RMs	Combination of 8	BP SQ VJ	9* 27*[b] 10*
O'Bryant, Byrd, and Stone 1988	19 M	11	3	3 × 6	81-97% of pre-training 1RM	SQ and 8 others	SQ WP	32* 6*
				Linear periodization wk 1-4: 5 × 10 wk 5-8: 3 × 5, 1 × 10 wk 9-11: 3 × 2, 1 × 10	70-117% of pre-training 1RM	SQ and 8 others	SQ WP	38*[a] 17*[a]
McGee et al. 1992	19-20 M	7	3	1 × 8-12	8- to 12RM	Combination of 7	Cycling to exhaustion SQ reps to exhaustion	12 46
				3 × 10	close to 10RM	Combination of 7	Cycling to exhaustion SQ reps to exhaustion	15* 71*
				Linear periodization wk 1 and 2: 3 × 10 wk 3-5: 3 × 5 wk 6 and 7: 3 × 3	close to RMs	Combination of 7	Cycling to exhaustion SQ reps to exhaustion	29* 74*
Willoughby 1992	20 M	12	2	3 × 10	10RM	BP and SQ	BP SQ	8* 13*
				3 × 6-8	6- to 8RM	BP and SQ	BP SQ	17*[c] 26*[c]
				Linear periodization wk 1-4: 5 × 8-10 wk 5-8: 4 × 5-7 wk 9-12: 3 × 3-5	RMs	BP and SQ	BP SQ	28*[d] 48*[d]
Willoughby 1993	20 M	16	3	5 × 10	79% of 1RM	BP and SQ	BP SQ	8* 14*
				6 × 8	83% of 1RM	BP and SQ	BP SQ	10* 22*[e]
				Linear periodization wk 1-4: 5 × 10 wk 5-8: 4 × 8 wk 9-12: 3 × 6 wk 13-16: 3 × 4	79% of 1RM 83% of 1RM 88% of 1RM 92% of 1RM	BP and SQ	BP SQ	23*[f] 34*[f]

Reference	Mean age (yr) and sex	Training length (wk)	Frequency per week	Sets × reps	Intensity	Exercises trained	Test	Percentage increase
Baker, Wilson, and Carlyon 1994a	19-21 M	12	3	5 × 6 core exercises 5 × 8 all others	RMs	Combination of 17	BP SQ VJ	12* 26* 9*
				Linear periodization wk 1-4: 5 × 10 core, 3 × 10 all others wk 5-8: 5 × 5 core, 3 × 8 all others wk 9-11: 3 × 3, 1 × 10 core, 3 × 6 all others wk 12: 3 × 3 core, 3 × 6 all others	RMs	Combination of 17	BP SQ VJ	12* 27* 4*
Herrick and Stone 1996	20-24 F	14	2	3 × 6	6RM	6	BP SQ	25* 46*
				Linear periodization wk 1-8: 3 × 10 wk 9: off wk 10-11: 3 × 4 wk 12: off wk 13 and 14: 3 × 2	RMs	6	BP SQ	31* 54*
Kraemer 1997	20 M	14	3	1 × 10, forced reps	8- to 10RM	9	BP HC VJ WP	3* 4* 3* 0
				Linear periodization wk 1-3: 2 or 3 × 8-10 wk 4 and 5: 3 or 4 × 6 wk 6 and 7: 5 × 1-4 repeat all weeks	50% of 1RM 70-85% of 1RM 85-95% of 1RM	12	BP HC VJ WP	11*ᵉ 19*ᵉ 17*ᵉ 14*ᵉ
Schiotz et al. 1998	24 M	10	4	4 × 6 core exercises 3 × 8 all others	Initially 80% of 1RM; then progressed at own pace	2 core and 5 assistance	BP SQ	5 11*
				Linear periodization wk 1 and 2: 5 × 10 core, 3 × 10 assistance wk 3: 3 × 10, 1 × 8, 1 × 6 core, 3 × 10 assistance wk 4: 2 × 8, 3 × 5 core, 3 × 8 assistance wk 5: 1 × 8, 1 × 6, 3 × 5 core, 3 × 8 assistance wk 6: 1 × 8, 4 × 5 core, 3 × 8 assistance wk 7: 1 × 8, 2 × 5, 1 × 3, 1 × 1 core, 3 × 6 assistance wk 8: 2 × 5, 1 × 3, 1 × 2, 1 × 1 core, 3 × 6 assistance wk 9 and 10: 2 × 3, 4 × 1 core, 3 × 4 assistance	Initially 50% of pretraining 1RM; then progressed at own pace	2 core and 5 assistance	BP SQ	8* 10*

>continued

TABLE 7.4 *>continued*

Reference	Mean age (yr) and sex	Training length (wk)	Frequency per week	Sets × reps	Intensity	Exercises trained	Test	Percentage increase
Stone et al. 2000	College M	12	3	5 × 6	6RM, mean 67% of pretraining 1RM	6	SQ	10
				Linear periodization wk 1-4: 5 × 10 major, 3 × 10 assistance wk 5-8: 5 × 5 major, 3 × 8 assistance wk 9-11: 3 × 3, 1 × 10 major, 3 × 6 assistance wk 12: 3 × 3 major, 3 × 6 assistance	RMs, mean 61% of pretraining 1RM	6	SQ	15*
				Linear periodization wk 1 and 2: 5 × 10 major, 3 × 10 assistance wk 3 and 4: 3 × 5, 1 × 10 major, 3 × 10 assistance wk 5: 3 × 3, 1 × 5 major, 3 × 10 assistance wk 6-8: 3 × 5, 1 × 5 major, 3 × 5 assistance wk 9: 5 × 5, 1 × 5 major, 3 × 5 assistance wk 10: 3 × 5, 1 × 5 major, 3 × 5 assistance wk 11: 3 × 3, 1 × 5 major, 3 × 5 assistance wk 12: 3 × 3 major, 3 × 5 assistance	Heavy and light days, heavy days use RM, mean 72% of pretraining 1RM	6	SQ	15*
Hoffman et al. 2009	20 M	15	4 (split body)	Nonpower exercises 3 or 4 × 6-8 Power exercises 4 or 5 × 3-4	RMs	Multiple per training session	SQ BP VJ Medicine ball throw	20* 9* 4 2
				Linear periodization wk 1-4: 3 or 4 × 9-12 wk 5-10: 3 or 4 × 3-8 wk 11-15: 3-5 × 1-5	RMs	Multiple per training session	SQ BP VJ Medicine ball throw	21* 8* 0 6*
Monteiro et al. 2009	27 M	12	4 (split body)	3 × 8-10	RMs	15	BP SQ	9 8
				Linear periodization wk 1-4: 3 × 12-15 wk 5-8: 3 × 8-10 wk 9-12: 3 × 4 or 5	RMs	15	BP SQ	9 16*

* = significant change pre- to posttraining.

a = significant difference from 3 × 6.

b = significant difference from 1 × 10 and 3 × 10 groups.

c = significant difference from 3 × 10.

d = significant difference from 3 × 10 and 3 × 6-8 groups.

e = significant difference from 5 × 10.

f = significant difference from 5 × 10 and 6 × 8 groups.

g = significant difference from 1 × 10.

BP = bench press 1RM, SQ = squat 1RM, HC = hang clean 1RM, VJ = vertical jump, WP = Wingate cycling power.

BOX 7.1 PRACTICAL QUESTION

How Are Training Zones Arranged in a Weekly or Biweekly Nonlinear Program?

Similar to all periodization models, weekly and biweekly nonlinear programs can differ substantially in training intensity and volume. However, both types vary their training intensity and volume using three training zones. Table 7.5 demonstrates how the typical three training zones of a nonlinear training plan could be arranged in a weekly and biweekly nonlinear program during six weeks of training. Note that, assuming the same number of sets, exercises, and training frequency for both programs, the total training intensity and volume are the same in the weekly and biweekly plans. The only difference is that changes in training intensity and volume are made after each week of training or after two weeks of training. If the training zones were arranged according to the increase in intensity, either weekly or biweekly nonlinear programs could be considered variations of linear periodization.

TABLE 7.5 **Example of Weekly and Biweekly Nonlinear Programs**

	Week 1	Week 2	Week 3	Week 4	Week 5	Week 6
Weekly nonlinear	12-15 reps/set	4-6 reps/set	8-10 reps/set	12-15 reps/set	4-6 reps/set	8-10 reps/set
Biweekly nonlinear	12-15 reps/set	12-15 reps/set	4-6 reps/set	4-6 reps/set	8-10 reps/set	8-10 reps/set

Although many variations in intensity and volume could be incorporated into a nonlinear program, the following are typical examples. All exercises, including both multi- and single-joint exercises, in a training session use three training zones in three training sessions per week. With three training sessions per week, only multijoint exercises use three training zones per week and single-joint exercises always use a training zone of 8- to 10RM. Some sessions composed of predominantly multijoint exercises use different training zones, and some sessions composed predominantly of single-joint exercises use only an 8- to 10RM training zone. For example, a nonlinear model using three training zones and two types of training sessions could be as follows: A Monday and Thursday session predominantly composed of multijoint exercises including power-type exercises, such as power cleans, would use all three training zones, and a session performed on Tuesday and Friday made up of predominantly single-joint exercises would always use an 8- to 10RM zone. With all variations of nonlinear periodization, if two training sessions are performed during one week, two training zones are used; the following week, one of the training zones used in the first week and a different training zone are

used. Obviously, many other nonlinear patterns of intensity and volume are possible.

Many patterns of training volume and intensity can be developed using periodization concepts, including combining various aspects of the linear and nonlinear models. For example, a linear model during the off-season and early preseason of a sport can ensure that strength and power peak immediately before the season. A nonlinear model during the late preseason and in-season can then help not only to maintain, but also to increase fitness during the season so that strength and power contribute maximally to success throughout the entire season. Other variations of the nonlinear model could include a model where the training zones gradually follow an increase in intensity and decrease in volume as training progresses and a model where exercise choice is varied to emphasize power development as training progresses.

Comparative Studies

When examining any comparison of weight training programs, we need to consider both the length of the study and the training status of the subjects (see chapter 2). This is true whether comparing nonvaried programs to each other, periodized programs to each other, or periodized programs to nonvaried programs. During the first four to six weeks of any realistic weight training program, substantial gains in strength occur because of neural adaptations. Other physiological adaptations, such as changes in the quality of the muscle proteins, can also be dramatic during the first several weeks of a training program. These very quickly occurring physical adaptations occur with any realistic training program and can result in substantial strength increases. Thus, in short-term studies, any significant difference between training programs in strength and power or short-term, high-intensity anaerobic endurance, such as measured by a Wingate cycling test, is difficult to achieve because these initial strength gains may mask any real difference between the training programs. This is especially true when untrained people are trained. Conversely, if a short-term study demonstrates the superiority of one training program over another, it may merely mean that the superior program brings about quicker neural adaptations or changes in the quality of protein, and any differences between programs may be nonexistent with longer-term training. This may be especially true if no gains in muscle fiber cross-sectional area or fat-free mass are demonstrated in the initial training period.

Another consideration in a discussion of comparative studies is that most studies use untrained or moderately trained subjects. This limits the applicability of the studies to highly trained people or athletes, because strength and power increases occur at a much slower rate in these people (Häkkinen et al. 1989). Thus, assuming that the magnitude of change and rate of change in variables, such as strength, from studies using untrained subjects are directly applicable to highly trained people is tenuous. It is also important to note that not all muscle groups will respond at the same rate or with the same magnitude after a specific resistance training program, including periodized programs (see tables 7.1, 7.4, and 7.6). For example, over 16 weeks of strength and power periodized training, the increase in strength shown in the bench press was substantially less than that shown in the squat after 4, 8, 12, and 16 weeks of training (Willoughby 1993). Thus, trainers should be cautious about assuming that a particular training program will result in the same rate and magnitude of adaptations in different muscle groups or different exercises. Nevertheless, a sufficient number of studies comparing period-

ization models to nonvaried training models have been performed so that we can form conclusions concerning the effectiveness of periodized models. This is not to imply, however, that further study of periodized models is not needed.

Comparisons of Linear Periodization and Nonvaried Programs

Comparative studies of linear periodization and single-set and multiple-set nonvaried programs demonstrate that periodization can result in significantly greater strength gains (see table 7.4). Most comparisons used healthy young males as subjects. However, one study did show greater percentage gains in strength in women with periodized training, but no significant difference between the periodized and multiple-set training program was shown (Herrick and Stone 1996). Several studies describing the subjects as moderately trained or trained people indicate that linear periodization does result in significantly greater strength gains than nonperiodized programs do. For example, defining trained as the ability to bench press 120% and squat 150% or greater of total body mass, it was shown in trained people that periodized training resulted in greater strength gains than nonvaried multiple-set programs did (Willoughby 1992, 1993). It has also been shown that high school (Stone, O'Bryant, and Garhammer 1981) and college American football players (Kraemer 1997) demonstrate greater strength gains with a periodized program than with a single-set nonvaried program. However, no significant difference in strength gains between linear periodization and nonvaried programs in college American football players (Hoffman et al. 2009) and resistance-trained (two years of training experience) males (Monteiro et al. 2009) has been shown. In this last study, although bench press 1RM increases were not different between the periodized and nonvaried programs, periodized training did cause a significantly greater increase in 1RM leg press ability.

Comparisons of gains in motor performance and local muscular endurance are less common than strength comparisons. Linear periodized programs have shown significantly greater gains in vertical jump ability, short-term cycling ability, and Wingate power than nonvaried single-set and multiple-set programs have shown. However, not all studies have shown significantly greater increases with periodized training, and relatively few studies have examined the training effects on these measures. Therefore, conclusions concerning motor performance must be viewed with caution. However, comparisons to date do favor linear periodized models over nonperiodized models in terms of motor performance.

Few studies have compared the total body mass and body composition changes of periodized and nonvaried training models. Some comparisons of a linear periodized program to a single-set program (McGee et al. 1992) and to nonvaried multiple-set programs (Hoffman et al. 2009; McGee et al. 1992; Monteiro et al. 2009: O'Bryant, Byrd, and Stone 1988; Schiotz et al. 1998; Stone, O'Bryant, and Garhammer 1981) show neither program causing a significant change in total body mass. Other comparisons show periodized training and multiple-set programs to result in significant, but identical, increases in total body mass (Baker, Wilson, and Carlyon 1994a) and a significantly greater increase in total body mass with a linear periodized program compared to a single-set program (Kraemer 1997).

Comparisons of body composition changes have shown linear periodized and multiple-set training programs to result in significant but identical increases in fat-free mass while total body fat showed a change with both types of training (Baker, Wilson, and Carlyon 1994a) and no significant change with either type of training (Hoffman et al. 2009; Monteiro et al. 2009). Comparisons have also shown nonsignificant increases in fat-free mass with both types of training, a small nonsignificant decrease with multiple-set training in body fat percentage, a small but significant decrease with periodized training in body fat percentage (Schiotz et al. 1998), and a significantly greater change in fat-free mass and percent body fat with periodized training compared to a nonvaried multiple-set program (Stone, O'Bryant, and Garhammer 1981). A comparison of a single-set nonvaried program to a linear periodized program reported a significantly greater decrease in body fat percentage with periodized training (Kraemer 1997). Although changes in fat-free mass were not reported in this study because periodized training also resulted in a significantly greater gain in total body mass, it can be concluded that periodized training also resulted in a greater increase in lean body mass than the single-set program did.

Because of the paucity of studies examining changes in total body mass, fat-free mass, and body fat, and the use of skinfolds to determine body composition in the majority of studies, conclusions concerning the superiority of one type of training over the other in bringing about changes in these variables must be viewed with caution. However, as with strength gains and motor performance changes, it is important to note that whenever a significant difference between training programs has been reported, it has always been in favor of the linear periodized programs.

Several studies do offer some insight into why strength and power periodized training may result in greater strength gains than nonperiodized training. For example, one unique aspect of the Willoughby 1993 study was that for the first 8 of 16 weeks of training there was no significant difference in total training volume between the periodized model and two multiple-set training models. After eight weeks of training all groups demonstrated significant, but identical increases in 1RM strength. Beginning at week 9, periodized training volume significantly decreased compared to that of the multiple-set programs, and it is after week 9 that significant differences in strength in favor of the periodized model become apparent. Thus, decreases in training volume present in linear periodized models as training progresses may in part explain the greater improvement in 1RM strength. Another aspect of this study was that subjects were at least moderately trained (able to squat 150% and bench press 120% or greater of total body weight). So the results also indicate that trained people may need at least eight weeks of training for periodized training to demonstrate superior results compared to nonvaried programs. This conclusion is supported by a meta-analysis indicating that periodized programs show greater improvement in strength compared to nonvaried programs when training is 9 to 20 weeks in length compared to when the programs are 8 weeks or less in length. Whether the programs are 9 to 20 weeks or 8 weeks or less in length, periodized programs are favored for increases in strength, but when the programs are 8 weeks or less in length, the periodized programs are less favored for increases in strength (Rhea and Alderman 2004).

The conclusion that changes in training volume may in part explain the differences between training programs is supported by other studies showing no significant difference in strength gains between linear periodized and nonvaried programs when training volume is equated (Baker, Wilson, and Carlyon 1994a; Hoffman et al. 2009). One of the studies, in addition to equating total training volume, equated training intensity between the linear periodized program and a multiple-set program. During a 12-week training period, training volume (total mass lifted) and relative training intensity were equated (Baker, Wilson, and Carlyon 1994a) and no significant difference in strength gains was shown. This indicates that greater increases in strength with periodized training may be due to greater training volumes, changes in training intensity, or both, in some comparisons.

Precisely what causes greater fitness gains from linear periodized training than from nonvaried models (when apparent) remains to be elucidated. However, the majority of studies do favor linear periodized models over nonvaried training models.

Comparisons of Nonlinear Periodization and Nonvaried Programs

As with linear periodization, studies that compare nonlinear periodization to single-set and multiple-set nonvaried programs demonstrate that periodization can result in significantly greater strength gains (see table 7.6). Studies that compared a single-set nonvaried model and a typical daily nonlinear model in which three training zones were used successively on a training session basis showed nonlinear training to cause greater percentages of strength gains in female college tennis players (Kraemer et al. 2000) and significantly greater strength gains in untrained college

females (Marx et al. 2001) compared to a one-set training model.

Comparisons of nonlinear training and multiple-set nonvaried training in female college tennis players (Kraemer et al. 2003) and college All-American football players (Hoffman et al. 2009) show no significant difference in strength gains between the two types of training. In the female tennis players percentage gains favored nonlinear training, whereas in the American football players percentage gains favored the nonvaried training. A variation of nonlinear periodization in a split-body training program in which two of three training zones were used per week of training, with a different combination of two of three zones used in successive weeks of training, showed the nonlinear training to result in significantly greater strength increases (Monteiro et al. 2009). Several studies testing strength at several points during the training program (12-36 weeks) do show more consistent strength gains with daily nonlinear periodization compared to nonvaried single-set training (Kraemer, Häkkinen et al. 2003; Marx et al. 2001) and multiple-set programs (Monteiro et al. 2009).

A variation of a nonlinear model employing three training zones has been shown to be as effective as a nonvaried multiple-set model in adults 66 to 77 years old (Hunter et al. 2001). The multiple-set model used a resistance equivalent to 80% of 1RM in all training sessions, whereas the nonlinear model used training zones equivalent to 80, 65, and 50% of 1RM. Subjects in both training models trained with two sets of 10 repetitions or repetitions to concentric failure, whichever occurred first. Thus, the nonlinear model did not use training RM or near-RM training zones in all training sessions. No significant differences in

TABLE 7.6   **Representative Daily Nonlinear Periodization Versus Nonvaried Training Studies**

Reference	Mean age (yr) and sex	Training length (wk)	Frequency per week	Sets and reps	Intensity	Exercises trained	Test(s)	Percentage increase
Kraemer et al. 2000	19 F	36	2 or 3	1 × 8-10	Close to 8- to 10RM	14	BP SP LP WP VJ	10* 14* 7* 1 5
			2 or 3	Daily nonlinear periodization 3 training zones: 2-4 × 4-6, 8-10, 12-15	Close to RMs	14	BP SP LP WP VJ	25* 28* 18* 14* 48*

Reference	Mean age (yr) and sex	Training length (wk)	Frequency per week	Sets and reps	Intensity	Exercises trained	Test(s)	Percentage increase
Marx et al. 2001	22-23 F	24	3	1 × 8-12	8- to 12RM	2 alternating groups of 10	BP LP BP reps at 80% of 1RM LP reps at 80% of 1RM WP Sit-ups in 1 min VJ 40 yd sprint	12* 11* 10* 19* 4 13* 10* +1
			4	Daily nonlinear periodization 2 sessions/wk used 3 training zones 2-4 × 3-5, 8-10, 12-15 2 sessions/wk always used 2-4 × 8-10	RMs	Nonvaried 1 × 8-12 RM	BP LP BP reps at 80% of 1RM LP reps at 80% of 1RM WP Sit-ups in 1 min VJ 40 yd sprint	47*a 32*a 24*a 64*a 27*a 42*a 40*a −6*a
Hunter et al. 2001	66-67 M and F	25	3	2 × 10	80% of 1RM	10	BP LP SP AC	34* 43* 42* 69*
			3	Daily nonlinear periodization 3 training zones: 50, 65, and 80% of 1RM	50, 65, and 80% of 1RM	10	BP LP SP AC	23* 31* 30* 59*
Kraemer, Häkkinen et al. 2003	19 F	36	2 or 3	3 × 8-10	RM	14	BP LP SP WP VJ 10 m sprint	17* 17* 23* 14* 37* -1
				Daily nonlinear periodization 3 training zones: 3 × 4-6, 8-10, 12-15	RM	14	BP LP SP WP VJ 10 m sprint	23* 19* 24* 12* 50*b −2
Hoffman et al. 2009	20 M	15	4 (split body)	Nonpower exercises: 3 or 4 × 6-8 Power exercises: 4 or 5 × 3 or 4	RMs	Multiple per training session	SQ BP VJ Medicine ball throw	20* 9* 4 2
				Daily nonlinear periodization 3 training zones: 3 or 4 × 9-12, 3 or 4 × 3-8, 3-5 × 1-5	RMs	Multiple per training session	SQ BP VJ Medicine ball throw	11* 8* 1 3
Monteiro et al. 2009	27 M	12	4 (split body)	3 × 8-10	RMs	15	BP LP	9 8
				Daily nonlinear periodization 3 training zones: 3 × 12-15, 8-10, 4 or 5	RMs	15	BP LP	28*b 39*b

* = significant change pre- to posttraining.

a = significant difference from 1 × 8-12 group.

b = significant difference from 3 × 8-10 group.

BP = bench press 1RM, SQ = squat 1RM, SP = shoulder press 1RM, LP = leg press 1RM, AC = arm curl 1RM, VJ = vertical jump, WP = Wingate cycling power.

strength between the two training programs were shown (see table 7.6). However, the nonvaried model showed a greater percentage of strength gains. This indicated that sets do not have to be carried to concentric failure (see chapter 6) and that high intensity (80% of 1RM) is not necessary in all training sessions with this age group. The nonlinear model did show some advantage over the nonvaried model: It had a significantly greater decrease in the difficulty of performing a carrying task.

Motor performance tasks have increased with nonlinear training; however, the increase is not always significantly greater than that which results from nonvaried training programs (see table 7.6). Nonlinear periodization has been shown to significantly increase motor performance in untrained college females (Marx et al. 2001) and female college tennis players (Kraemer et al. 2000) compared to nonvaried single-set training. Of particular interest is the 30% increase in serve velocity with nonlinear training compared to a 4% increase with single-set training. Percentage increase in serve (29 vs. 16%), forehand (22 vs. 17%), and backhand (36 vs. 14%) ball velocity has also been shown to increase significantly more with nonlinear periodization than with a multiple-set nonvaried training program (Kraemer, Häkkinen et al. 2003).

Nonlinear models have also been shown to be effective in bringing about body composition changes, although the changes are not consistently significantly different from those that result from nonvaried training programs. The studies training collegiate American football players (Kraemer 1997), female collegiate tennis athletes (Kraemer et al. 2000; Kraemer, Häkkinen et al. 2003), and previously untrained college-age females (Marx et al. 2001) all demonstrate the nonlinear models to bring about significant decreases in percent body fat and significant increases in fat-free mass. However, only in untrained college females did the nonlinear model show a significantly greater decrease in percent fat and increase in fat-free mass than nonvaried one-set training (Marx et al. 2001). In this study the difference in body composition could be due to the increased training volume performed in the nonlinear compared to the single-set training model. No significant change in body mass and body composition has also been shown with nonlinear training (Hoffman et al. 2009; Monteiro et al. 2009). A weakness of all of these reports is the use of skinfolds to determine

body composition changes. A variation of the nonlinear model, previously described, showed that a multiple-set high-intensity program and a nonlinear model cause significant but similar increases in fat-free mass and decreases in percent body fat (air plethysmography) in older adults but no significant change in total body mass (Hunter et al. 2001). Thus, the comparisons of nonlinear to nonvaried training concerning body composition changes are mixed.

Nonlinear periodization is an effective program for increasing strength and motor performance and changing body composition in both trained and untrained people. This type of training may also produce more consistent changes in strength than nonvaried training does. Thus, nonlinear periodization is a viable training program for both the fitness enthusiast and the athlete.

Comparisons of Types of Periodization

Most comparisons of periodization models are between daily nonlinear and linear periodization (see table 7.7). Within these training models a wide variety of training volumes (number of exercises, number of sets and repetitions) and intensities have been used. For example, the number of repetitions per set in the comparisons shown in table 7.7 ranges between 4 and 25. Program choices involving volume and intensity can affect training outcomes, such as increases in maximal strength, and thereby affect the outcome of a training model comparison. This is especially true if training volume and intensity are not equated between training models. All of the comparisons depicted in table 7.7 have similar training volumes and intensities in both training models. The major difference is that the daily nonlinear training volume and intensity vary substantially within a week of training, whereas the linear training volume and intensity change substantially after several weeks of training.

Some of these comparisons show significantly greater strength gains with the daily nonlinear model in college-age males (Monteiro et al. 2009; Rhea et al. 2002; Simão et al. 2012). Others show nonsignificant differences between the two training models, but favor the nonlinear model (Kok, Hamer, and Bishop 2009; Prestes, Frollini et al. 2009) or the linear model (Bufford et al. 2007; Hartman et al. 2009; Hoffman et al. 2009) for percentage or effect size in maximal strength gains. One of these studies compared a linear to a mixed training model (Simão et al. 2012). The mixed model (see table 7.7) consisted of a linear program for six weeks followed by six weeks of a daily nonlinear program. Strength increases favored the mixed model. Some of these comparisons show no significant differences among linear, daily nonlinear, and weekly nonlinear training models (Bufford et al. 2007) and linear, biweekly linear, and nonvaried programs. However, there were differences in maximal strength percentage gains among the programs (see tables 7.4, 7.6, and 7.7).

The majority of these comparisons involved healthy young males and females with limited or no resistance training experience; one involved trained collegiate American football players (Hoffman et al. 2009). The training duration in these comparisons range between 9 and 15 weeks. Collectively, these studies indicate that the daily nonlinear model is as effective as, or possibly more effective than, the linear model for maximal strength gains.

The limited information on motor performance and power increases with training over these same training durations shows no significant difference between daily nonlinear and linear training models (Hartman et al. 2009; Hoffman et al. 2009). Additionally, body mass and body composition changes with these two training models are similar and did not significantly change over the training durations investigated (Bufford et al. 2007; Hoffman et al. 2009; Kok, Hamer, and Bishop 2009; Monteiro et al. 2009; Prestes, Frollini et al. 2009; Rhea et al. 2002). However, skinfolds, which may not be sensitive enough to determine body composition changes between training programs, were used to estimate body composition changes in all but one of these studies (Rhea and colleagues used plethysmography). Muscle thickness changes due to a mixed model as described earlier, of linear and daily nonlinear models compared to a linear model are not significantly different between the linear model and the mixed model, but favor the mixed model (Simao et al. 2012).

Weekly and biweekly nonlinear training patterns in which a different training zone is used for one or two weeks before changing training zones, respectively, has been compared to linear periodization (see table 7.7). These comparisons show

TABLE 7.7 Representative Nonlinear Versus Linear Periodization Studies

Reference	Mean age (yr) and sex	Training length (wk)	Frequency per week	Sets and reps	Intensity	Exercises trained	Test	Percentage increase
Baker, Wilson, and Carlyon 1994b	19-21 M	12	3					
				Linear periodization wk 1-4: 5 × 10 core, 3 × 10 all others wk 5-8: 5 × 5 core, 3 × 8 all others wk 9-11: 3 × 3, 1 × 10 core, 3 × 6 all others wk 12: 3 × 3 core, 3 × 6 all others	RMs	Combination of 17	BP SQ VJ	12* 27* 4*
				2 wk nonlinear wk 1 and 2: 5 × 10 core, 3 × 10 all others wk 3 and 4: 5 × 6 core, 3 × 8 all others wk 5 and 6: 5 × 8 core, 3 × 10 all others wk 7 and 8: 5 × 4 core, 3 × 6 all others wk 9 and 10: 5 × 6 core, 3 × 8 all others wk 11 and 12: 4 × 3 core, 3 × 6 all others	RMs	Combination of 17	BP SQ VJ	16* 28* 10*

>continued

TABLE 7.7 >*continued*

Reference	Mean age (yr) and sex	Training length (wk)	Frequency per week	Sets and reps	Intensity	Exercises trained	Test	Percentage increase
Rhea et al. 2002	21 M	12	3	Linear wk 1-4: 3 × 8 wk 5-8: 3 × 6 wk 9-12: 3 × 4	RMs	5	LP BP	14* 26*
				Daily nonlinear day 1: 3 × 8 day 2: 3 × 6 day 3: 3 × 4	RMs	5	LP BP	29*[a] 56*[a]
Rhea et al. 2003	21-22 M and F	15	2	Linear wk 1-5: 3 × 25 wk 6-10: 3 × 20 wk 11-15: 3 × 15	RMs	KE	KE KE local muscular endurance	9* 56*
				Daily nonlinear sessions repeated for entire training duration session1: 3 × 25 session 2: 3 × 20 session 3: 3 × 15			KE KE local muscular endurance	10* 55*
				Reverse linear wk 1-5: 3 × 15 wk 6-10: 3 × 20 wk 11-15: 3 × 25			KE KE local muscular endurance	6* 73*
Buford et al. 2007	22 M and F	9	3	Linear wk 1-3: 3 × 8 wk 4-6: 3 × 6 wk 7-9: 3 × 4	RMs	6 per session	LP BP	24* 85*
				Daily nonlinear day 1: 3 × 8 day 2: 3 × 6 day 3: 3 × 4	RMs	6 per session	LP BP	17* 79*
				Weekly nonlinear wk 1, 4, and 7: 3 × 8 wk 2, 5, and 8: 3 × 6 wk 3, 6, and 9: 3 × 4	RMs	6 per session	LP BP	24* 100*
Monteiro et al. 2009	27 M	12	4 (split body)	Linear wk 1-4: 3 × 12-15 wk 5-8: 3 × 8-10 wk 9-12: 3 × 4 or 5	RMs	15	BP LP	9 16*
				Daily nonlinear 3 training zones repeated: 3 × 12-15, 8-10, 4 or 5	RMs	15	BP LP	28*[a] 39*[a]
Hoffman et al. 2009	20 M	15	4 (split body)	Linear wk 1-4: 3 or 4 × 9-12 wk 5-10: 3 or 4 × 3-8 wk 11-15: 3-5 × 1-5	RMs	Multiple per training session	SQ BP VJ Medicine ball throw	21* 8* 0 6*
				Daily nonlinear 3 training zones repeated: 3 or 4 × 9-12, 3 or 4 × 3-8, 3-5 × 1-5	RMs	Multiple per training session	SQ BP VJ Medicine ball throw	11* 8* 1 3

Reference	Mean age (yr) and sex	Training length (wk)	Frequency per week	Sets and reps	Intensity	Exercises trained	Test	Percentage increase
Hartman et al. 2009	24 M	14	3	Linear wk 1-10: 5 × 8-12 wk 11-14: 5 × 3-5	RMs	BP	BP Vmax MVC MRFD	15* 8* 4 7
				Daily nonlinear day 1: 5 × 3-5 day 2: 5 × 8-12 day 3: 5 × 20-25	RMs	BP	BP Vmax MVC MRFD	10* 6* 1 2
Prestes, J., Frollini et al. 2009	18-25 M	12	4	Linear wk 1, 5, and 9: 3 × 12 wk 2, 6, and 11: 3 × 10 wk 3, 7, and 11: 3 × 8 wk 4, 8, and 12: 3 × 6	RMs	9 per session	BP LP AC	18* 25* 14*
				Daily nonlinear wk 1, 3, 5, 7, 9, and 11: days 1 and 2: 3 × 12 days 3 and 4: 3 × 10 wk 2, 4, 6 ,8, 10, and 12: days 1 and 2: 3 × 8 days 3 and 4: 3 × 6	RMs	9 per session	BP LP AC	25* 41* 24*
Kok, Hamer, and Bishop 2009	20 F	9	3	Linear wk 1-3: BP and SQ 3 × 10, other exercises 3 × 10 wk 4-6: BP and SQ 3 or 4 × 6, other exercises 3 × 6 wk 7-9: BP and SP 3 or 4 × 8, other exercises 3 × 8	wk 1-3: BP and SQ, 75-80% of 1RM; other exercises, RMs wk 4-6: BP and SQ, 85-90% of 1RM; other exercises, RMs wk 7-9: BP and SQ, 30-40% of 1RM; other exercises, 30-40% of 1RM[b]	10	BP SQ BP throw power SQ jump power	22* 35* 11* 10*
				Nonlinear wk 1-9: BP, SQ, and other exercises 1 session/wk from wk 1-3, 4-6, and 7-9 of linear program	wk 1-9: BP, SQ, and other exercises, 1 session/wk from wk 1-3, 4-6, and 7-9 of linear program	10	BP SQ BP throw power SQ jump power	28* 41* 14* 9*
Simao et al. 2012	29 M	12	2	Linear wk 1-4: 2 × 12-15 wk 5-8: 3 × 8-10 wk 9-12: 4 × 3-6	RMs	BP, lat pull-down, biceps curl, triceps extension	BP lat pull-down biceps curl triceps extension	12a 12* 16*a 25*
				Nonlinear wk 1 and 2: 2 × 12-15 wk 3 and 4: 3 × 8-10 wk 5 and 6: 4 × 3-5 wk 7-12: day 1: 2 × 12-15 day 2: 3 × 8-10 day 3: 4 × 3-5	RMs	BP, lat pull-down, biceps curl, triceps extension	BP lat pull-down biceps curl triceps extension	21* 9* 18* 27*

* = significant change pre- to posttraining.

a = significant difference between nonlinear and linear periodization.

Vmax = maximal velocity in bench press throw.

MVC = maximal voluntary contraction in isometric bench press.

MRFD = maximal rate of force development in isometric bench press.

BP = bench press 1RM, SQ = squat 1RM, LP = leg press 1RM, AC = arm curl 1RM, KE = knee extension 1RM, VJ = vertical jump.

no significant difference in maximal strength, vertical jump ability, body mass, or body composition between training models. One of these comparisons (Baker, Wilson, and Carlyn 1994b) also shows that a biweekly nonlinear periodization, linear periodization, and nonvaried training model (three sets of six repetitions) all result in significant increases in maximal strength, vertical jump ability, and fat-free mass; the comparison shows no significant differences among the training models.

Comparisons of various daily nonlinear and linear periodization models show both training models to produce significant increases in maximal strength; however, some comparisons demonstrate significantly greater gains in maximal strength with the daily nonlinear model. Although both training models likely produce significant changes in body composition and measures of motor performance, no significant difference appears to exist between training models in these measures. All of these conclusions need to be viewed with some caution because more comparisons of periodized training models are needed, especially long-term comparisons in well-trained people and athletes.

Flexible Daily Nonlinear Periodization

Flexible daily nonlinear periodization involves changing the training zone used in a nonlinear model based on the trainee's readiness to perform in a specific training zone. The information needed for making the decision to change the training zone in a specific training session can be gathered in several ways. A test, such as a maximal vertical jump, standing long jump, or medicine ball throw test, can be performed immediately prior to a training session to determine the physical readiness of the trainee. The initial sets of the first few exercises in a training session can also be monitored to determine readiness to perform the session.

Consider a trainee who performs a vertical jump immediately prior to a training session; if she cannot achieve at least 90% of her previous maximal vertical jump, she may be fatigued. Likewise, if someone could previously perform six repetitions of an exercise with a specific resistance and at the start of a training session can perform only three repetitions with this resistance, fatigue is also indicated. Fatigue or another physiological factor, such as delayed-onset muscle soreness, could be

due to previous resistance training sessions or other types of training. Psychological stress due to schoolwork or job-related stresses could also keep a trainee from performing up to previously demonstrated abilities. In any case, in this example, if a high-intensity, low-volume (e.g., four sets of 4-6 repetitions) training zone were scheduled for that session, the intensity of the training zone could be lowered (e.g., three sets of 12-15 repetitions).

It is also possible to change from a low-intensity, high-volume training zone to a higher-intensity and lower-volume zone. Consider a trainee who performs at 100% of his best vertical jump, or 12 repetitions per set when only 8 to 10 repetitions are planned, in the first exercise of a training session. Rather than continuing with a training zone of 8 to 10 repetitions, the trainee could perform in a higher-intensity zone and do four to six repetitions. Flexible daily nonlinear periodization and training zone changes have been previously extensively discussed (Kraemer and Fleck 2007). Anecdotally, many coaches change training sessions to better match the physical readiness of their athletes. For example, if an intense interval training session is planned and the athlete is clearly unable to perform the session close to her previously demonstrated ability, the coach may lower the intensity of the session.

Flexible daily nonlinear periodization has been employed to maintain and increase physiological markers in collegiate Division I soccer players throughout a 16-week season (Silvester et al. 2006). Resistance training sessions were changed to meet the players' degree of readiness to perform a specific type of training session based on the strength and conditioning coaches' subjective evaluations and athlete heart rates during soccer practices and games. The flexible nonlinear periodized program resulted in the maintenance of vertical jump ability, short sprint ability, and maximal oxygen consumption throughout the season. However, significant increases in total lean tissue, leg lean tissue, trunk lean tissue, total body power (17% increase in repeat push-press power), and lower-body power (11% increase in repeat squat jumps followed by a short sprint) were shown pre- to postseason. Although no comparison to another training model was made, the results indicate that a flexible nonlinear model does maintain or increase physical fitness throughout a soccer season.

A comparison of a flexible daily nonlinear and a nonlinear model demonstrates that the flexible nonlinear model offers some advantage (McNamara and Stearne 2010). Male and female students in a college weight training class performed either a flexible nonlinear or a planned (had to perform the planned training session on a specific day) nonlinear periodized program two times per week for 12 weeks. Prior to a training session those performing the flexible nonlinear program could choose, based on fatigue, which of three training zones (10, 15, or 20 repetitions per set) to perform. However, by the end of the 12 weeks of training, those in the flexible nonlinear program had to perform the same number of training sessions in each training zone as those in the planned nonlinear program did.

Pre- to posttraining maximal chest press ability (1RM) and maximal standing long jump ability significantly increased with both training plans; no significant difference was shown between them. However, maximal leg press ability (see figure 7.2) increased significantly more with the flexible nonlinear program. This indicates that the flexible nonlinear plan did not offer any advantage for upper-body strength, but did offer an advantage for lower-body strength.

Flexible daily nonlinear periodization is an extension of what some coaches already do; that is, change planned training sessions based on the physical readiness of their athletes to perform that session. This type of training may offer advantages over the course of the season to maintain and improve physiological markers of performance and to increase maximal strength.

Reverse Linear Periodization

Reverse linear periodization refers to a resistance training program that changes from lower volume and higher intensity training to higher volume and lower intensity as training progresses. Thus, training volume and intensity progressively change in a pattern that is opposite to that of linear periodization. This type of training may offer some advantages for increasing such factors as local muscular endurance at the end of a periodized training plan compared to a linear periodized plan.

A comparison of linear and reverse linear periodization indicates that linear periodization results in greater maximal strength and hypertrophy gains (Prestes, Frollini et al. 2009). The number of repetitions per set with each training plan is depicted in table 7.8. Note that training intensity and volume over several weeks of training move in opposite directions with the linear and reverse linear periodized plans. Women (20-35 years) training

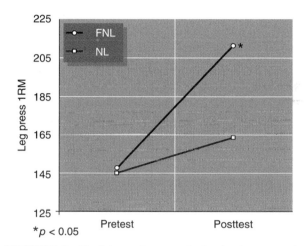

FIGURE 7.2 Flexible nonlinear periodization increases in leg press 1RM are significantly greater than with nonlinear periodization.

FNL = flexible nonlinear periodization; NL = nonlinear periodization.

Adapted, by permission, from J.M. McNamara and D.J. Stearne, 2010, "Flexible nonlinear periodization in a beginner college weight training class," *Journal of Strength and Conditioning Research* 24:17-22.

TABLE 7.8 Repetitions per Set in Linear and Reverse Linear 12-Week Training Plans

Weeks	Weeks of training											
	1	2	3	4	5	6	7	8	9	10	11	12
Linear periodization reps per set	12-14	10-12	8-10	12	5-12	8-10	6-8	12	8-10	6-8	4-6	12
Reverse linear periodization reps per set	4-6	6-8	8-10	12	6-8	8-10	10-12	12	8-10	10-12	12-14	12

Based on Prestes et al., 2009.

three days per week with each plan demonstrated significant increases in maximal strength (1RM) in the bench press, lat pull-down, arm curl, and knee extension. However, the increases were significantly greater with the linear plan for the arm curl and lat pull-down. Repetitions to failure using 50% of body mass in the arm curl and knee extension, a measure of local muscular endurance, showed no significant increase with either training plan. Significant body composition (skinfolds) changes of increased fat-free mass and decreased percent body fat occurred only with the linear periodized plan. Overall, the results indicate that the classic periodized plan resulted in greater strength and body composition changes.

A comparison of linear, daily nonlinear, and reverse linear periodization is presented in table 7.7 (Rhea, Phillips, et al. 2003). Within this comparison the number of repetitions per set are always relatively high (over 25 repetitions); thus, considering the repetition continuum (see chapter 5), all programs emphasized local muscular endurance more so than maximal strength gains. Because trainees were initially untrained and performed only the knee extension exercise, the application of the results to other exercises and trained people needs to be considered carefully. None of the programs showed a significantly greater increase in maximal strength or local muscular endurance. However, the linear and daily nonlinear programs showed substantially greater percentage increases in maximal strength, and the reverse linear program showed a substantially greater percentage increase in local muscular endurance.

Past training history and the training level of the athlete may determine the type of periodized plan that is most effective. A study of collegiate rowers performing either a traditional linear periodized program or a reverse linear periodized program indicates that the training level of the athlete affects which training plan is most effective (Ebben et al. 2004). The linear periodized plan progressed from sets of 12 repetitions to 5 repetitions over the course of eight weeks; the reverse linear periodized plan progressed from 15 repetitions per set to 32 repetitions per set over the same time period. Both types of periodized training significantly increased physiological markers of fitness (e.g., maximal oxygen consumption and power output while rowing) equally. However, more experienced rowers (University varsity) performing the linear periodized plan demonstrated a greater decrease in time to row 2,000 m in an ergometry test com-pared to experienced rowers performing the reverse linear periodized plan (–7 vs. –4 seconds). Less experienced rowers performing the reverse linear periodized plan demonstrated a greater decrease in time to row 2,000 m compared to those performing the linear periodized plan (–15 vs. –10 seconds). Results indicate that more experienced rowers show greater improvement with a linear periodized plan, whereas less experienced rowers show greater improvement with a reverse linear periodized plan. It is important to note that training intensity was greater and training volume less with the linear plan compared to the reverse linear plan (12-5 vs. 15-32 repetitions per set). So results also indicate that more experienced rowers benefit more from a lower-volume, higher-intensity resistance training plan, whereas less experienced rowers benefit more from a higher-volume, lower-intensity plan.

Significant advantages in local muscular endurance gains are not apparent with reverse linear periodization. Likewise, consistently greater increases in maximal strength with linear and daily nonlinear periodization are not apparent compared to reverse linear periodization. However, these conclusions must be viewed with caution because few studies have compared reverse linear periodization with other training models.

Power Development

Power development is thought to be intimately related to the performance of most daily life activities, such as climbing stairs, as well as sport tasks, such as throwing a ball or dunking a basketball. This is in part due to correlational data showing significant correlations between measures of power and performance. However, such correlations generally leave a large portion (unexplained variance) of the test performance unexplained. For example, maximal power measured with a stair-climbing test (Margaria-Kalamen step test) shows significant correlations to sprint and agility performance when power is expressed relative to body mass. However, these correlations leave a large portion (50-81% unexplained variance) of the sprint and agility performance unexplained (Mayhew et al. 1994). Thus, although power may be a characteristic related to performance training, other factors related to power, such as rate of force development and time to reach a specific force output, may be just as important as maximal power development to increasing performance in a specific task (Cronin and Sleivert 2005). Additionally, the relationship of power or some other factor related to power may be different among various tasks. For example, an upper-body task such as a bench throw, a lower-body task such as a vertical jump or squat jump, or a total-body task such as throwing a shot put show correlations of different strengths to various measures of power (Cronin and Sleivert 2005). Other factors, such as whether a power test includes a stretch-shortening cycle (countermovement vs. squat jump) or the resistance used when measuring power may also affect the strength of the correlation between a measure of power and a specific task. Despite these factors it is generally believed that when power or some factor related to power improves, performance in many tasks also improves. The relationship of power to force, the distance an object is moved, and the time involved in performing a movement is shown by the following equation:

$$\text{power} = \text{force} \times \text{distance} / \text{time}$$

This fundamental equation reveals the multiple ways power can be improved. The numerator of the equation is "work," and power can be increased by either increasing force development or the distance an object is moved. The denominator of the equation indicates the importance of the time used to perform a task in the calculation of power;

a decrease in time results in an increase in power. Training programs dedicated to the development of power require both high-force training and fast movements, which affects the time to perform a movement, to maximally increase power.

In most activities power depends on concentric force and velocity of movement. The classic concentric force–velocity curve indicates that as the speed of a muscle action increases, the force produced decreases. However, the power output peaks at an intermediate velocity between zero and the maximal velocity of movement. Viewing it from another perspective, at very fast velocities, low force results in low power output. However, slow velocities at which high force is generated also result in low power output. In fact, when force is maximal, velocity is zero (isometric action), which results in zero power output. High power results from a combination of intermediate velocity and an intermediate force output. The relationships among force, velocity of movement, and power can be seen in figure 7.3.

Training for power production in various movements or tasks should take these concepts into consideration. The success of a power training program is related to the specificity of the training activity and the ability to optimize physiological function for high-power movements at the velocity necessary to increase performance in a specific task

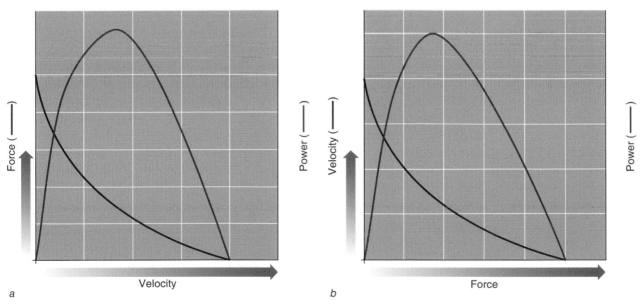

a

b

FIGURE 7.3 *(a)* The relationship of force generation and power generation to velocity of shortening in maximal concentric actions. *(b)* The relationship of velocity shortening and power generation to force development in maximal concentric actions. All muscular actions are concentric except those at zero velocity, which are isometric.

Adapted, by permission, from H.G. Knuttgen and W.J. Kraemer, 1987, "Terminology and measurement in exercise performance," *Journal of Applied Sport Science Research* 1: 1-10.

or in a spectrum of velocities or tasks. The necessity to increase power in a variety of tasks or velocities is apparent in many team sports in which the ability to accelerate at the start of a sprint, perform a vertical jump, kick a ball, or throw a ball may be necessary for success.

Ballistic resistance training refers to exercises in which a high rate of force development is needed and in which the mass being accelerated, such as body mass or an external weight, can be projected into the air (Newton and Wilson 1993b). Such exercises include the squat jump (assuming a squat or semi-squat position and then jumping into the air), stretch-shortening cycle exercises such as medicine ball throwing plyometrics, and weighted and unweighted jumping plyometric exercises. Other power-type exercises, such as the clean and snatch pull and other variations of the Olympic lifts, require acceleration of the weight and have a ballistic component, although the resistance is not actually thrown into the air. Ballistic resistance training creates specific increases in muscle activation and rates of force development (Häkkinen and Komi 1985c). These types of exercises do not have a deceleration (see the section Deceleration Phase and Traditional Weight Training later in this chapter) of the resistance at the end of the range of motion (Newton et al. 1996). When a "normal" bench press was performed explosively (e.g., speed reps) with a light resistance (e.g., 30% of 1RM), power decreased during approximately the last 50% of the range of motion because the lifter had to hold on to the bar and reach zero velocity when the bar was at arm's length (Newton et al. 1996). When the weight could be released into the air at the end of the range of motion with the use of a specialized testing device (i.e., a ballistic exercise), power output and acceleration were enhanced throughout the range of motion. The reduction in power and decreased rate of acceleration when the bar was "held on to" was due to decreased agonist activation and increased antagonist activation of muscles of the upper back, which resulted in deceleration of the bar because it had to be at zero velocity at arm's length (see figure 7.4). It is theorized that this effect was needed to protect the joints from a sudden deceleration at the end of the range of motion when the weight was not released. The deceleration was not needed when the weight could be released at the end of the bench press's range of motion. This demonstrates why speed reps may be counterproductive to power

development in some exercises (e.g., bench press, shoulder press, knee extension) and supports the proper use of resistance training equipment that allows the release of the weight, such as medicine ball throws, or exercises in which deceleration does not occur, such as plyometric jumping exercises or variations of the Olympic lifts.

With many exercises, when attempting to lift the maximal amount of weight possible (e.g., a resistance close to 1RM), movement velocities are just higher than zero. Thus, maximal force is generated, but because of the slow velocity of movement, power output is very low. Pure 1RM strength is required in the sport of powerlifting because there is no requirement for maximal or near-maximal power development (thus, the name of the sport is inappropriate) given that lifters must move heavy weights slowly.

Many strength and conditioning specialists believe that if slow-velocity strength increases, power output and dynamic performance will also improve. This is true to a certain extent because maximal strength, even at slow velocities, is a contributing factor to explosive power because this affects the force in the power equation. All explosive movements start from zero, or slow velocities, and it is at these phases of the movement that slow-velocity strength can contribute to power development. However, as the muscles begin to achieve high velocities of shortening, slow-velocity strength capacity has a reduced impact on the ability to produce high force at rapid shortening velocities (Duchateau and Hainaut 1984; Kanehisa and Miyashita 1983a; Kaneko et al. 1983; Moss et al. 1997). This fact becomes increasingly important when already strong people attempt to train specifically for optimal power development. Negative correlations between increases in motor performance tasks (vertical jump and short sprint ability) and pretraining 1RM caused by normal weight training 1RM (Wilson, Murphy, and Walshe 1997) support this concept. These negative correlations indicate that stronger people showed smaller increases in motor performance as a result of normal weight training. So to improve motor performance in already strong people, training strategies other than increasing maximal strength need to be employed.

Improved performance in power activities, such as vertical jump (Adams et al. 1992; Bauer, Thayer, and Baras 1990; Clutch et al. 1983; Wilson et al. 1993) and sprint ability (Harris et al. 2008) after

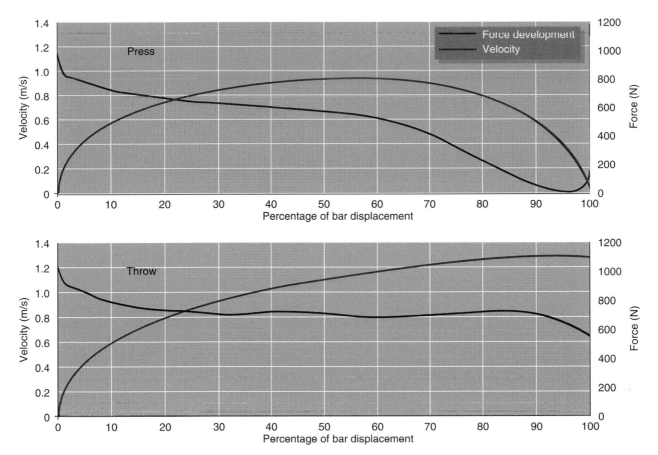

FIGURE 7.4 The top panel shows the relationship of velocity and force development during a normal bench press with 45% of 1RM. The bottom panel shows the relationship of velocity and force development during a bench press throw with 45% of 1RM.

Adapted, by permission, from R.U. Newton et al., 1996, "Kinematics, kinetics, and muscle activation during explosive upper body movements: Implications for power development," *Journal of Applied Biomechanics* 13: 31-43.

a strength training program have been shown. For example, a study by Häkkinen and Komi (1985a) showed a 7% improvement in vertical jump ability after 24 weeks of intense weight training. Comparisons of heavy resistance training and ballistic training show significantly greater increases in power-type activities with ballistic training (Cronin and Sleivert 2005). For example, comparing heavy resistance training (6- to 10RM squats) to ballistic training (jump squats with 30% of maximal isometric force), both resulted in significant increases in countermovement jump ability, but the increase from ballistic training was significantly greater than that from heavy resistance training (18 vs. 5%) (Wilson et al. 1993). Such comparisons, however, may show greater increases in power-type activities from ballistic training because of a difference in total training volume when the power training exercises are added to a traditional strength training program (Cronin and

Sleivert 2005). Substituting some ballistic exercises for heavy resistance exercises produces greater increases in power-type activities, such as a squat jump (+5 vs. –3%), than does heavy resistance training alone (Mangine et al. 2008). This substitution helps to maintain equal training volumes in the total training program, which indicates that ballistic training, and not an increase in training volume, causes the increase in power.

Initial strength level may affect the results of heavy resistance and ballistic training programs. Men who could perform a back squat with approximately 1.3 times body mass show significant, but not significantly different, improvement in power activities (sprint and vertical jump ability) as a result of either a resistance or ballistic-type training (Cormie, McGuigan, and Newton 2010b). However, squat 1RM strength improvement was significantly greater with the heavy resistance training (31 vs. 5%). A comparison of relatively strong men and relatively weak men (squat 1RM times body mass 1.97 vs. 1.32) training with weighted and unweighted jump squats showed a tendency (greater effect sizes) for larger increases in vertical jump, but not short sprint ability, in the stronger men (Cormie, McGuigan, and Newton 2010a). Combined, these results indicate that heavy resistance training will result in greater increases in maximal strength and similar increases in power-type activities in relatively weak men, whereas ballistic-type training may result in greater increases in some power-type activities in relatively strong men. Thus, ballistic training may not be necessary to produce optimal increases in power-type activities in the initial stages of training. However, some studies indicate that when strength plateaus, specialized power training appears to be important to optimize power development (Baker 2001a; Newton, Kraemer, and Häkkinen 1999).

Resistance- and velocity-specific training adaptations have been shown with training (Kaneko et al. 1983; Moss et al. 1997). Training the elbow flexors of various groups with resistances of 90, 35, and 15% of 1RM (all groups trained for maximal power by attempting to move the resistance as fast as possible during each repetition) showed interesting results concerning power (Moss et al. 1997). Power was tested with resistances of 2.5 kg (5.5 lb) and 15, 25, 35, 50, 70, and 90% of pretraining 1RM. The group training with 15% of 1RM showed significant increases in power at resistances equal to or less than 50% of 1RM and no significant increases above resistances greater than 50% of 1RM. No significant difference in power increase was shown between groups at resistances equal to or less than 50% of 1RM. The 35 and 90% groups showed no significant differences between each other at any resistance but did demonstrate significantly greater power increases than the 15% group at resistances of 70 and 90% of 1RM. However, the 90% group showed the greatest power increases at the heaviest two resistances, and the 35% group showed the most consistent power gains across all resistances.

Velocity-specific effects for a task that involved lifting a weight as quickly as possible have also shown training specificity (Kaneko et al. 1983). Subjects who trained with a resistance of 0, 30, 60, or 100% of maximal isometric strength demonstrated a classic resistance-specific training effect. The groups training with the heavier resistances showed the greatest increases in isometric strength,

and the group training with 0% resistance showed the greatest increase in unloaded movement velocity. Perhaps the most interesting finding was that the 30% resistance produced the greatest increase in force and power over the entire concentric velocity range and also resulted in the greatest increase in maximal mechanical power. The results of these studies demonstrate some training specificity for power.

However, no training specificity has also been shown between jump squat training at 80 and 30% of 1RM squat (McBride et al. 2002). Training was equated for overall intensity and volume between programs. Both programs showed significant increases in 1RM strength, short sprint ability (5, 10, and 20 m), and agility (T-test). The only significant difference among the training programs was that the 30% of 1RM training showed a greater increase in 10 m sprint performance. The percentage increase in 1RM squat ability favored the 80% of 1RM training, and generally, the percentage increase in weighted (30, 55, and 80% squat 1RM) jump squat ability favored the 30% of 1RM training.

Thus, performance changes are not always consistent with the principle of training specificity. The conflict results from the complex nature of explosive muscle actions and the integration of slow and fast force production requirements within a specific movement. Another confounding influence is that most of the preceding studies trained previously untrained people, in whom a wide variety of training interventions will produce increases in both strength and power and the force part of the power equation may dominate power increases until a stable base of strength is attained (Baker 2001c). Additionally, as discussed earlier, depending on the training status of the person, the response to training may not always follow the specificity of training principle (Komi and Häkkinen 1988). However, if a person already has an adequate level of strength, then increases in explosive power performance in response to traditional strength training will be poor; more specific power training interventions are required to further improve power output (Baker 2001c; Häkkinen 1989; Newton, Kraemer, and Häkkinen 1999). Thus, improvement in power-oriented activities in trained athletes may require complex combinations of strength and power exercises (Baker 2001a; Newton, Kraemer, and Häkkinen 1999; Wilson et al. 1993).

Rate of Force Development

In some activities, because the time to develop force and power is limited (e.g., foot contact time during sprinting), the muscle needs to exert as much force as possible in a short period of time (Häkkinen and Komi 1985b). For this reason, **rate of force development** (RFD), or the rate at which force is developed or increases, is an important consideration in the performance of some activities. Training-induced changes in RFD may explain to some extent why heavy resistance training has not always increased power performance, especially during movements requiring very little time (e.g., 100-200 ms). Squat training with heavy resistances (70-120% of 1RM) has been shown to improve maximum isometric strength; however, it did not improve the maximal RFD (Häkkinen, Komi, and Tesch 1981) and may even reduce the muscle's ability to develop force rapidly (Häkkinen 1989). However, activities during which an attempt is made to develop force rapidly, such as explosive jump training with light resistances, increase the ability to develop force rapidly (Behm and Sale 1993; Häkkinen, Komi, and Tesch 1981).

Explosive-type resistance training increases the slope of the early portion of the force–time curve (see figure 7.5). Although heavy resistance training increases maximal strength, it does not improve

RFD appreciably, especially in athletes who have already developed a strength training base (i.e., have had more than six months of training). This is because the movement time during explosive activities is typically less than 300 ms. So if RFD is not increased, the majority of maximal force increases due to heavy resistance training cannot be realized and power-type activity performance is not improved.

In the preceding discussion of RFD, heavy resistance training refers to lifting the weight in an exercise, but not attempting to lift the weight as fast as possible or in an explosive manner. Trainees can increase RFD during heavy resistance training by attempting to lift the weight as fast as possible (Behm and Sale 1993; Crewther, Cronin, and Keogh 2005; Cronin and Sleivert 2005). Thus the intent to move the weight as fast as possible, even if the resistance is heavy, can result in an increase in RFD. So if the goal of training is to increase RFD and power development no matter what resistance is being lifted, the trainee should attempt to lift the resistance as fast as possible.

Deceleration Phase and Traditional Weight Training

The **deceleration phase** of a repetition occurs when the resistance's movement slows in the last part of the concentric phase of a repetition even though there is an attempt to increase or maintain movement speed. The deceleration phase is necessary in many exercises because the resistance must come to a complete stop at the end of the concentric repetition phase. This deceleration of the resistance over the last part of the concentric phase of a repetition results in an exercise that will contribute less than optimally to power production (see box 7.2). This phenomenon has been frequently observed (Berger 1963c; Wilson et al. 1993; Young and Bilby 1993). For example, when someone lifts 1RM in the bench press, the bar is decelerating for the last 24% of the concentric movement (Elliott, Wilson, and Kerr 1989). The deceleration phase increases to 52% when the person performs the lift with a lighter resistance (e.g., 81% of 1RM) (Elliott, Wilson, and Kerr 1989). Additionally, if an attempt is made to lift the weight at a fast velocity, the duration of the deceleration phase increases (Newton and Wilson 1993a).

Plyometric jump and medicine ball training avoid this problem by allowing the person to

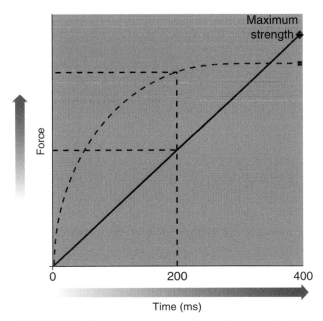

FIGURE 7.5 With power training, force developed in 200 ms or less is increased compared to training to increase predominantly maximal strength levels.

Dotted line = power training; solid line = strength training.

BOX 7.2 RESEARCH

Effects of the Deceleration Repetition Phase on Strength and Power

Whether a difference in strength and power gains exists between training with a controlled velocity and training with a fast velocity is an important practical consideration. Such a comparison can be made by having some subjects perform the concentric and eccentric phases of repetitions using a controlled velocity and having others perform the eccentric phase using a controlled velocity and the concentric phase using a fast velocity.

Training inexperienced males in this fashion with the half squat (knees to a 90-degree angle) for 7.5 weeks, three times per week with four sets of 8 to 12 repetitions does result in various training adaptations (Young and Bilby 1993). The fast concentric training resulted in a significantly greater increase in rate of force development of 69% compared to the controlled velocity increase of 24%. The controlled velocity resulted in a significantly greater increase in absolute isometric strength of 31% compared to the fast concentric training increase of 12%. No significant differences were shown between the fast concentric and the controlled velocity training for squat 1RM (21 vs. 22%, respectively), vertical jump (5 vs. 9%, respectively) or muscle thickness (ultrasound) measured at several sites of the quadriceps. Thus, training with different concentric velocities does make a difference in some training outcomes.

Young, W.B., and Bilby, G.E. 1993. The effect of voluntary effort to influence speed of contraction on strength, muscular power, and hypertrophy development. *Journal of Strength and Conditioning Research* 7: 172-178.

accelerate throughout the movement to the point of load projection, such as the takeoff in jumping, ball release in throwing, or impact in striking activities. It could be argued that traditional weight training promotes the development of the deceleration action. The deceleration results from a decreased activation of the agonists during the later phase of the lift and may be accompanied by considerable activation of the antagonists, particularly when using lighter resistances and trying to lift the weight quickly (Kraemer and Newton 2000). This is undesirable when attempting to maximize power performances. The problem of the deceleration phase can be overcome with ballistic resistance training in which the resistance is thrown, such as throwing a medicine ball, or jumping into the air with or without added resistance, such as in plyometric jump training.

A comparison of training using traditional back squats and two types of ballistic training (loaded jump squats and plyometric, or stretch-shortening cycle, training, or drop jumps) on vertical jump performance favored the loaded jump squat training for increases in power (Wilson et al. 1993). The loaded jump squats were completed using a resistance of 30% of 1RM. This allowed the subjects to produce a high mechanical power output. All training groups showed increases in vertical jump performance; however, the loaded-jump-squats group showed significantly greater increases (18%) than the other two groups (traditional back squats, 5%; stretch-shortening cycle training, 10%). These results were similar to those obtained by Berger (1963c), who also found that performance of jump squats with a resistance of 30% of maximum resulted in greater vertical jump ability increases compared with traditional weight training, plyometric training, or isometric training.

Although ballistic resistance training improves power performance, it does result in high eccentric forces when landing from a jump or catching a falling weight in some exercises, such as a bench throw, which typically involves throwing the bar into the air at the end of the concentric repetition phase, on a Smith machine (Newton and Wilson 1993a). However, weight training equipment can be adapted to reduce the eccentric resistance (Newton and Wilson 1993a).

A comparison of weighted jump squat training (30% of half squat 1RM) shows some differences between training with and without an eccentric braking system (Hori et al. 2008). The eccentric braking system removed virtually all of the resistance used in the jump squat training during the landing phase of a jump. Both types of training resulted in significant increases in countermovement jump and squat jump ability, and no significant differences were shown between groups. The braking group did show a significantly greater increase than did the nonbreaking group (11.5

vs. 7.4%) in squat jump ability relative to body mass (W · kg^{-1}). However, the nonbraking group showed a significantly greater increase in concentric isokinetic hamstring torque at 300 degrees per second (8.1 vs. –4.5%). Other measures of strength and power showed significant increases by both groups, but no significant differences between groups. So eccentric braking resulted in the same changes in performance measures as no braking. To minimize the chance of injury with weighted jump squats and other types of ballistic-type training, trainees should use a progression from the unloaded or light resistance to heavier resistances.

Ballistic Training and Neural Protective Mechanisms

Neural protective mechanisms can affect force output. Plyometric, or stretch-shortening cycle, training (Schmidtbleicher, Gollhofer, and Frick 1988) and ballistic weighted jump squat training (McBride et al. 2002) result in an increase in the overall neural stimulation of the muscle and thus force output. There are, however, indications that neural protective mechanisms are active during this type of training. Subjects unaccustomed to intense jumping-type plyometric training experienced a reduction in electromyographic activity starting 50 to 100 ms before ground contact and lasting for 100 to 200 ms (Schmidtbleicher, Gollhofer, and Frick 1988). This protective mechanism has been attributed to the Golgi tendon organ reflex acting during a sudden, intense stretch to reduce the tension in the tendomuscular unit during the peak force of the stretch-shortening cycle (Gollhofer 1987). After a period of plyometric training, the inhibitory effects are reduced (this is termed disinhibition), and increased plyometric performance results (Schmidtbleicher, Gollhofer, and Frick 1988).

Quality of Training Repetitions

The effectiveness of a power training program may be related to the quality of repetitions. In other words, if a repetition does not achieve a high percentage (e.g., 90% or greater) of the maximal power output or maximal velocity possible, its impact on training adaptations may be negligible. Thus, if a person performs any type of power training when fatigued or when not ready to exercise maximally, a truly effective power training session may not be possible. An exception may be in the

area of power development under conditions of extreme fatigue, such as a wrestler performing a throw at the end of a match when fatigue and blood lactate concentrations are high (20 mmol · L^{-1}) or a vertical jump in volleyball at the end of a match. Training power when fatigued may enhance performance in a sport in which fatigue does occur.

Power is one measure of repetition quality. Figure 7.6 depicts sets of squat jumps performed prior to a normal practice and after a normal practice with a resistance of 30% of squat 1RM. A person who performs sets of one repetition prior to practice may not be able to achieve 90% of maximal power output or greater. However, performing three repetitions per set results in a much greater likelihood of reaching 90% of peak power in at least one of the repetitions. After practice, power of the best of three repetitions per set is decreased. However, further information concerning quality of repetitions and the interaction of repetition quality with rest periods between sets is needed.

Guidelines have been developed for training power (see box 7.3) and are briefly described in chapter 2. However, some caveats concerning these

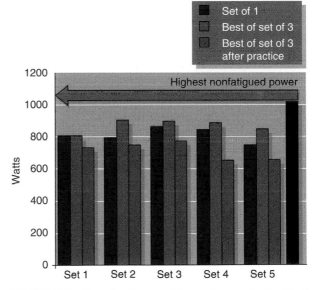

FIGURE 7.6 Data for the squat jump demonstrating that a greater quality of repetitions, as indicated by at least 90% of peak power, is achieved in at least one repetition per set in sets of three repetitions. In sets of one repetition the chance of achieving at least 90% of peak power is decreased, whereas performing three repetitions per set under conditions of fatigue, such as after practice, diminishes power production. Resistance equals 30% of 1RM. See text for further explanation.

Unpublished data, Dr. William J. Kraemer, Department of Kinesiology, University of Connecticut, Storrs, CT.

BOX 7.3 PRACTICAL QUESTION

What Are the Guidelines for Training for Power?

Training for power can increase power, maximal strength, and motor performance. Following are guidelines for the inclusion of power training in a resistance training program based on research (American College of Sports Medicine 2009):

- Power- or ballistic-type resistance training should be incorporated into the typical strength training program if one goal of training is to increase power.
- Exercises should be performed in an explosive manner.
- For upper-body exercises, use 30 to 60% of 1RM for one to three sets per exercise of three to six repetitions per set not to failure.
- For lower-body exercises, use 0 to 60% of 1RM for one to three sets per exercise of three to six repetitions per set not to failure.
- For advanced training, heavier resistances (85-100% of 1RM) may also be incorporated in a periodized manner using three to six sets per exercise of one to six repetitions per set.

American College of Sports Medicine. 2009. Progression models in resistance training for healthy adults. *Medicine & Science in Sports & Exercise* 41: 687-708.

power training guidelines are worth mentioning. The resistances used for upper- and lower-body exercises are different. This difference is in part due to the fact that, with most lower-body power exercises, body mass must be moved in addition to the resistance being used. With upper-body exercises, on the other hand, typically only a small percentage of body mass is moved during the exercise. Sets are typically not carried to failure in part because, when they are, power increases with training may be lower (see chapter 6 for a more in-depth discussion of the effect of carrying sets to failure).

Because of the resistance specificity of power training, as discussed earlier, a variety of resistances, or a mixed model, should be used when power training (Newton and Kraemer 1994). The use of multiple training resistances results in greater maximal power increases (Toji and Kaneko 2004). Training with of a combination of 30, 60, and 100% of maximal force; 30 and 60% maximal force; or 30 and 100% of maximal force result in significant increases in maximal power of 53, 41, and 24%, respectively, even though gains in maximal strength were not significantly different.

Another consideration is that trained athletes who have performed both strength and power training may express maximal power outputs at higher percentages (47-63%) of 1RM strength (Baker, Nance, and Moore 2001a, 2001b) than

the typical percentage of 1RM strength (30-45%) at which maximal power is expressed. So trained people may need to incorporate higher percentages of 1RM into their periodized training plans when performing power training. Power increases due to training normally occur when the same resistance is used to measure power (Crewther, Cronin, and Keogh 2005; Cronin and Sleivert 2005). However, if any percentage of 1RM is used when testing power, little or no change in power due to training occurs because as 1RM strength increases so does the resistance at any percentage of 1RM. Thus, normally, when testing power changes due to training, the same resistance pre- and posttraining, and not a percentage of pre- and posttraining 1RM, should be used.

Plyometrics

Perhaps the oldest and most frequently used power-type training is **plyometrics**. This type of training is typically thought of as performing body weight jumping-type exercises and throwing medicine balls. Synonymous with the term *plyometrics* is the term *stretch-shortening cycle exercise*, a term that more accurately describes body weight jumps and medicine ball throws.

The **stretch-shortening cycle** refers to a natural part of most movements. As an example, when the foot hits the ground during walking, the quadriceps first go through an eccentric action, then a brief isometric action, and finally a concentric action. If the reversal of the eccentric action to an isometric and then a concentric action is performed quickly, the muscle is stretched slightly. This entire sequence of eccentric, isometric, and concentric actions resulting in a slight stretching of the muscles prior to muscle shortening is called a stretch-shortening cycle.

The stretching stores elastic energy that can be released during the shortening phase, resulting in a more powerful concentric action. The addition of the elastic energy to the force of a normal concentric action, where no stretching occurs, is one of the reasons commonly given to explain why a more powerful concentric action results after a stretch-shortening cycle. The other common explanation for the more forcible concentric action is that a neural reflex results in the quicker recruitment of muscle fibers or a recruitment of more muscle fibers.

The more powerful concentric action following the stretch-shortening cycle is easy to demonstrate. During a normal vertical jump (a countermovement jump), the jumper bends at the knees and hips (eccentric action of the extensors), quickly reverses direction, and jumps (an isometric action followed by a concentric action). Thus, a countermovement jump involves a stretch-shortening cycle. A jump performed by bending at the knees and hips, stopping for three to five seconds in the bent-knee and bent-hip position, and then jumping is termed a noncountermovement jump, or squat jump; it does not involve a stretch-shortening cycle and results in a lower jump than a countermovement jump (a jump involving a stretch-shortening cycle). It is also possible to demonstrate the effect of a stretch-shortening cycle by throwing a ball for distance. Throwing a ball with a normal overhand throwing motion, which involves a stretch-shortening cycle, results in a longer throw than throwing a ball without a windup, or starting the throwing motion from the end of the windup position (no stretch-shortening cycle).

Stretch-shortening cycle exercises can be performed with both the upper and lower body. Many medicine ball exercises for the upper body involve a stretch-shortening cycle. The depth jump (stepping off a bench and immediately jumping upon hitting the ground) is the exercise perhaps most frequently associated with the stretch-shortening cycle, but virtually all jumping exercises and throwing motions in which no pause is taken in the movement involve the stretch-shortening cycle.

Mechanisms Causing Greater Force With a Stretch-Shortening Cycle

The ability to use stored elastic energy and neural reflexes are the most common explanations of why stretch-shortening cycle training increases force output (Markovic 2007; Saez-Saez de Villarreal et al. 2009). Research supports the use of stored elastic energy during a stretch-shortening cycle (Biewener and Roberts 2000; Bosco et al. 1987; Bosco, Tarkka, and Komi 1982; Farley et al. 1991). Bosco and colleagues (1987) estimated that elastic energy may account for 20 to 30% of the difference between a countermovement and noncountermovement jump. Elastic energy can be stored in tendons, other connective tissues, and the myosin crossbridges (Biewener and Roberts 2000). If elastic energy were stored during a prestretch in the myosin crossbridges, it would be lost as soon as the crossbridges detached from active sites. Therefore, the elastic energy stored in this fashion would have to be recovered very quickly. The average attachment time of a crossbridge to an active site is 30 ms. Because the enhancement of force from a prestretch lasts longer than this, other mechanisms must be at work. Thus, although it is possible to store elastic energy at the myosin crossbridge level, the majority of elastic energy is probably stored in connective tissues. An adaptation in connective or muscle tissue may take place with training to enhance storage and therefore the use of more elastic energy; this is implicated in studies showing changes in muscle stiffness as a result of plyometric training (Cornu, Almeida Silveira, and Goubel 1997; Hunter and Marshall 2002).

Another mechanism involved in creating greater force with a stretch-shortening cycle is muscle or fascicle length. During plyometric-type exercise in humans, the vastus lateralis generates more force when a prestretch is used, yet no difference in electromyographic activity occurs between the prestretch and no-prestretch condition (Finni, Ikegawa, and Komi 2001). The force enhancement may be related to longer fascicle length before the concentric action in the prestretch condition. This would place the muscle in a more advantageous position on the length–tension diagram to produce force.

Reflex recruitment of additional motor units, or an increased rate of firing by already recruited motor units, may result in increased force as a result of a stretch-shortening cycle. However, electromyographic activity does not change significantly in muscle that performs an isometric action and is then stretched (Thompson and Chapman 1988). Electromyographic activity has been reported to be not significantly different between a prestretch and a nonprestretch muscle action (Finni, Ikegawa, and Komi 2001). This indicates that reflex activity does not account for the increased force caused by the stretch-shortening cycle. Clearly, some type of force potentiation is caused by the stretch-shortening cycle. However, the mechanisms responsible are not completely elucidated, and more than a single mechanism may be involved.

Long and Short Stretch-Shortening Cycle Training Exercises

Stretch-shortening cycle actions have been classified as either long or short based on the ground contact time (Schmidtbleicher 1994). A **long stretch-shortening cycle** action has a ground contact time greater than 250 ms (e.g., a countermovement jump or a block jump in volleyball). A long stretch-shortening cycle action is also characterized by large angular displacements at the hip, knee, and ankle joints. A **short stretch-shortening cycle** action has a ground contact time of less than 250 ms (e.g., a drop jump in which an attempt is made to minimize ground contact time, sprinting, and takeoff in the high and long jumps). A short stretch-shortening cycle action is also characterized by small angular displacements at the hip, knee, and ankle joints. Correlations between countermovement jump height and drop jump height with minimum ground contact time are low, indicating that these tests measure different movement characteristics (Hennessy and Kilty 2001; Schmidtbleicher 1994). Therefore, these two types of stretch-shortening cycle actions should be considered different training modalities, and this difference should be considered when planning a stretch-shortening cycle training program for different activities.

Meta-analyses support the existence of a difference between these two types of stretch-shortening cycle jumps and note that plyometric training generally tends to increase performance more in the long than the short stretch-shortening cycle jumps. However, the differences are not statistically significant (Markovic 2007; Saez-Saez de Villarreal et al. 2009). With plyometric training, increases in countermovement jump ability using a long stretch-shortening cycle jump, without (hands on hips) and with an arm swing are 8.7 and 7.5%, respectively (Markovic 2007). Short stretch-shortening cycle jumps, such as a drop jump, increase 4.7% with plyometric training. These percentage differences must be viewed with caution because most training studies do not differentiate between the types of stretch-shortening cycle jump used in training, and many use more than one type of jump in the training program.

The concept that long and short stretch-shortening cycle actions are related differently to performance is supported by correlation data. For example, in nationally ranked American female sprinters and hurdlers, correlations between long and short stretch-shortening cycle tests and sprint ability at varying distances do vary (Hennessy and Kilty 2001). Correlations between 30 m (–.79 and –.60), 100 m (–.75 and –.64), and 300 m (–.49 and –.55) sprint ability and performance in a drop jump with minimal ground contact time and a countermovement jump, respectively, vary. All correlations were significant except for 300 m sprint performance and performance in a drop jump with minimal ground contact time. The drop jump with minimal ground contact time was the primary variable related to 30 m sprint performance; this variable and ground contact time explain 70% of the variance in 30 m sprint performance. For the 100 m sprint, 61% of the variance was explained by countermovement jump height and drop jump height with minimal ground contact time. This suggests that both long and short stretch-shortening cycle actions are related to 100 m sprint performance. Countermovement jump ability explained 30% of the variance in 300 m sprint performance, and drop jump ability with minimal ground contact time was not significantly related to 300 m sprint performance. It has also been reported that sprint ability (maximal velocity) shows the highest correlation ($r = .69$) to a drop jump compared to other plyometric jumps (Kale et al. 2009). These results indicate that trainers should consider the differences between short and long stretch-shortening cycle actions when planning stretch-shortening cycle training programs for athletes in particular activities or sports.

Efficacy of Stretch-Shortening Cycle Training

Training studies support the contention that performing only stretch-shortening cycle training can improve performance in motor performance tasks such as vertical jumping, sport-specific jumping, sprinting, sprint cycling, long jumping, and distance running, as well as running economy (Berryman, Maurel, and Bosquet 2009; Lockie et al. 2012; Markovic 2007) and foot velocity in a soccer kick (Young and Rath 2011). Studies ranging in length from 6 to 12 weeks have shown improvements in the motor performance tasks of subjects using only one or two types of plyometric exercises (Bartholomeu 1985; Blackey and Southard 1987; Gehri et al. 1998; Matavulj et al. 2001; Miller 1982; Scoles 1978; Steben and Steben 1981). The effect of a single type of plyometric exercise on upper-body performance also shows positive effects. Performing only plyometric push-ups (three sessions per week for six weeks) resulted in significant improvement in upper-body power using a medicine ball throw (Vossen et al. 2000). A plyometric push-up involves performing a normal push-up and then propelling the body upward so that the hands leave the ground; the person must then catch his body weight upon returning to the ground before performing another plyometric push-up. These studies demonstrate that stretch-shortening cycle training using only one or two types of plyometric exercises can improve motor performance in both the upper and lower body.

Studies using a variety of plyometric exercises for 6 to 12 weeks have also shown significant improvements in motor performance tasks (Adams et al. 1992; Bartholomeu 1985; Bosco and Pittera 1982; Diallo et al. 2001; Fatouros et al. 2000; Ford et al. 1983; Hawkins, Doyle, and McGuigan 2009; Lockie et al. 2012; Potteiger et al. 1999; Rimmer and Sleivert 2000; Wagner and Kocak 1997; Young and Rath 2011). These studies used combinations of depth jumps, countermovement jumps, alternate-leg bounding, hopping, and other plyometric exercises. Untrained subjects were trained in the majority of studies using only one or two types of plyometric exercises or a combination of plyometric exercises. Some studies of trained athletes (basketball, field sport, and soccer players) have also shown positive improvements in motor performance (Diallo et al. 2001; Lockie et al. 2012; Matavulj et al. 2001; Wagner and Kocak 1997). Plyometric training results not only in increased jumping ability, but also improved sport-specific ability, such as decreased 10 m sprint time (– 2%), decreased agility test time (9.6%), and increased kicking speeds of the dominant (11%) and nondominant (13%) legs in soccer players (Meylan and Malatesta 2009; Sedano Campo et al. 2009). One meta-analysis concluded that jumping ability increases equally in both athletes and nonathletes (Markovic 2007); however, another meta-analysis indicated that plyometric training increases vertical jump ability more so in international-level athletes than in regional-level athletes and that athletes with more experience obtain greater increases in vertical jump ability with plyometric training (Saez Saez de Villarreal et al. 2009). Thus, plyometric training does increase motor performance in athletes and may be of more importance as experience increases.

The preceding studies indicate that a variety of plyometric training frequencies and durations can be used. Plyometric training volume is measured as the number of plyometric repetitions, such as jumps or throws, per training session. In jumping-type plyometric exercises, foot contacts are a measure of volume. A foot contact consists of a foot or both feet together contacting the ground. Therefore, if a person performs 2×10 depth jumps, 20 total foot contacts occur. A meta-analysis and other research gives some insight into the optimal design of a jumping plyometric program (see box 7.4).

Height of Depth Jumps and Drop Jumps

Depth jumps and drop jumps are popular types of plyometric training, and increases in jumping ability have resulted from their performance from a wide range of heights. Depth jumps involve dropping from a box, hitting the floor, and jumping onto another box. Drop jumps involve dropping from one box and only jumping. The height from which a trainee drops is an important consideration because the ground reaction forces increase with both types of jumps as height increases (Wallace et al. 2010); jumping from high heights could increase the risk of injury and possibly affect the optimal number of jumps needed to bring about maximal gains in jumping ability.

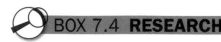

BOX 7.4 **RESEARCH**

Designing a Jumping Plyometric Program

A meta-analysis (Saez Saez de Villarreal et al. 2009) and other research (Saez Saez de Villarreal, Gonzalez-Badillo, and Izqueirdo 2008) offer some guidance for designing a jumping plyometric training program.

Frequency: To bring about positive benefits, a training frequency of two times per week for at least 10 weeks is needed.

Training efficiency: The percentage of increase in performance per plyometric jump is a measure of training efficiency. Training two days per week may also be more efficient than higher training frequencies. Training two and four days per week both result in a significant increase in jumping ability (12 and 18%, respectively), but no significant difference exists between frequencies. However, training two days per week results in greater training efficiency (0.014 vs. 0.011% per jump, respectively) than training four days per week. Similar enhancements of 20 m sprint times and training efficiency were shown with both training frequencies. Thus, training two days per week resulted in similar increases in motor performance but with greater training efficiency.

Foot contacts: At least 50 foot contacts are needed per training session to bring about positive effects from plyometric training.

Variety of plyometric exercises: A variety of plyometric jumps is needed to bring about the greatest increase in jumping ability, and higher-intensity plyometric exercises result in greater increases in vertical jump ability.

Saez Saez deVillarreal, E., Gonzalez-Badillo, J.J., and Izquierdo, M. 2008. Low and moderate plyometric training frequency produces greater jumping and spending gains compared with high frequency. *Journal of Strength and Conditioning Research* 22: 715-725.

Saez Saez de Villarreal, E., Kellis, E., Kraemer, W.J., and Izquierdo, M. 2009. Determining variables of plyometric training for improving vertical jump height performance: A meta-analysis. *Journal of Strength and Conditioning Research* 23: 495-506.

The possible effect of the height of the drop on jumping ability was recognized as early as 1967. Verhoshanski (1967) stated that depth jumps from a height greater than 110 cm (43.3 in.) are counterproductive because the change from eccentric to concentric action takes place too slowly. Schmidt-bleicher and Gollhofer (1982) later suggested that the height should not be so great that the trainee cannot keep her heels from touching the ground. This is in part because of the increased chance of injury from the high-impact forces encountered when the heels do touch the ground.

Training by dropping from various heights (40-110 cm, or 15.7-43.3 in.) alone or in combination with weight training has resulted in increased vertical jump ability, leg strength, and motor performance; however, no significant difference is shown among drop heights (Bartholomeu 1985; Blackey and Southard 1987; Clutch et al. 1983; Matavulj et al. 2001). It has been suggested that drop jumps from heights greater than 40 cm (15.7 in.) offer no advantage because mechanical efficiency is not increased compared to lower heights, and that

drop jumps in excess of 60 cm (23.6 in.) are not recommended because of a lack of mechanical efficiency and an increased chance of injury (Peng 2011). A meta-analysis concluded that drop height has no significant effect on vertical jump ability increases due to training (Saez Saez de Villarreal et al. 2009). Thus, presently it appears there is no optimal drop height for this type of training.

Weighted Lower-Body Plyometric Exercises

The use of a weight vest, a weight belt, or a barbell supported on the back while performing stretch-shortening cycle exercises has resulted in greater and no significant difference from the same training with no additional resistance (Saez Saez de Villarreal et al. 2009). This type of exercise is similar to the power-type training described in the previous section. A meta-analysis concluded that vertical jump height with body weight only is not enhanced by plyometric training using additional resistance (Saez Saez de Villarreal et al. 2009).

However, additional resistance may enhance performance when carried (e.g., body pads or other equipment) during a motor task. Thus, the use of additional resistance during plyometric training may be warranted in some situations or when training for specific sports.

Concurrent Strength and Stretch-Shortening Cycle Training

Performance of both strength and stretch-shortening cycle exercises two or three times per week for 4 to 10 weeks of training results in increased vertical jump ability, countermovement jump ability, and leg strength (Adams et al. 1992; Bauer, Thayer, and Baras 1990; Blackey and Southard 1987; Clutch et al. 1983; Fatouros et al. 2000; Hunter and Marshall 2002). Increases in vertical jump ability have ranged from 3.0 to 10.7 cm (1.2 to 4.2 in.) with this type of training. This type of training has also been shown to significantly increase standing long jump ability in males but not females, to significantly decrease 40 yd sprint time (Polhemus et al. 1981), to significantly increase the velocity when kicking a soccer ball (Young and Rath 2011), and to significantly increase performance in a sprint stair-climbing task (Blackey and Southard 1987).

In general, the positive changes in motor performance tests with concurrent strength and stretch-shortening cycle training are greater than with either training type alone (Adams et al. 1992; Bauer, Thayer, and Baras 1990; Fatouros et al. 2000; Polhemus et al. 1981). For example, vertical jump ability improved 3.3, 3.8, and 10.7 cm (1.3, 1.5, and 4.2 in.) with squat-only, plyometric-only, and combination training, respectively (Adams et al. 1992) and 11, 9, and 15% with lower-body weight training only, plyometric training only, and combination training, respectively (Fatouros et al. 2000). Those in the combination group improved significantly more than did those in either type of training alone in these studies.

Concurrent strength and stretch-shortening cycle training is also of value in specific training situations. Adolescent baseball players performing a periodized strength training program or the same training program plus medicine ball plyometric training consisting of medicine ball throws, including throws involving torso rotation, significantly increased measures of torso rotational and hip-torso-arm rotational strength and power (Szymanski et al. 2007). However, concurrent training resulted in significantly greater increases in these measures. Increases in rotational strength and power are of value in swinging a baseball bat and throwing. Thus, both types of training should be included in resistance training programs when gains in motor performance are desired.

Stretch-Shortening Cycle Training Effect on Strength

Stretch-shortening cycle training does increase maximal strength. The isometric force of the knee extensors, but not the knee flexors, is significantly increased by performing only stretch-shortening cycle jump training (Bauer, Thayer, and Baras 1990). Jump rope training with a weighted rope has resulted in significant increases in 1RM leg press and bench press ability (Masterson and Brown 1993). Drop jumps have also been shown to increase hip extensor strength (Matavulj et al. 2001), squat 1RM (Hawkins, Doyle, and McGuigan 2009; MacDonald, Lamont, and Garner 2012), and leg press 1RM (Saez Saez de Villarreal, Gonzalez-Badillo, and Izqueirdo 2008). For example, a plyometric training program including a variety of stretch-shortening cycle jumps significantly increases 1RM squat ability 28% (Hawkins, Doyle, and McGuigan 2009) and 3RM squat ability 7% (Lockie et al. 2012).

Plyometric push-up training significantly increases seated 1RM bench press ability, but not to a greater extent than training with normal push-ups does (Vossen et al. 2000). As would be expected, the combination of strength and plyometric training also increases strength (Blackey and Southard 1987; Fatouros et al. 2000). Interestingly, one of the studies reports squat ability to be enhanced significantly more (29, 12, and 22%, respectively) with combination training than with plyometric or strength training alone (Fatouros et al. 2000). The increase shown by the weight-only group was significantly greater than that shown by the plyometric-only group, and the increase shown by the combination group was significantly greater than that of either type of training alone. Although the subjects in this study were not weight trained, they could squat 1.5 times their body weight.

Thus, whether plyometric training only will increase 1RM strength in highly weight-trained people is speculative. With adolescent baseball players, the addition of medicine ball plyometric throwing exercises to a periodized weight training program does not result in significantly greater increases in bench press 3RM than a weight training program alone (17 vs. 17%, respectively) or 3RM squat (27 vs. 30%). As described in the previous section, greater increases in torso and hip-torso-arm rotational strength and power were found with concurrent training.

Thus, whether concurrent strength and stretch-shortening cycle training result in greater strength increases than weight training alone depends on the specific stretch-shortening cycle exercises added to the total training program and the movement in which strength is measured. However, stretch-shortening cycle training in and of itself can increase strength.

Effect of Stretch-Shortening Cycle Training on Body Composition

Studies examining the effects of stretch shortening cycle-only training on body composition and muscle fiber size are inconclusive. The performance of only jump-type stretch-shortening cycle training in females resulted in no significant change in percent body fat or fat-free mass (Bauer, Thayer, and Baras 1990). In boys aged 12 to 13 years, stretch-shortening cycle training performed along with normal soccer training resulted in a significant decrease in percent body fat (Diallo et al. 2001). Performance of normal soccer training and plyometric training resulted in no significant body composition changes in adult female athletes (Sedano Campo et al. 2009). Performance of stretch-shortening cycle jump-type training and some normal resistance training resulted in no significant type I or II muscle fiber hypertrophy or change in percent body fat or fat-free mass (Häkkinen et al. 1990). However, Potteiger and colleagues (1999) reported that stretch-shortening cycle training resulted in a significant increase in both type I and type II fiber hypertrophy. As with any type of training the effect on body composition and muscle fiber size may depend on initial training status, the length of training, the volume of training, and whether other types of training were performed concurrently.

Compatibility of Stretch-Shortening Cycle Training With Other Training Types

Other training types seem quite compatible with stretch-shortening cycle training. As previously discussed, combining stretch-shortening cycle

training with weight training may actually result in greater motor performance and strength gains compared to either type of training performed alone. Both stretch-shortening cycle training with 20 minutes of aerobic training (70% of maximal heart rate) and stretch-shortening cycle training only result in significant gains in vertical jump ability, but no significant difference exists between groups (Potteiger et al. 1999). It is interesting to note that significant increases in both type I and type II muscle fiber cross-sectional area occurred with both training programs, but no significant difference was noted between programs. Additionally, stretch-shortening cycle training of the legs decreases the cost of running or increases running economy in distance runners; the decrease in the cost of running due to stretch-shortening cycle training is greater than that due to traditional resistance training (Berryman, Maurel, and Bosquet 2010; Spurrs, Murphy, and Watsford 2003).

Weight and stretch-shortening cycle training two days per week for the lower body and flexibility training four days per week for the lower body show no incompatibility (Hunter and Marshall 2002). Both groups significantly improved in countermovement vertical jump ability as well as drop jump ability from 30, 60, and 90 cm (11.8, 23.6, and 35.4 in.), but no significant difference between groups was noted. Although data are limited, stretch-shortening cycle training shows no incompatibility with strength, aerobic, or flexibility training.

Injury Potential of Stretch-Shortening Cycle Training

As with any type of physical training, stretch-shortening cycle training does have inherent injury risks; anecdotal evidence indicates that injuries have occurred as a result of stretch-shortening cycle training. However, some of these injuries appear to be related to such factors as performing depth jumps from too great a height or improper flooring or landing areas. Several authors of stretch-shortening cycle training studies explicitly state that no injuries occurred from the training (Berryman, Maurel, and Bosquet 2010; Polhemus et al. 1981), even in untrained people (Bartholomeu 1985; Blattner and Nobel 1979). As an injury prevention measure, some have suggested that anyone performing stretch-shortening cycle lower-body exercises should first be capable of performing a back squat with at least 1.5 to 2 times body weight. This might preclude many people from ever performing stretch-shortening cycle training even after a significant amount of weight training, and a meta-analysis indicates that initial fitness level has no effect on increases in jumping ability due to stretch-shortening cycle training (Saez Saez de Villarreal et al. 2009).

Stretch-shortening cycle training can result in significant muscle fiber damage and neuromuscular fatigue (Chatzinkolaou et al. 2010; Nicol, Avela, and Komi 2006). Typically, after a stretch-shortening cycle training session is a reduction in performance lasting one to two hours followed by a second reduction approximately 24 hours later as a result of muscle soreness and damage (delayed-onset muscle soreness). Full recovery from a training session can take up to eight days depending on the intensity and volume of the stretch-shortening cycle training session. Fatigue from other types of training prior to stretch-shortening cycle training may increase the chance of injury during a stretch-shortening cycle training session. Fatigue induced by treadmill running significantly alters the biomechanics of a drop jump (increased peak impact acceleration and knee flexion peak angular velocity) on landing during drop jumps from as low as 15 and 30 cm (5.9 and 11.8 in.) (Moran et al. 2009).

As previously discussed, impact on landing increases as the height of a drop jump increases (Peng 2011; Wallace et al. 2010). Thus, performing plyometric training in a fatigued state or drop jumps or depth jumps or depth jumps from increasing heights may increase the chance of injury. Because of the stresses encountered during this type of training, stretch-shortening cycle training should be introduced into the training program slowly and should begin with a relatively low training volume.

Comparisons With Other Types of Strength Training

The increase in 1RM squat ability with six weeks of normal weight training is greater, but not significantly so, compared to stretch-shortening training (MacDonald, Lamont, and Garner 2012). Another comparison showed that plyometric-only, resistance training–only, and complex training all significantly increased 1RM squat, calf raise, and Romanian deadlift ability, but no significant dif-ferences existed among the programs (MacDonald, Lamont, and Garner 2012).

Because few studies have compared stretch-shortening cycle training to other types of strength training, conclusions must be viewed with caution. Training resulted in no significant difference in increasing vertical jump ability between stretch-shortening cycle and normal dynamic constant external resistance training (Adams et al. 1992). The normal weight training consisted of back squats using a variation of the linear periodized training model, whereas stretch-shortening cycle training consisted of a periodized program of depth jumps, double-leg hops, and split jumps. The squat and stretch-shortening cycle training resulted in similar increases in vertical jump ability of 3.3 and 3.8 cm (1.3 and 1.5 in.), respectively. Training with either a stretch-shortening cycle or dynamic constant external resistance training program resulted in significant, but similar, gains in vertical jump height in both groups (Fatouros et al. 2000). However, significant differences in favor of the dynamic constant external resistance training program in leg press (9 vs. 15%) and squat (12 vs. 22%) 1RM strength were shown.

A comparison of weight training, weightlifting, and stretch-shortening cycle training showed all groups to significantly increase countermovement jump, squat jump, and 1RM squat ability (Hawkins, Doyle, and McGuigan 2009). The weight training program consisted of total-body resistance exercises with no attempt to accelerate the resistance while training. The weightlifting program predominantly used variations of the Olympic lifts. The stretch-shortening cycle training program included a variety of stretch-shortening cycle exercises for the lower body. Although all programs significantly increased all variables measured, the weight training program was favored (greater effect size) over the other two groups for increases in 1RM squat, countermovement jump, and squat jump ability. However, the weight training program was less effective than the other two training types in increasing vertical jump ability.

Another comparison showed that stretch-shortening cycle training only, resistance training only, and complex training all significantly increased 1RM squat, calf raise, and Romanian deadlift ability; no significant difference existed among the programs (MacDonald, Lamont, and Garner 2012). However, the increases shown by the resistance training only and the complex training were greater than that shown by the stretch-shortening cycle–only training in all three measures of strength.

A comparison of stretch-shortening cycle and isokinetic training showed no significant difference in increases of vertical jump ability between these two training methods (Blattner and Noble 1979). Both resulted in increased vertical jump ability of 4.8 and 5.1 cm (1.9 and 2.0 in.), respectively. As with any comparison of training programs, the results in part depend on the efficacy of the programs.

Other Considerations

Stretch-shortening cycle training is effective in increasing performance (25% increase in vertical jump ability) in women (Ebben et al. 2010), and a meta-analysis indicates that it results in equivalent increases in vertical jump ability in males and females (Saez Saez de Villarreal et al. 2009). Although stretch-shortening cycle training is normally associated with training for anaerobic activities such as sprints and jumping, it may also play a role in training for longer-duration sport activities. Distance in a plyometric leap test consisting of three consecutive leaps of jumping from one foot to the opposite foot and landing on both feet after the last leap explained 74% of the variance in a 10K race (Sinnett et al. 2001). Subjects in this study were recreationally trained distance runners. Additionally, as previously discussed (Berryman, Maurel, and Bosquet 2010; Spurrs, Murphy, and Watsford 2003), stretch-shortening cycle training decreases the cost of running, or increases running economy, in distance runners. This indicates that stretch-shortening cycle training should be included in the total training program of distance runners.

Typically, the goal of stretch-shortening cycle training is to increase maximal power. Normally, relatively long recovery periods are allowed with this type of training so that near-maximal power can be expressed during each repetition. In some programs this means allowing rest periods after every repetition with some types of stretch-shortening cycle training. A study comparing 15-, 30-, and 60-second rest periods between depth jumps in a set of 10 jumps showed no significant difference in jump height or ground reaction force (Read and Cisar 2001). Although it is generally believed that sufficient recovery must be allowed during a stretch-shortening cycle training session,

excessively long rest periods between repetitions do not seem necessary.

Body weight and body composition may be a consideration in the stretch-shortening cycle exercise prescription. The majority of these types of exercises, especially lower-body exercises, use body mass as the resistance to overcome. A person with a higher percentage of body fat must perform the exercises with greater resistance (body mass) with a smaller relative fat-free mass. Thus, to avoid injury and possibly optimize training, heavy people may need to use smaller training volumes (i.e., total number of foot contacts) than those with lower percentages of body fat.

Two Training Sessions in One Day

Two or more resistance training sessions on the same day are becoming relatively common. Some trainees may have started this practice because of time and schedule constraints. Others may want to accumulate a greater total training volume. However, training at a relatively high volume twice a day is not recommended for the beginning trainee. As with all physical training, time must be allowed to adapt to increases in intensity or volume.

When elite Olympic-style weightlifters perform a training session in the morning and one in the afternoon on the same day, strength measures decrease after the first training session, but recover by the second session (Häkkinen 1992; Häkkinen, Pakarinen et al. 1988c). Strength measures of Olympic-style weightlifters also recover between training sessions when two training sessions per day are performed on four out of seven days (Häkkinen, Pakarinen et al. 1988b). These well-conditioned resistance-trained athletes appear to be able to tolerate two training sessions per day, at least for short periods of time.

When elite Olympic-style weightlifters performed two training sessions on the same day for two days, no significant change in maximal snatch ability occurred (Kauhanen and Häkkinen 1989). However, the angular velocity of the knee in the drop under the bar decreased, and the barbell was pulled to a slightly lower height. After one day of rest, angular velocity of the knee increased, and the maximal height of the pull returned to normal. After one week of two training sessions per day, maximal leg isometric force production was unchanged in these elite weightlifters (Kauhanen and Häkkinen 1989). However, the time needed to reach maximal isometric force or rate of force development did increase. After two weeks of two or three training sessions per day, vertical jump ability decreased in junior elite Olympic-style weightlifters (Warren et al. 1992). These studies and anecdotal evidence indicate that elite strength-trained athletes can tolerate two sessions per day at least for short periods of time, but that changes in exercise technique and decreased power output can occur. Possible indications that the athlete is not tolerating two training sessions per day are small changes in exercise or sport technique and decreases in power-oriented tasks, such as vertical jump ability.

One reason for performing two training sessions per day is to increase total training volume. Another reason is to split a training session into two half sessions to allow almost complete recovery between half sessions. This allows the athlete to maintain intensity during each half session and achieve a higher intensity in the second half of the training. This schedule was investigated, and the results indicate that when total training volume is equal, two half-volume training sessions per day are advantageous (Häkkinen and Pakarinen 1991).

In a two-week period trained bodybuilders and powerlifters performed one training session per day. In another two-week period they performed the same training exercises with the same volume, but divided the volume into two sessions on the same day. Thus, total training volume was equal in the two-week periods; the only difference was the number of sessions per day. Each two-week training period was followed by one week at a reduced training volume. Isometric force during a squat-type movement was unchanged after each two-week training period. Isometric force was also unchanged after the week of reduced training volume after the one-session-per-day period. However, isometric force significantly increased after the week of reduced training volume after the two-sessions-per-day period.

In a similar study female competitive athletes performed a two-week training period during which their normal training volume was equally distributed between two training sessions on the same day followed by a one-week period of reduced training volume (Häkkinen and Kallinen 1994).

Compared to subjects in a normal one-session-per-day program over three weeks, the subjects in the two-sessions-per-day group demonstrated significant increases in maximal isometric strength and quadriceps cross-sectional area. These results indicate that dividing total training volume into two sessions a day may result in greater strength increases after a short recovery period.

Summary

Advanced training strategies, such as periodization, power training, stretch-shortening cycle training, and two sessions per day, may be necessary to optimize training adaptations in advanced lifters. More research concerning advanced training strategies is needed, especially with advanced lifters and elite athletes. However, the information presently available does indicate that advanced training strategies do work and can be more effective than training strategies not including an advanced strategy. Therefore, advanced strategies should be used, especially when developing resistance training programs for well-trained people and athletes.

SELECTED READINGS

Cronin, J., and Sleivert, G. 2005. Challenges in understanding the influence of maximal power training on improving athletic performance. *Sports Medicine* 35: 213-234.

Fleck, S.J. 2002. Periodization of training. In *Strength training for sport*, edited by W.J. Kraemer and K. Häkkinen, 55-68. Oxford, UK: Blackwell Science.

Häkkinen, K. 2002. Training-specific characteristics of neural muscular performance. In *Strength training for sport*, edited by W.J. Kraemer and K. Häkkinen, 20-36. Oxford, UK: Blackwell Science.

Kraemer, W.J., and Fleck, S.J. 2007. *Optimizing strength training: Designing nonlinear periodization workouts.* Champaign, IL: Human Kinetics.

Kraemer, W.J., and Newton, R.U. 2000. Training for muscular power. *Physical and Medical Rehabilitation Clinics of North America* 11: 341-368.

Nicol, C., Avela, J., and Komi, P.V. 2006. The stretch-shortening cycle: A model for studying naturally occurring neuromuscular fatigue. *Sports Medicine* 36: 977-999.

Saez Saez de Villarreal, E., Kellis, E., Kraemer, W.J., and Izquierdo, M. 2009. Determining variables of plyometric training for improving vertical jump height performance: A meta-analysis. *Journal of Strength and Conditioning Research* 23: 495-506.

8

Detraining

After studying this chapter, you should be able to

1. describe under what circumstances detraining would occur,
2. describe the typical timeline of physical ability loss during detraining,
3. discuss the physiological mechanisms resulting in detraining,
4. discuss the effects of detraining in season in different sports and what factors effect in-season detraining,
5. discuss why detraining at the end of a career is important to a bulked-up athlete, and
6. recommend training practices for the bulked-up athlete after their career.

The classic definition of detraining is the "cessation of exercise training." However, detraining may also occur with a planned cessation, such as in a periodized training program, or with an unplanned cessation as a result of injury, reduced training volume, or reduced intensity. **Detraining** is a deconditioning process that occurs when training is reduced or ceases completely; it affects performance because of diminished physiological capacity. Whenever strength and power performance decrements occur or when muscle mass is lost, some type of detraining may have occurred. Detraining can take place after several weeks or over many years, as a result of no exercise training with aging or the end of an athletic carrier. Short-term (weeks to months) detraining is typically more relevant to resistance training program design. The goals of resistance training maintenance or in-season programs are to prevent detraining from occurring while allowing more time to train other fitness or performance components.

Detraining in athletes can occur in several situations including complete cessation of weight training (e.g., due to an injury), decreased volume of weight training or complete cessation of weight training (e.g., as a planned part of a training program such as an in-season or off-season resistance training program), and long periods of no weight training or reduced volume and intensity of resistance training (e.g., following completion of an athletic career). The general effects of detraining are depicted in figure 8.1. It is important to note that detraining will not occur unless training resulted in physiological adaptations or changes in performance. An understanding of detraining will facilitate the design of optimal resistance training programs for improving performance and maintaining strength and power during periods in which resistance training is reduced.

Mujika and Padilla (2001) reviewed the time course of detraining responses. From a cardiovascular perspective, detraining has been characterized by decreased capillary density, which may take place after two to three weeks of inactivity, with arterial-venous oxygen difference decreases if training is stopped for three to eight weeks. Rapid declines in some oxidative enzymes bring about reduced mitochondrial ATP production. These are related to a reduction in peak oxygen consumption and are important for cardiorespiratory fitness. Athletes who have greater cardiorespiratory fitness levels have greater reductions in

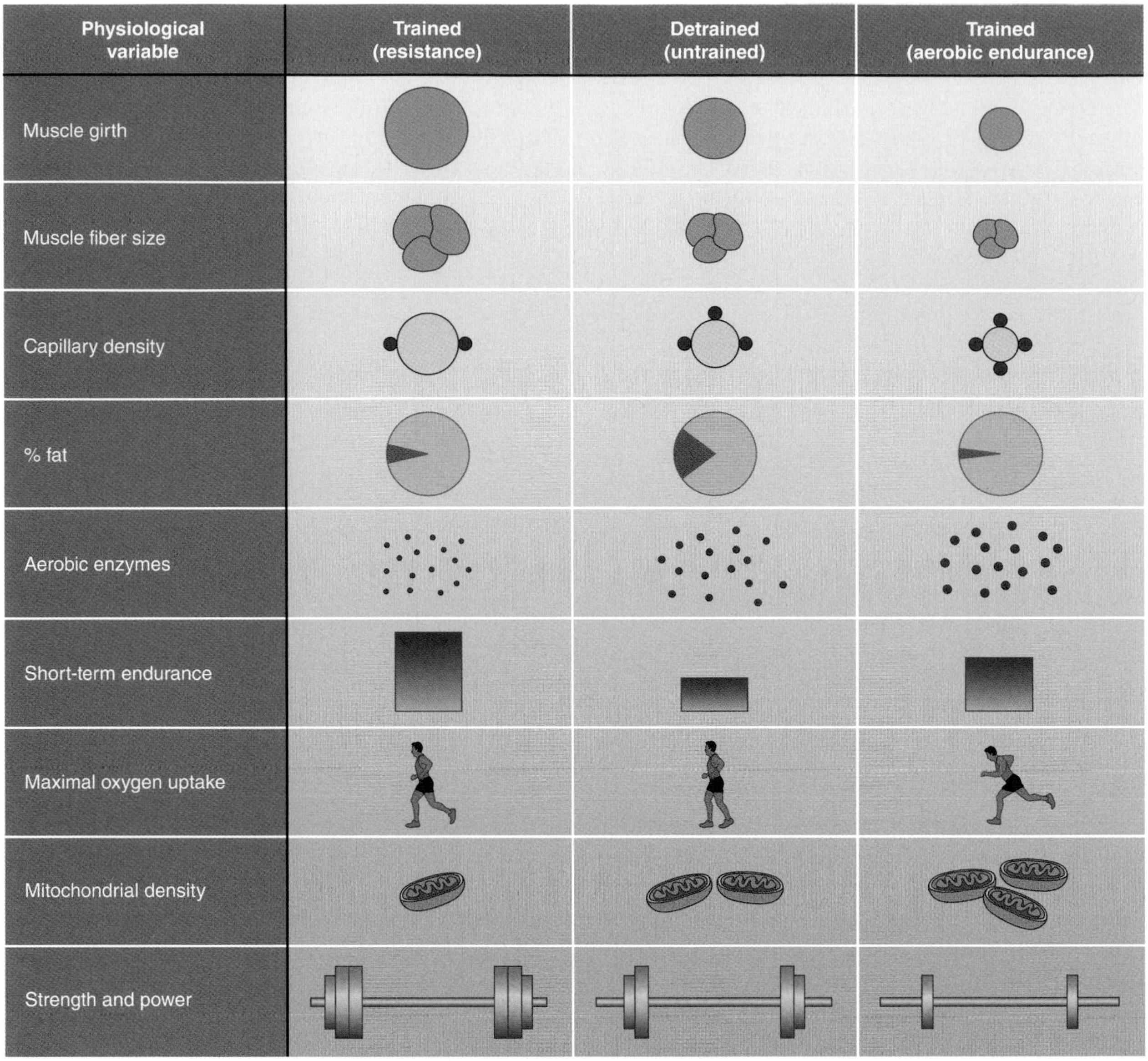

Physiological variable	Trained (resistance)	Detrained (untrained)	Trained (aerobic endurance)
Muscle girth			
Muscle fiber size			
Capillary density			
% fat			
Aerobic enzymes			
Short-term endurance			
Maximal oxygen uptake			
Mitochondrial density			
Strength and power			

FIGURE 8.1 The general effects of detraining are a return toward the untrained state.

physiological factors related to the transport and use of oxygen for energy generation. However, following a short period of detraining, athletes still have values for such variables that are higher than those in untrained, sedentary subjects, and their physiological functions return quickly with retraining after a short detraining period. However, cardiorespiratory fitness may be lost more quickly than high force and power production.

With detraining strength may be maintained for up to two weeks in power athletes (Hortobagyi et al. 1993) and in general up to four weeks (Mujika and Padilla 2001). In recreationally trained people, because of lower initial strength levels, strength loss may take up to six weeks or longer to occur

compared to highly trained people (Kraemer et al. 2002). However, even in previously untrained people short detraining periods, such as two weeks, can cause decreases in maximal strength. For example, after four weeks of weight training, isometric strength increased 31%, and after two weeks of no weight training, isometric strength had decreased to a level that was 24% greater than the pretraining level (Herrero et al. 2010a).

Eccentric force and sport-specific power may decrease with short detraining periods of several weeks in trained athletes (Mujika and Padilla 2001). However, following three months of training, previously untrained people maintained eccentric force but not concentric force during three months of detraining (Andersen et al. 2005). The slow loss of maximal strength with detraining is mirrored by a decrease in EMG activity (Andersen et al. 2005; Mujika and Padilla 2001). Power appears to decrease more rapidly than maximal strength during detraining (Izquierdo et al. 2010; Kraemer et al. 2002). Other physiological adaptations change toward the untrained state during detraining: muscle fiber size (Blazevich 2006), muscle fiber pennation angle (Blazevich 2006), satellite cell number (Kadi et al. 2004), left ventricular hypertrophy (Kawano, Tanaka, and Miyachi 2006), and tendon stiffness (Kubo et al. 2010) all decrease with detraining. However, arterial compliance generally increases with detraining after resistance training (Kawano, Tanaka, and Miyachi 2006). Additionally, resting blood hormonal concentrations change (e.g., a decrease in growth hormone and increase in cortisol; Kraemer and Ratamess 2005) indicating less of an anabolic state during detraining. Collectively, the preceding studies indicate that, during detraining, virtually all training adaptations return toward the untrained state, although the time line of this return varies.

Types of Detraining

Detraining typically occurs in several situations. The first is complete cessation of all types of training. This type of detraining may occur at the end of a season or at the termination of an athletic career. Complete cessation of training is seldom desirable because of negative physical performance as well as health implications. A reduction in weight training volume or intensity can occur in several situations. One is a situation in which only weight training was performed and training is reduced. This situation might occur as part of a research project or following an injury. Another situation is a planned reduction in weight training volume or intensity with continued performance of other types of physical training. This occurs in many in-season sport weight training programs.

Cessation of Resistance Training

Early studies indicate that when training ceases completely or is drastically reduced, strength gains decline at a slower rate than the rate at which strength increased as a result of training (McMorris and Elkins 1954; Morehouse 1967; Rasch 1971; Rasch and Morehouse 1957; Waldman and Stull 1969). The decrease in strength with the cessation

of resistance training may be quite large (see table 8.1). For example, the squat ability of Olympic weightlifters (see figure 8.2) shows a decline of approximately 10% in a four-week period after cessation of weight training. However, after a two-week detraining period active males showed a slight increase in isometric force (see figure 8.3).

Although short periods of detraining may result in decreased maximal strength, levels are still higher than pretraining levels (Herrero et al. 2010a, 2010b; Izquierdo et al. 2010). A nonsignificant change in strength may also occur after a short-term detraining period (Prestes, Frolini et al. 2009; Terzis et al. 2008). For example, 1RM strength in several exercises during one week of detraining after a linear periodization or reverse linear periodization program shows nonsignificant changes; some exercises show small increases (Prestes, Frolini et al. 2009).

Thus, the direction and magnitude of strength or power changes during a short detraining period may vary depending on the initial level of conditioning or the test used to determine maximal strength or power. However, as the detraining period increases in duration, a significant decrease in strength and power will eventually take place.

Longer periods of detraining (up to 24 weeks) result in a significant decrease in strength (see table 8.1), although strength is still greater after the detraining period than it was before beginning resistance training. Whether an initial decrease in strength occurs during a detraining period after the first several weeks of detraining strength shows a slow decline toward untrained values as the detraining period increases in duration (Häkkinen et al. 2002; Ishida, Moritani, and Itoh 1990; Ivey et al. 2000; Lo et al. 2012).

Some studies show a better maintenance of strength during the first weeks of detraining compared to later weeks of detraining. However, the magnitude of strength loss as a detraining period increases in length may be affected by age; older subjects lose more strength than younger subjects as a detraining period increases in length (see box 8.1).

In general, older and younger people show a similar pattern of strength decrease with detraining (Ivey et al. 2000): Although they lose strength with detraining, strength remains above pretraining levels. For example, Kalapotharakos and colleagues (2007) showed that after six weeks of detraining, senior males (aged 68) experienced a decrease in

TABLE 8.1 Representative Strength and Power Changes With Detraining

Reference	Subjects	Length of training (wk)	Type of training	Days/ wk	Sets × reps	Length of detraining (wk)	Type of strength test	% above pretrained Trained	% above pretrained Detrained
Häkkinen et al. 1989	Male strength athletes	10.5	Weightlifting	3.5	70-100% of 1RM	2	Maximal isometric knee extension	8*	5
	Males	10.5	Weightlifting	3.5	70-100% of 1RM	2		13*	15*
	Females	10.5	Weightlifting	3.5	70-100% of 1RM	2		19*	18*
Kraemer et al. 2002	Resistance-trained males	2+ years	Total-body periodization	3 or 4	3-5 × 1- to 12RM	6	1RM squat 1RM bench press 1RM shoulder press	? ? ?	−3.2 −4.7 −0
Hortobagyi et al. 1993	Powerlifters and football players	8.1 year	Weightlifting	3.4	2-5 × 1-12	2	1RM squat 1RM bench press Wingate power	? ? ?	−1.7 −0.9 −8.7
Terzis et al. 2008	Males	14	Total body	2 or 3	2 wk: 2 × 8- to 10RM 12 wk: 3 × 6RM	4	1RM squat 1RM leg press 1RM bench press	28* 34* 22*	22* 25* 17*
Izquierdo et al. 2010	Males	16	Total body periodized + ballistic training	2	Progressed 3 × 10 at 80% of 10RM to 3 × 2-4 at 90% of RM	4	1RM bench press 1RM squat	17* 22*	4 16*
Dudley et al. 1991	Males	19	Leg press Knee extension	2	4-5 × 6-12	4	3RM leg press 3RM knee extension	26* 29*	20* 20*
Herrero et al. 2010a	Males	4	Knee extension	4	8 × 8 at 70% of 1RM	2	Isometric knee extension	31*	26*
Narici et al. 1989	Males	8.6	Isokinetic, 120 deg/ sec	4	6 × 10	5.7	Isometric	21*	3 wk = 10 5.7 wk = 4
Häkkinen and Komi 1983	Males	16	Squat	3	15 reps at 80-100% of 1RM 5 reps eccentrically at 100-120% of 1RM	8	Isometric squat	30*	19*
Ishida et al. 1990	Males	8	Calf raise	3	3 × 15 at 70% of 1RM	8	Isometric	32*	4 wk = 20* 8 wk = 16*
Häkkinen et al. 1985a	Males	24	Squat	3	18-30 reps at 70-100% of 1RM, 3-5 reps eccentrically at 100-120% of 1RM	12	Isometric squat	27*	12*
Häkkinen et al. 1985b	Males	24	Squat	3	18-30 reps at 70-100% of 1RM, 3-5 reps eccentrically at 100-120% of 1RM	12	Squat 1RM	30*	15*
Houston et al. 1983	Males	10	Leg press, knee extension	4	3 × 10 RM	12	Knee extension, 0-270 deg/sec	39-60*	4 wk = 29-52* 12 wk = 15-29*
Andersen et al. 2005	Males	12	Leg press, back squat, knee extension and flexion	3	Linear periodization 10-12RM progress to 4RM	12	Knee extension Eccentric 30 deg/sec Eccentric 240 deg/sec Concentric 30 deg/sec Concentric 240 deg/sec	50* 25* 19* 11*	20* 24* 5 1

								% above pretrained	
Reference	Subjects	Length of training (wk)	Type of training	Days/wk	Sets × reps	Length of detraining (wk)	Type of strength test	Trained	Detrained
Häkkinen et al. 1985c	Males	24	Jump training with 10-60% of 1RM squat	3	100-200 jumps per session	12	Isometric squat	6.9*	2.6*
Lo et al. 2011	Males	24	Total body	3	Linear periodization	48	1RM chest press 1RM knee extension	32* 71*	2* 30*
Taaffe and Marcus 1997	Elderly males	24	Upper and lower body	3	3 × 8 at 75% of 1RM (+GH)	12	1RM knee extension	40.4*	10.5*
Häkkinen et al. 2000	Middle-aged males and females	24	Leg press/ extension	2	3 or 4 × 8-15 at 50-80% of 1RM	3	1RM knee extension	27*	27*
	Elderly males and females	24	Leg press/ extension	2	3 or 4 × 8-15 at 50-80% of 1RM	3	1RM knee extension	29*	29*
	Middle-aged males and females	24	Leg press/ extension	2	3 or 4 × 8-15 at 50-80% of 1RM	24	1RM knee extension	29*	23*
	Elderly males and females	24	Leg press/ extension	2	3 or 4 × 8-15 at 50-80% of 1RM	24	1RM knee extension	23*	19*
Prestes, De Lima et al. 2009	Females	12	Linear periodized	3	Progressed 12- to 14RM to 4- to 6RM	1	1RM bench press 1RM knee extension	15* 37*	17* 37*
			Reverse linear		Progressed 4- to 6RM to 12- to 14RM		1RM bench press 1RM knee extension	16* 30*	17* 32*
Lemmer et al. 2000	Young males and females	99	Knee extension	3	5 × 5-10	31	1RM knee extension	34*	26*
	Elderly males and females		Knee extension	3	5 × 5-10	31	1RM knee extension	28*	14*
LeMura et al. 2000	Females	16	Total-body weightlifting	3	2 wk: 2 × 8-10 at 60-70% of 1RM 14 wk: 3 × 8-10 at 60-70% of 1RM	6	1RM mean of several upper-body exercises 1RM mean of several lower-body exercises	29* 38*	19* 24*
Staron et al. 1991	Females	20	Leg press, squat, leg extension	2	3 × 6- to 8RM one session, 3 × 10- to 12RM	30-32	1RM squat 1RM knee extension 1RM leg press	67* 70* 70*	45* 105* 61*
Tsolakis et al. 2004	Male children	8	Total body	3	3 × 10RM	8	Isometric elbow flexion	17*	6*
Faigenbaum et al. 1996	Male and female children	8	Weightlifting	2	4 wk: 2 × 6- to 8RM 4 wk: 3 × 6- to 8RM	8	6RM knee extension 6RM chest press	53* 41*	17 19*
Blimkie et al. 1989	Male children	20	Total body	3	3 × 15 at 70% of 1RM	8	Bench press Leg press Isometric knee extension Isometric elbow flexion 1RM knee extension	35* 22* 21* 31* 70*	34* 17* 14* 30* 61

* = significantly different from pretrained, +GH = growth hormone supplementation.

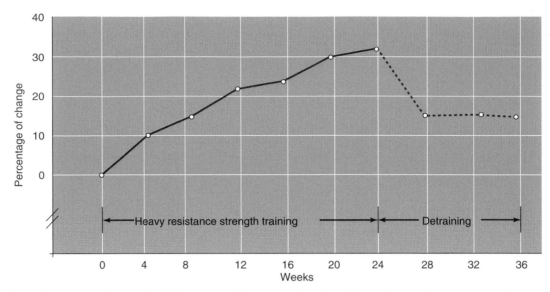

FIGURE 8.2 Percentage changes in 1RM squat of Olympic-style weightlifters with training and detraining.

Adapted, by permission, from K. Häkkinen and P.V. Komi, 1985, "Changes in electrical and mechanical behavior of leg extensor muscles during heavy resistance strength training," *Scandinavian Journal of Sports Science* 7: 55-64.

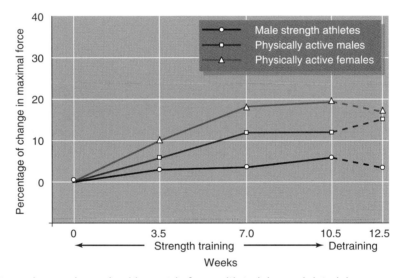

FIGURE 8.3 Percentage changes in maximal isometric force with training and detraining.

Reprinted from *Journal of Biomechanics*, Vol. 8, K. Häkkinen et al., "Neuromuscular adaptations and hormone balance in strength athletes, physically active males, and females, during intensive strength training," pp. 889-894, Copyright 1989, with permission from Elsevier.

1RM strength of approximately 15% in several exercises, although their levels were still above their pretraining levels. Older women appear to be more susceptible to detraining (Ivey et al. 2000). One difference between seniors and younger people is that, eventually, seniors experience greater strength losses as the detraining increases in duration (see box 8.1). In children or adolescents, detraining (6-12 weeks) also results in a decrease in strength, although strength after detraining is greater than pretraining values (Ingle, Sleap, and Tolfrey 2006;

Tsolakis, Vagenas, and Desssypris 2004). Children's natural growth and increases in strength may partially offset strength decreases due to long periods of detraining.

Collectively, the information available on both short (two to four weeks) and long periods of detraining indicates that strength decreases do occur, but the loss is quite variable in magnitude. The rate of strength loss may depend in part on the length of the training period prior to detraining, the type of strength test used (e.g., bench press,

BOX 8.1 **RESEARCH**

Effects of Age on Strength Loss With Detraining

Age does appear to affect strength loss during the detraining period. Both young (20- to 30-year-old) and older (65- to 75-year-old) men and women showed a significant increase in 1RM strength of 34 and 28%, respectively, after nine weeks of training the knee extensors (Lemmer et al. 2000). The gains made by the younger subjects were significantly greater than those made by the older subjects. During 31 weeks of detraining, the older and younger subjects showed significant decreases in strength of 14 and 8%, respectively. The loss shown by the older people was significantly greater than that of the younger people. Interestingly, both the older (13%) and younger (6%) people showed the majority of strength loss from weeks 12 to 31. The young men, older men, and older women all showed significant strength decreases from week 1 to week 12 and from week 12 to week 31 of the detraining period. The younger women showed a similar pattern of strength loss, except that the loss from weeks 12 through 31 was not significant. The results indicate that both young and old people maintain strength better during the first 12 weeks of detraining compared to the later weeks of detraining, but that older people in particular lose strength rapidly after 12 weeks of detraining. The greater strength loss in older people is in part due to the natural loss of strength with aging.

Lemmer, J.T., Hurlbut, D.E., Martel, G.F., Tracy, B.L., Ivey, F.M., Metter, E.J., Fozard, J.L., Fleg, J.L., and Hurley, B.F. 2000. Age and gender responses to strength training and detraining. *Medicine & Science in Sports & Exercise* 32: 1505-1512.

eccentric, concentric), and the specific muscle group examined. However, age may also affect the magnitude of strength losses, especially with longer detraining periods.

The vast majority of detraining research used normal resistance training, with concentric and eccentric actions during each repetition, prior to detraining. Some research indicates that performing this type of training prior to detraining may result in a slower loss of strength during four weeks of detraining than would occur with concentric-only training (Dudley et al. 1991). In this study normal resistance training and concentric-only training (only lifting and not lowering a weight) consisted of three sets of 10 to 12 repetitions at a 10- to 12RM resistance. Double-volume concentric training consisted of six sets of 10 to 12 repetitions at the normal resistance training of 10- to 12RM resistance. Thus, with double-volume concentric training, the number of concentric-only muscle actions was equal to the number of concentric and eccentric actions performed during the normal resistance training. Training consisted of the leg press and knee extension exercises performed three days per week for 19 weeks. Strength increases (3RM) for both exercises were tested with concentric-only and normal weight training. All groups improved significantly in concentric-only leg press ability (see figure 8.4).

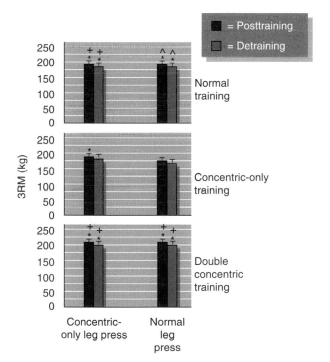

FIGURE 8.4 Changes in 3RM leg press with normal resistance training, concentric-only training, and double-volume concentric training.

* = increase over pretraining; + = greater increase than concentric-only group; ^ = increase greater than concentric-only and double-volume concentric groups

Adapted, by permission, from G.A. Dudley et al., 1991, "Importance of eccentric actions in performance adaptations to resistance training," *Aviation, Space, and Environmental Medicine* 62: 543-550.

in a smaller decrease in strength than no training at all, did not maintain strength at the levels achieved by the previous two years of training at a higher intensity. However, in this group of seniors decreased strength due to aging probably also affected the results as evidenced by the decrease in strength shown by the control group.

In-Season Detraining

In-season detraining refers to losses of performance, power, or strength when people stop training completely or reduce resistance training volume while undertaking other sport-type training. This type of detraining is important to consider because it occurs in many sports during an entire season or a portion of a season. How much strength or performance is lost during a season depends on several factors, such as how much playing time the person receives during the season, other types of conditioning drills performed, and the strength or power requirements of the sport or activity.

The preceding sections make it clear that cessation of resistance training results in strength loss. It is also clear that cessation of resistance training eventually results in a decrease of motor performance. However, short detraining periods may not affect motor performance. For example, plyometric training that significantly increased countermovement jump ability (25%) and countermovement jump peak power showed no significant change during a detraining period of 10 days (Ebben et al. 2010). Twenty-four weeks of primarily squat-type movements using 70 to 100% of 1RM three times per week significantly increased vertical jump ability 13% (Häkkinen and Komi 1985c). With 12 weeks of detraining vertical jump ability significantly decreased, but was still 2% above the pretraining value. Similarly, 24 weeks of plyometric training increased vertical jump ability 17%, and after 12 weeks of detraining vertical jump ability decreased but was still 10% above the pretraining value (Häkkinen and Komi 1985a). During both of these studies decreases in squat jump ability (jump with no countermovement) during the detraining period also occurred.

Two weeks of detraining in strength-trained athletes (powerlifters and American football players) resulted in small, nonsignificant increases in vertical jump (2.3%) and squat jump (3.6%) ability (Hortobagyi et al. 1993). However, even though

changes in strength and motor performance may be correlated (Terzis et al. 2008), they are distinctly different factors. This is indicated by a decrease in strength that may occur in a short detraining period (four weeks) without a significant decrease in a motor performance task, such as shot put ability (Terzis et al. 2008). This appears to be true in older people as well. During a 24-week detraining period, levels of performance of motor performance tasks and explosive jumping and walking actions remain elevated above pretraining levels in middle-aged and elderly people even though muscle atrophy and strength loss occur (Häkkinen et al. 2002).

During in-season training, even if resistance training stops, athletes are still performing other types of training. Elite downhill, freestyle, and speed skiers show some change in strength during a season even though performance in these sports requires a high level of strength and power (Koutedakis et al. 1992). Three months into the season, isokinetic knee extension strength at 60 degrees per second decreased significantly by 6% and knee flexion strength nonsignificantly by 7%. After seven months knee extension strength at 60 degrees per second decreased significantly by 14% and knee flexion strength by 16%. Isokinetic knee flexion and knee extension strength at 180 degrees per second after three and seven months of detraining showed small, nonsignificant decreases, and power output during a 30-second maximal cycling test (Wingate test) also showed nonsignificant changes. Thus, skiers may lose strength at very slow velocities, but not intermediate velocities, during a season. However, because no loss of power output occurs, the effect on performance may be minimal.

A lack of resistance training during the season of some ball sports appears to have small effects on strength or motor performance. Detraining periods during a basketball season have little effect on strength or motor performance. A resistance training program of five weeks preceding the season of a collegiate Division I men's season significantly increased 1RM squat 18% and resulted in nonsignificant changes in 1RM bench press, 27 m sprint time, and vertical jump ability of 4, 2, and 0%, respectively (Hoffman et al. 1991). Performing no resistance training during the 20-week season resulted in nonsignificant changes in 1RM bench press, 1RM squat, and vertical jump ability (−1 to +5%), whereas 27 m sprint ability declined significantly (3%). Adolescent (14.5 years) male basketball players performing a 10-week plyometric (jumps and medicine ball throws) program two times per week along with normal basketball practice showed significant increases in the squat jump, countermovement jump, depth jump, and seated medicine ball throw of 9 to 16% (Santos and Janeira et al 2011). During the next 16 weeks, performing no plyometric training while continuing normal basketball training resulted in no significant changes in these same measures (+2-7%). In a similar project (Santos and Janeira et al. 2009) male adolescent (14-15 years) basketball players performed complex training two times per week for 10 weeks. During the next 16 weeks of performing normal basketball training but no complex training, nonsignificant changes in the squat jump, countermovement jump, depth jump, and seated medicine ball throw were shown (see box 8.3).

Similar results have been shown for tennis players and team handball players. Women collegiate Division I tennis players performing no resistance training during a nine-month season showed that playing tennis and participating in tennis drills does maintain fitness (Kraemer et al. 2000; Kraemer, Häkkinen et al. 2003). However, although fitness was maintained, no improvement in fitness measures or sport-specific performance measures, including serve, forehand, and backhand ball velocity, occurred. After performing a 12-week total-body weight training program, elite male team handball players show significant increases of 13% in countermovement jump and 6% in ball-throwing velocity (Marques and Gonzalez-Badillo 2006). During a seven-week detraining period in which no weight training was performed, countermovement jump showed a nonsignificant decrease (–2%); ball-throwing velocity showed a significant decrease (–3%).

Collectively, the preceding indicates that, generally, strength and motor performance can be maintained during the course of a season or portion of a season by playing a sport and performing associated drills with training, especially if such training requires the development of high force or power. However, some decrements in strength and performance measures may occur.

In-Season Resistance Training Programs

The goal of an **in-season program** is to further increase or at least maintain strength, power, and motor performance during a competitive season. Results of in-season programs, however, can be quite variable.

 BOX 8.3 PRACTICAL QUESTION

Does Normal Sport Training Maintain Motor Performance In-Season?

Whether motor performance gains can be maintained in some sports with normal training is an important question. In 14- and 15-year-old male basketball players, normal basketball training does maintain motor performance in-season, and performing one weight training session per week has little effect (Santos and Janeira 2009). Prior to the season a 10-week weight training program was performed. Stopping weight training or performing one weight training session per week for 16 weeks in-season both generally maintained motor performance. However, there was a gradual decrease in motor performance as the 16-week detraining period progressed. For example, after four weeks of detraining, nonsignificant increases occurred in the squat jump, countermovement jump, and medicine ball throw when weight training was stopped (+7, +3, and +8%, respectively) or training volume was reduced (+7, +4, and +3%, respectively). However, after 16 weeks of detraining, nonsignificant decreases were generally shown in the squat jump, countermovement jump, and medicine ball throw when weight training was stopped (–8, 0, and –3%, respectively) or training volume was reduced (–4, +6, and –6%, respectively). Although the changes in motor performance were nonsignificant, motor performance levels generally decreased as the season progressed whether weight training was stopped completely or performed one time per week.

Santos, E.J.A.M., and Janeira, M.A.A.S. 2009. Effects of reduced training and detraining on upper and lower body explosive strength in adolescent male basketball players. *Journal of Strength and Conditioning Research* 23: 1737-1744.

Rowing in and of itself has high strength and aerobic requirements. After 10 weeks of resistance training three times per week, rowers demonstrate increased strength (see figure 8.5; Bell et al. 1993). Six weeks of resistance training at a reduced frequency of either one or two times per week resulted in either no significant change or an increase in strength. All training sessions consisted of approximately three sets of each of the six exercises shown in figure 8.5 at an intensity of approximately 75% of maximal. These results indicate that strength can be maintained or increased for a period of six weeks in rowers who do not weight train but continue rowing.

Two studies, described in the previous section, of male adolescent basketball players demonstrate the variability in fitness maintenance with an in-season program. Adolescent male basketball players performing a 10-week plyometric program two times per week along with normal basketball practice showed significant increases in the squat jump, countermovement jump, depth jump, and seated medicine ball throw (Santos and Janeira 2011). During the next 16 weeks, performing no plyometric training while continuing normal basketball training resulted in no significant changes in these same measures. However, performing one plyometric training session per week during the 16-week detraining period showed significant increases (8-15%) in three of these four measures. Thus, performing no plyometric training maintained performance in motor performance measures; however, performing plyometric training at a reduced training volume generally resulted in significant increases in motor performance measures.

In a similar project male adolescent basketball players showed nonsignificant changes (–5 to +8%) in the squat jump, countermovement jump, depth jump, and seated medicine ball throw after performing complex training two times per week for 10 weeks followed by 16 weeks with either no complex training or complex training one time per week (Santos and Janeiro 2009). No difference was shown between performing no or one complex training session per week. However, it should be noted that the 10-week complex training program prior to the detraining period did not significantly increase performance in any of the motor performance tasks tested.

During a 22-week basketball season in which female players performed resistance training once or twice a week, vertical jumping ability

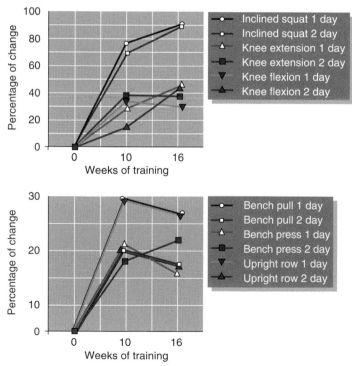

FIGURE 8.5 Changes in strength during 10 weeks of resistance training three days per week followed by six weeks of resistance training one or two days per week in oarswomen.

Data from Bell et al. 1993.

significantly increased by 6% (Häkkinen 1993). Maximal isometric leg extension force remained unchanged. The in-season training consisted of one or two lower-extremity exercises per session of three to eight repetitions per set at 30 to 80% of maximal. Subjects performed 20 to 30 repetitions per training session, and once every two weeks they undertook a jump training session consisting of 100 to 150 horizontal and vertical jumps. This in-season program maintained strength and increased vertical jumping ability.

An in-season program for professional soccer players indicates that one session per week, but not one session every two weeks, maintains fitness during the season (Ronnestad, Nymark, and Raastad 2011). After a 24-week preseason weight training program, the half squat, 40 m sprint time, and squat jump all showed significant improvement (19, 2, and 3%, respectively). Countermovement jump ability was not significantly affected. Twelve weeks of an in-season weight training program that consisted of one session per week resulted in no significant change in half squat ability and 40 m sprint time. Training only one time every two weeks resulted in significant performance decreases in half squat ability (10%) and 40 m sprint time (1%). Squat jump and countermovement jump ability was unchanged in-season with both training frequencies, indicating that one session per week maintains fitness more so than one session every two weeks. Fitness maintenance, however, showed

substantial individual variation with both training frequencies.

In-season programs for American football players also show variable results. Both college linemen and nonlinemen (Schneider et al. 1998) performing an in-season weight training program twice a week during a 16-week season showed either significant decreases or small, nonsignificant decreases in typical measures of motor performance as well as flexibility and strength (see figure 8.6). A total of 68 college football players performing a program of reduced training volume (i.e., decreased training frequency) showed maintenance of strength during a season (Kraemer, unpublished data). The subjects performed an in-season program (see table 8.4) two times per week during the 14-week season; 1RM strength was assessed preseason, midseason, and postseason. Prior to the season during winter and summer resistance training programs, players performed resistance training four or five days per week with a higher training volume and more exercises per session than the in-season program. The entire group exhibited no significant decreases in 1RM for any of the exercises tested during the season (see figure 8.7). A separate evaluation of backs and linemen showed similar results.

A comparison of a multiple-set nonlinear program and a single-set program (described in more detail in chapter 7) performed by female tennis players for nine months, including the

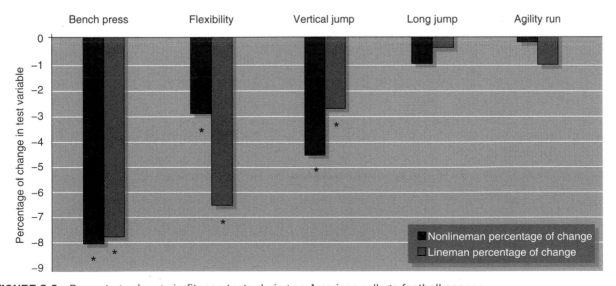

FIGURE 8.6 Percentage change in fitness tests during an American college football season.

* = significant decrease from start to end of 16-week season.

Data from Schneider et al. 1998.

tennis season, shows some interesting results (Kraemer et al. 2000). Both programs were performed two or three times per week for the entire nine months depending on the match schedule. Generally, the nonlinear program resulted in consistent and significant gains in fitness measures, including serve velocity, throughout the period. The single-set program generally resulted in no change in fitness measures or a significant change during the first three months and then a plateau in fitness for the remaining six months. The single-set program resulted in no significant change in serve ball velocity throughout the nine months. The nonlinear program generally resulted in greater fitness gains than the single-set program did. A similar study (described in more detail in chapter 7) compared a two- or three-set nonlinear program to a two- or three-set nonvaried program (Kraemer, Häkkinen et al. 2003). This comparison showed results similar to those of the first study on female tennis players except that the differences in strength and performance gains between the nonlinear and multiple-set programs were much closer. However, during the entire season, overall, the nonlinear program resulted in greater strength, power, and motor performance increases compared to the multiple-set program. The comparison also indicated that the nonlinear program resulted in significantly greater increases in forehand and backhand ball velocity. The results of these two studies indicate that fitness gains can be made in-season, but the magnitude and whether a gain is achieved at all depends on the total volume and type of program performed.

TABLE 8.4 Fourteen-Week In-Season Training Program for American College Football Players

Exercise	Reps per set
Bench press	8, 5, 5, 8
Squat	5, 5, 5, 5
Single-leg knee extension	10, 10
Single-leg knee curl	10, 10
Military press	8, 8, 8
Power clean	8, 8, 8

Note: Two-minute rest periods occurred between sets and exercises. Training frequency was two times per week.

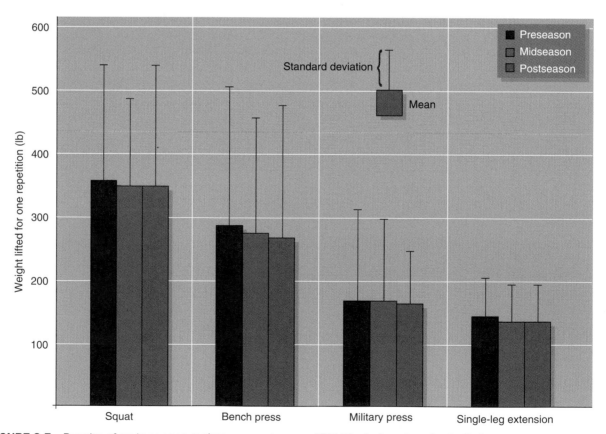

FIGURE 8.7 Results of an in-season resistance program on 1RM lifts in American football players.

Collectively, the studies described here indicate that in-season programs can maintain or increase strength, power, and motor performance during a season. It appears that one or two resistance training sessions per week can maintain strength and power in-season. However, the volume and intensity of training as well as the type of program can influence whether fitness gains are maintained or increased. It is also important to note that if the goal of an in-season program is to maintain motor performance, the motor performance task should be included in the training program. This, however, is typically not a concern because the motor performance tasks of a sport (tennis serve, jumping, sprinting) are typically performed as part of playing the game and in various conditioning and sport skill drills performed during the season.

Long Detraining Periods

Long detraining periods (i.e., several months or years in duration) have received less study than shorter detraining periods have. Detraining in this context refers to no resistance training at all. In older people (mean ages 58 and 70, respectively), two and six months of detraining results in a decline of strength, but strength remains above pretraining levels (Elliott, Sale, and Cable 2002; Fatouros et al. 2006). As previously described (see box 8.2), in this same population strength losses during detraining are affected by the intensity of the training preceding detraining; greater losses occur after less intense (40% > 60% > 80% of 1RM) training (Fatouros et al. 2006).

Several case studies give some insight into the effect of long-term detraining in younger people after long periods of resistance training. Table 8.5 depicts the effects of seven months of detraining and dieting on an elite powerlifter. The results suggest that detraining results in a physiological shift from a strength profile to an improved aerobic profile (Staron, Hagerman, and Hikida 1981). Three observations reflected this shift: the improvement of peak oxygen consumption ($\dot{V}O_2$peak), increased mitochondrial density, and improved oxidative enzyme profile of the muscle fibers. These changes occurred without any aerobic training stimulus during the seven-month detraining period. The large weight loss (27.5 kg, or 60.6 lb) and reduction in body fat during this period may have accounted for some of these changes; the decrease in muscle fiber area contributed to the decrease in thigh girth. These observations

TABLE 8.5 Physiological Changes After Seven Months of Detraining

Variable	Trained	Detrained
Ht (cm)	170.0	170.0
Wt (kg)	121.5	94.0
% body fat	25.2	14.8
Thigh girth (cm)	82.5	66.5
BP (systolic/diastolic)	146/96	137/76
$\dot{V}O_2$peak (ml/kg/min)	32.6	49.1
HRmax	200	198
% volume of mitochondria Type I (slow twitch) Type II (fast twitch)	3.04 1.76	4.41 2.46
Fiber type SO (%) FG (%) FOG (%)	31.2 53.2 15.6	38.1 43.7 27.2
Cross-sectional area (μm²) SO FG FOG	5,625 8,539 9,618	3,855 5,075 5,835

BP = blood pressure; HR = heart rate; SO = slow oxidative; FG = fast glycolytic; FOG = fast oxidative glycolytic. SO fibers are smaller than fast-twitch fibers and FOG fibers.

Adapted from *Journal of Neurological Sciences*, Vol. 51, R.S. Staron, F.C. Hagerman, and R.S. Hikida, "The effects of detraining on an elite power lifter," pgs. 247-257, Copyright 1981, with permission from Elsevier.

are consistent with changes normally attributed to muscle atrophy.

The loss of muscle fiber area with long periods of detraining in previously highly resistance-trained athletes is also shown in a case study of a world-class male shot-putter (Billeter et al. 2003). At the end of his competitive career, the shot-putter's type II mean fiber area was substantially greater than that of his untrained brother. After three years of detraining, type II mean fiber area of the former shot-putter had decreased to a value much closer to that of his untrained brother. Type I mean fiber area increased slightly during the three years of detraining and approached that of his untrained brother.

A third case study examined two men who performed resistance training for eight weeks and then detrained for five months (Thorstensson 1977). The initial training period consisted of various exercises for the leg extensors and weighted and unweighted jumping exercises. After the initial training period, one man performed resistance training at a reduced volume two or three days per week and did not perform any jumping exercises.

The other man performed no training at all for the five-month detraining period. The man training at a reduced volume during the detraining period showed increases compared to immediately after the eight-week training period in 1RM squat and isokinetic torque at 60 degrees per second and faster, but not at slower velocities. However, decreases in isometric leg extension force, vertical jump ability, and horizontal jump ability occurred. After detraining all measures were still above pretraining values. The man not training showed decreases in all of the measures; only the level of 1RM squat ability was still greater than the pretraining level after the detraining period. Fat-free mass continued to increase in the man training at a reduced volume and decreased to slightly below pretrained levels in the man not training. The ratio of type II to type I fiber area decreased in both men during the detraining period, but was still above pretraining values for both, indicating a greater loss of type II fiber area than of type I fiber area. Thus, after five months of detraining, virtually all increases in strength and muscle mass from an eight-week training period are lost if no resistance training is performed. However, resistance training at a reduced volume for five months can maintain or even increase gains in strength and muscle mass following an eight-week training program.

Physiological Mechanisms of Strength Loss

As with strength gains during training, several mechanisms could result in strength and power changes during periods of detraining. Knowledge of these mechanisms will help the practitioner design better in-season programs. One mechanism, atrophy, does occur during detraining. For example, three months of training resulted in a significant increase of 10% in quadriceps cross-sectional area; after three months of detraining, cross-sectional area returned to the pretraining value (Andersen et al. 2005).

Electromyographic (EMG) changes during muscular actions after training and detraining indicate changes in motor unit firing rate and motor unit synchronization. EMG changes have been followed during detraining periods ranging from 2 to 12 weeks. During short periods of detraining, decreases and no change in strength and power measures have been accompanied by no significant

changes in EMG activity (Häkkinen et al. 1990; Häkkinen and Komi 1985c; Hortobagyi et al. 1993). However, decreases in EMG activity due to short periods of detraining have also been shown (Häkkinen and Komi 1986; Häkkinen, Komi, and Alen 1985; Narici et al. 1989), and decreased EMG activity has shown significant correlations to decreases in strength (Andersen et al. 2005; Häkkinen, Alen, and Komi 1985; Häkkinen and Komi 1985a, 1986). When strength decreased in concentric actions, decreased EMG activity was shown, and during eccentric actions showing no strength loss, no significant change in EMG activity was shown (Andersen et al. 2005). Decreased EMG activity may occur in some muscles (vastus lateralis), but not others (vastus medialis, rectus femoris) with detraining (Häkkinen, Alen, and Komi 1985). Thus, the initial strength loss, when it does occur during the first several weeks of detraining, is due to neural mechanisms; further strength loss as the detraining duration increases is in part the result of muscle atrophy (Häkkinen and Komi 1983).

During periods of detraining, positive adaptations in fiber size that occurred as a result of training regress toward the untrained or pretrained state (see table 8.6). During short periods (two to eight weeks) of detraining in men, type I and type II fiber area (Häkkinen, Komi, and Alen 1985; Häkkinen, Komi, and Tesch 1981; Hather, Tesch et al. 1991; Hortobagyi et al. 1993) may decrease compared to the posttrained state, but it is still greater than the untrained fiber size. However, no change also has been reported (Hather et al. 1992; Hortobagyi et al. 1993). In older people (65 to 77 years) the return to pretraining cross-sectional area type I and type II muscle fiber sizes may be more rapid than in younger people even when accompanied by recombinant hGH therapy (Taaffe and Marcus 1997). This may be due in part to differences in spontaneous activity and lifestyle in younger and older people. Interestingly, training resulted in a 40% increase in strength, of which only 30% was lost during detraining despite muscle fiber areas returning to pretraining levels, suggesting that neural mechanisms account for part of the strength retention (Taaffe and Marcus 1997).

Decreases in the ratio of type I to type II fiber area have been shown during periods of detraining in men (Häkkinen, Komi, and Tesch 1981; Hather et al. 1992), which indicates a selective atrophy of type II fibers. However, no change compared

TABLE 8.6 Fiber Changes With Detraining

Reference	Length of training (wk)	Length of detraining (wk)	Type of training	Type of detraining	Fiber atrophy (µm²)	Type I/ type II ratio	Fiber transformation
Häkkinen, Komi, and Tesch 1981	16	8	Squat, concentric, 1-6 reps/set at 100-120% of 1RM	No training	Type I* Type II*	Decrease*	FT % decrease*
Houston et al. 1983	10	12	Knee extension, leg press 8RM, 4/wk, 3 sets	No training	Type IIx*	—	None
Staron, Hagerman, and Hikida 1981	36	28	Powerlifter, case study	No training	FOG*, FG*, SO*	—	FG to FOG
Thorstensson 1977	8	20	2 to 32 to 2 sessions/ wk, weights and jumping	No training	Type II* Type I*	Decrease*	FT only
Hather et al. 1991	19	4	Leg press, knee extension 4 or 5 sets, 2/wk 6-12 reps, concentric/ eccentric Concentric/ concentric Concentric	No training	Type II	Decrease*	None
Staron et al. 1991	20	30-32	Squat, knee extension, leg press	No training	Type IIa + type IIx*	Decrease*	—
Andersen and Aagaard 2000	12	12	Heavy load, lower body	No training	Type I and type II*	Decrease*	Type IIa to type IIx
Billeter et al. 2003	15 years	36	Competitive shot-putter	Unclear	Type II	Decrease	FT % decrease

1RM = one-repetition maximum; RM = repetition maximum; * = p <.05; FG = fast twitch glycolytic; SO = slow oxidative; FOG = fast oxidative.

to the trained state has also been shown (Hather et al. 1992). In women, small but nonsignificant decreases in type I fiber area accompanied by a significant decrease in the combined areas of type IIax and IIx fibers has been shown (Staron et al. 1991). No change in either type I or type II fiber area has also been reported during eight weeks of detraining; however, this study showed no increase in fiber area as a result of the stretch-shortening cycle–type (plyometric) training performed prior to the detraining period (Häkkinen et al. 1990).

Collectively, this information indicates that type II fibers may atrophy to a greater extent than type I fibers during short periods of detraining in both men and women. This, of course, can only occur if the training induced an increase in fiber area.

A case study of a former male world champion shot-putter supports the assertion that detraining results in the selective atrophy of type II fibers (Billeter et al. 2003). After a 15-year competitive career, three years of detraining resulted in a 25% decrease in type II fiber area and a small increase (5%) in type I fiber area. However, opposite of what might be expected, at the end of his competitive career 40% of all fibers were type II and 60% were type I. After three years of detraining only 27% of all fibers were type II and 73% were type I. However, at the end of his career, as a result of the extreme hypertrophy of the type II fibers, 67% of the muscle cross-sectional area was type II fibers. After detraining the atrophy of the type II fibers resulted in 43% of the muscle cross-sectional area being type II fibers. Type II and I muscle fiber size and the percentage of muscle cross-sectional area occupied by type II fibers after detraining were similar to values shown in the subject's untrained brother, indicating that during detraining muscle fibers return toward the untrained state.

In addition to atrophy and changes in fiber type, detraining also affects myosin heavy and light chains. Three months of detraining results in increased myosin heavy chain IIx content and decreased myosin heavy chain IIa content (Andersen and Aagaard 2000). The detraining resulted in myosin heavy chain IIx values that were higher than before resistance training, or an "overshoot" in the myosin heavy chain IIx values compared to before training. However, no such effect after three months of detraining has been shown in obese diabetics (Gjøvaag and Dahl 2009). In a former world champion male shot-putter, myosin light chains also showed a change with three years of detraining from faster to slower isoforms (Kadi et al. 2004). Thus, changes in myosin heavy and light chains may show a pattern of moving toward the slower isoforms with detraining.

The response of the hormonal system to detraining may vary drastically, and individual hormones may respond differently (Kraemer, Dudley et al. 2001; Kraemer and Ratamess 2005). Generally, short detraining periods of several weeks in men (Häkkinen et al. 1989, 1985; Häkkinen and Pakarinen 1991; Kraemer et al. 2002) and women (Häkkinen et al. 1990, 1989) have shown no significant changes in a large number of hormones including resting growth hormone, testosterone, cortisol, adrenocorticotropin, luteinizing hormone, progesterone, estradiol, follicle-stimulating hormone, and sex hormone–binding globulin. With detraining periods of eight weeks or longer, decreases in

the testosterone/cortisol ratio that are correlated to decreases in strength have been shown (Alen et al. 1988; Häkkinen et al. 1985). However, two weeks of detraining in trained powerlifters and American football players resulted in significant increases in resting growth hormone, testosterone, and the testosterone/cortisol ratio (Hortobagyi et al. 1993). The authors suggested that this might be an initial compensatory response to combat muscle atrophy. Thus, past training history or the duration of resistance training prior to detraining and the duration of detraining may affect the hormonal response to detraining.

The possible effect of acute training variables on the hormonal response to detraining is demonstrated by a study by Häkkinen and Pakarinen (1991). After two weeks of daily training followed by a one-week period of reduced training volume, no significant changes in testosterone, free testosterone, cortisol, or the testosterone/cortisol ratio occurred. However, when the same training volume was performed but divided into two training sessions per day for one week followed by a one-week period of reduced training volume, testosterone and the testosterone/cortisol ratio significantly decreased while cortisol significantly increased after the one week of reduced training.

Thus, generally, the hormonal response to short periods of detraining is minimal. However, it probably depends on the volume, intensity, and duration of training prior to the detraining period as well as the past training history, and shows some variation. The long-term hormonal response to detraining, on the other hand, is probably related to strength and muscle size loss with detraining (Kraemer and Ratamess 2005).

During short periods of detraining, fat-free mass and percent body fat show small, nonsignificant changes (Häkkinen et al. 1990; Häkkinen, Komi, and Alen 1985; Häkkinen, Komi, and Tesch 1981; Hortobagyi et al. 1993; Izquierdo et al. 2007; Prestes, De Lima et al. 2009; Staron et al. 1991) including in 58-year-old women (Elliot, Sale, and Cable 2002) and 12-year-olds (Ingle, Sleap, and Tolfrey 2006). Although muscle cross-sectional areas show either nonsignificant (Häkkinen et al. 1989) or significant decreases (Andersen et al. 2005; Narici et al. 1989), the lack of a significant change in fat-free mass is probable due to the gross nature of this measurement and the short duration of the detraining period. However, changes in fat-free mass and percent body fat do occur with detraining in the direction that would negatively affect performance. For example, after 16 weeks of weight training, fat-free mass increased 1.3 kg (2.9 lb) (from 48.1 to 50.3 kg [106 to 110.9 lb]) and percent fat decreased 2.6% (24.8 to 22.2%) in young women. During six weeks of detraining, fat-free mass decreased (48.5 kg [107 lb]) and percent fat increased (23%) back toward pretraining values (LeMura et al. 2000). None of the changes in body composition were significant at any point in the training or detraining period, but the changes are in the direction that would negatively affect performance during the detraining period.

Effects of Muscle Action Type

Previously described studies (Dudley et al. 1991; Hather et al. 1992) indicate that both normal resistance training, which includes an eccentric repetition phase, and double-volume concentric-only training result in greater retention of training adaptations during a short (four-week) detraining period compared to concentric-only training (see figure 8.4). In addition, when using concentric-only repetitions, detraining may result in greater maximal isometric strength losses than loses of dynamic 1RM strength over eight weeks of detraining (Weir et al. 1997).

In one of these studies (Dudley et al. 1991), normal resistance training (concentric and eccentric repetition phases), concentric-only training, and double-volume concentric training resulted in an increase in the percentage of type IIa fibers and a corresponding decrease in type IIx fibers. These changes were maintained during the detraining period. The normal resistance training and the double-volume concentric training resulted in an increase in mean fiber area, but only the normal resistance training resulted in the maintenance of this increase after the detraining period. The concentric-only training resulted in no increase in mean fiber area. Only the normal resistance training resulted in an increased fiber area and the maintenance of this increase in both type I and II fibers during the detraining period. The double-volume concentric training resulted in an increased size of only the type II fibers and the maintenance of this increase after detraining. The concentric-only training resulted in no significant size increase of either the type I or type II fibers. This could be interpreted to indicate that normal resistance training and high-volume training result

in the greatest maintenance of fiber size during a short detraining period.

The number of capillaries per fiber increased following all three types of training and remained above pretraining values after the detraining period. However, only the double-volume concentric and concentric-only training resulted in an increase of capillaries per cross-sectional area as a result of training and the maintenance of capillaries per cross-sectional area during detraining. This was due in part to a slightly greater fiber size increase following normal resistance training and a slightly greater increase in capillaries per fiber following double-volume concentric and concentric-only training. This change could be interpreted to indicate that concentric-only training may be appropriate for athletes needing to maintain aerobic fitness.

Detraining Effects on Bone

Little is known about the effects of detraining on bone even though this has potentially important implications, especially if the normal sedentary lifestyle of many people is viewed as detraining. Bone metabolism, structure, and status are sensitive to loading with weight training and unloading with detraining. The neuromuscular system appears to mediate much of what happens in bone, and this may be due to the resultant hormonal changes that occur with resistance exercise training. The time course of changes in bone and the influence of various types of resistance training programs on bone during detraining remain unclear. In addition, the length of the detraining period may be important, because changes in some bone parameters occur at a much slower rate than changes in muscle force production.

It is apparent that increased physical activity increases bone mineral density (BMD) and that detraining results in a loss of BMD in both male and female athletes (Nordstrom, Olsson, and Nordstrom 2005; Snow et al. 2001). For example, the effect of two years of gymnastics training in women (18 years old) demonstrates that bone is responsive to training and detraining (Snow et al. 2001). In both years bone mineral density (BMD) increased during the eight-month competitive season and decreased during the four-month off-season, which can be considered a form of detraining. During the first and second competitive seasons total-body BMD increased 1.2 and

1.6%, respectively, and showed decreases in the off-season of 0.3 and 0.4%, respectively. The net result was a total gain in total-body BMD of 2.1% over the two years. However, not all bones demonstrated the same pattern of increases and decreases in BMD. For example, lumbar spine BMD during the two competitive seasons showed increases of 3.5 and 3.7%, respectively, and decreases of 1.5 and 1.3% in the off-season, respectively. This resulted in an increase in lumbar spine BMD over the two years of 4.3%. Femoral neck BMD increased 2.0 and 2.3%, respectively, during the first and second competitive seasons and decreased 1.5 and 2.1%, respectively, during the first and second off-seasons. This resulted in an increase over the two-year period of only 0.6%. Thus, the BMD of different bones responded in the same manner by increasing during the competitive season and decreasing during the off-season. However, the magnitude of the response varied substantially, and at some sites the losses of BMD during the off-season canceled out the increases during the competitive season resulting in no net gain over the two-year period. At other sites the increase in BMD during the competitive season was greater than the loss during the off-season resulting in a net gain in BMD.

Women 30 to 45 years old (Winters and Snow 2000) who completed a 12-month program of lower-body resistance training and maximal unloaded and loaded (10-13% of body mass) jumps showed dramatic increases in strength and power (13-15% above controls) along with increases in bone mineral density (1-3% above controls). After six months of detraining, BMD, muscle strength, and power all decreased significantly toward baseline values, whereas those of the control subjects did not change. Results indicate the importance of maintaining a training program to keep not only muscle force performance elevated, but bone mineral density as well. Conversely, resistance training of the arms in younger women (23.8 ± 5 years) resulted in an increase in arm flexion and extension strength, but no dramatic changes in BMD or bone geometry (Heinonen et al. 1996). With eight months of detraining, strength decreased, but no changes occurred in bone.

Collectively, the preceding studies indicate that bone can be affected by detraining, but the effect may depend in part on age, inherent normal activity, and the bone site. Additionally, in many situations in which unloading or detraining may occur, such as space flight or bed rest, resistance training may be an important intervention to improve or protect against bone mineral loss.

Detraining the Bulked-Up Athlete

A bulked-up athlete is an athlete who has gained substantial amounts of body weight through resistance training and dietary practices. The weight gain is related to the increased muscle mass and total body weight necessary for successful participation in sports such as American football, track and field throwing events, and powerlifting. It is well known that obesity and a sedentary lifestyle contribute to an increased risk of cardiovascular disease, and chronic detraining, especially in such athletes, may lead to health problems following an athletic career.

Many athletes who exercise to increase muscle mass and strength do not know how to exercise for health and recreation using other types of training, such as aerobic or circuit weight training. The retired athlete needs to start training again with new objectives and to examine dietary habits to avoid large weight gains. This is especially true for strength- and power-type athletes, because an aptitude for these types of athletic events, including weightlifting, does not offer protection against cardiovascular disease after retirement from competitive sport. However, an aptitude for athletic events requiring endurance and the continuation of vigorous physical activity after retirement from competitive sport does offer protection against cardiovascular disease (Kujala et al. 2000).

Comparisons of nonathletes and former athletes reveal that athletes have an advantage in cardiorespiratory fitness (Fardy et al. 1976). This advantage did not exist in a comparison of nonathletes and former athletes who engaged in strenuous leisure-time activities. However, one comparison (Paffenbarger et al. 1984) concluded that postcollege physical activity is more important than participation in college athletics in avoiding coronary artery disease. Endurance athletes in particular (see box 8.4) have an advantage in terms of total life span (Ruiz, Moran et al. 2011). A survey of former Finnish world-class athletes concluded that they have a longer-than-normal life expec-

BOX 8.4 **RESEARCH**

Effect of Being an Athlete on Life Expectancy

Many factors other than participation in sport affect life expectancy. Factors related to lifestyle during and after an athletic career also affect life expectancy. For example, smoking, a poor diet, and physical inactivity after a competitive career may reduce life expectancy. Genetics also plays a part. Following are the life expectancies of former male Finnish world-class athletes (Sarna et al. 1993):

- Nonathletes: 69.9 years
- Endurance sport athletes (long-distance running, cross-country skiing): 75.6 years
- Team sport athletes (soccer, ice hockey, basketball, track and field sprinting): 73.9 years
- Power sports (boxing, wrestling, weightlifting, track and field throwing): 69.9 years

Sarna, S., Sahi, T., Koskenvuo, M., and Kaprio, J. 1993. Increase life expectancy of world-class male athletes. *Medicine & Science in Sports & Exercise* 25: 237-244.

tancy; the authors hypothesized that recreational aerobic activity and infrequent smoking after athletic retirement may in part explain the longer life expectancy (Fogelholm, Kaprio, and Sarna 1994). However, athletes who require substantial body weight gains to succeed in their sport careers may be at greater risk for cardiovascular diseases. To reduce this risk, retired athletes require the proper prescription of exercise, along with dietary changes and weight control.

Retired strength-trained athletes should feel that they can still enjoy resistance training. Periodization of training and the development of new training goals are important for facilitating this feeling. More than anything, the continuation of training is of paramount importance, because many athletes drop out of their exercise routines during retirement. Healthy detraining of the resistance-trained athlete necessitates new training goals such as improving health and fitness by participating in aerobic exercise programs to improve cardiovascular function, reducing body weight, and performing resistance training to maintain muscular fitness. In addition, nutritional counseling may be important to deal with aberrant calorie intake behaviors (e.g., American football players ingest from 5,000 to 10,000 calories a day) adopted over an athletic career to gain body mass. As an ex-competitive athlete ages, training goals should be consistent with those of the general population: to improve health and fitness and reduce risk factors for chronic diseases (e.g., cardiovascular disease, cancer, diabetes).

Those with a number of risk factors for cardiovascular disease have an increased risk of developing those diseases (see table 8.7). Management of these risk factors helps to reduce the risk of cardiovascular disease. It is easy to perform a risk factor analysis; this procedure has been described extensively (American College of Sports Medicine 2008).

The role of teachers and coaches is to educate everyone, including athletes, about lifelong health and fitness and to expose people to exercise other than heavy resistance training (Kraemer 1983a). This adds variation to the total training program and also contributes to a healthy transition for athletes whose careers end after high school, college, or professional participation in sports. It is up to conditioning professionals to help athletes make the transition from competitive sports to lifetime sports and exercise for health.

TABLE 8.7 Cardiovascular Disease Risk Factors

Controllable risk factors	Noncontrollable risk factors
Smoking tobacco	Heredity (family history)
Blood lipid level	Male gender
High LDL cholesterol level	Advancing age
Low HDL cholesterol level	
High triglyceride level	
Hypertension	
Physical inactivity	
Obesity and overweight	
Diabetes mellitus	

Summary

Detraining can occur in several situations including complete cessation of weight training, decreased volume of weight training (e.g., during an in-season resistance training program), and long periods of no weight training or reduced volume of resistance training (e.g., following the completion of an athletic career). The exact resistance, volume, and frequency of resistance training or the type of program needed to maintain training gains in a decreased resistance training situation, such as in-season, has not been determined. However, to maintain strength gains or slow strength losses during a detraining period, people should maintain the intensity but reduce the volume and frequency of training. In many sports, especially those requiring high force or power, performance of and normal training for the sport maintain strength during the season. Likewise, in-season resistance training programs also maintain strength gains.

SELECTED READINGS

Andersen, L.L., Andersen, J.L., Magnusson, S.P., and Aagaard, P. 2005. Neuromuscular adaptations to detraining following resistance training in previously untrained subjects. *European Journal of Applied Physiology* 93: 511-518.

Billeter, R., Jostarndt-Fogen, K., Gunthor, W., and Hoppeler, H. 2003. Fiber type characteristics and myosin light chain expression in a world champion shot putter. *International Journal of Sports Medicine* 4: 203-207.

Blazevich, A.J. 2006. Effects of physical training and the training, mobilization, growth and aging on human fascicle geometry. *Sports Medicine* 36: 1003-1017.

Fatouros, I.G., Kambas, A., Katrabasas, I., Leontsini, D., Chatzinikolaou, A., Jamurta, A.Z., Douroudos, I., Aggelousis, N., and Taxildaris, K. 2006. Resistance training and detraining effects on flexibility performance in the elderly are intensity-dependent. *Journal of Strength and Conditioning Research* 20: 34-642.

Izquierdo, M., Ibanez, J., Gonzalez-Badillo, J.J., Ratamess, N.A., Kraemer, W.J., Häkkinen, K., Granados, C., French, D.N., and Gorostilaga, E.M. 2007. Detraining and tapering effects of hormonal responses and strength performance. *Journal of Strength and Conditioning Research* 1: 768-775.

Lemmer, J.T., Ivey, F.M., Ryan, A.S., Martel, G.F., Hurlbut, D.E., Metter, J.E., Fozard, J.L., Fleg, J.L., and Hurley, B.F. 2001. Effect of strength training on resting metabolic rate and physical activity: Age and gender comparisons. *Medicine & Science in Sports & Exercise* 33: 532-541.

LeMura, L.M., Von Duvillard, S.P., Andreacci, J.A., Klebez, J.M., Chelland, S.A., and Russo, J. 2000. Lipid and lipoprotein profiles, cardiovascular fitness, body composition, and diet during and after resistance, aerobic and combination training in young women. *European Journal of Applied Physiology* 82: 451-458.

Mujika, I., and Padilla, S. 2000a. Detraining loss of training-induced physiological and performance adaptations. Part I. Short term insufficient training stimulus. *Sports Medicine* 30: 79-87.

Mujika, I., and Padilla, S. 2000b. Detraining loss of training-induced physiological and performance adaptations. Part II. Long term insufficient training stimulus. *Sports Medicine* 30: 79-87.

Mujika, I., and Padilla, S. 2001. Muscular characteristics of detraining in humans. *Medicine & Science in Sports & Exercise* 33: 1297-1303.

Ruiz, J.R., Moran, M., Arenas, J., and Lucia A. 2011. Strenuous endurance exercise improves life expectancy: It's in our genes. *British Journal of Sports Medicine* 45: 159-161.

9

Women and Resistance Training

After studying this chapter, you should be able to

1. understand the performance differences between men and women,
2. identify sex differences between men and women in upper- and lower-body strength from both a relative and absolute perspective,
3. understand sex differences related to hormonal function and responses to resistance exercise,
4. identify the key sex differences between men and women in muscle fiber morphology,
5. understand the effects of different resistance training programs for women,
6. understand the different phases of the menstrual cycle and factors related to menstrual dysfunction,
7. identify factors related to injury prevention in women and the role of resistance training, and
8. develop a resistance training program for women.

Women of all ages have realized the benefits of resistance exercise and an overall active lifestyle. Resistance exercise is common among women, particularly those who are fitness enthusiasts, soldiers, and other tactical professionals (e.g., police officers and firefighters). Whether for health and fitness benefits or strength, power, and performance (or both), resistance training is a necessary component of a total conditioning program (see figure 9.1).

This chapter addresses an array of issues related to training for women. With few exceptions, women can perform almost identical programs as men because few major sex differences exist that affect resistance training program design. Women experience the same physiological acute and chronic responses to resistance training as men. In fact, from a health perspective, women may benefit more from resistance training because of its positive effects on bone health and osteoporosis risk.

Physiological and Performance Differences Between Sexes

The sex differences between men and women are often obvious. Underscoring these differences is a fundamental fact of biology. The impact of testosterone on muscle cells during growth phases, along with the androgenic changes that occur in both boys and girls as they grow, lead to differences in physiological response and performance differences related to strength, power, and hypertrophy. Even at the highest level of competition in weightlifting and powerlifting, when matched for body weight classifications, men are stronger than women in lifting performance. However, the stimulus of resistance training to various aspects of physiology and performance is remarkably similar in both sexes; only the magnitude of the responses differs between them. Understanding

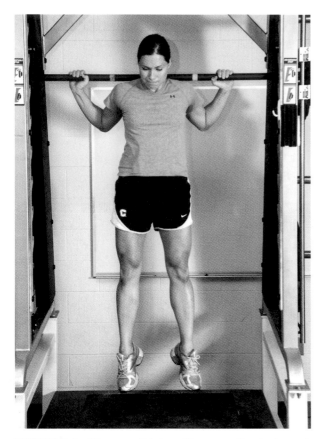

FIGURE 9.1 Women athletes, fitness enthusiasts, soldiers, and other tactical athletes all use advanced resistance training programs to improve strength and power to enhance performance and prevent injury.

Courtesy of Dr. William J. Kraemer, Department of Kinesiology, University of Connecticut, Storrs, CT.

these differences, which have been documented for decades, is important for designing resistance training programs for women.

Physical Activity Participation

As a result of social perceptions, sex stereotyping, and misconceptions regarding women and exercise, many women have been hesitant to incorporate resistance training into their activities and have not been encouraged to do so. The fear of "getting big" still prompts many women to avoid heavy lifting, believing it is a "guy thing." Because of this fear, many women use resistance training programs that are inferior to those used by men, even though we now know that the benefits of training cannot be achieved without heavy loading. Moreover, women of all ages tend to be less physically active than men to this day despite substantial research evidence supporting the benefits of resistance training for women (discussed in the

Training in Women section). Historically, more boys participate in sports than girls, and men have typically taken part in more vigorous exercise than women have (Barnekow-Bergkvist et al. 1996). In schoolchildren, 42% of boys meet the guideline of at least one hour of moderate-intensity physical activity a day, whereas only 11% of girls meet this guideline (Metcalf et al. 2008).

Whether we are making progress in the promotion of physical activity in men and women, and in the promotion of resistance training in particular, is still not clear. Data from the U.S. Centers for Disease Control and Prevention (CDC) show that only 17.5% of American women and 20% of university-age women meet the aerobic and strength training recommendations of the CDC. Men do not show much more improvement; only 23% of men and 37% of university-aged men have attained the CDC levels of fitness and participation in physical activity. One study found that 21% of American adults strength train at least two days a week, but differences exist based on sex, ethnicity, marital status, level of education, and census region. In women, participation is lower as they get older, but here again, education level affects these percentages (Chevan 2008). Thus, although strength training may be more present in the public eye given all of the commercial fitness programs and infomercials today, participation could be much greater. Progress has been made, but exercise strength and conditioning professionals still have much work to do to increase resistance exercise participation in women of all ages.

Childhood levels of physical activity may have long-ranging effects on health, neurological development, and performance later in life. More active children of both sexes display better metabolic composite scores (based on insulin resistance, triglycerides, blood pressure, and other measures), indicating that inactivity at a young age may place both sexes at a metabolic health disadvantage (Metcalf et al. 2008). Even in athletic populations at a young age (9-10 years), boys show greater isokinetic strength than girls (Buchanan and Vardaxis 2009). Furthermore, unlike boys, girls do not tend to show a clear pattern of strength gain with age; 12- and 13-year-old girls at times show less strength than 9- and 10-year-old girls. This disparity in physical activity may be the reason for compromised bone density, strength, and physical performance in women compared to men, clearly indicating the importance of resistance exercise for women. Women's lower levels of exercise participation than men's appear to have serious repercussions for women's lifelong health.

The rest of this section reviews the differences between women and men in a variety of parameters including strength, power, and muscle fiber makeup. It is important to note that the differences in activity levels starting from childhood, but also exposure to resistance training and equipment (e.g., health clubs, fitness clubs, YMCA/YWCA), may play various roles in many of the sex differences discussed. Increases in physical exercise among women of all ages may decrease the gap between men and women in physical performance.

Differences in Muscle Fiber Size, Type, and Composition

Prior to describing the sex differences in physical performance parameters (strength and power) between men and women, it is important to understand any underlying differences in muscle fibers. First, although men and women both possess the same types of muscle fibers, some of the profiles might be different in some comparisons. From one person to the next, muscle fiber characteristics can vary according to total muscle and muscle fiber cross-sectional area, number, type, and recruitment patterns. Fiber number and the percentage of type II and type I fibers do not appear to differ by sex;

however, few studies have been done to verify this fact, which runs counter to anecdotal observations, embryonic cell cycle development, and changes with adolescence. Many of the differences that do exist in fiber morphology may be due to women being less physically active or not participating in any progressive resistance training programs consistently throughout life.

As might be expected, levels of characteristics of trained muscle, such as total muscle cross-sectional area, muscle fiber size, and relative type II/type I ratios, are lower in women. In a recent study, cross-sectional area (CSA) of type I and type II fibers were 10.4 and 18.7% smaller, respectively, in women than in men (Claflin et al. 2011). Further, type II fibers from female subjects generated 17.8% less force and 19.2% less power than those from male subjects, indicating an underlying difference in muscle form and function. Overall, women have smaller muscle fiber areas than men do (see figure 9.2). Given that the absolute size of the muscle dictates force and power production, these differences in muscle size will be pertinent when discussing performance (Patton et al. 1990).

Whether differences exist between men and women in the number of fibers in various muscles is still not clear; differences may depend on the type of muscle and the type of comparison. However, anecdotal data suggest that women

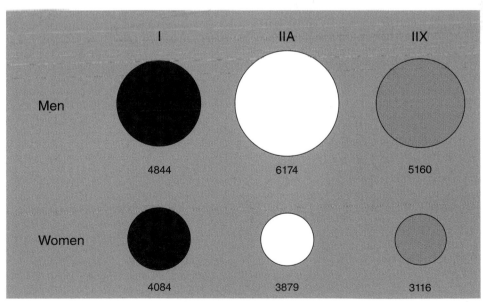

Cross-sectional area (μm²)

FIGURE 9.2 Graphic comparisons of physically fit (non-resistance-trained) women's and men's cross-sectional area muscle fiber sizes (μm²) for the various muscle fiber types. Note the greater cross-sectional area of the men's fibers compared to the women's fibers and the size relationships among the fibers.

Data from Staron et al. 2000.

have lower numbers of muscle fibers, especially in upper-body musculature. The number of muscle fibers in the average woman's biceps brachii has been reported to be less than (Sale et al. 1987) or the same as (Miller et al. 1992) the average man's. Female bodybuilders have been reported to have the same number of muscle fibers in the biceps brachii as male bodybuilders (Alway, Grumbt et al. 1989). Women's tibialis anterior has been reported to have fewer muscle fibers than men's (Henriksson-Larsen 1985), whereas women's triceps brachii and vastus lateralis have the same number of muscle fibers as men's (Schantz et al. 1983, 1981). Thus, depending on the level of training and muscle comparison made, sex differences might exist in the number of muscle fibers in a given muscle; women have a lower number. Based on maturation characteristics during adolescence, women's upper bodies do have lower numbers of muscle fibers than men's, which is confirmed by the differences in upper-body strength performances between men and women.

There is no consistent evidence that the percentage of type I to type II muscle fibers varies by sex because men and women have similar arrays of muscle fiber types (Drinkwater 1984; Staron et al. 2000). In one investigation, the untrained starting point for muscle fiber type in young men and women (approximately 21 years) was characterized (Staron et al. 2000). Using a biopsy analysis (see chapter 3) of the vastus lateralis of 55 young women and 95 young men, the investigators conducted a histochemical analysis in which muscle fiber types I, Ic, IIc, IIa, IIax, and IIx and cross-sectional areas of I, IIa, and IIx fibers were measured. Myosin heavy chain content was also analyzed. Both men and women demonstrated fiber types of about 41% type I, 1% type Ic and IIc, 31% IIa, 6% IIax, and 20% IIx. No differences in the percentages of fiber types were detected.

In the studies that have been done with biopsy measurements, women have smaller type II fibers than men do. In the investigation mentioned earlier, the cross-sectional area of all of the major fiber types was larger in men than in women. In men, the type IIa muscle fiber was the largest; in women, however, the type I fiber tended to be the largest, larger than IIa or IIx, indicating a lack of use of the type II motor units. Myosin heavy chain fiber type characterization followed the same pattern. Despite these differences, men and women both had a high percentage of IIx fibers, which convert to IIa and are not present after a heavy resistance training program (see chapter 3). Women's type I and II muscle fibers both have smaller cross-sectional areas than men's do (Alway et al. 1992; Alway, Grumbt et al. 1989; Miller et al. 1992; Ryushi et al. 1988; Staron et al. 2000), and the type II muscle fibers have a smaller cross-sectional area relative to men than do the type I muscle fibers (Alway et al. 1992; Alway, Grumbt et al. 1989). For example, female bodybuilders' average type I fiber cross-sectional area is 64% that of male bodybuilders, whereas their average type II fiber cross-sectional area is 46% that of male bodybuilders (Alway et al. 1992).

Given that women have smaller type II muscle fibers than men do, it follows that the total area occupied in a muscle by type II muscle fiber types is far smaller in women. From the greatest area to smallest area of a muscle, the descending order of muscle fiber type area in males is type IIa, IIx, and I, whereas in females the order is type I, IIa, and IIx. This results in a smaller type II/type I muscle fiber area ratio in women and may explain their slower fatigue rate in some high-intensity types of exercise (Kanehisa et al. 1996; Pincivero et al. 2000). For example, fatigue rate during 50 consecutive isokinetic knee extension actions is significantly less (48 vs. 52%) in females than in males (Kanehisa et al. 1996). The smaller type II/type I muscle fiber area ratio in females than in males may result in reduced performance on strength and power tasks compared to men.

In summary, women may have lower numbers of fibers in some muscles; however, they do possess smaller cross-sectional areas in all muscle fibers compared to men, and the percentages are almost the same in similar group comparisons (e.g., untrained men and untrained women). However, women do have lower total muscle cross-sectional area and a lower type II/type I muscle fiber size ratio. These muscle attributes may make it difficult to compare men and women directly in terms of performance and will certainly result in performance differences on an absolute basis. Ultimately, sex differences need to be placed into proper context and are based on the groups compared and their similarities or lack thereof (e.g., untrained women vs. untrained men or trained women vs. untrained men).

Sex Absolute Strength Differences

Absolute strength refers to the maximal amount of strength or force (i.e., 1RM) generated in a movement or exercise without adjusting for height, weight, or body composition. In general, the absolute strength of women is lower than that of men, and although some changes appear to be closing the sex difference gap, this fact remains true for appropriate comparisons. A woman's average maximal mean whole-body strength is 60.0 to 63.5% of the average man's (Laubach 1976; Shephard 2000a). A woman's upper-body strength averages 55% of a man's, and her lower-body strength averages 72% of a man's (Bishop, Cureton, and Collins 1987; Knapik et al. 1980; Laubach 1976; Sharp 1994; Wilmore et al. 1978). Strength ranges between normally active men and women show that men still have greater absolute strength than women (see figure 9.3). For example, differences are seen in the percentages of men's strength in single-joint (e.g., elbow flexion, shoulder extension, hip extension) and multijoint (e.g., bench press, squat, shoulder press) movements in both the upper and lower body. Additionally, the use of different types of maximal strength tests also contributes to these findings. For example, the knee extension strength of women (as determined by 1RM on a machine) (Cureton et al. 1988), maximal isometric strength (Maughan et al. 1986), and concentric isokinetic peak torque at 150 degrees per second (Colliander and Tesch 1989) have been reported to be 50, 68, and 60% of men's, respectively. Regardless of the measure, women's absolute strength tends to be lower than men's.

Although training may decrease the differences in absolute strength, it does not always do so. For example, women's total-body, lower-body and upper-body strength have been reported to be 57.4, 58.6, and 54.1%, respectively, of men's (Lemmer et al. 2007). After both men and women participated in a 24-week resistance training program, women's total-body strength increased to 63.4% of men's, and lower-body strength increased to 67.3% of men's (Lemmer et al. 2007). However, surprisingly, upper-body strength in women decreased slightly to 53.1% of men's, which raises questions about the training program's progression and effectiveness.

The potential disparity in upper-body strength gains between women and men, as noted, may be due to women's lower numbers of muscle fibers. In another study sex differences in maximal strength and large variations in these differences are still apparent in young male and female adults after 24 weeks of weight training three days per week (Lemmer et al. 2001) (see table 9.1). However, when women perform a total-body periodized resistance training program for six months, three days per week, dramatic increases in upper-body bench press and squat strength (1RMs) and power (W) result suggesting the potential importance of using a periodized training program (Kraemer, Mazzetti et al. 2001). Thus, training may decrease the absolute gap in strength between men and women somewhat; however, absolute strength alone does not account for body size, and therefore may not be the best measure of strength when comparing men and women.

Relative Strength Differences

Measures of absolute strength may place women at a disadvantage compared to men in terms of body size, muscle mass, and starting fitness level. On average, adult women 20 years of age and older are shorter in height than men (162.2 ± 0.16 cm [63.9 ± 0.06 in.] compared to 176.3 ± 0.17 cm [69.4 ± 0.07 in.) and lighter in body mass (74.7 ± 0.53 kg [164.7 ± 1.17 lb] compared to 88.3 ± 0.46 kg [194.7 ± 1.0 lb]) (McDowell 2008). Total body weight and fat-free mass may explain in part the sex differences in absolute strength. To account for differences in body size, investigators may use **relative strength**, which refers to absolute strength divided by, or expressed relative to, total body weight or fat-free mass.

We have known for quite some time that women's strength is more equivalent to men's when expressed relative to total body weight or fat-free mass. In a classic study, women's 1RM bench

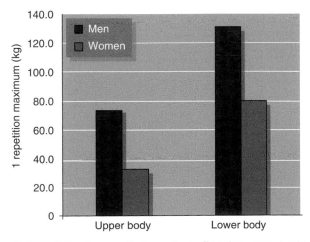

FIGURE 9.3 A compilation of studies for upper-body (bench press) and lower-body (squat) mean 1RM strength performances in recreationally active American college-age men and women.

Courtesy of Dr. William J. Kraemer, Department of Kinesiology, University of Connecticut, Storrs, CT.

TABLE 9.1 Changes in 1RM Strength by Sex Before (Pre) and After (Post) Training

	Men (n = 21)		Women (n = 18)	
	Pre	Post	Pre	Post
Biceps curl	31.2	40.5†	15.0	22.2†
Chest press*	58.3	70.9†	30.7	37.5†
Lat pull-down*	62.0	76.7†	31.7	39.5†
Shoulder press*	47.4	57.3†	29.0	31.6†
Triceps push-down*	65.9	88.0†	37.1	46.5†
Knee extension*	97.4	123.4†	58.0	73.2†
Leg press	613.4	747.4†	385.6	513.5†

*The increase in strength was significantly influenced by sex.

†The exercise showed a significant increase in strength after 24 weeks of resistance training.

Data from Lemmer et al. 2007.

press was 37% that of men's (Wilmore 1974). If expressed relative to total body weight and fat-free mass, women's 1RM bench press was 46 and 55%, respectively, that of men's. Similarly, women's maximal isometric force in a leg press movement was 73% that of men's. However, if expressed relative to total body weight and fat-free mass, women's isometric leg press strength was 92 and 106%, respectively, that of men's. Similarly, women's maximal absolute isokinetic bench press and leg press strength is 50 and 74% that of men's, respectively (Hoffman, Stauffer, and Jackson 1979). When adjusted for height and fat-free mass, women's bench press strength is 74% that of men's, but women's leg press strength is 104% that of men's. Thus, relative measures of strength place women about equivalent to men in terms of lower-body strength but not upper-body strength.

Relative measures of eccentric to concentric strength also reveal differences between men and women. Eccentric isokinetic peak torque relative to fat-free mass may be more similar between the sexes than concentric isokinetic peak torque (Colliander and Tesch 1989; Shephard 2000a). Women's concentric isokinetic peak torque relative to fat-free mass of the quadriceps and hamstrings at 60 degrees per second, 90 degrees per second, and 150 degrees per second averaged 81% of men's (see table 9.2). Women's eccentric isokinetic peak torque relative to fat-free mass at the same velocities averaged 93% of men's. Interestingly, other research has indicated that women's eccentric strength in relation to their concentric strength is greater than men's (Hollander et al. 2007). The ratio of concentric to eccentric strength was found to be greater using dynamic resistance exercises,

TABLE 9.2 Women's and Men's Quadriceps and Hamstrings Eccentric and Concentric Isokinetic Peak Torque

	Percentage of women's strength to men's relative to body mass	
	Eccentric	Concentric
Quadriceps		
60 deg · s⁻¹	90	83
90 deg · s⁻¹	102	81
150 deg · s⁻¹	99	77
Hamstrings		
60 deg · s⁻¹	84	84
90 deg · s⁻¹	90	80
150 deg · s⁻¹	92	81

Data from Colliander and Tesch 1989.

rather than the isokinetic exercises used in previous research. Furthermore, the ratios were even greater in upper-body exercises than in lower-body exercises.

It is possible that women store elastic energy to a greater extent than men do (Aura and Komi 1986) or that women are not able to recruit as many of their motor units during concentric muscle actions as during eccentric muscle actions compared to their male counterparts. More recent research has agreed with this earlier explanation, and no new theories have been put forward in the scientific literature, which has not really provided any significant amount of data on this question.

In summary, women's lower-body eccentric strength relative to fat-free mass is almost equal to men's, whereas concentric strength is not. However, the ratio of eccentric to concentric strength may be greater in women than in men, and the measures may vary by modality.

Training may help to reduce or eliminate differences in relative strength between men and women. For example, a recent study compared the relative strength of trained men and women both at baseline and after a 12-week nonlinear periodized strength training program. In accordance with the earlier research, men were shown to have greater relative strength than women in upper-body exercises (bench press, shoulder press, lateral pull-down), but not in the squat exercise (Kell 2011). Interestingly, despite the fact that the men and women were already previously trained, women still showed less relative strength in upper-body exercises. However, after 12 weeks of a nonlinear periodized program, differences in relative strength in the bench press exercise were no longer observed. However, a difference in rel-

ative strength was still seen in the shoulder press and lateral pull-down exercises. This suggests that optimal strength training programs might be able to reduce the difference in relative strength seen between men and women, in some upper-body exercises.

One difficulty in comparing strength in men and women is the underlying differences in training status that may inevitably exist even in untrained or recreationally trained people. One comparison between men and women that may reduce this complication would be within the context of highly trained people (see figure 9.4). For example, the 2011 world records in powerlifting of the International Powerlifting Federation for the 114 lb (51.7 kg) body weight class for women were 518.1 lb (235.0 kg) for the squat, 319.7 lb (145.0 kg) for the bench press, and 446.4 lb (202.5 kg) for the deadlift. The men's world records in the

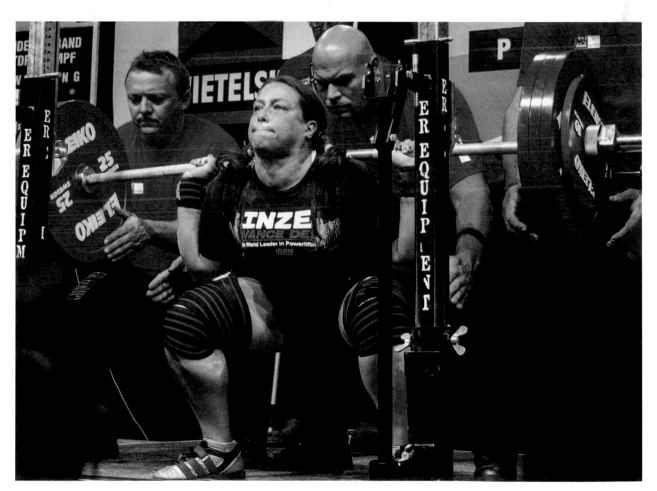

FIGURE 9.4 Even elite female powerlifters show sex-related differences in relative and maximal strength compared to their male counterparts.

Photo courtesy of Dr. Disa L. Hatfield, University of Rhode Island, Kingston, RI.

114 lb weight class were 662.5 lb (300.5 kg) for the squat, 402.3 lb (182.5 kg) for the bench press, and 573.2 lb (260 kg) for the deadlift. Thus, women's world records for the squat, bench press, and deadlift were 78.2, 79.5, and 77.9% those of the men. Women naturally carry more body fat than men do, and thus a better relative measure may be lean body mass. With that said, even highly trained women are not as strong as highly strength-trained men when adjusted for body weight.

Generally, data indicate that women's upper-body strength is less than men's in absolute terms and relative to either total body weight or fat-free mass. Women's absolute lower-body strength is less than men's, but may be equivalent relative to fat-free mass. Some of the discrepancies in the previously cited studies in strength expressed relative to fat-free mass may be related to fat-free mass distribution differences between the sexes. Generally, men do have a larger fat-free mass, and the greatest regional difference is in the upper body (Janssen et al. 2000). When strength is expressed relative to fat-free mass, women's values are over-corrected for the lower body and under-corrected for the upper body. Thus, upper-body strength relative to fat-free mass will not be equivalent between the sexes, but lower-body strength relative to fat-free mass will be higher in females than in males. Therefore, lower-body strength appears comparable with relative strength measures, but the upper body does not appear as strong in women. It appears that relative measures of strength would benefit from some indication of the muscle mass in the specific area of interest, such as regional fat-free mass or muscle cross-sectional area.

Strength Relative to Muscle Cross-Sectional Area

Generally, men have a greater skeletal muscle mass than women do, and regional differences in skeletal muscle mass between the sexes are greatest in the upper body (Janssen et al. 2000; Nindl et al. 2000). The large variation is in total muscle mass, and its distribution in the body may account for much of the difference in strength by sex. The previous discussion of relative measures of strength, including body mass or fat-free body mass, is based on the idea that a person who is physically larger (more specifically, with more muscle mass) would be stronger. In other words, these measures are attempts to correct for muscle

size or muscle cross-sectional area under the assumption that strength depends primarily on muscle mass. Indeed, strength relative to muscle cross-sectional area is significantly correlated to maximal strength (Castro et al. 1995; Miller et al. 1992; Neder et al. 1999) (see figure 9.5). Thus, relative strength between the sexes may be best expressed relative to muscle cross-sectional area.

Over the years, research has clearly and repeatedly demonstrated that normalizing maximal strength (using relative equations per total body weight, fat-free mass, or muscle size) closes the gap between the differences of men and women, especially in the lower body (Kanehisa et al. 1994, 1996). The percentage difference between men and women in concentric isokinetic knee extension torque (60 degrees per second) is gradually reduced when expressed in absolute terms (54% difference), relative to body weight (30% difference), relative to fat-free mass (13% difference), and relative to bone-free lean leg mass (7% difference). The difference between the sexes is statistically significant until peak torque is expressed relative to bone-free lean leg mass (Neder et al. 1999). In the upper arms (elbow flexor plus elbow extensor divided by total muscle cross-sectional area) and thighs (knee flexor plus knee extensor divided by total muscle cross-sectional area) of both trained and untrained people, maximal isometric force

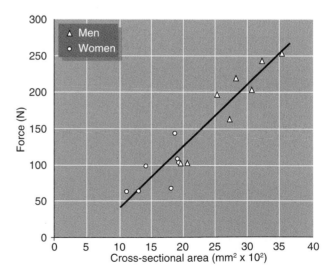

FIGURE 9.5 Elbow flexor strength is significantly correlated to the cross-sectional area of the elbow flexors (r = .95) in a group composed of both sexes.

Adapted, by permission, from A.E.J. Miller et al., 1992, "Gender differences in strength and muscle fiber characteristics," *European Journal of Applied Physiology* 66: 254-264. © Springer-Verlag.

shows a similar pattern when expressed in absolute terms, relative to body weight, relative to fat-free mass, and relative to muscle cross-sectional area (see table 9.3). Women's 1RM knee extension and elbow flexion have been reported to be 80 and 70%, respectively, of men's when expressed relative to fat-free mass (Miller et al. 1992). However, when expressed relative to muscle cross-sectional area, no significant difference is demonstrated between the sexes (Miller et al. 1992). Thus, muscle cross-sectional area may account for most of the difference in strength between men and women.

Some investigations have demonstrated sex differences in strength despite its being expressed relative to cross-sectional area. These investigations demonstrated significant percent differences in muscle cross-sectional area, either in young adults (6% greater in men) or competitive bodybuilders (10% greater in men) (Alway, Grumbt et al. 1989; Kent-Braun, Ng, and Young 2000). Both studies showed a significant relationship between maximal force and muscle size, but the strength differences between the sexes could not be entirely accounted for by muscle cross-sectional area alone. The differences could be related to lower integrated electromyographic activity during maximal voluntary muscle actions in women, longer electrical-mechanical delay time, or both (Kanehisa et al. 1994). It is possible that the method of determining muscle cross-sectional area affected the results, because these studies used ultrasound to determine muscle cross-sectional area. Regardless, any difference in maximal force relative to muscle size is unlikely to be related to noncontractile tissue within a muscle, because no significant differences in noncontractile tissue between the sexes have been observed. Thus, in some investigations, women have displayed lower strength relative to muscle cross-sectional area than men. Again, this area of research begs for more attention.

Sex Differences in Power Output

Sex differences are also seen in power output, a major determinant of success in many sports and activities. In terms of the Olympic-type lifts, power capability plays a crucial role in performance. The untrained woman's average in the clean high pull is 54% of the average man's, whereas after 24 weeks of weight training, the average woman's high pull increases to 66% of the average untrained man's (Kraemer et al. 2002). As of 2012, the world records for Olympic weightlifting in the 63 kg (138.9 lb) weight class for women were 143 kg (315.3 lb) in the clean and jerk and 117 kg (257.9 lb) in the snatch, whereas for men in the 62 kg (136.7 lb) weight class the records were 182 kg (401.2 lb) in the clean and jerk and 153 kg (337.3 lb) in the snatch. The women's world records were 79 and 76% of the men's in the clean and jerk and snatch lift, respectively. Thus, in the competitive world of weightlifting, women seem to be achieving a higher percentage of men's performances. However, a woman's maximal performance in Olympic-type lifts, although impressive, is less than that of her male counterparts in absolute terms as well as relative to total body weight.

Power output during jumping tasks appears to differ between men and women if not corrected for relative fat-free mass. The average woman has been reported to have 54 to 79% of the maximal vertical jump and 75% of the maximal standing long jump of the average man (Colliander and Tesch 1990b; Davies, Greenwood, and Jones 1988; Maud and Shultz 1986; Mayhew and Salm 1990). Even in American Division I volleyball players, men have been shown to have a 48% higher

TABLE 9.3 **Relationship of Maximal Isokinetic Torque at 30 Degrees per Second Relative to Body Weight, Lean Body Mass, and Muscle Cross-Sectional Area**

	Absolute torque		Torque/BW		Torque/FFM		Torque/CSA	
	Elbow flexors	Knee flexors	Elbow flexors	Knee flexors	Elbow flexors	Knee flexors	Elbow flexors	Knee flexors
Untrained females (% of males)	52	73	68	97	74	105	95	101
Trained females (% of males)	66	79	84	102	92	112	98	98

BW = body weight; FFM = free-fat mass; CSA = cross-sectional area.

Data from Castro et al. 1995.

vertical jump than women (McCann and Flanagan 2010), suggesting that even in highly trained athletes a substantial discrepancy is still seen in maximal power. The power generated by women during the standing long jump per unit of lean leg volume is significantly less than that generated by men (Davies, Greenwood, and Jones 1988). If fat-free mass is accounted for, women's short-sprint running and maximal stair-climbing ability (Margaria-Kalamen test) are 77% and 84 to 87%, respectively, of men's (Maud and Shultz 1986; Mayhew and Salm 1990). However, vertical jump ability when expressed relative to fat-free mass shows only small (0-5.5%) differences between the sexes (Maud and Shultz 1986; Mayhew and Salm 1990). Thus, sex differences in power output during jumping tasks, as discussed, may be greatly diminished with the use of relative corrections of the absolute values.

Relative tests of lower-body power output using the Wingate cycling test have shown mixed results in terms of whether men are more powerful than women. Cycling short-sprint ability (30-second Wingate test) is not significantly different (2.5% difference) between the sexes if expressed relative to fat-free mass (Maud and Shultz 1986). A strong correlation ($r = .73$) between mean power assessed by the Wingate test and overall fat-free mass in elite male and female wrestlers has been observed (Vardar et al. 2007). These data indicate, as expected, that greater amounts of fat-free mass would be associated with enhanced power performances and that men, because they have greater fat-free mass than women, would have greater power. However, the study was not able to normalize power by fat-free mass because of the small study population. In a much larger subject population of 1,585 Division I college athletes, men averaged 11.65 (W $\times$ kg^{-1}) relative peak power, whereas women averaged 9.59 (W $\times$ kg^{-1}) (Zupan et al. 2009), showing a large sex difference and contradicting the findings of the earlier study (Maud and Shultz 1986). Thus, although results from Wingate tests have been mixed, men appear to have higher lower-body power output than women in one large investigation.

Women have lower isokinetic power than men except when expressed in terms of relative power. Women's concentric isokinetic knee extension power (300 degrees per second) when expressed in absolute terms, relative to body weight, relative to fat-free mass, and relative to bone-free lean leg mass is 62, 34, 18, and 13% lower than men's, respectively (Neder et al. 1999). This difference is statistically significant until expressed relative to bone-free lean leg mass. Corrections for relative muscle size may eliminate sex differences in isokinetic power. One factor that may affect isokinetic power is how long it takes to reach peak velocity. Brown and colleagues (1998) reported that during isokinetic knee extension, women require a greater portion of the range of motion than men to achieve maximal velocity.

The absolute maximal power output also shows some subtle sex differences when examined as a percentage of 1RM in men and women soccer athletes (Thomas et al. 2007). In the bench press men showed the highest maximal power output at 30% of 1RM, whereas in women the maximal power output was no different between 30 and 50% of 1RM. In the squat jump exercise, maximal power occurred at a larger percentage range of 1RM for women (30-50% of 1RM squat) than men (30-40% of 1RM squat). However, in the hang pull exercise, no sex differences were seen. A number of factors could account for this difference, including training status or absolute strength. Regardless, it appears that women may produce peak power at a higher percentage of 1RM, therefore making power output appear relatively lower compared to men when using a low percentage of 1RM.

Although these data are not consistent, the rationale as to why women may generate less power per unit volume of muscle is often raised. Nevertheless, the amount of directed research on this question is limited. Power at faster velocities of movement would be affected if women's force–velocity curve were different from men's. However, it appears that the drop-off in force as the concentric velocity of movement increases is similar in both sexes (Alway, Sale, and MacDougall 1990; Griffin et al. 1993) and that peak velocity during knee extension is not different between the sexes (Houston, Norman, and Froese 1988). Skeletal muscle rate of force development is slower for the average woman than for the average man (Komi and Karlsson 1978; Ryushi et al. 1988), but that is itself a measure of power, not an answer to the primary question. As previously described, differences in the type II/type I fiber area ratio likely produce differences in power between the sexes. This disparity may also be related to neural differences between the sexes that affect muscle fiber recruitment, some of which could be attributed to decreased activation through physical activity in childhood.

Women appear to produce less power than men on a relative basis in Olympic lifts and Wingate tests, but not in all jumping or isokinetic tasks. As discussed in the earlier section Relative Strength Differences, normalizing by fat-free mass tends to overcorrect for the lower-body measures. This means that relative to total fat-free mass, a normalized measure for lower-body power would be higher in females than in males; despite this, differences in power were seen in some measures. It is apparent, however, that the appropriate correction must be made, and the closer the correction is to muscle fiber cross-sectional area (which does not overcorrect in this manner), the more likely significant differences between the sexes will be observed. In addition, other factors such as the percentage of 1RM that power is tested at or the range of motion permitted may have a large impact on differences seen. Thus, similar to maximal strength, differences in muscle size may account for differences in maximal power output between the sexes.

Pennation Angle

Muscle fiber pennation angle and length are associated with muscle fiber force and velocity shortening capabilities. **Pennation angle** refers to the angle of the muscle fiber's direction of pull relative to the direction of pull of the entire muscle or the direction of pull needed to produce movement at a joint (see chapter 3 and figure 3.13). Larger pennation angles may permit a greater degree of muscle fiber packing, which results in a greater force exerted on a tendon for the same muscle volume. Ultrasonography revealed larger pennation angles in males than in females, but the difference varied by muscle group. For example, male and female pennation angles were as follows: in the tibialis anterior, 9.4 and 8.7 degrees; in the lateral gastrocnemius, 14.1 and 11.8 degrees; in the medial gastrocnemius, 18.6 and 15.8 degrees; and in the soleus, 20.0 and 15.2 degrees, respectively, in males and females (Manal, Roberts, and Buchanan 2008). Unfortunately, statistical significance was not reported. These differences also appeared to increase as the subjects reached maximal voluntary contraction.

Sex differences have also been observed in vertical jump performance in volleyball players, which have been explained by differences in muscle morphology. Muscle architecture of the vastus lateralis, gastrocnemius medialis, and gastrocnemius lateralis were analyzed at rest by ultrasonography. The investigator reported significant relationships between the vastus lateralis muscle size and jump performance ($r = .49-.50$), and nonlinear relationships between muscle size parameters and pennation angles ($R^2 = .67-.77$) (Alegre et al. 2009). Again, more study is needed for gaining a more definitive understanding of the role of muscle fiber pennation angles on sex differences in performances.

In terms of muscle fiber length, longer muscle fibers have more sarcomeres arranged in series, thus permitting greater muscle excursion and contraction velocity. Only a few studies have examined the effect of sex on this muscle fiber characteristic. In the gastrocnemius (medialis and lateralis) and soleus muscles, females are reported to have greater average muscle fiber length and greater variation in fiber length (Chow et al. 2000), whereas males have greater pennation angles in these same muscles. Conversely, no significant sex differences have been reported in fascicle length of the triceps (long head), vastus lateralis, and gastrocnemius (medialis) (Abe et al. 1998), although another study has reported women to have longer fascicle lengths in the vastus lateralis (Kubo et al. 2003). Pennation angle in these same muscles, however, is greater in males. Muscle thickness also appears to be significantly greater in men than in women (Kubo et al. 2003).

Significant positive correlations have been shown between pennation angle and muscle thickness (pennation angle increases as muscle thickness increases) (Abe et al. 1998; Ichinose et al. 1998). The greater muscle thickness in males (Abe et al. 1998; Chow et al. 2000) may account for their greater pennation angle. Because relatively few studies have examined these characteristics, no firm conclusions concerning sex differences in muscle fiber length and pennation angles can be reached. However, regardless of sex, increases in muscle size as a result of resistance training would likely result in increases in pennation angle.

Training in Women

The debate as to whether women can benefit from resistance training appears to have pretty much disappeared in the scientific community. More attention has been placed on the type of programs that are most effective (Kraemer 1993,

2005; Marx et al. 2001; Nichols 2007; Schuenke et al. 2012; Staron 1989). At present research has demonstrated only positive benefits of a properly designed and implemented program for women, as for men. Women experience significant strength gains, muscle fiber–type conversions (Kraemer 1993, 2005; Staron 1989), and increases in bone mineral density (Nichols 2007) from properly designed resistance training programs. Research to date indicates that resistance training is generally at least as beneficial for women as for men, if not more so, because relative gains may be greater as a result of a greater window of potential adaptation.

Strength Gains

When performing the identical resistance training program as men, women generally gain strength at the same rate as, or faster than, men (Cureton et al. 1988; Lemmer et al. 2000, 2007; Wilmore 1974; Wilmore et al. 1978). Over the course of a 24-week (see figure 9.6) and a 16-week (see figure 9.7) resistance training program, women generally gained strength at a rate equal to or greater than that of men. Men may demonstrate greater absolute increases in strength than women, but women generally demonstrate the same or greater relative increases as men. After 24 weeks of resistance training, both younger (20-30 years) and older (65-75 years) women were able to improve strength in the upper and lower body as measured by 1RM. In comparison with men, there was no difference

in the overall gain in strength in the lower body when the results from the leg extension, leg curl, and leg press tests were combined. However, upper-body strength gains seen in the chest press, lateral pull-down, shoulder press, and triceps push-down were significantly lower in the women than in the men (Lemmer et al. 2007). Despite the substantial increases in maximal strength apparent in women with training, the average woman's maximal strength (1RM back squat, bench press, clean high pull) is still significantly lower than the average untrained man's after six months of resistance training (Kraemer, Mazzetti et al. 2001).

It has been proposed that women's strength gains may plateau after three to five months of training and may not progress as quickly as men's after this point (Häkkinen 1993; Häkkinen et al. 1989). When apparent, such a plateau may be related to the type of training program performed. Periodized multiple-set programs performed by women have not shown plateaus in strength, power, and body composition during six to nine months of training (Kraemer et al. 2000; Kraemer, Mazzetti et al. 2001; Marx et al. 2001), whereas nonvaried single-set programs have shown plateaus in strength, power, and body composition after three to four months of training (Kraemer et al. 2000; Marx et al. 2001). This indicates that, as in men, either periodized programs or higher-volume programs may help women avoid training plateaus. Thus, one important chronic training

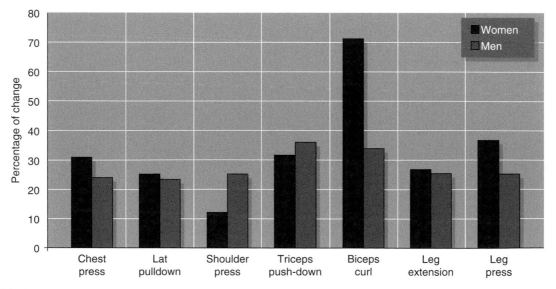

FIGURE 9.6 Male and female strength changes after a 24-week resistance training program.

Data from Lemmer et al. 2001.

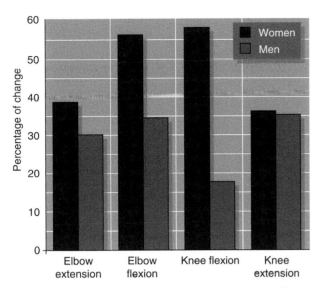

FIGURE 9.7 Male and female strength changes after a 16-week resistance training program.

Data from Cureton et al. 1988.

requirement for women as well as men would be the use of periodization to optimize intensity, volume, and recovery over long-term training programs.

Hypertrophy

Some women do not perform heavy resistance training because they believe their muscles will hypertrophy excessively and that they may look less feminine. This type of fear can limit the use of heavy weights and thereby limit collateral health benefits such as bone and tendon development and other connective tissue adaptations, physical function, and performance. Heavy loading must be included in a training program to recruit the entire motor unit pool. Although hypertrophy of type I and two major type II (types IIa and IIx) muscle fibers can occur in women performing resistance training (Staron et al. 1989, 1991), the average woman's muscles do not hypertrophy excessively most of the time, apparently because of a low number of muscle fibers.

Women do hypertrophy from properly designed resistance training programs that use moderate to heavy loading (e.g., 10RM and lower RM zones). Light weight, however, results in limited changes in muscle fiber hypertrophy. This was demonstrated in a study of untrained women in their 20s that implemented different loading schemes in a lower-body resistance training program that used leg press, squat, and knee extension exercises

(Schuenke et al. 2012). With resistance training zones of 6- to 10RM and 20- to 30RM performed two days a week for the first week and three days a week for the next five weeks, only the 6- to 10RM zone produced hypertrophy of the type I and II muscle fibers. This showed that even in the early phase of training, heavier resistances result in more dramatic changes in muscle fiber hypertrophy. The lighter resistance training group did not result in any changes in muscle fiber hypertrophy. Too often in today's fitness world, light weights and high repetitions are promoted, again playing on women's fears of becoming too muscular. This limits the benefits gained from the programs.

Men and women had their isometric and dynamic elbow flexor strength and biceps brachii cross-sectional area (CSA) measured via MRI before and after 12 weeks of progressive, DCER training. As a result of resistance training, men gained significantly more absolute biceps brachii CSA (4.2 ± 0.1 cm^2 vs. 2.4 ± 0.1 cm^2 in women), and they had significantly greater relative gains in biceps brachii CSA (20.4 ± 0.6 vs. $17.9 \pm 0.5\%$). Although men had greater absolute gains in 1RM elbow flexor strength (4.3 ± 0.1 kg [9.5 ± 0.2 lb] vs. 3.6 ± 0.1 kg [7.9 ± 0.2 lb]), the women had significantly greater relative gains in 1RM strength (64.1 ± 2.0 vs. $39.8 \pm 1.4\%$). Similarly, men had greater absolute gains in isometric strength but significantly lower gains in relative isometric strength (9.5 ± 0.6 kg [20.9 ± 1.3 lb] vs. 6.1 ± 0.3 kg [13.4 ± 0.7 lb] and 22.0 ± 1.1 vs. $15.8 \pm 1.1\%$, respectively).

Women generally experience small yet significant increases in muscle size as indicated by increases in limb circumference in upper-arm and thigh muscle musculature after six months of weight training (Kraemer et al. 2002; Nindl et al. 2000). Starting from an untrained status, women see the largest gains in the arms compared to the thighs when using MRI analyses of the cross-sectional areas of muscle (Kraemer et al. 2004). Although many women worry about circumference measurements, the largest increase in various body circumferences in women after 10 weeks (Wilmore 1974), 12 weeks (Boyer 1990), or 20 weeks (Staron et al. 1991) of resistance training was 0.6, 0.4, and 0.6 cm (0.2, 0.16, and 0.2 in.), respectively. After a six-month resistance training program, a group of female athletes exhibited increases of 3.5, 1.1, and 0.9 cm (1.4, 0.4, and 0.35 in.) (5, 4, and 2%) in shoulder, upper-arm, and thigh circumferences, respectively (Brown and Wilmore 1974). Larger-than-average increases in fat-free mass and limb circumferences in some women are probably related to other factors such as genetic disposition, number of muscle fibers, or higher circulating concentrations of adrenal androgens. With the 10-week program hip, thigh, and abdomen circumferences actually decreased 0.2 to 0.7 cm (0.08 to 0.3 in.). During three different 12-week programs, abdomen circumference decreased 0.2 to 1.1 cm (0.08 to 0.4 in) (Boyer 1990). The finding that resistance training in women results in no change or small changes in body circumferences is supported by other studies (Capen, Bright, and Line 1961; Häkkinen et al. 1989; Staron et al. 1994; Wells, Jokl, and Bohanen 1973). Given that muscle takes up less room than fat, studies really show women becoming leaner rather than larger (i.e., more muscular). Thus, women are not at risk of excessive hypertrophy, as indicated by limb circumference changes, with properly designed progressive heavy resistance training programs.

One outcome of large gains in muscle hypertrophy can be increased body circumferences. However, body circumferences may not change because of decreases in adipose tissue in the limb or body part, which conceals any circumference increase due to increased muscle mass (Mayhew and Gross 1974). Because muscle tissue is denser than adipose tissue, an increase in muscle mass accompanied by a decrease in adipose tissue equaling the gain in muscle mass will result in a slight decrease in body circumferences. The 10-, 12-, and 16-week training studies discussed earlier all demonstrated decreases in skinfold thickness, indicating a decrease in subcutaneous fat. There may, however, be regional body differences in the ability to lose adipose tissue and gain muscle mass (Fleck, Mattie, and Martensen 2006; Nindl et al. 2000). For example, after six months of a periodized weight training program and endurance training, women showed a significant loss in fat mass but no change in lean mass in the arms and trunk. This resulted in a reduction in arm and trunk circumferences.

Using linear periodization over a six-month period of training resulted in significantly greater increases in the cross-sectional area of the arms than of the thighs in women; magnetic resonance image analysis (MRI) was used in this study (Kraemer et al. 2004) (see figure 9.8). Furthermore, with

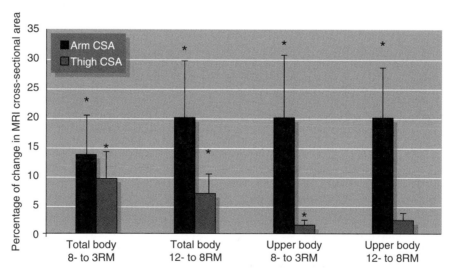

FIGURE 9.8 Percentage increases in a magnetic resonance image analysis (MRI) of the upper arms and thighs of women who participated in a periodized resistance training program for only the total body or upper body. Different periodization ranges were used, with one group in each range going from 8RM to 3RM and the other going from 12RM to 8 RM in a linear periodization model over six months of training. Exercise specificity clearly exists; women who did not train the lower body had no changes in thigh cross-sectional area. In addition, the arms of these women were more responsive to training potentially because of a lack of significant arm training in their typical activity programs.

*$P \leq .05$ from pretraining value. Arm values were significantly higher than thigh values in the groups that trained the total body.

Data from Kraemer et al. 2004.

the use of the 8- to 3RM sequence of loading, more of the muscles of the thigh saw individual increases in cross-sectional area. Obviously, as a result of the lack of prior arm training of any significant amount in the non-resistance-trained women, the arm musculature made dramatic increases because of the larger window of adaptational potential. The lack of increases or even small decreases in body circumferences are encouraging for women who want increased strength and the fit-firm look of trained muscle without increased body circumferences.

Men and women display similar relative changes in hypertrophy with resistance exercise. Increased muscle cross-sectional area (determined by computerized tomography) after isometric training (Davies, Greenwood, and Jones 1988) and after dynamic constant external resistance training (Cureton et al. 1988; O'Hagan et al. 1995b) show the same relative increases in both sexes. After eight weeks of resistance training, all fiber types in both sexes showed similar gradual increases in cross-sectional area, although these were not statistically significant (Staron et al. 1994). This information indicates that changes in both whole muscle and fiber cross-sectional area during an initial short-term training period are similar between the sexes. When a focused short-term (six to eight weeks) resistance training program is implemented in untrained men and women, dramatic increases are seen with moderate and heavy (3- to 11RM) resistance training programs in all muscle fiber cross-sectional areas but not when using very light weights (>20RM) (Campos et al. 2002; Schuenke et al 2012). One difference between the sexes is that the transformation of myosin heavy chains from type IIx to type IIab to type IIa takes place at a faster rate in women than in men (Staron et al. 1994). As discussed in the previous section, the cross-sectional area of type II muscle fibers of untrained women is less than that of men (Alway et al. 1992; Alway, Grumbt et al. 1989). This difference in untrained muscle fiber cross-sectional area between the sexes may result in a greater potential for type II fiber hypertrophy in women. Such a tendency has been shown in women performing weight training for the lower body (Staron et al. 1994); they demonstrated muscle fiber hypertrophy (vastus lateralis) of 25, 23, and 11% in types IIa, IIx, and I fibers, respectively. Men demonstrated a less dramatic difference in fiber type hypertrophy of 19, 20, and 17% in types IIa, IIx, and I fiber types, respectively, after performing the identical resistance training program (Staron et al. 1994). However, relative increases in type II fiber cross-sectional area in the upper body (biceps) appear to be similar between the sexes (O'Hagan 1995b). Thus, some differences between the sexes may exist in the hypertrophy response of muscle fibers to various resistance training programs.

Peak Oxygen Consumption

Women's relative peak oxygen consumption (mL · kg^{-1} · min^{-1}) increases 8% on average as a result of 8 to 20 weeks of circuit weight training, and men's increases an average of 5% over the same time period (Gettman and Pollock 1981). The average woman's cardiorespiratory endurance capabilities therefore increase more than those of the average man after circuit weight training. The reason women's peak oxygen consumption increases more than men's is unclear, but it may be related to the average man's higher cardiorespiratory fitness level before beginning a circuit weight training program. Surprisingly, despite previous studies showing women having a more favorable response to circuit weight training, recent findings indicate that men have higher acute responses in absolute and relative oxygen uptake, systolic blood pressure, and respiratory exchange ratio when compared with women (Ortego et al. 2009). However, the higher acute responses are not entirely clear at this time and do not necessarily indicate that this difference between the sexes affects long-term adaptations.

Women can realize even greater gains in relative peak oxygen consumption ($\dot{V}O_2$peak) if they perform an aerobic circuit weight training program, which consists of resistance training exercises interspersed with short periods of aerobic training. This type of program, when performed using five groups of five resistance and callisthenic exercises separated by five 3-minute periods of aerobic exercise, results in a 22% increase in peak oxygen consumption in previously untrained women over 12 weeks of training (Mosher et al. 1994). Care must be taken not to use it as the only type of workout in a training program, though, because circuit training has limitations in addressing other neuromuscular training goals due to the exclusive use of lighter weights. Also, if done too frequently as a type of "extreme metabolic" training without recovery days, overreaching syndromes may occur (Bergeron et al. 2011).

Body Composition

Body composition changes are a goal of many women and men performing resistance training. Increases in fat-free mass and decreases in percent body fat from short-term (8 to 20 weeks) resistance training programs are of the same magnitude in both sexes. Men and women performing identical short-term weight training programs have both shown significant decreases in percent body fat with no significant difference shown between the sexes (Staron et al. 2000). It has also been reported that both sexes show a significant increase in fat-free mass and no change in percent body fat when performing the identical weight training program for 24 weeks (Lemmer et al. 2001). In this study only men showed a significant reduction in fat mass, indicating that women may have a more difficult time losing body fat during resistance training.

Body composition changes in various regions of the body after training may also be an important consideration in women (Nindl et al. 2000). After six months of performing a periodized weight training program and endurance training exercise, women showed a 31% loss in fat mass with no change in lean mass in the arms. They also showed a 5.5% gain in lean mass in the legs, but no change in fat mass. These results indicate that women may have more difficulty increasing lean mass in the upper body than in the lower body. However, other data dramatically contradict this assertion. After performing several weight training programs for six months, untrained women demonstrated upper-arm muscle cross-sectional area increases from approximately 15 to 19% and increases in thigh muscle cross-sectional area from approximately 5 to 9% (Kraemer et al. 2004). This indicates that the upper-arm musculature undergoes greater hypertrophy than the thigh (again, see figure 9.8).

This conclusion is supported by another report of increased lean tissue in the upper but not lower bodies of women performing 14 weeks of resistance training (Fleck, Mattie, and Martensen 2006). This suggests the possibility of large gains in the upper body in women who may not expose their arms to the same intensity of recruitment as their lower body musculature in everyday and recreational activities. Thus, the need for resistance training may even be greater to reduce the dramatic loss of muscle in women's upper bodies that occurs with aging (see chapter 11).

Women's Hormonal Responses to Resistance Training

The acute and chronic hormonal responses to resistance training affects the anabolic/catabolic environment to which muscle tissue is exposed. This is true for both sexes and may partly explain gains in muscle size and strength from resistance training. When interpreting a woman's hormonal response to training, the potential effects of the menstrual cycle must be considered, because hormone concentrations can fluctuate depending on the phase of the menstrual cycle. It must also be remembered that a low concentration of a hormone does not necessarily mean that the hormone does not have an active role in controlling a bodily function or process, such as tissue growth. Hormones at low concentrations may still affect a bodily function as a result of increased interaction with receptors, higher rates of use, or both. The possible effect of a low hormone concentration is discussed in box 9.1.

Testosterone

At rest, men normally have 10 to 40 times more testosterone in circulation than women do (Kraemer et al. 1991; Vingren et al. 2010; Wright 1980). This may account in part for the larger muscle mass of men compared to women because testosterone affects the developmental cell cycle, is an acute signal to make protein, and interacts with a variety of cell-signaling processes including the activation of satellite cells and neurons. However, as noted in chapter 3, testosterone responses to resistance exercise depend on several factors, including the amount of muscle mass activated and the manipulation of the acute program variables—specifically, intensity and the volume of the exercise protocol (Fragala et al. 2011a; Kraemer et al. 1991).

Even though the resting testosterone concentrations of women are low compared to those of men, small changes in its concentration may affect muscle tissue growth. Women's serum testosterone has been reported to increase significantly in response to one session of resistance training (Cumming et al. 1987; Nindl, Kraemer, Gotshalk et al. 2001). However, acute testosterone increases in women in response to one training session are variable and low compared to those of men (see figure 9.9) (Fragala et al. 2011a; Kraemer et

The Anabolic Environment for Muscle Hypertrophy in Women

Hormonal responses to resistance training in men and women are varied. One of the most profound differences between the sexes is in the anabolic hormone testosterone. Women have 20 to 40 times lower concentrations than men of this so-called male hormone. In men, testosterone is an important hormone that signals anabolic processes in a host of target cells and tissues including skeletal muscle (Vingren et al. 2010). Circulating concentrations of testosterone are known to increase significantly in men in response to resistance exercise or, for that matter, exercise stress in general. It is important to emphasize here that only activated muscle fibers experience androgen receptor upregulation and subsequent testosterone signaling that eventually interacts with the cell's DNA. Thus, the signal for testosterone in response to stress is only realized when a receptor binds to the hormone to create the start of a signal cascade. Interestingly, although aerobic exercise can increase testosterone in both men and women, the type I motor units used to perform such oxidative submaximal aerobic exercise cause the associated fibers to downregulate the androgen receptor and binding, along with subsequent signaling, does not occur. This demonstrates a difference in aerobic and resistance exercise in terms of growth stimulus for both sexes.

Women have a dramatically attenuated testosterone response to acute resistance exercise, yet interestingly enough, a woman's androgen receptors upregulate in response to these small changes in hormone with acute resistance exercise. Despite lower testosterone levels, women do experience increases in muscle cross-sectional area as a result of resistance exercise. Interestingly, research has shown that in women, growth hormones and insulin-like growth factor (IGF)-I appear to compensate for the attenuated testosterone response to signal muscle tissue growth and therefore may play a more central role in muscle hypertrophy than they do in men.

Vingren, J.L., Kraemer, W.J., Ratamess, N.A., Anderson, J.M., Volek, J.S., and Maresh, C.M. 2010. Testosterone physiology in resistance exercise and training: The up-stream regulatory elements. *Sports Medicine* 40: 1037-1053.

al. 1991; Kraemer, Fleck et al. 1993; Nindl, Kraemer, Gotshalk et al. 2001). In the study depicted in figure 9.9, the testosterone concentration of women was not affected by the exercise session of three sets of 10RM with one minute rest. In comparison, men's serum testosterone concentrations consistently increased in response to the identical resistance training session. Although most studies in women have demonstrated no significant increases in testosterone in response to resistance exercise, interestingly, some studies have reported transient and significant elevations in testosterone in response to resistance exercise (Nindl, Kraemer, Gotshalk et al. 2001).

Further research is required to determine the underlying factors contributing to this difference in hormonal response in women and the combination of acute exercise variables that stimulate a change in testosterone response. However, it is obvious that despite the lower response to the acute resistance exercise stress, women's androgen receptors show a similar response pattern and interactions with testosterone as men's, demonstrating an active interface with testosterone signaling in women (Vingren et al. 2009).

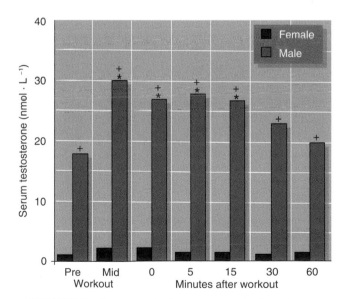

FIGURE 9.9 Serum testosterone concentrations in men and women caused by performing the same resistance training session of three sets of eight exercises at 10RM with one-minute rests between sets and exercises.

* = significantly different from preexercise value of same sex; + = significantly different from female value at the same time point.

Adapted, by permission, from W.J. Kraemer et al., 1991, "Endogenous anabolic hormonal and growth factor responses to heavy resistance exercise in males and females," *International Journal of Sports Medicine* 12: 231.

Another known factor affecting resistance training–induced elevations is the time of day at which training occurs. It appears that men experience greater testosterone spikes when resistance training occurs later in the day. This may be due to higher resting concentrations at other times of the day, which may not allow dramatic spikes in circulating or saliva concentrations. This effect in the saliva has been observed in a weightlifting competition (Crewther and Christian 2010). Women do not appear to experience the same magnitude of time-dependent testosterone response to exercise, which is likely due to lower resting concentrations of testosterone in all biocompartments of the body including blood and saliva.

Interestingly, resting serum testosterone concentrations are not significantly different between untrained and highly competitive women Olympic weightlifters (Stoessel et al. 1991). This again attests to the fact that testosterone is a signal hormone and not an accumulating entity that tracks gains in strength or tissue mass. Eight weeks of resistance training (Staron et al. 1994) and 16 weeks of power training (Häkkinen et al. 1990) have both been reported not to alter resting serum testosterone concentrations in women. However, other studies have demonstrated that eight weeks of resistance training by women does significantly increase resting testosterone concentrations as well as the immediate postexercise response compared to the exercise response in the untrained state. This is most likely the body's attempt to establish a new higher resting homeostatic concentration and optimize the acute response to exercise (Kraemer, Staron et al. 1998). Nevertheless, a potential confounding factor is that none of the aforementioned studies controlled for menstrual cycle phase. When menstrual cycle phase was controlled (serum obtained in early follicular phase), increases in resting testosterone concentrations from six months of resistance training occurred. As with the aforementioned study, this is most likely an attempt to establish a higher resting baseline in the trained state (Enea et al. 2009; Marx et al. 2001). Additionally, training volume did affect the resting testosterone concentration response. Women performing a multiple-set periodized program demonstrated a small but significantly greater increase in resting testosterone concentration after three and six months of training than did women performing a nonvaried single-set program (Kraemer et al.

1998; Marx et al. 2001). The testosterone response of women has also been shown to be related to regional body fat distribution. Women having a higher degree of upper-body fat show an accentuated response, and the underlying mechanisms for this remain speculative (Nindl, Kraemer, Gotshalk et al. 2001).

Cortisol

Cortisol plays several regulatory roles in metabolism and has catabolic effects on protein metabolism (see chapter 3). Women's serum cortisol concentrations, when menstrual cycle phase is controlled, can increase in response to a resistance training session (Cumming et al. 1987; Kraemer, Fleck et al. 1993; Mulligan et al. 1996); the same can occur when menstrual cycle phase is not controlled (Kraemer, Staron et al. 1998). Additionally, higher training volumes (one vs. three sets of exercises) result in an increased cortisol response in women (Kraemer, Fleck et al. 1993; Mulligan et al. 1996). Similarly, the cortisol response of men also depends in part on training volume.

It appears that an athlete's level of training affects the hormonal response (Nunes et al. 2011) that may occur as a result of exercise stress, such as high-intensity resistance exercise. Additionally, an athlete's emotional state can also influence the magnitude of the cortisol response, regardless of sex. Significant cortisol increases have been observed in both men and women athletes immediately before a competition and up to one hour postcompetition (Crewther et al. 2011; McLellan et al. 2011). It has been hypothesized that this anticipatory spike in cortisol may actually have performance-enhancing effects by heightening arousal and creating enough "positive" stress to drive athletic performance.

No changes were observed in resting serum cortisol concentrations after eight weeks of resistance training (Staron et al. 1994) or 16 weeks of power-type resistance training in women (Häkkinen et al. 1990) when menstrual cycle phase was not controlled. However, resting cortisol concentrations have also decreased after eight weeks of resistance training when menstrual cycle phase was not controlled, and the response immediately after a resistance training session is decreased after eight weeks of resistance training compared to the untrained state. This indicates a reduction in total stress from some combination of factors (Kraemer, Staron et al. 1998).

Training volume may be an important factor in determining whether resting cortisol concentrations will decrease in response to resistance training. After six months of a multiple-set periodized resistance training program in women (~30 years) in which menstrual cycle phase was controlled, resting concentrations of cortisol decreased significantly, whereas no significant change occurred following a six-month single-set program (Marx et al. 2001). Reductions in cortisol concentrations at rest appear to reduce the total physiological stress. However, in resistance-trained men and women the glucocorticoid receptor content in muscle was not altered by an acute resistance exercise stress using six sets of a 10RM squat protocol with two-minute rest periods (Vingren et al. 2009). However, women did demonstrate a much higher concentration of glucocorticoid receptors than men at all time points, potentially demonstrating a more dramatic influence of cortisol in resistance-trained women than resistance-trained men for catabolic signaling to the muscle cell target. More research will be needed to clarify this observed difference. The lack of any up- or downregulation of glucocorticoid receptors in muscle in response to acute exercise stress or over the 70-minute time period from rest through recovery indicates a saturation of receptors with any catabolic signals to muscle from acute cortisol increases are potentially more impactful on other cell targets such as immune cells (Fragala et al. 20011a; Fragala et al. 2011c). Such data again demonstrate the need to look at multiple targets for hormonal signaling with resistance exercise stress. Again, during acute exercise and recovery phases other cells may see differential regulation of their glucocorticoid receptors. With six sets of 5RM and three-minute rest periods in the squat exercise, men have significantly higher B-lymphocyte glucocorticoid receptor content before exercise than women do. However, with heavy resistance exercise both sexes show significant decreases in B-lymphocyte glucocorticoid receptor content followed by significant increases at both one and six hours into recovery (Fragala et al. 2011c). Thus, the receptor targets available for cortisol to bind with can vary with sex and both the type of cells and the time frame when receptors are measured.

Growth Hormones

As discussed in considerable detail in chapter 3, different forms of growth hormone (GH) exist from the original 22 kD 191 amino acid polypeptide derived from the DNA in the anterior pituitary somatotrophs to higher- and lower-molecular-weight aggregates or combinations of GH and binding proteins. Research has demonstrated in women that resistance exercise–induced acute elevations in growth hormone depend on the molecular weight fraction examined as well as the type of assay used (Hymer et al. 2001; Kraemer, Gordon et al. 1991; Kraemer, Vingren et al. 2009; Kraemer, Nindl et al. 2006; Kraemer, Fleck et al. 1993; Kraemer and Spiering 2006; Kraemer, Staron et al. 1998; Mulligan et al. 1996). Unless otherwise noted in this section, we will define GH as the 22 kD form because this has been the primary form studied.

Similar to men, women respond to resistance training sessions (see figure 9.10) with an increase in serum human 22 kD GH. Additionally, the GH response to resistance exercise, much like the response of other hormones (testosterone and cortisol), also depends on the manipulation of the acute program variables (Kraemer et al. 2010; Kraemer and Spiering 2006). As in men, the acute increase in GH in women is responsive to the total

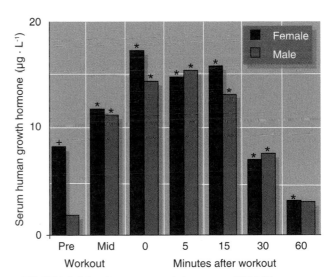

FIGURE 9.10 Serum growth hormone (22 kD) concentrations as measured by radioimmunoassay in men and women performing the same resistance training session of three sets of eight exercises and a 10RM with one-minute rests between sets and exercises.

* = significantly different from preexercise value of same gender; + = significantly different from female value at the same time point.

Adapted, by permission, from W.J. Kraemer et al., 1991, "Endogenous anabolic hormonal and growth factor responses to heavy resistance exercise in males and females," *International Journal of Sports Medicine* 12: 232.

volume of a session; a significantly higher response is observed with sessions of greater volume (one vs. three sets of each exercise) compared to sessions of lower volume (Kraemer et al. 1991; Kraemer, Fleck et al. 1993; Mulligan et al. 1996). Higher-volume sessions are especially effective at increasing the human GH response in both sexes when short rest periods (approximately one minute) are used between sets and exercises because the release of the 22 kD GH is linked to the low pH and high H+ concentrations as reflected by the blood lactate concentrations (Kraemer et al. 2010). As mentioned in box 9.1, growth hormones may play a greater role in signaling muscle tissue hypertrophy in women than in men (Kraemer et al. 2010).

Training status may also affect women's acute human growth hormone response. Women with at least one year of weight training experience exhibited a longer time period of growth hormone elevation above resting values (resulting in a greater magnitude of growth hormone response) compared to women with no regular weight training experience (Kraemer, Vingren et al. 2009; Kraemer, Nindl et al. 2006; Kraemer and Spiering 2006; Taylor et al. 2000). Women's resting serum human growth hormone concentration is unaffected by eight weeks (Kraemer, Staron et al. 1998) and six months (Marx et al. 2001) of resistance training. However, it has been reported that women with at least one year of weight training experience had a lower resting serum growth hormone concentration immediately before a resistance training session than women with no regular weight training experience (Taylor et al. 2000). But this may well be due to homeostatic changes in the larger-molecular-weight forms (Kraemer et al. 2010). In other words, several isoforms of growth hormone exist, and the decrease could be related to a shift in the 22 kD form to aggregate a form(s) that is not picked up by the typical GH assay. However, to date, the acute growth hormone response and the resting chronic response of no change appear to be quite similar between the sexes for aggregate bioactive GH.

The acute and chronic responses to resistance training of various hormones create the anabolic environment to which skeletal muscle, bone, and other tissues are exposed. The hormonal response to resistance training is responsible in part for both sexes' strength and muscle hypertrophy increases following resistance training. Although women's testosterone response to resistance training appears to be lower than that of their male counterparts, the growth hormone response to resistance training is quite similar between the sexes. Although not discussed here, other hormones, such as IGF-I, luteinizing hormone, follicle-stimulating hormone, and estradiol (see box 9.2) may also be responsive to resistance training and thus affect women's long-term adaptations to resistance training. Each hormone has specific targets, and these targets can be diverse; together they interact to optimize the physiological environment for the development of cells spanning from those of the

 ## BOX 9.2 **RESEARCH**

The Role of Estradiol in Exercise-Induced Endocrine Responses

Compared to men, women have an attenuated inflammatory response to muscle damage and also fatigue more slowly than men do in response to acute exercise stress (Fragala et al. 2011a). These differences are generally in part attributed to sex-specific circulating hormone levels—primarily estradiol in women and testosterone in men. In women, estradiol functions as an antioxidant and membrane stabilizer during exercise, particularly exercise that induces high levels of oxidative stress, such as intense aerobic and resistance exercise. The protective role of estradiol appears to be a primary factor in mitigating muscle damage due to exercise stress and is evident in the smaller inflammatory response seen in women. Even at rest, women have lower levels of circulating creatine kinase, one of the most commonly measured markers of muscle damage, in the blood than do men. Although estradiol response to resistance exercise must be further researched, the protective role of estradiol indicates that it has important implications for women in terms of muscle tissue fatigability and recovery from exercise stress.

Fragala, M.S., Kraemer, W.J., Denegar, C.R., Maresh, C.M., Mastro, A.M., and Volek, J.S. 2011. Neuroendocrine-immune interactions and responses to exercise. *Sports Medicine* 41: 621-639.

immune system to connective tissues (e.g., bone and tendon) to skeletal muscle. Thus, signaling hormones elevate in response to a stressor, are circulated in the blood, and attach to a target cell receptor to deliver a signal; they then decrease in concentration and the signal ends (Fragala et al. 2011a; Kraemer et al. 2010).

Menstrual Cycle

The menstrual cycle is an important topic in women's health. Understanding the basics is vital for exercise conditioning professionals working with women because it has physiological relevance to a host of issues from nutritional status to performance.

Oligomenorrhea and Secondary Amenorrhea

Differences in menstrual cycle patterns among women can be considerable, and it can therefore be difficult to determine what constitutes a regular, as opposed to an irregular, menstrual cycle for a particular woman. Regardless, some women engaged in physical training, including resistance training, experience variations in their menstrual cycles. Irregularities include shortening of the luteal (postovulatory) phase to less than 10 days; lack of ovulation (release of an egg); **oligomenorrhea,** an irregular menstrual cycle (more than 36 days between menstrual flows) in women who previously had a normal menstrual pattern or a cycle; and **secondary amenorrhea,** the absence of menstruation for 180 days or more in women who previously menstruated regularly.

Although such irregularities may be seen in athletic women, exercise is typically secondary to the primary issue of low energy availability (i.e., inadequate food or caloric intake) (Ducher et al. 2011; Loucks, Kiens, and Wright 2011). Menstrual disorders in active women are often related to the female athlete triad (disordered eating, amenorrhea, and osteoporosis) and are more frequently seen in sports emphasizing low body mass or subjective scoring systems, such as gymnastics and figure skating. In fact, energy deficiency in active women can be accurately predicted by a psychological test of the drive for thinness (DeSouza et al. 2007). Thirty-one percent of women in so-called thin-build sports have disordered eating patterns as compared to 5.5% of the regular population (Byrne and McLean 2002). Primary amenorrhea

is seen in 1% of the regular population and 22% of women participating in cheerleading, diving, and gymnastics, all of which are judged subjectively. Secondary amenorrhea, seen in 2 to 5% of the regular population, is seen in 69% of women engaged in ballet training (Abraham et al. 1982).

Out of 199 Olympic-style weightlifters with an average age of 16 years, 25% reported having irregular menses; only three of these athletes aged 13 to 15 had not yet begun to menstruate (Liu, Liu, and Qin 1987). The prevalence of oligomenorrhea and secondary amenorrhea in women not taking oral contraceptives was 20 and 2%, respectively, in a group of recreational resistance trainers; 71 and 14%, respectively, in a group of women who had competed in at least one bodybuilding contest (which emphasizes very low body mass and subjective judging); and 9 and 4% in a group of sedentary women (Walberg and Johnston 1991). Thirty-three percent of women who competed in a bodybuilding contest and did not take oral contraceptives reported oligomenorrhea or secondary amenorrhea (Elliot and Goldberg 1983). Thus, some sports or activities are associated with an increased risk of menstrual irregularities.

In distance runners, greater training volume, intensity, frequency, and training session duration have all been implicated as factors that increase the risk of menstrual irregularities (Cameron, Wark, and Telford 1992; Gray and Dale 1984; Loucks and Horvath 1985). Athletes who train for long periods of time, daily or over years, at high intensities appear to be at greater risk of experiencing oligomenorrhea and secondary amenorrhea. In female recreational resistance trainers who do not use oral contraceptives, the incidence of either oligomenorrhea or amenorrhea is 22%, whereas it is 85% in competitive bodybuilders (Walberg and Johnston 1991). Thus, greater resistance training intensity or volume seems to result in a greater risk of menstrual irregularities likely because of the increased energy requirement. Even in eumenorrheic athletes (those who menstruate normally), anovulation or luteal phase deficiency was seen in 78% of runners (DeSouza et al. 1998). That said, not all athletes performing high-volume, high-intensity training experience menstrual irregularities. Also, it is important to note that amenorrhea and other menstrual disorders are often the result of inadequate caloric intake to meet the demands of the athlete rather than the level of physical activity alone.

The incidence of amenorrhea is higher in younger than in older women. In runners, 85% of those experiencing secondary amenorrhea were under 30 years of age (Speroff and Redwine 1980). Several researchers have also proposed that physical training at an early age delays menarche and that late menarche is associated with a greater chance of experiencing amenorrhea (Gray and Dale 1984; Loucks and Horvath 1985; Nattiv et al. 1994). A previous pregnancy has been associated with a decreased risk of amenorrhea (Loucks and Horvath 1985). Insufficient caloric intake, psychological stress, abrupt changes in body composition, and previous menstrual irregularities have all been associated with increased risk of menstrual irregularities (Lebenstedt, Platte, and Pirke 1999; Loucks and Horvath 1985; Nattiv et al. 1994; Shepard 2000b). All of these factors may be associated with hormonal disturbances resulting in menstrual irregularities. For example, insufficient caloric intake while performing physical training may predispose women to hormonal disturbances (luteinizing hormone secretion) associated with menstrual cycle disturbances (Williams et al. 1995), whereas sufficient caloric intake may prevent these changes.

Amenorrhea is serious in terms of health consequences (Roupas and Georgopoulos 2011). The restoration of energy is the first priority with exercise-induced amenorrhea (Kopp-Woodroffe et al. 1999). In today's environment, seeking assistance to manage such conditions has lost much of its former, unfounded social stigma. Screening for eating disorders should be conducted, and if appropriate, psychological treatment should be arranged (Nattiv et al. 2007). Increases in weight typically restore normal menstrual function and alleviate, in part, the decreased bone density often seen in this population (Mendelsohn and Warren 2010).

Premenstrual Symptoms and Dysmenorrhea

One of the first adaptations to an exercise program is a decrease in normal premenstrual symptoms (Prior, Vigna, and McKay 1992), such as breast enlargement, appetite cravings, bloating, and mood changes. Active, athletic women have fewer difficulties with premenstrual symptoms than sedentary women do (Prior, Vigna, and McKay 1992). If training is decreased, premenstrual symptoms

may increase, especially if weight gain is concurrent with a decrease in training (Prior, Vigna, and McKay 1992). Thus, athletes with excessive premenstrual symptoms who are decreasing training should not do so abruptly and should try to avoid large weight gains.

Dysmenorrhea, or painful menstruation, may accompany premenstrual symptoms (Prior, Vigna, and McKay 1992). Increased production of the hormone prostaglandin is associated with uterine cramping and is thought to be the cause of dysmenorrhea (Dawood 1983). Dysmenorrhea is reported by 60 to 70% of adult women, and increases with chronological and gynecological age (Brooks-Gunn and Rubb 1983; Widholm 1979). Like other premenstrual symptoms, dysmenorrhea occurs less frequently and is less severe in athletes than in the general population (Dale, Gerlach, and Wilhite 1979; Timonen and Procope 1971). The reduced frequency and severity of premenstrual and dysmenorrhea symptoms in athletes could be caused by differences in hormonal concentrations or in pain tolerance. In either case, physical training appears to decrease the incidence of premenstrual symptoms and dysmenorrhea. Some studies have reviewed treatment strategies for athletes with dysmenorrhea and other premenstrual symptoms (Prior, Vigna, and McKay 1992). Oral contraceptives have also been used as a treatment for dysmenorrhea (Lebrun 1994).

Menstrual Cycle Phase Effects on Strength and Weight Training

Surprisingly, little information is available on the effect of menstrual cycle phase on maximal strength, as differences in training cycles, sport competition, birth control, and individual differences among women's responses make definitive findings difficult to determine. Lebrun (1994) reported no differences in strength measures between the follicular phase (menstrual flow to approximately 14 days after menstrual flow) and the luteal phase (approximately 14 days after the menstrual flow to the beginning of the next menstrual flow). However, women vary greatly in the effect of menstrual cycle phase on maximal strength.

The explanation of why strength or physical performance may vary during different phases of the menstrual cycle is normally explained by hormonal variations. For example, progesterone is supposed to have a catabolic effect on muscle and reaches its highest blood concentrations during the luteal phase. Cortisol, which also has catabolic effects, also reaches higher concentrations during the luteal phase than during the follicular phase. Testosterone remains at a relatively constant concentration throughout the entire menstrual cycle, except for an increase during ovulation. Such increases in catabolic hormones can be offset by a disinhibition of receptors to anabolic hormones. Thus, receptors may not interact with catabolic hormones even though their concentrations have increased.

These hormonal changes that occur during the phases of the menstrual cycle have led some to suggest that strength training should vary according to the menstrual cycle phases. The varying hormone concentrations result in conditions for muscle growth and repair being better in the follicular compared to the luteal phase (Reis, Frick, and Schmidbleicher 1995). Thus, resistance training intensity or volume may need to be reduced during the luteal phase and increased during the follicular phase (Reis, Frick, and Schmidbleicher 1995). Comparing such a training plan to a traditional resistance training plan over two consecutive menstrual cycles (approximately eight weeks) has been done (Reis, Frick, and Schmidbleicher 1995). Normal training consisted of performing resistance training every third day throughout the menstrual cycle. "Menstrual cycle–triggered training" consisted of performing training every second day during the follicular phase and about once a week during the luteal phase. Maximal isometric leg strength increased 33% following menstrual cycle–triggered training and 13% with the normal training. Muscle cross-sectional area increases of the quadriceps femoris were equivalent (approximately 4%) between the two groups; however, maximal strength per muscle cross-sectional area was significantly greater with the menstrual cycle–triggered training (27 vs. 10%). Significant correlations among hormone, strength, and muscle cross-sectional area increases were shown. For example, estradiol in the training period correlated with increased muscle cross-sectional area ($r = .85$), and changes in progesterone concentrations between the first and second luteal phases in the training period correlated with maximal strength increases ($r = .77$).

Not all information supports the rationale of the menstrual cycle–triggered training plan that hormonal conditions during the follicular phase are more conducive to muscle tissue growth and repair than those during the luteal phase. In untrained women a higher acute growth hormone response to resistance training is apparent in the luteal phase compared to the follicular phase (Kraemer, Fleck et al. 1993). Thus, although varying training with the phases of the menstrual cycle is an attractive hypothesis, more study of this subject is needed.

Performance During the Menstrual Cycle and Menstrual Problems

Lebrun (1994) noted little or no difference in aerobic and anaerobic performance at various times during the menstrual cycle. No differences in anaerobic capacity were seen between the midluteal and midfollicular phases with cycle sprints (Shaharudin, Ghosh, and Ismail 2011). However, decrements in performance during the premenstrual or menstrual phase have been shown; the best performances occur during the immediate postmenstrual period and the 15th day of the menstrual cycle (Allsen, Parsons, and Bryce 1977; Doolittle and Engebretsen 1972; Lebrun 1994). Likewise, peak power, anaerobic capacity, and fatigue rate (Wingate test) have been shown to be negatively affected during the follicular phase compared to the luteal phase (Masterson 1999). Individual variations in the effects of menstrual cycle phase on performance can be substantial; some athletes even notice an improvement in performance during menstruation (Lebrun 1994).

Reasons for decreased performance during the premenstrual or menstrual phase may be associated with many factors, including self-expectancies, negative attitudes toward menstruation, and weight gain. Although the effect of controlling premenstrual symptoms and dysmenorrhea with oral contraceptives is unclear, some anecdotal and retrospective studies have reported increases in performance with the use of oral contraceptives (Lebrun 1994). The possible detrimental effect on athletic performance of premenstrual symptoms or dysmenorrhea has led some researchers to recommend the use of oral contraceptives or progesterone injections to ensure that menses does not occur during major competitions (Liu, Liu, and Qin 1987). However, Olympic medal–winning performances have taken place during all phases of the menstrual cycle. The effect of the menstrual cycle on performance is therefore unclear and is probably very specific to the individual. Oligomenorrhea and amenorrhea, although having potential long-term health effects such as bone loss, should have no effect on performance. However, menstrual cycle disturbances accompanied by low estradiol and progesterone serum concentrations show an attenuated growth hormone response to a resistance training session (Nakamura et al. 2011). This could affect long-term adaptations to resistance training. Overall, participation in physical training and athletic events during menstruation or any other phase of the menstrual cycle has no detrimental effect on health and should not be discouraged.

Bone Density

Changes in bone mass or density relate to two major types of bone, cancellous and cortical. Cancellous, or trabecular, bone has a high turnover rate and responds to changes in hormonal concentrations to a greater extent than it does to exercise. Cortical bone has a slower turnover rate and is influenced more by mechanical strain than cancellous bone is (Rico et al. 1994; Young et al. 1994). In the female athlete triad, with sedentary aging, and as a result of medical conditions, decreased bone density and mass can occur both in the lumbar spine, composed predominantly of cancellous bone (Cameron, Wark, and Telford 1992; Prior, Vigna, and McKay 1992; Tomten et al. 1998), and in the axial skeleton or vertebral column, composed primarily of cortical bone (Nyburgh et al. 1993; Tomten et al 1998). Thus, the entire skeleton of amenorrheic women, including amenorrheic athletes (Nyburgh et al. 1993), can experience a decrease in bone density. Over one year, healthy runners with an average luteal phase greater than 11 days showed no significant change in lumbar cancellous bone mineral density, whereas runners with an average luteal phase of less than 10 days showed a significant 3.6% lumbar cancellous bone mineral density loss (Petit, Prior, and Barr 1999). This indicates that variations in the menstrual cycle may affect bone density.

With appropriate energy availability, women can experience increased bone density with physical activity (Chilibeck, Sale, and Webber 1995; Dalsky et al. 1988; DeCree, Vermeulen, and Ostyn 1991; Jacobson et al. 1984), including weight training (Chilibeck, Sale, and Webber 1995). Increased bone density with training was shown in women aged 20 to 23 (Hawkins et al. 1999) and 40 to 50 (Dornemann et al. 1997). Significant correlations of fat-free mass, regional lean tissue, and strength to bone density support the contention that weight training can increase bone density (Aloia et al. 1995; Hughes et al. 1995; Nichols et al. 1995). However, no significant change in bone mineral density with resistance training in women 28 years of age (Nindl et al. 2000) and 54 years of age (Pruit et al. 1992) has also been shown. Many factors, including the weight training program design, duration of training, and site at which bone density is measured may affect whether bone density changes occur after weight training. In a series of case studies of elite women powerlifters, middle-aged women's bone density was shown to be dramatically higher than that of their age- or sex-matched peers (48-54 years); this suggests that long-term weight training using heavy weights has dramatic effects on the aging process of bone in women (Walters, Jezequel, and Grove 2012). Well-designed weight training programs appear to offer a good possibility of increasing bone density in women, or at least slowing bone density loss as women age. This is true even after menopause (see box 9.3).

Menstrual Cycle Dysfunction and Bone Density

Menstrual dysfunction is related to decreased bone density and an increased risk of osteoporosis (Cameron, Wark, and Telford 1992; Constantini 1994; DeCree, Vermeulen, and Ostyn 1991; Nyburgh et al. 1993; Shepard 2000b; Tomten et al. 1998). It has been reported that amenorrheic athletes have greater bone density than amenorrheic nonathletes (Cameron, Wark, and Telford 1992). The effect of menstrual dysfunction on bone density may be dramatic. Women who have never had regular menstrual cycles show on average a 17% deficit in bone density compared to their normally menstruating peers (Shephard 2000b). The loss of bone mass may occur predominantly during the first three to four years of amenorrhea (Cann et al. 1984). Age at menarche, age at menarche with subsequent amenorrhea, duration of oligomenorrhea, and duration of menstrual dysfunction have all been correlated with reduced bone density compared to normal values (Cameron, Wark, and Telford 1992; Drinkwater, Bruemner, and Chestnut 1990; Lloyd et al. 1987;

? BOX 9.3 PRACTICAL QUESTION

Can Strength Training Be Beneficial to Menopausal Women?

With an increasing life span, more females are living longer after menopause. Menopause leads to many physiological changes that increase the risk of many diseases, such as diabetes, obesity, and hypertension as well changes in body composition. Diet and exercise are recommended to combat these changes. Menopause is associated with sarcopenia and osteopenia (Leite et al. 2010). Because resistance training has been shown to increase bone and muscle mass as well as strength, it appears to be an appropriate treatment for some of the changes that occur during menopause. However, despite the potential benefits, studies examining the effects of resistance training on menopausal women are lacking. Studies are needed for elucidating the precise molecular and intracellular mechanisms that lead to the negative responses of the body during menopause, and to establish a better dose–response for the prescription of resistance training for menopausal women.

Leite, R.D., Prestes, J., Pereira, G.B., Shiguemoto, G.E., and Perez, S.E.A. 2010. Menopause: Highlighting the effects. *International Journal of Sports Medicine* 31: 761-767.

Nyburgh et al. 1993). Young amenorrheic women may therefore be losing bone mass at a point in their lives when bone mass should be increasing. Athletes who were amenorrheic and then regained menses for 15 months showed an increase in bone density, whereas athletes who did not regain menses showed no change or a continued loss of bone density (Cameron, Wark, and Telford 1992). How readily normal bone density can or may be restored in amenorrheic women once a normal menstrual cycle resumes is yet to be determined (Drinkwater, Bruemner, and Chestnut 1990).

Highly trained women in any activity who do not take in sufficient calories to achieve sufficient energy levels appear to have a greater-than-normal risk for menstrual problems (as previously discussed) and therefore may also be at risk for osteoporosis. Women performing recreational activity, including weight training, over two years showed a positive effect on total-body bone mineral content. However, oral contraceptives had a negative impact on total-body bone mineral content even when exercise was performed (Weaver et al. 2001).

Hormonal Mechanisms of Menstrual Cycle Disturbances and Bone Density Loss

Bone mass, or density, in healthy women generally increases as a result of physical activity. Menstrual cycle disturbances are related to factors that stimulate bone resorption (bone loss) and formation. Stressors such as physical stress from training, psychological stress, inadequate caloric intake, and

other dietary deficiencies may result in menstrual cycle disturbances (Chilibeck, Sale, and Webber 1995; Prior, Vigna, and McKay 1992). These stressors cause an increase in corticotropin-releasing hormone from the hypothalamus (see figure 9.11), causing a decrease in gonadotropin-releasing hormone, which in turn results in a decrease in the pituitary hormones, luteinizing hormone and follicle-stimulating hormone. The decrease in the pituitary hormones may result in menstrual cycle disturbance. These disturbances decrease the ovarian hormones progesterone and estrogen, which in turn eventually affect osteoclasts and osteoblasts, which result in resorption and bone formation, respectively. The net result is a decrease in bone mass or density.

Decreased concentrations of the ovarian hormones estrogen and progesterone are the hormonal factors most frequently associated with osteoporosis and bone loss. Some have suggested that estrogen may reduce bone resorption but that it has little impact on bone formation, resulting in a net loss of bone (Cameron, Wark, and Telford 1992; DeCree, Vermeulen, and Ostyn 1991). Receptors for estrogens, androgens, progesterone, and corticosteroids have been found in bone (Bland 2000; Quaedackers et al. 2001). It is also possible that a hormone such as estrogen has an indirect effect on bone by acting through another hormone (DeCree, Vermeulen, and Ostyn 1991).

Corticotropin released from the anterior pituitary stimulates cortisol release from the adrenal cortex; this may result in bone loss and be related to menstrual cycle disturbances (DeSouza and

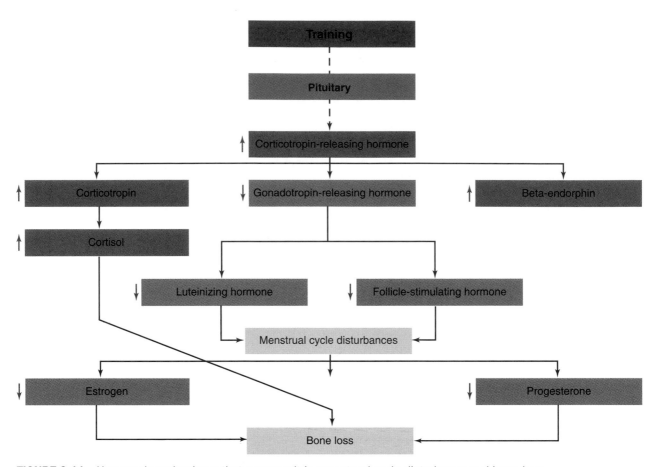

FIGURE 9.11 Hormonal mechanisms that may result in menstrual cycle disturbance and bone loss.

Metzger 1991; Prior, Vigna, and McKay 1992). Increased beta-endorphin may also be associated with menstrual cycle disturbances (Cameron, Wark, and Telford 1992; DeCree, Vermeulen, and Ostyn 1991; Prior, Vigna, and McKay 1992). Increases in beta-endorphin have been shown to occur in women in response to resistance training, especially when accompanied by a negative caloric balance, and this could be responsible in part for menstrual cycle disturbances in these women (Walberg-Rankin, Franke, and Gwazdauskas 1992). Many other hormones, such as growth hormone, testosterone, estradiol, progesterone, corticosteroids, insulin, and calcitonin, are also probably involved to varying degrees with menstrual cycle disturbances and bone loss in active women (Bland 2000; Cameron, Wark, and Telford 1992; Prior, Vigna, and McKay 1992).

Local factors are also involved in bone resorption and formation. Prostaglandin, which stimulates osteoblasts, is released from bone itself and is implicated in the early response of bone formation to mechanical loading (Chilibeck, Sale, and Webber 1995; Chow 2000). Insulin-like growth factor I, which stimulates bone formation, is produced by many cells in response to growth hormone and may be released from bone itself in response to mechanical loading from exercise and prostaglandin stimulation (Chow 2000; Snow, Rosen, and Robinson 2000). Collectively, hormonal responses result in decreased bone mass or density in women with menstrual cycle disturbances.

Knee Injuries

In sports that require jumping and cutting, women are four to six times more likely to sustain a serious knee injury than their male counterparts in the same sports (Hewett 2000). The greater knee injury rate in women compared to men is likely multifactorial. Anatomical, neuromuscular, and hormonal differences are all thought to affect knee injuries in women.

One anatomical difference between men and women relates to the **Q-angle**. The Q-angle is the angle between a line connecting the anterior superior iliac crest to the midpoint of the patella and a line connecting the midpoint of the patella to the tibia tubercle. Women tend to have a wider pelvic structure and their lower-extremity alignment results in a greater Q-angle than men's. Researchers have reported Q-angle to be both associated and not associated with incidence of knee injury (Hewett 2000; Lathinghouse and Trimble 2000). Women also have smaller femoral notch widths relative to the anterior cruciate ligament than men, but evidence that this accounts for the increased injury rates in women is inconclusive (Hewett 2000). If the femoral notch theory were valid, no conditioning program could reduce the knee injury rate in women.

Neuromuscular differences between the sexes have also been proposed to explain the differential knee injury rate between the sexes. This theory hypothesizes that differences in muscle recruitment patterns and longer reaction times or longer time to generate maximum force during cutting or landing predisposes women to knee injury. Some differences in recruitment patterns, such as female athletes relying more on their quadriceps muscle in response to anterior tibial translation as compared to males, have been shown (Huston and Wojtys 1996). Likewise, longer reaction times and longer times to generate maximal force have also been shown in females compared to males (Hewett 2000; Huston and Wojtys 1996). Other studies have reported no difference between the sexes in these measures.

Hormonal variations throughout the menstrual cycle have also been theorized to predispose women to knee injury (Hewett 2000). The hormones estrogen, progesterone, and relaxin have been reported to increase joint laxity, slow muscle relaxation, affect tendon and ligament strength, and decrease motor skills (Hewett 2000). Joint laxity does increase and decrease during the menstrual cycle (Shultz et al. 2012). Increased knee laxity is associated with increased knee valgus and external rotation, which are associated with an increased risk of injury. These factors could predispose women to knee injury at various phases within the menstrual cycle. A study examining younger women at three different phases of their menstrual cycle linked estrogen to a chronic,

rather than an acute, impact on tendon behavior. The scientists suggested that in terms of the properties of tendons, the menstrual cycle phase does not necessarily need to be considered because no significant differences were observed in tendon properties over the three phases (Burgess, Pearson, and Onambélé 2010).

Physical conditioning programs, including plyometrics and weight training, have been shown to drastically reduce the knee injury rate in women (Hewett 2000). American high school female athletes who participated in a six-week conditioning program had a knee injury rate 1.3 times higher than that of a control group of high school male athletes (Hewett et al. 1999), whereas female athletes who did not participate in the conditioning program had a knee injury rate 4.8 times higher than that of the male athletes and 3.6 times higher than that of the female athletes participating in the conditioning program. Those with the worst starting scores from the Landing Error Score System (LESS), a clinical movement assessment tool used for identifying improper movement patterns during jump-landing tasks, appear to benefit most from such interventions (DiStefano et al. 2009). One investigation found that a nine-month intervention was more effective than a three-month intervention in terms of long-term retention of improvements in movement assessed by LESS (Padua et al. 2012). These studies do not address the mechanism by which injury rate is reduced. However, they do demonstrate that physical conditioning programs can reduce the knee injury rates in women (see box 9.4).

General Needs Analysis

The needs analysis for a woman in a particular sport or activity or for general strength and fitness is conducted using the outline presented in chapter 5. What it takes to be successful in a particular sport or activity is generally dictated by the sport or activity and not by the sex of the participant. The training program for the particular sport is based on the requirements for successful participation in that sport and the athlete's individual weaknesses, training history, and injury history. So the process of designing a resistance training program for a sport or activity is essentially the same for both sexes. The absolute strength differences between the sexes make it apparent that the key difference

❓ BOX 9.4 PRACTICAL QUESTION

Can Strength Training Reduce the Risk of Knee Injury?

When quadriceps strength is significantly greater than the strength of the hamstrings, both the hamstrings and anterior cruciate ligament (ACL) become more susceptible to injury because they are responsible for preventing anterior translation of the tibia on the femur. If the quadriceps can produce more anterior translation than the hamstrings and ACL can tolerate, injury is likely. Therefore, increasing the strength of the hamstrings in relation to the quadriceps could theoretically reduce the risk of ACL injury in women.

Six weeks of emphasizing hamstring-strengthening exercises in the strength training regimen of 12 NCAA Division I female soccer players showed a possible reduction of knee injury risk. In addition to other strength and conditioning exercises, the straight-leg deadlift, good morning, trunk hyperextension, resistance machine single-leg curl, resisted sled walking, and exercise ball leg curl were performed twice per week. All of these exercises involve the hamstring muscle group. Over the six weeks of training the functional ratio increased from 0.96 to 1.08 (Holcomb et al. 2007). Functional ratio was calculated as eccentric hamstring isokinetic torque divided by concentric quadriceps isokinetic torque. This ratio when greater than 1.0 indicates a decrease in the risk of anterior cruciate ligament injury (Li et al. 1996). Therefore, strength training may be beneficial in reducing ACL injuries, which are particularly common in females.

Holcomb, W.R., Rubley, M.D., Lee, H.J., and Guadagnoli, M.A. 2007. Effect of hamstring-emphasized resistance training on hamstrings: Quadriceps strength ratios. *Journal of Strength and Conditioning Research* 21: 41-47.

Li, R.C., Maffulli, N., Hsu, T.C., and Chan, K.M. 1996. Isokinetic strength of the quadriceps and hamstrings and functional ability of anterior cruciate deficient knees in recreation athletes. *British Journal of Sports Medicine* 30: 161-164.

---

between programs for men and those for women is the total amount of resistance used for particular exercises.

The higher incidence of knee injuries in women should be considered in the program design. A preseason conditioning program, including lower-body plyometrics and weight training, can be performed to help decrease the knee injury rate in at-risk sports. Continuing an in-season conditioning program may also be advisable so that any physiological adaptations with potentially positive effects on the incidence of knee injury are maintained throughout the season.

Women's generally smaller upper-body muscle mass and reduced upper-body performance compared to men may limit their performance in sports or activities that require upper-body strength and power. The training program for such sports or activities therefore may need to stress upper-body exercises to increase total upper-body strength and power. This can be accomplished in several ways. If the program is relatively low in total training volume, one or two upper-body exercises may be added to the program. Perhaps the most effective way to address this need is to lengthen the preseason weight training program to provide additional time for physiological adaptations.

Women's weaker upper-body musculature can also cause difficulties in the performance of structural exercises, such as power cleans and squats. In these types of exercises, women may find it very difficult or impossible to support with their upper bodies the resistances their lower bodies can tolerate. Practitioners should not allow lifters to use incorrect technique, in any exercise including structural exercises, for the purpose of lifting slightly greater resistances; doing so can cause serious injury. Instead, the program should stress exercises to strengthen the upper-body musculature over time.

All women, including those interested in improving health and appearance, benefit from heavier weights that increase bone density. Incorporating loads of over 80% of the person's 1RM once every one to two weeks is appropriate for all ages (even elderly women as discussed in chapter 11). Unless contraindicated, exercises should emphasize loading at the spine, hip, and wrist and with structural exercises such as the squat. Heavy weights with fewer repetitions should stimulate bone growth and improve both performance and functional health. Jumping exercises may also improve bone density as a result of the ground reaction forces on the body, which is encouraging due to the benefits of plyometric training for the prevention of knee injuries.

Summary

Although women's absolute strength is less than men's, the difference is greatly reduced or nonexistent if expressed relative to fat-free mass or muscle cross-sectional area. Women's lower-body strength relative to fat-free mass is more equivalent to men's than is their upper-body strength because of a greater relative distribution of women's fat-free mass in the lower body. Women's adaptations to resistance training programs are generally of the same magnitude or even slightly greater than men's for some variables. This emphasizes that, in general, resistance training programs for women do not need to be different from those for men, except that the absolute resistance used by women will be less. A focus on the use of more upper-body exercises to stimulate and maximize the use of all available motor units might be one important aspect to optimize upper-body development. In addition, the use of periodized training seems paramount to ensure long-term resistance training adherence and adaptational effectiveness.

In most cases, physical activity has beneficial impacts on the menstrual cycle and premenstrual syndrome in women. Menstrual irregularities such as amenorrhea may be more prevalent in women performing strenuous activity than in the normal population, particularly in sports emphasizing lean body mass and subjective scoring systems. These menstrual irregularities typically indicate an energy imbalance and may be associated with the female athlete triad of amenorrhea, disordered eating, and osteoporosis. In the case of disordered eating, screening for eating disorders and psychological follow-up, if necessary, is essential. Once energy level is restored, menstrual anomalies typically disappear and bone density often improves, although the person should be monitored for long-term health issues.

Resistance training can result in many of the fitness characteristics desired by many women including a fit appearance and increased strength and power for daily life, occupational demands, and sport activities. Often, the slender and fit appearance women seek through cardiorespiratory training alone is only possible when cardiorespiratory training is paired with resistance exercise. However, excessive cardiorespiratory exercise can lead to compatibility issues in muscular development and performance (see chapter 4). Women should not be afraid to use heavier resistances and plyometric exercises in their training programs. They should also avoid becoming victims of marketing ploys and adopting unfounded fears that are detrimental to optimal training results for all women.

SELECTED READINGS

Burgess, K.E., Pearson, S.J., and Onambélé, G.L. 2010. Patellar tendon properties with fluctuating menstrual cycle hormones. *Journal of Strength and Conditioning Research* 24: 2088-2095.

De Souza, M.J., Hontscharuk, R., Olmsted, M., Kerr, G., and Williams, N.I. 2007. Drive for thinness score is a proxy indicator of energy deficiency in exercising women. *Appetite* 48: 359-367.

DiStefano, L.J., Padua, D.A., DiStefano, M.J., and Marshall, S.W. 2009. Influence of age, sex, technique, and exercise program on movement patterns after an anterior cruciate ligament injury prevention program in youth soccer players. *American Journal of Sports Medicine* 37: 495-505.

Drinkwater, B.L. 1984. Women and exercise: Physiological aspects. In *Exercise and sport science reviews*, edited by R.L. Terjung, 21-52. Lexington, KY: MAL Callamore Press.

Harbo, T., Brincks, J., and Andersen, H. 2012. Maximal isokinetic and isometric muscle strength of major muscle groups related to age, body mass, height, and sex in 178 healthy subjects. *European Journal of Applied Physiology* 112: 267-275.

Kraemer, W.J., Mazzetti, S.A., Nindl, B.C., Gotshalk, L.A., Volek, J.S., Bush, J.A., Marx, J.O., Dohi, K., Gómez, A.L., Miles, M., Fleck, S.J., Newton, R.U., and Häkkinen, K. 2001. Effect of resistance training on women's strength/power and occupational performances. *Medicine & Science in Sports & Exercise* 33: 1011-1025.

Kraemer, W.J., Nindl, B.C., Ratamess, N.A., Gotshalk, L.A., Volek, J.S., Fleck, S.J., Newton, R.U., and Häkkinen, K. 2004. Changes in muscle hypertrophy in women with periodized resistance training. *Medicine & Science in Sports & Exercise* 36: 697-708.

Kraemer, W.J., Nindl, B.C., Volek, J.S., Marx, J.O., Gotshalk, L.A., Bush, J.A., Welsch, J.R., Vingren, J.L., Spiering, B.A., Fragala, M.S., Hatfield, D.L., Ho, J.Y., Maresh, C.M., Mastro, A.M., and Hymer, W.C. 2008. Influence of oral contraceptive use on growth hormone in vivo bioactivity following resistance exercise: Responses of molecular mass variants. *Growth Hormone and IGF Research* 18: 238-244.

Laubach, L.L. 1976. Comparative muscular strength of men and women: A review of the literature. *Aviation, Space and Environmental Medicine* 47: 534-542.

Lester, M.E., Urso, M.L., Evans, R.K., Pierce, J.R., Spiering, B.A., Maresh, C.M., Hatfield, D.L., Kraemer, W.J., and

Nindl, B.C. 2009. Influence of exercise mode and osteogenic index on bone biomarker responses during short-term physical training. *Bone* 45: 768-776.

Loucks, A.B., Kiens, B., and Wright, H.H. 2011. Energy availability in athletes. *Journal of Sports Science* 29: S7-15.

Nattiv, A., Loucks, A.B., Manore, M.M., Sanborn, C.F., Sundgot-Borgen, J., and Warren, M.P. 2007. American College of Sports Medicine position stand. The female athlete triad. *Medicine & Science in Sports & Exercise* 39: 1867-1882.

Puthucheary, Z., Skipworth, J.R., Rawal, J., Loosemore, M., Van Someren, K., and Montgomery, H.E. 2011. Genetic influences in sport and physical performance. *Sports Medicine* 41(10): 845-859.

Ratamess, N.A., Chiarello, C.M., Sacco, A.J., Hoffman, J.R., Faigenbaum, A.D., Ross, R.E., and Kang, J. 2012. The effects of rest interval length manipulation of the first upper-body resistance exercise in sequence on acute performance of subsequent exercises in men and women. *Journal of Strength and Conditioning Research* 26: 2929-2938.

Singh, J.A., Schmitz, K.H., and Petit, M.A. 2009. Effect of resistance exercise on bone mineral density in premenopausal women. *Joint Bone Spine* 76: 273-280.

Staron, R.S., Hagerman, F.C., Hikida, R.S., Murray, T.F., Hostler. D.P., Crill, M.T., Ragg, K.E., and Toma, K. 2000. Fiber type composition of the vastus lateralis muscle of young men and women. *Journal of Histochemistry and Cytochemistry* 48: 623-629.

Staron, R.S., Karapondo, D.L., Kraemer, W.J., Fry, A.C., Gordon, S.E., Falkel, J.E., Hagerman, F.C., and Hikida, R.S. 1994. Skeletal muscle adaptations during the early phase of heavy-resistance training in men and women. *Journal of Applied Physiology* 76: 1247-1255.

Volek, J.S., Forsythe, C.E., and Kraemer, W.J. 2006. Nutritional aspects of women strength athletes. *British Journal of Sports Medicine* 40: 742-748.

von Stengel, S., Kemmler, W., Kalender, W.A., Engelke, K., and Lauber, D. 2007. Differential effects of strength versus power training on bone mineral density in post-menopausal women: A 2-year longitudinal study. *British Journal of Sports Medicine* 41: 649-655.

Walberg, J.L., and Johnston, C.S. 1991. Menstrual function and eating behavior in female recreational weight lifters and competitive body builders. *Medicine & Science in Sports & Exercise* 23: 30-36.

Walters, P.H., Jezequel, J.J., and Grove, M.B. 2012. Case study: Bone mineral density of two elite senior female powerlifters. *Journal of Strength and Conditioning Research* 26 (3): 867-872.

Warren, M., Petit, M.A., Hannan, P.J., and Schmitz, K.H. 2008. Strength training effects on bone mineral content and density in premenopausal women. *Medicine & Science in Sports & Exercise* 40: 1282-1288.

10

Children and Resistance Training

After studying this chapter, you should be able to

1. outline training adaptations in preadolescents and adolescents,
2. discuss acute and chronic injuries due to training in preadolescents and adolescents,
3. describe the steps in developing a safe, effective weight training program for preadolescents and adolescents,
4. describe resistance training program differences in children of varying ages,
5. develop a periodized resistance training program for preadolescents and adolescents, and
6. describe equipment modifications that may be needed when children perform resistance training, including appropriate resistance increases during the program.

The popularity of resistance training among prepubescents and adolescents has increased dramatically. The acceptance of youth resistance training by qualified professional organizations is becoming universal. The following organizations have produced statements indicating that youth resistance training is both effective and safe when properly supervised: American Academy of Pediatrics (2008), American College of Sports Medicine (2008), American Orthopedic Society for Sports Medicine (1988), Australian Strength and Conditioning Association (2007), British Association of Exercise and Sport Sciences (2004), Canadian Society for Exercise Physiology (2008), International Federation of Sports Medicine (1998), International Olympic Committee (2008), National Association for Sport and Physical Education (2008), National Strength and Conditioning Association (2009), and South African Sports Medicine Association (2001).

Despite these statements, youth resistance training still raises some important issues and concerns. Can resistance training harm a child's skeletal system? What type of weight training program is appropriate for prepubescent males (prior to the growth spurt) and females (prior to first menstruation)? What type of weight training program is appropriate for a pubescent, and how should this program differ from a prepubescent program? How can resistance training be safely adapted for youth? All of these questions have answers based on research. However, some misconceptions and misunderstandings still exist.

When evaluating information concerning injuries, such as skeletal muscle injuries, one needs to consider the difference between resistance training and the sports of Olympic weightlifting, powerlifting, and bodybuilding. Resistance training does not have to involve the use of maximal (1RM) or near-maximal resistances. On the other hand, competitive Olympic weightlifting and powerlifting, by their very nature, involve lifting maximal resistances, and bodybuilding emphasizes the development of hypertrophy, which, in children, is typically less than that shown by adults.

As with all physical activity, injuries as a result of resistance training will occur. However, the risk to children of injury from weight training may not be as dramatic as perceived (Caine, DiFiori, and Maffulli 2006; Hamil 1994; Meyer et al. 2009;

Meyer et al. 2010). Paradoxically, many of the competitive sporting activities children participate in carry much greater risk of injury than resistance training. It is now apparent that the benefits from a properly designed and supervised resistance training program for children outweigh the risks (Miller, Cheathman, and Patel 2010).

Training Adaptations

Statements or position stands from the organizations listed earlier indicate that children can benefit from participation in a properly prescribed and supervised resistance training program. The major benefits include the following:

- Increased muscular strength, power, and local muscular endurance (i.e., the ability of a muscle or muscles to perform multiple repetitions against a given resistance)
- Decreased cardiovascular risk
- Improved performance in sports and recreation
- Increased resistance to sport-related injuries

In addition, resistance training of youths improves psychological well-being and helps promote and develop lifelong exercise habits. To confer these benefits, however, resistance training programs for youth must be properly designed and progressed, stress correct exercise technique, and be competently supervised. All of these areas are paramount for safe and effective programs. Although greater understanding has diminished the unrealistic fears about youth and resistance training, further research is needed concerning all aspects of youth resistance training.

Strength Gains

Research clearly demonstrates that resistance training confers significant strength increases in children (see table 10.1) (National Strength and Conditioning Association 2009). Meta-analyses demonstrate that boys younger than 13 years and older than 16 years as well as girls younger than 11 years and older than 14 years (Payne et al. 1997) and boys and girls under the ages of 12 and 13, respectively, demonstrate significant strength gains following resistance training (Falk and Tenenbaum 1996). Additionally, strength gains due to resistance training increase with maturity in both prepubertal and postpubertal children (see box

10.1). Strength gains as great as 74% have been shown after eight weeks of progressive resistance training (Faigenbaum et al. 1993), although more typically gains of approximately 30% are found after short-term resistance training programs (8 to 20 weeks) in children (National Strength and Conditioning Association 2009). Relative (percent improvement) strength gains in prepubescents are equal to or greater than those shown by adolescents (National Strength and Conditioning Association 2009). Adolescents' absolute strength gains are greater than prepubescents' gains and generally less than adults' gains, and there is no clear evidence that strength gains between preadolescent girls and boys are different (National Strength and Conditioning Association 2009). It is important to note that many studies report that no injuries occurred in preadolescents or adolescents from performing resistance training (National Strength and Conditioning Association 2009; Sgro et al. 2009).

Some early weight training studies reporting no strength gains in children resulted in the belief that strength or muscle size gains above normal growth would not occur in children performing weight training as a result of an immature hormonal system (Legwold 1982; Vrijens 1978). In untrained subjects, resting testosterone and growth hormone levels increase from age 11 to age 18 in boys, but not in girls (Ramos et al. 1998). Despite this sex difference, a significant positive correlation ($r = .64$, boys; $r = .46$, girls) in both sexes is found between testosterone concentration and absolute muscle strength. This indicates that hormonal changes are in part responsible for increased strength from age 11 to age 18 in both sexes. Increases in the resting blood concentrations of hormones (testosterone, growth hormone) indicative of a more anabolic environment can occur as a result of resistance training in prepubertal (11-13 years) and pubertal (14-16 years) boys (Tsolakis et al. 2000). Additionally, insulin sensitivity increases in adolescent (15 years) males and females with short-term (12-20 weeks) resistance training (Shaibi et al. 2006; Van Der Heijden et al. 2010). Thus, although more research is definitely needed, changes in resting hormonal concentrations may in part explain increased strength from resistance training in prepubertal and pubertal boys and girls.

Training history may also play a part in hormonal changes, and therefore strength and hypertrophy increases, over time in young people. Male

TABLE 10.1 Representative Strength Training Studies in Prepubescent Children

Reference	Age or grade	Sex	Training mode	Testing mode	Duration (wk)	Training description	Frequency (per wk)	Control group	Strength increase
Nielson et al. 1980	7-19	F	Isometric	Isometric	5	24 maximal actions	3	Yes	Yes
Blanksby and Gregory 1981	10-14	M and F	Weights	Isometric	3	2 × 8- to 12RM	3	Yes	Yes
Baumgartner and Wood 1984	Grades 3-6	M and F	Calisthenics	Calisthenics	12	1 × to fatigue	3	Yes	Yes
Pfeiffer and Francis 1986	8-11	M	Weights	Isokinetic	8	3 × 10 at 50, 75, and 100% of 10RM	3	Yes	Yes
Sewall and Micheli 1986	10-11	M and F	Weight machines	Isometric	9	3 × 10-12 at 50%, 80%, and 100% 10- to 12RM	3	Yes	Yes
Weltman et al. 1986	6-11	M	Isokinetic	Isokinetic	14	3 × 30 sec	3	Yes	Yes
Docherty et al. 1987	12.6	M	Isokinetic		4-6	2 × 20 sec	3	No	No
Rains et al. 1987	8.3	M	Hydraulic concentric	Hydraulic concentric	14	Max number of reps in 30 sec	3	Yes	Yes
Sailors and Berg 1987	12.6	M	Free weights	Free weights	8	3 × 5 at 65, 80, and 100% of 5RM	3	Yes	Yes
Siegal, Camaione, and Manfredi . 1988	8.4	M and F	Weights, calisthenics	Isometric, calisthenics	12	30-45 sec exercise, 15 sec rest	3	Yes	Yes
Ramsay et al. 1990	9-11	M	Free weights and machines	Weights, isokinetic, isometric	20	3 × 10- to 12RM, 1 × to fatigue	3	Yes	Yes
Fukunaga, Funato, and Ikegawa 1992	Grades 1, 3, and 5	M and F	Isometric	Isometric, isokinetic	12	3 × 10 sec max isometric action, 2 times/day	3	Yes	Yes
Faigenbaum et al. 1993	10.8	M and F	Weights	Weights	8	3 × 10-15	2	Yes	Yes
Ozmun, Mikesky, and Surburg 1994	9.8-11.6	M and F	Free weights	Free weights and isokinetic	8	3 × 7- to 10RM	3	Yes	Yes
Falk and Mor 1996	6-8	M	Calisthenics and weight exercises	Body weight exercises	12	3 × 1-15	2	Yes	Yes
Faigenbaum et al. 1996	7-12	M and F	DCER machines	DCER machines	8	4 wk: 1 × 10 and 2 × 6 4 wk: 3 × 6	2	Yes	Yes
Faigenbaum et al. 2001	8.1	M and F	DCER machines	DCER machines	8	1 × 6- to 8RM	2	Yes	No
Faigenbaum et al. 2001	8.1	M and F	DCER machines	DCER machines	8	1 × 13- to 15RM	2	Yes	Yes
Faigenbaum et al. 2002	12.3	M and F	Machines	Machines	8	1 × 15	2	Yes	Yes
Pikosky et al. 2002	8.6	M and F	DCER	DCER machines	6	1 or 2 × 10- to 15RM	2	No	Yes
Faigenbaum et al. 2007	13.9	M			9		2	No	Yes
Naylor, Watts et al. 2008	12	M and F	Machines	Machines	8	2 × 8 at 75-90% of 1RM	5	Yes	Yes
McGuigan et al. 2009	9.7	M and F	Machines and free weights	Machines	8	3 × 3- to 12RM	3	No	Yes

DCER = dynamic constant external resistance.

Adapted, by permission, from A. Faigenbaum, 1993, "Strength training: A guide for teachers and coaches," *National Strength and Conditioning Association Journal* 15(5): 20-29.

BOX 10.1 RESEARCH

Puberty and Maximal Strength Gains

It is generally believed, and some research supports this belief, that during puberty maximal strength significantly increases. However, this does not mean that resistance training of postpubertal children results in greater strength gains than training of prepubertal children. A meta-analysis indicates that the maturity of both prepubertal and postpubertal children significantly affects strength gains as a result of weight training (Behringer et al. 2010). However, there is no significant increase in strength gains due to resistance training during puberty compared to prepuberty or postpuberty. This meta-analysis also concluded that longer-duration studies and increased training frequency significantly affect strength gains. The conclusion that longer-duration studies result in greater strength gains indirectly supports the belief that hypertrophy contributes to strength gains in youth. Although the conclusion that increased frequency (e.g., two or three sessions per week) is optimal for strength gains, the meta-analysis also showed that strength increases are related to the increased number of sets performed.

Behringer, M., Heede, A., Yue, Z., and Mester, J. 2010. Effects of resistance training in children and adolescents: A meta-analysis. *Pediatrics* 125: 999-1000.

Olympic weightlifters 14 to 17 years old with less than two years of training experience did not show an acute increase in serum testosterone after a training session; however, lifters with more than two years of training experience did (Kraemer et al. 1992). This indicates that past training experience affects the response to training.

Similar to women, prepubescent children do not show an increase in serum testosterone concentration after an exercise bout (see figure 10.1). Yet both women and prepubescent children clearly can experience strength increases from resistance training. Neural factors and other hormonal changes are in part responsible for increased strength and hypertrophy in women (see chapter 9) and may also play a role in strength increases in prepubescent boys and girls (National Strength and Conditioning Association 2009). Although the exact mechanisms resulting in strength increases in prepubescent and pubescent girls and boys are not completely elucidated, resistance training clearly increases strength in both.

Muscle Hypertrophy

Weight training in adults brings about strength increases in part as a result of neural adaptations and hypertrophy. However, the majority of evidence indicates that strength gains in prepubescents are related much more to neural mechanisms than to hypertrophy (Blimkie 1993; National Strength and Conditioning Association 2009).

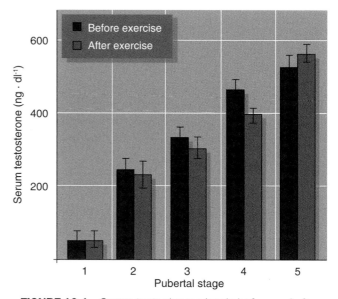

FIGURE 10.1 Serum testosterone levels before and after an exercise bout in pubescent children. Pubertal stages 1 through 5 refer to the maturity of the subject: 1 = immature and 5 = fully mature.

Adapted, by permission, from T.D. Fahey et al., 1989, "Pubertal stage difference in hormonal and hematological responses to maximal exercise in males," *Journal of Applied Physiology* 46: 825.

Some early studies showed increases in muscle size with resistance training (Fukunaga, Funato, and Ikegawa 1992), but the majority of early studies ranging in length from 8 to 20 weeks did not show an increase in the muscle size of preadolescents with resistance training (Blimkie 1993;

National Strength and Conditioning Association 2009; Ramsay et al. 1990). Many of these studies used skinfolds to determine body composition, which may not be sensitive enough to detect small yet significant changes in fat-free mass. More recent studies using predominantly dual-energy X-ray absorptiometry (DEXA) have shown small, but significant, increases in lean body mass in preadolescents and adolescents. Training of boys and girls 8 to 10 years old for 8 to 24 weeks resulted in significant increases of lean body mass at 8, 16, and 24 weeks ranging from 5 to 11% (Sgro et al. 2009). Training boys and girls aged 9.7 years (McGuigan et al. 2009) and 12 years (Naylor, Watts et al. 2008) for eight weeks resulted in significant increases in lean body mass of 5 and 2%, respectively. In adolescents (15 years) increases in lean body mass of 4 and 7.4% over 12 and 16 weeks of training, respectively, have been shown (Shaibi et al. 2006; Van Der Heijden et al. 2010). All of these studies trained overweight or obese preadolescents and adolescents. There is, however, good reason to believe that if lean body mass increased in these subjects, it would in youngsters who are not overweight as well. It is also important to note that the increase in lean body mass (see box 10.2) can be greater than that due to normal growth in a group of nonexercising children (Naylor, Watts et al. 2008).

Although hypertrophy does occur in younger people, neural adaptations are also very important for increases in strength with training, especially when minimal or no significant hypertrophy occurs. Many other adaptations in the muscle, nerve, and connective tissue of children may still be occurring, such as changes in muscle protein (i.e., myosin isoforms), recruitment patterns, and connective tissue, all of which could contribute to improved strength and sport performance, as well as injury prevention.

In males, starting at puberty, the influence of testosterone on muscle size and strength is dramatic without any training. Figure 10.2 presents a group of physiological variables that ultimately contribute to the ability to exhibit strength. Dramatic progress in each of the variables is observed during adolescence, indicating that strength increases with physiological age as a result of normal growth. Younger boys sometimes envy the better-defined, larger muscles of older boys (16- and 17-year-olds) and may believe that by merely lifting weights they can have their muscle size and physique in a few months. Although small muscle mass gains beyond normal growth are possible in younger children, muscle hypertrophy should not be a major goal of their training programs. Only after a child has entered adolescence is it realistic to expect gains in muscle mass similar to those of adults. However, because of differences in maturation rates among children, care must be taken to evaluate this goal individually, especially in younger boys and girls.

 BOX 10.2 PRACTICAL QUESTION

To Cause Muscle Hypertrophy, Does the Resistance Training Program Need to Be Unique?

Weight training programs do not need to be unique to bring about significant hypertrophy in children. For example, overweight children (pretraining BMI of 32.5) performing eight weeks of circuit training with 10 machine exercises for two circuits of eight repetitions per exercise, beginning with 70% of 1RM and progressing to 90% of 1RM, with one minute of rest between exercises showed a significant increase in total lean body mass of 2% (Naylor, Watts et al. 2008). This increase was significantly greater than the change shown in a group of nonexercising children. The children performing weight training showed a nonsignificant decrease in fat mass. The combination of an increase in total lean body mass and decrease in fat mass resulted in a significant decrease of percent body fat of 1% (49.6 to 48.5%). Programs used in other studies showing a significant increase in lean body mass are also not unique from a program design perspective.

Naylor, N.H., Watts, K., Sharpe, J.A., Jones, T.W., Davis, E.A., Thompson, A., George, K., Ramsay, J.M., O'Driscoll, G., and Green, D.J. 2008. Resistance training and diastolic myocardial tissue velocities in obese children. *Medicine & Science in Sports & Exercise* 40: 2027-2032.

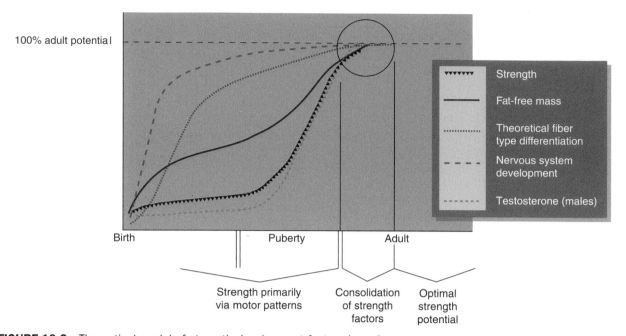

FIGURE 10.2 Theoretical model of strength development factors in males.

Adapted, by permission, from W.J. Kraemer et al., 1993, "Resistance training and youth," *Pediatric Exercise Science* 1(4): 336-350.

Motor Performance

Similar to strength, motor performance will improve with a child's age (see box 10.3). However, resistance training can also improve motor performance in prepubescent children and adolescents. Resistance training with free weights or weight training machines and plyometric training have all been reported to increase motor performance (National Strength and Conditioning Association 2009). Additionally, resistance training alone in preadolescents and adolescents has been shown to increase short sprint ability, vertical jump ability, medicine ball throwing ability, and agility (Channell and Barfield 2008; Christou et al. 2006; DiStefano et al. 2010; Gabbett, Johns, and Riemann 2008; McGuigan et al. 2009; Santos et al. 2012; Sgro et al. 2009; Wong, Chamari, and Wisloff 2010). For example, in 48 boys and girls (aged 9.7 years), countermovement jump height increased 8% after eight weeks of nonlinear resistance training (McGuigan et al. 2009). However, 14-year-old male soccer players who performed resistance training using linear periodization for 12 weeks experienced significant increases of 6, 2, and 5% in countermovement jump, 30 m sprint, and ball-kicking velocity, respectively (Wong, Chamari, and Wisloff 2010). In all cases these increases were significantly greater than those of soccer players performing only soccer-specific training.

Plyometric training also has been shown to increase motor performance in preadolescents and adolescents (Bishop et al. 2009; Kotzamanidis 2006; Meylan and Malatesta 2009). Eleven-year-old boys after 10 weeks of plyometric training significantly increased 30 m sprint and countermovement jump ability 3 and 34%, respectively (Kotzamanidis 2006). Thirteen-year-old boy and girl soccer players significantly increased countermovement jump, 10 m sprint, and performance in an agility test 8, 2, and 10%, respectively, after performing an in-season eight-week plyometric program (Meylan and Malatesta 2009). In both of these studies the performance increase was significantly greater than that of children not performing plyometric training. Plyometric training also increases start ability in 13-year-old swimmers (Bishop et al. 2009).

A combination of both traditional resistance training and plyometric training also increases motor performance. Complex training of 15-year-olds that involves resistance training, plyometric jump drills, and medicine ball throwing drills significantly increases vertical jump, squat jump, and medicine ball throwing ability (Santos and Janeira 2008). Although not all reports show significant increases in motor performance with resistance or plyometric training, it is clear that both can significantly increase general as well as

BOX 10.3 **RESEARCH**

Motor Performance Improvements as a Child's Age Increases

Changes in mean motor performance of adolescent soccer players indicate that sprint performance improves in the early teenage years, whereas vertical jump performance improves at a more constant rate throughout the teenage years (Williams, Oliver, and Faulkner 2010). It is important to note that this information is longitudinal, and not cross-sectional, which makes it more reliable in terms of improvement from year to year. Even though mean changes can be calculated, large individual variations in motor performance test improvements do exist. The total percentage of improvement in the 10 m sprint, 30 m sprint, and vertical jump from under 12 years to under 16 years was 11, 15, and 28%, respectively (see table 10.2).

TABLE 10.2 **Motor Performance Changes From 12 to 16 Years of Age**

Age (years)	Mean 10 m sprint (sec)	10 m sprint % improvement from previous year	Mean 30 m sprint (sec)	30 m sprint % improvement from previous year	Vertical jump (cm)	Vertical jump % improvement from previous year
Under 12	1.98	—	5.04	—	44.9	—
Under 13	1.97	0	4.97	1	47.9	4
Under 14	1.89	4	4.71	5	50.5	5
Under 15	1.79	5	4.46	5	53.1	6
Under 16	1.77	1	4.29	4	57.3	8

Data from Williams, Oliver, and Faulkner 2010.

sport-specific motor performance in preadolescents and adolescents.

Bone Development

Resistance training can have a favorable effect on bone mineral density in prepubescents and adolescents of both sexes (National Strength and Conditioning Association 2009; Naughton et al. 2000). Moreover, weight training has no detrimental effect on linear growth in children and adolescents (National Strength and Conditioning Association 2009; Malina 2006). However, not all studies report an effect on bone mineral density in children. It has been hypothesized that mechanical loading of bone has a threshold that must be met to have a positive effect on factors related to bone health, such as bone mineral density (Twisk 2001). Thus, studies that report no effect on bone mineral density as a result of resistance training may not have reached the threshold of mechanical loading needed to affect bone mineral density. The mechanical loading caused by resistance training is a result of exercise choice, sets, repetitions per set, resistance used, and training duration.

Unfortunately, the minimal mechanical loading necessary to bring about changes in bone health is not known.

Increased bone density from resistance training may be one of the primary mediating factors involved in empirical observations that resistance training prevents injury in young athletes (Hejna et al. 1982). Prepubescence and adolescence may be an opportune time to increase bone mineral density and periosteal expansion of cortical bone (compact bone) through physical activity (Bass 2000; Khan et al. 2000; National Strength and Conditioning Association 2009). This is an important consideration for long-term bone health, because training increases in bone health are lost over time when physical activity is decreased (National Strength and Conditioning Association 2009). Athletes who increase bone mineral density in adolescence appear to suffer less bone loss in later years despite reduced physical activity (Khan et al. 2000; Nordstrom, Olsson, and Nordstrom 2005). Thus, any increase in bone mineral density above normal growth during the prepubertal and adolescent years may help prevent osteoporosis later in life.

Detraining

The examination of detraining in adolescents and prepubescents is complicated by the fact that natural growth processes result in increased strength and hypertrophy even without resistance training. Moreover, few studies have examined detraining in children. However, as in adults, detraining in children results in strength loss so that strength regresses toward untrained control values (National Strength and Conditioning Association 2009). For example, complete detraining (performance of no resistance training) for eight weeks in children who previously completed 20 weeks of weight training results in strength loss: After the detraining period no significant strength differences between the previously weight-trained children and untrained children exist (Blimkie 1993). How quickly strength loss occurs with complete detraining may vary by muscle group (Faigenbaum et al. 1996). During an eight-week detraining period children (mean age 10.8 years) showed a decrease of 28% in leg extension strength and 19% in bench press strength. Leg extension strength after the detraining period was not significantly different from that of a control group of children who performed no weight training, whereas bench press strength was still significantly greater than that of the control group.

Motor performance losses during detraining may be minimal in short detraining periods (Santos et al. 2012). Boys (mean age 13.3 years) after weight training for eight weeks showed improvements in 1 and 3 kg (2.2 and 6.6 lb) medicine ball throwing ability (approximately 10%), countermovement vertical jump and standing long jump ability (approximately 4%), and 20 m sprint ability (11.5%). All of these motor performance tasks showed small but not significant decreases in a 12-week detraining period when no structured training was performed.

Although disagreement exists, a training frequency of one or two sessions per week appears to maintain strength and power gains in prepubescents and adolescents during short periods of detraining (DeRenne et al. 1996; National Strength and Conditioning Association 2009). Thus, although information is limited, the response of children to complete detraining and reduced-volume detraining appears to be similar to that of adults (see chapter 8). Strength and power gains achieved with plyometric training in prepubescents (Diallo et al. 2001) and adolescents (Santos and Janeira 2009) as well as in adolescents after complex training (Santos and Janeira 2011) are maintained (8 or 16 weeks) by normal soccer and basketball training without additional resistance training. So, also similar to adults, children's participation in sport training maintains strength and power gains for some period of time.

Because of natural growth, the advantage in strength gains that children achieve from weight training is only maintained with continued training. Cessation of training for a three-month period equalizes strength between children in a training group who detrained and those who did not perform any weight training (Blimkie 1992, 1993).

Injury Concerns

The chance of injury in children performing resistance training is less than 1%, which is lower than in many other sports, such as American football, basketball, and soccer (National Strength and Conditioning Association 2009). Resistance and plyometric training or a combination of both appear to help prevent sport-related injuries in adolescent athletes, and it is possible this is also true in prepubescent athletes (Hejna et al. 1982; National Strength and Conditioning Association 2009). For example, high school male and female athletes who performed resistance training had an injury rate of 26% compared to 72% in athletes who did not perform resistance training (Hejna et al. 1982). Additionally, the rehabilitation time required for those who were injured was only two days for the athletes performing resistance training compared to 4.8 days for athletes who did not perform resistance training. Preseason resistance and plyometric training also appear to reduce the risk of knee injury in young female athletes, a risk that is much higher than in their male counterparts (National Strength and Conditioning Association 2009). Female adolescent athletes performing resistance training had an injury rate of 14% compared to 33% in those who did not perform resistance training; they also had fewer knee and ankle injuries (Heidt et al. 2000). Overall, stronger athletes may be less susceptible to certain types of injury (Moskwa and Nicholas 1989). Thus, one goal of a resistance training program for child athletes should be to prepare them physically for their sport or activity.

Despite the possible positive effects of resistance training on injury prevention, the possibility of acute and chronic injuries to children is a valid concern (Dalton 1992; Markiewitz and Andrish 1992; National Strength and Conditioning Association 2009; Naughton et al. 2000). A resistance training program for children should not focus primarily on lifting maximal or near-maximal resistances because this is when many injuries occur. Children's resistance training programs should focus on proper exercise technique because many injuries in resistance exercise are related to improper technique. In fact, many weight training injuries in children are related to poorly designed equipment, equipment that does not fit children, use of excessive resistance, unsupervised access to the equipment, or lack of qualified adult supervision.

Like adults, children need time to adapt to the stress of resistance training; thus, training progression should be gradual. Children who find training difficult or do not enjoy resistance training at a particular age should not be forced to participate. Interest, growth, physical maturity, psychological maturity, and understanding all influence children's views of exercise training and their adoption of proper safety precautions. All of these factors need to be considered on an individual basis to ensure a safe and effective resistance training program.

Acute Injuries

Acute injury refers to a single trauma that causes an injury. Acute injuries do occur in children performing weight training; however, skeletal system injuries, such as growth cartilage damage and bone fractures, are rarely caused by weight training.

Accidental Injury

Accidental injuries account for 77% of all injuries sustained by 8- to 13-year-old children during a weight training session (see figure 10.3). Two-thirds of these injuries are to the hands and feet; common descriptions of the cause of injury include "dropping" and "pinching" (Meyer et al. 2009). This high percentage of accidental injury in 8- to 13-year-old children decreases with age (8-13 > 14-18 > 19-22 = 23-30 years). Thus, stressing weight room safety when training children is an important aspect of the training program.

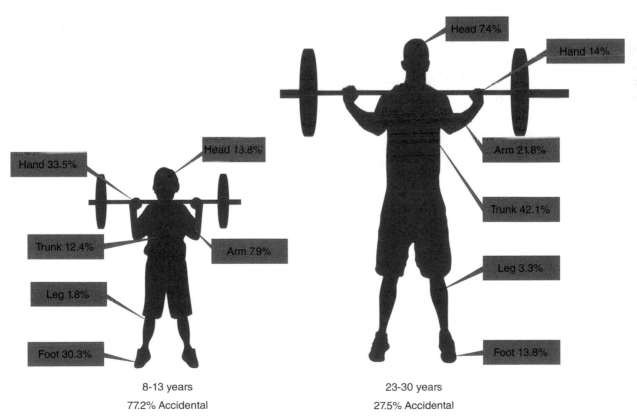

Head 13.8%

Hand 33.5%

Trunk 12.4%

Arm 7.9%

Leg 1.8%

Foot 30.3%

8-13 years

77.2% Accidental

Head 7.4%

Hand 14%

Arm 21.8%

Trunk 42.1%

Leg 3.3%

Foot 13.8%

23-30 years

27.5% Accidental

FIGURE 10.3 Percentage of injuries to various body parts in children and adults.

Adapted, by permission, from G.D. Meyer et al., 2009, "Use versus adult 'weightlifting' injuries presenting to United States emergency rooms: Accidental versus non-accidental injury mechanisms," *Journal of Strength and Conditioning Research* 23: 2054-2060.

Muscle Strains and Sprains

Muscle strains and sprains are common injuries in all age groups (Meyer et al. 2009). Strains and sprains account for 18, 44, 60, and 66% of all injuries in 8- to 13-, 14- to 18-, 19- to 22-, and 23- to 30-year-olds (Meyer et al. 2009). The risk of sprains and strains significantly increases with increasing age. Strains and sprains can be the result of not warming up properly before a training session. Trainees should perform several sets of exercise before beginning the actual training sets of a workout. Other common causes of muscle strain or sprain are attempting to lift too much weight for a given number of repetitions and improper exercise technique. Children should understand that the suggested number of repetitions is merely a guideline, and that they can perform fewer repetitions than prescribed in the training program. The incidence of this type of injury, as with all injury types, can be reduced by taking proper safety precautions.

Growth Cartilage Damage

Growth cartilage damage is historically a traditional concern for children performing weight training. **Growth cartilage** is located at three sites: the **epiphyseal plates**, or growth plates, at the end of long bones; the **epiphysis**, or cartilage on the joint surface; and the **apophyseal insertion**, or tendon insertion (see figure 10.4). The

long bones of the body grow in length from the epiphyseal plates. Damage to the epiphyseal plates, but not to the other types of growth cartilage, can decrease linear bone growth. Normally, because of hormonal changes, the epiphyseal plates ossify after puberty. Once this happens, the growth of long bones, and therefore increased height, is no longer possible.

The epiphyseal plate is weakest during phases of rapid growth during pubescence (Caine, DiFiori, and Maffulli 2006). Additionally, bone mineralization may lag behind linear growth making the bone more susceptible to injury (Caine, DiFiori, and Maffuli 2006). The cartilage of the epiphysis acts as a shock absorber between the bones that form a joint. Damage to this cartilage may lead to a rough articular surface and subsequent pain during joint movement. The growth cartilage at apophyseal insertions of major tendons ensures a solid connection between the tendon and bone. Damage to apophyseal insertions may cause pain and also increase the chance of separation between the tendon and bone, resulting in an **avulsion fracture**. It has also been proposed that during the growth spurt muscle tendon tightness around joints increases resulting in a decrease in flexibility. If excessive muscular stress occurs because the growth cartilage is weak during the growth spurt, injury to the growth cartilage may occur (Caine et al. 2005). This injury mechanism, however, is controversial.

Epiphyseal Plate Fractures

The epiphyseal plate is prone to fractures in children because it is not yet ossified. Thus, it is not surprising that epiphyseal plate fractures in preadolescent and adolescent weight trainees have occurred (Caine, DiFiori, and Maffuli 2006; National Strength and Conditioning Association 2009). However, this type of injury is rare. The majority of epiphyseal plate fracture cases result from lifting near-maximal resistances, improper exercise technique, or lack of qualified supervision (National Strength and Conditioning Association 2009). Two appropriate precautions for prepubescent and adolescent resistance training programs are (1) to discourage maximal or near-maximal lifts (1RM), especially in unsupervised settings, and (2) because improper form is a contributing factor to many injuries, to emphasize appropriate increases in resistance and proper technique in all exercises to young resistance trainees.

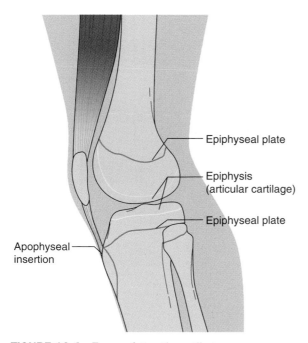

FIGURE 10.4 Types of growth cartilage.

- Epiphyseal plate
- Epiphysis (articular cartilage)
- Epiphyseal plate
- Apophyseal insertion

Fractures

Because the metaphysis, or shaft, of the long bones is more elastic in children and adolescents than in adults, green stick fractures, which occur from a bending of the shaft, occur more readily in children and adolescents (Naughton et al. 2000). Peak fracture incidence in boys occurs between the ages of 12 and 14 and precedes the age of peak height increase, or the growth spurt (Blimkie 1993). The increased fracture rate appears to be caused by a lag in cortical bone thickness and mineralization in relation to linear growth (Blimkie 1993). Therefore, controlling the resistance that boys between the ages of 12 and 14 use during weight training may be important. The same line of reasoning may apply to girls between the ages of 10 and 13.

Lumbar Problems

Acute trauma can cause lumbar spine problems in adults as well as prepubescents and adolescents. Low back problems, whether from acute or chronic injuries, are the most frequent type of injury reported by high school athletes performing weight training (National Strength and Conditioning Association 2009). Low back injury accounts for 50% of all injuries in adolescent powerlifters (National Strength and Conditioning Association 2009). These problems may be caused by lifting maximal or near-maximal resistances or attempting to perform too many repetitions with a given resistance (see figure 10.5). In many cases back pain is associated with improper form, especially in exercises such as the squat and deadlift. When performing these exercises, as well as others, trainees should use proper exercise technique, which involves maintaining as upright a position as possible to minimize the stress on the low back.

Chronic Injuries

The terms chronic injury and *overuse injury* refer to injury caused by repeated microtraumas. Shin splints and stress fractures are examples of these injuries. Using improper exercise technique over long periods of time can result in overuse injuries (e.g., improper bench press technique can cause shoulder problems and pain).

Growth Cartilage Damage

Repeated physical stress can cause damage to all three growth cartilage sites. As an example, repeated mechanical stresses to the shoulder and

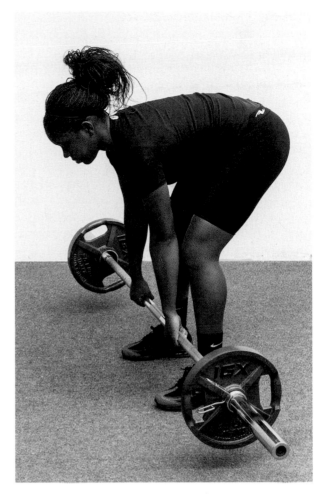

FIGURE 10.5 Incorrect technique, such as rounding the low back in the deadlift, which places undue stress on the low back, can result in injury.

elbow from baseball pitching as well as other throwing or hitting motions, such as in the sports of volleyball and tennis, result in inflammation and irritated ossification centers in the elbow and epiphyseal plate of the humerus. This causes pain with shoulder and elbow movement and is a probable cause of shoulder and elbow pain in prepubescent and adolescent baseball pitchers (Barnett 1985; Caine, DiFiori, and Maffulli 2006; Lyman et al. 2001).

The growth cartilage on the articular surface of prepubescent joints, especially at the ankle, knee, and elbow, may be more prone to injury than that of adult joints. Repeated microtrauma from pitching appears to be responsible in part for elbow and shoulder pain in young (9- to 12-year-old) pitchers (Lyman et al. 2001) and ankle pain in young runners (Conale and Belding 1980). In many cases joint pain in adolescents and prepubescents is caused by **osteochondritis** (inflammation of growth cartilage) or **osteochondritis dissecans** (a condition in which a piece of bone or cartilage, or both, inside a joint loses blood supply and dies, often resulting in separation of a portion of the joint surface from the bone). Tiny avulsions of the growth cartilage at the site of the patellar tendon insertion onto bone may be related to the pain associated with Osgood-Schlatter disease (Caine, DiFiori, and Maffulli 2006; Micheli 1983). Although damage to growth cartilage is a concern, incidences of this type of injury as a result of weight training appear to be very rare (Blimkie 1993; Caine, DiFiori, and Maffulli 2006; National Strength and Conditioning Association 2009).

Lumbar Problems

As in adults, lumbar spine problems may be one of the most common types of injury in adolescents and prepubescents performing weight training. Lumbar problems constituted 50% of the total number of injuries reported in adolescent powerlifters who presumably trained with maximal or near-maximal resistances (Brady, Cahill, and Bodnar 1982). Although this report involved adolescents, the potential for similar injuries in prepubescents needs to be recognized. Adolescents may be at a greater risk than adults for spondylitis (inflammation of one or more vertebrae) and stress-related pain. The incidence of this abnormality in adolescents is 47% percent, whereas in adults it is only 5% (Micheli and Wood 1995).

Lordosis is an anterior bending of the spine, usually accompanied by flexion of the pelvis. Many children during the growth spurt have a tendency to develop lordosis of the lumbar spine. Several factors contribute to lordosis, including enhanced growth in the anterior portion of the vertebral bodies and tight hamstrings that cause the hips to assume a flexed position (Micheli 1983). Lordosis may contribute to low back pain. However, low back soft-tissue injuries are also often associated with low back pain in adolescents (Blimkie 1993).

Although many factors may result in lower back pain, insufficient strength and muscular endurance, as well as instability, are associated with low back pain in adolescents (National Strength and Conditioning Association 2009). Back pain from resistance training may be minimized by performing exercises that strengthen the abdominal and low back musculature. Strengthening these areas

will help maintain proper exercise technique, thus reducing the stress on the lumbar area.

Program Considerations

The development of a prepubescent or adolescent resistance training program should follow the same steps as that of an adult program. Although a medical examination before beginning a resistance training program is not mandatory for apparently healthy children, it is recommended for youth with signs or symptoms suggestive of a disease or with a known disease (Miller, Cheathman, and Patel 2010; National Strength and Conditioning Association 2009). The following questions need to be considered before a child begins a resistance training program:

- Is the child psychologically and physically ready to participate in a resistance exercise training program?
- What type of resistance training program should the child follow?
- Does the child understand the proper lifting techniques for each exercise in the program?
- Do spotters understand the safety spotting techniques for each exercise in the program?
- Does the child understand the safety concerns for each piece of equipment used in the program?
- Does the resistance training equipment fit the child properly?
- Does the child's exercise training program include aerobic and flexibility training to address total fitness needs?
- Does the child participate in other sports or activities in addition to resistance training?

These last two questions need to be considered in the context of the total training stress to which the child is exposed. For example, in young baseball pitchers weight training during the season is associated with elbow but not shoulder pain (Lyman et al. 2001). However, the total number of pitches thrown and pitching arm fatigue are also associated with elbow and shoulder pain. This does not necessarily indicate that young pitchers should not perform weight training during the season, but that the total training stress placed on children may be associated with some types of injuries. As with all resistance training programs, individual differences need to be considered in the program design.

Developmental Differences

Developmental differences in children of the same age need to be considered when developing a resistance training program. Preadolescents and adolescents of the same age differ from each other physically and psychologically. Some children are tall for their chronological age and others are short, some are fast sprinters and others are slow, and some become upset when they make a poor play in a game whereas others seem unconcerned. Physical and psychological differences are the result of differences in genetics and growth rates. Adults must realize that children are not miniature adults. Understanding some of the basic principles of growth and development will help adults have more realistic expectations of children. This understanding will also help when developing goals and exercise progressions for resistance training programs.

There are many aspects of children's growth and development besides height. These include body mass gains, fitness gains, genetic potential, nutrition, and sleep patterns. Also included in discussions of children's development is maturation, which has been defined as progress toward adulthood. Maturation of children involves the following areas:

- Physical size
- Bone maturity
- Reproductive maturity
- Psychological maturity

Each of these areas can be evaluated clinically, generally by the family physician. Physicians recognize that each person has a chronological age as well as a physiological age for each of the preceding areas. Because physiological age determines the functional capabilities and performance of the person, it is an important factor to consider when developing a resistance training program.

When strength increases occur relative to the growth spurt is not entirely clear. Both prepubescent males and females may show peak strength gains, as a result of normal growth, in the year following the growth spurt, or peak increase in height (De Ste Croix, Deighan, and Armstrong 2003). In prepubescent males the velocity of strength gain appears to peak following the growth spurt (Naughton et al. 2000), whereas many girls peak in strength before or during the growth spurt. In either case, generally, girls experience the growth spurt and so peak strength increase prior to boys. Whatever the developmental stage at which peak strength gain occurs, it is consistently greater in boys than in girls. The possible difference in the magnitude of strength gains should be considered when developing training goals for boys and girls and during the needs analysis.

Needs Analysis and Individualization

The needs of each child, like those of adults, are unique. Prepubescents and adolescents need to develop their total health and fitness, which involves cardiorespiratory fitness, flexibility, body composition, and motor skills as well as strength and power. A resistance training program should not be so time consuming as to ignore these other aspects of total fitness or interfere with a child's play time. Prepubescents as well as many adolescents should not be expected to perform adult training programs or those of successful adult athletes. To ensure compliance with the training program, adults should allow children to set their own goals and monitor their physical and psychological tolerance of the program. Children's comments such as, "I don't want to do this," "This program is too hard," "Some of these exercises are hurting me," "I am just too tired after a workout," or "What other exercises can I learn?" may indicate that the program needs to be evaluated and appropriate alterations made.

Most of the dangers of resistance training are related to inappropriate exercise demands being placed on the prepubescent or adolescent. Although general guidelines can be offered and should be followed, sensitivity to the special needs that arise in each child is necessary. The program must be designed for each child's needs, and proper exercise techniques and safety considerations must be employed. A properly designed and supervised resistance training program provides many positive physical and psychological benefits. Perhaps the most important outcome is the behavioral development of an active lifestyle in the prepubescent or adolescent. Good exercise behaviors contribute to better health and well-being over a lifetime.

With the increasing popularity of youth sports, from American football and gymnastics to soccer and T-ball, children need better physical preparation to prevent sport-related injuries. The American College of Sports Medicine (1993) estimated that over 50% of the overuse injuries diagnosed in adolescents are preventable. A total fitness training program that includes resistance training to prepare the child for the stresses of sport competition, along with preparticipation screening and regular visits to sports medicine health professionals, has great potential to reduce the number of athletic and overuse injuries.

Another consideration for all children is upper-body strength. The recent decline in upper-body strength in boys and girls (Hass, Feigenbaum, and Franklin 2001) represents a significant weakness in prepubescent and adolescent fitness profiles. Upper-body strength limits many sport-specific tasks even at the recreational level. The general lack of upper-body strength in many prepubescent and pubescent children indicates the need for exercises for the upper body in resistance training programs for these groups.

The general goals of all youth resistance training programs could include the following:

- Conditioning of all fitness components (aerobic, flexibility, strength)
- Generally balanced choice of exercises for upper- and lower-body development (although as the child ages, some sport-specific exercises may be added)
- Balanced choice of exercises for the agonists and antagonists of all major joint movements to promote muscle balance
- Increased strength and power of specific muscle groups
- Increased local muscular endurance of specific muscle groups
- Increased motor performance (increased ability to jump, run, or throw)
- Increased total body weight (age dependent)
- Increased muscle hypertrophy (age dependent)
- Decreased body fat

Some goals of resistance training programs, such as muscle hypertrophy, change with the age of a child. The training goals may also change depending on the sports or other activities in which a child is participating. Individualization of the program should take place based on the child's progress, desire to train, other sports or activities, current or previous injuries, how long resistance training has been performed, as well as other factors. Individualized, proper program progression is necessary for bringing about the physiological adaptations needed for continued fitness gains.

Program Progression

Regardless of the type of program progression used for youth resistance training (i.e., resistance increases, training volume increases, exercise choice), it should occur slowly. Slow progression helps to ensure safety, allows time to adapt to training stress, develops exercise tolerance, and aids in the mastery of exercise technique. The progression in exercise choice, resistance, volume, or other factors used for one child may be too advanced for another child of the same age or training experience. Thus, program progression should always occur on an individual basis.

Age Group Progression

Although resistance training has been performed safely by very young children (National Strength and Conditioning Association 2009), this does not mean that all children should or must perform resistance training at a young age. Physiological and psychological maturity vary greatly in youth of the same age; therefore, the progression guidelines presented in table 10.3 need to be adapted to accommodate individual needs and training situations. Regardless of the age of the child, the training program should be conducted in an atmosphere conducive to both the child's safety and enjoyment. The training environment should present appropriate information in the form of posters, goal charts, and pictures that reflect the goals and expectations of the resistance training program.

Resistance, or Intensity, Progression

Training intensity, or the resistance used when performing an exercise, should be progressed in small increments of 5 to 10% (National Strength

TABLE 10.3 Basic Guidelines for Resistance Exercise Progression for Children

Age (yr)	Considerations
5-7	Introduce child to basic exercises with little or no resistance; develop the concept of a training session; teach exercise techniques; progress from body-weight calisthenics, partner exercises, and lightly resisted exercises; keep volume low.
8-10	Gradually increase the number of exercises; practice exercise technique for all lifts; start gradual progress of loading the exercises; keep exercises simple; increase volume slowly; carefully monitor tolerance to exercise stress.
11-13	Teach all basic exercise techniques; continue progressive loading of each exercise; emphasize exercise technique; introduce more advanced exercises with little or no resistance.
14-15	Progress to more advanced resistance exercise programs; add sport-specific components; emphasize exercise techniques; increase volume gradually.
16 or older	Entry level into adult programs after all background experience has been gained.

If a child at a particular age level has no previous weight training experience, progression must start at previous levels and move to more advanced levels as exercise tolerance, exercise technique, and understanding permit.

Adapted, by permission, from W.J. Kraemer and S.J. Fleck, 2005, *Strength training for young athletes* (Champaign, IL: Human Kinetics), 13.

and Conditioning Association 2009). With free weights this is not difficult because small weight plates are readily available. However, the resistance increments on some weight training machines are too large to allow smooth resistance progression as the child becomes stronger. Many machines' weight stacks increase in increments of 10 to 20 lb (4.5 to 9.1 kg). If a child can bench press 30 lb (13.6 kg), a weight stack increment of 10 lb (4.5 kg) represents a 30% increase in resistance, which is too large for a safe and smooth progression in resistance. This problem is remedied on some machines by built-in small resistance increases. On other machines this can be remedied by using weights, usually 2.5 lb (1.1 kg) and 5 lb (2.3 kg), that are specially designed to be easily added and removed from the machine's weight stack. On machines designed for children, the initial resistance and increases in resistance are appropriate. Use of such small increases in resistance will not hinder strength gains (see Small Increment Technique in chapter 6).

On some adult machines the starting resistance is too great for a prepubescent to perform even one repetition. In this case the child will have to perform an alternate exercise for the same muscle group using either a free weight, body-weight, or partner-resisted exercise until he is strong enough to perform the desired number of repetitions using the machine. For example, if the child cannot perform a machine leg press because the starting resistance is too great, he could perform body-weight squats and then squats holding light dumbbells in each hand until he is strong enough to perform the leg press at the starting resistance on the machine.

Plyometrics

Plyometrics, or exercises that emphasize training of the stretch-shortening cycle, (see chapter 7), can be included in preadolescent and adolescent programs. This type of training is a safe and effective conditioning that increases functional ability and reduces sport-specific injuries in preadolescents and adolescents (National Strength and Conditioning Association 2009). Conveniently, children regularly perform plyometric actions when at play. Examples of these actions include hopscotch, skipping, jumping, and jumping rope (see figure 10.6). Thus, it is not surprising that plyometric training is a safe training method for children if training volume is controlled. Injuries have, however, been reported with excessive plyometric training, such as exertional rhabdomyolysis in a 12-year-old boy after performing more than 250 squat jumps in a physical education class (Clarkson 2006).

A literature review concludes that plyometric training is effective in 5- to 14-year-olds as a means to increase sprinting, jumping, kicking distance, balance, and agility (Johnson, Salzberg, and Stevenson 2012). Guidelines for an effective program include two sessions per week, 50 to 60 foot contacts per session, and a duration of at least eight weeks (Johnson, Salzberg, and Stevenson 2012). As with all types of resistance training for children, plyometrics training volume and intensity must be

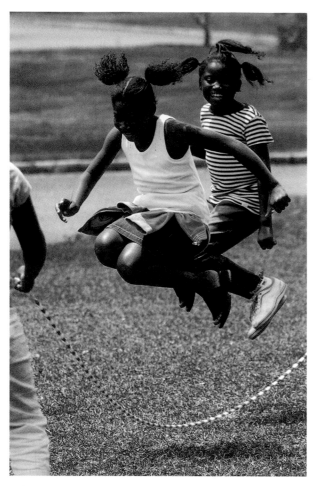

FIGURE 10.6 Many childhood activities include plyometric-type actions.

Zuma Press/Icon SMI

controlled and progressed slowly for this to be a safe and effective training methodology.

Strength and Power Progression

Strength and power can be progressed throughout a program by increasing the training volume and intensity, or by varying the exercises used. Initially, low-volume and low-intensity programs do cause fitness gains. A well-organized and well-supervised basic training program for children can be as short as 20 minutes per training session. During the initial training period a frequency of two sessions per week in children (8-11 years old) does bring about significant strength gains and changes in body composition (Faigenbaum et al. 1993, 1999). Also, during the initial training period higher numbers of repetitions (13 to 15) per set may produce greater gains in strength and local muscular endurance than lower numbers (6 to 8) of repetitions per set (Faigenbaum et al. 1999, 2001). Like adults, children can realize significant changes in strength and body composition from low-volume, single-set programs. Thus, a program for children may be composed initially of one set of approximately 10 to 15 repetitions per set with at least one exercise for all the major muscle groups of the body (see box 10.4). As with adults, sets do not need to be carried to failure to produce significant fitness gains; this reduces total training stress while also promoting the learning of proper exercise technique. As a child gets older, more

 BOX 10.4 PRACTICAL QUESTION

What Are Recommendations for a Beginning Resistance Training Program for Adolescents?

Weight training program recommendations for a beginning adolescent lifter include the following (Miller, Cheathman, and Patel 2010):

- Primary training goal: increase strength

- Number of sets: one to three

- Repetitions per set: 10-15, depending on previous weight training experience

- Resistance: one that allows the performance of the desired number of repetitions per set

- Training frequency: two or three sessions per week on nonconsecutive days

- Exercises: involve all the major muscle groups—chin-up, bench press, lat pull-down, leg press, knee flexion, knee extension, abdominal crunch, biceps curl, triceps extension, calf raise, rowing, stability or ball exercises

Miller, M.G., Cheathman, C.C., and Patel, N.D. 2010. Resistance training for adolescents. *Pediatric Clinics of North America* 57:671-682.

advanced programs that resemble adult programs can be introduced gradually.

A suggested progression for youth programs with the goal of increasing maximal strength is presented in table 10.4. The suggestions include typical resistance training exercises (concentric and eccentric repetition phases) and progressions for the major acute training program variables. The definition of novice, intermediate, and advanced refers to children with less than 3 months of resistance training experience, 3 to 12 months of resistance training experience, and more than 12 months of resistance training experience, respectively.

Performance of variations of the Olympic weightlifting movements and plyometrics is safe for children (Faigenbaum et al. 2010, 2007; National Strength and Conditioning Association 2009). Performance of these types of exercises is part of the progression of increasing power (see table 10.5). Different from the suggestions for increasing strength, power training predominantly involves multijoint exercises, generally uses lower

percentages of 1RM to allow fast velocities of movement and fewer repetitions per set so that fatigue does not affect exercise technique or result in significant slowing of the movement velocity. Sets of power training exercises should not be carried to failure because this may increase the risk of injury as well as cause significant slowing of the movement velocity. As with all types of program progression, sufficient time must be allowed to learn proper exercise technique when power exercises are performed, and increases in training volume or intensity should be made slowly.

Periodization

Periodization, which is discussed in more detail in chapter 7, is a popular way of varying the training volume and intensity of workouts in adult athletes and fitness enthusiasts. The effects of periodization on prepubescents and adolescents have received less study than the effects on adults. However, as in adults, periodization in children optimizes long-term training gains and helps reduce boredom and the risk of overuse injuries (Miller,

TABLE 10.4 Guidelines for Strength Development

	Novice	Intermediate	Advanced
Muscle action	Eccentric and concentric	Eccentric and concentric	Eccentric and concentric
Exercise choice	Single-joint and multijoint	Single-joint and multijoint	Single-joint and multijoint
Intensity	50-70% of 1RM	60-80% of 1RM	70-85% of 1RM
Volume	1 or 2 sets × 10-15 reps	2 or 3 sets × 8-12 reps	>3 sets × 6-10 reps
Rest intervals	1 min	1-2 min	2-3 min
Velocity	Moderate	Moderate	Moderate
Frequency per week	2 or 3	2 or 3	3 or 4

Adapted, by permission, from National Strength and Conditioning Association, 2009, "Youth resistance training: Updated position statement paper from the National Strength and Conditioning Association," *Journal of Strength and Conditioning Research* 23: S60-S79.

TABLE 10.5 Guidelines for Power Development

	Novice	Intermediate	Advanced
Muscle action	Eccentric and concentric	Eccentric and concentric	Eccentric and concentric
Exercise choice	Multijoint	Multijoint	Multijoint
Intensity	30-60% of 1RM	30-60% of 1RM velocity 60-70% of 1RM strength	30-60% of 1RM velocity 70->80% of 1RM strength
Volume	1 or 2 sets × 3-6 reps	2 or 3 sets × 3-6 reps	>3 sets × 1-6 reps
Rest intervals	1 min	1-2 min	2-3 min
Velocity	Moderate/fast	Fast	Fast
Frequency per week	2	2 or 3	3 or 4

Adapted, by permission, from National Strength and Conditioning Association, 2009, "Youth resistance training: Updated position statement paper from the National Strength and Conditioning Association," *Journal of Strength and Conditioning Research* 23: S60-S79.

Cheathman, and Patel 2010; National Strength and Conditioning Association 2009). Both linear and nonlinear periodization have been used to train prepubescents and adolescents (Faigenbaum et al. 2007; Foschini et al. 2010; McGuigan et al. 2009; Sgro et al. 2009; Stone, O'Bryant, and Garhammer 1981; Szymanski et al. 2004). Both of these types of periodization can be varied by doing the following:

- Increasing the resistance for an exercise by increasing the percentage of 1RM or the resistance used for an RM or RM training zone
- Varying the RM training zone or percentage of 1RM used
- Varying the number of sets per exercise
- Varying the exercises for the same muscle groups
- Including power-type exercises

Programs can also be varied based on the lifting experience of children (see tables 10.3, 10.4, and 10.5). As with any type of training progression, children's tolerance of the program needs to be carefully monitored.

Copying Elite Athlete Programs

Prepubescents, pubescents, and young adolescents should not perform programs designed for collegiate or professional athletes, whether those programs are periodized or not. The ability of older athletes to improve strength and power using advanced programs is in part a result of their years of resistance training experience. Often, elite programs involve training intensities and volumes that are inappropriate for children and may result in injury. Forcing youths to perform programs designed for mature, gifted athletes can result in overuse or acute injuries.

Exercise Tolerance

Regardless of the type of resistance training program, the importance of the child's ability to tolerate the exercise stress cannot be overemphasized. For a program to work optimally, parents, teachers, and coaches need to hear from the prepubescents and adolescents performing the program concerning how they are tolerating it. Adults should encourage discussion and feedback of the children's concerns and fears. Most important, adults must take steps to address the concerns children

express. Trainers need to use common sense in providing exercise variation, active recovery periods, total rest from training, and individualized training programs for children. They must also be careful not to fall into the trap of believing that more training is always better.

The general guidelines for program design offered in this chapter are only suggestions. No single optimal program exists. Prepubescents and adolescents should start with a program that is individually tolerable but becomes more advanced as they grow older. Dramatic changes in the tolerance of resistance training programs can reflect the increased maturity of the trainee. Trainers should be careful, however, not to overestimate the child's ability to tolerate the total amount of physical activity being performed, which may include resistance training, aerobic training, and sport participation. It is better to start the child out conservatively than to overestimate exercise tolerance and reduce the child's enjoyment of participation. Using the proper resistance training principles, the program designer can create a program that reflects the child's developmental stage and particular needs. All adults associated with a program must remember that they are not the ones for whom the program is developed; their job is to provide a positive environment that protects and serves the children participating. Children should be free to participate or not participate in any exercise or sport program.

Sample Sessions

Two sample sessions are outlined in this section. One involves the use of no weight training equipment, and the second requires resistance training equipment in the form of free weights or typical weight training machines. Both sessions are meant to provide a total-body workout and can be modified to provide exercise variation and increases or decreases in the difficulty of an exercise, and to use available equipment. Additionally, these sessions can be modified based on past lifting experience. All weight training sessions should be preceded by a warm-up and followed by a cool-down (Miller, Cheathman, and Patel 2010; National Strength and Conditioning Association 2009).

Workouts Using Little Equipment

This workout session uses either the child's body weight, self-resistance using one muscle group

TABLE 10.6 Resistance Training Workout for Children Using Body Weight and Self-Resistance

Exercise	Sets × repetitions
Push-up	1-3 × 10-20
Bent-leg sit-up	1-3 × 15-20
Parallel squat	1-3 × 10-20
Self-resistance arm curl using opposite arm as resistance	1-3 × 10 actions 6 sec in duration
Toe raise	1-3 × 20-30
Partner-resisted lateral arm raise	1-10 reps of 10 sec duration
Lying-back extension	1-3 × 10-15

against another muscle group, resistance provided by another child, or another child's body weight as resistance (see table 10.6). It can be performed as a circuit, moving from one exercise to the next, or in a set–repetition manner, performing all sets of an exercise with a rest between sets before moving on to the next exercise. The resistance used in all of the exercises can be increased or decreased in some manner. For example, the difficulty of push-ups can be decreased by doing knee push-ups and increased by placing the feet on a chair. The self-resistance and partner-resisted exercises are meant to be performed in a dynamic manner; each concentric and eccentric repetition phase should take approximately 5 seconds to complete for a total of 10 seconds per repetition. Exercises can also be modified. For example, self-resisted arm curls could be replaced by partner-resisted arm curls using a towel. The goal is to provide some form of resistance training for all of the major muscle groups using little or no equipment.

Session Using Equipment

This session can be performed with a variety of either free weights or typical weight training machine exercises using either a circuit or a set–repetition protocol. The session as outlined emphasizes strength and is designed for a novice child lifter (see table 10.7). If adult-size machines are used, trainers should make sure that each child is properly fitted to the machine to ensure proper exercise technique. Initially, the resistance used for each exercise should be such that the trainee can perform at least the minimum recommended number of repetitions with correct technique. When the maximum recommended number of repetitions can be performed, the resistance

TABLE 10.7 Resistance Training Workout for Children Using Equipment

Exercise	Sets × repetitions
Squat or leg press	1-3 × 10-15RM zone
Bench press	1-3 × 10-15RM zone
Knee curl	1-3 × 10-15RM zone
Arm curl	1-3 × 10-15RM zone
Knee extension	1-3 × 10-15RM zone
Overhead press	1-3 × 10-15RM zone
Crunch	1-3 × 15-20RM zone
Back extension	1-3 × 10-15RM zone

is increased so that the trainee can perform the minimum number of repetitions per set. Children should perform all exercises in a controlled manner to prevent injury, learn proper exercise technique, and know how to prevent damage to equipment. Trainers should continually stress the importance of correct exercise and spotting techniques for all exercises.

Equipment Modification and Organizational Difficulties

Children require more individualized help than adults. Moreover, trainers often encounter organizational problems with children that are not present with adults (e.g., adult machines may need to be modified with pads or blocks to fit the smaller bodies of children). If dumbbells or barbells are used, lighter weights may be needed to provide an alternate exercise when a machine does not fit or cannot provide the proper resistance for some children in a group. Trainers must also be aware of the fact that equipment may need to be modified as the child grows. Typically, exercise machines made for adults require more modifications than free weight exercises. If machines designed for children are available, equipment fit is much less of a problem (see figure 10.7). Proper equipment fit may need to be checked as frequently as every month, especially during the growth spurt of the child.

The organizational problems created by having to accommodate children need not be difficult to solve. Two solutions are to mark needed modifications or machine adjustments on each child's workout card to keep track, or to teach children to make their own equipment modifications or machine adjustments. However, adults need to carefully check that equipment modifications and adjustments are done properly. Although effective, these solutions may be impractical with a large group of children. With timed workouts (specific exercise periods and rest periods), the time needed for equipment modifications and

adjustments must be considered, especially when many children are training and modifications or adjustments are needed on an individual basis.

Program designers may want to perform the training session to find out how long a particular equipment modification or adjustment takes. Rest period alterations, if needed, can then be made to account for the time needed for equipment modifications. Although one-minute rest periods in a particular training session may be preferred, organizational problems such as equipment modifications or adjustments may make this impossible. In such cases, the safety of the children and correct exercise technique are the priorities rather than maintaining the desired rest period. Organizational problems must be resolved without sacrificing safety, correct exercise technique, or the effectiveness of the training session.

The most important equipment consideration when training children is whether the resistance training equipment fits each child properly. With free weights, body-weight exercises, or partner-

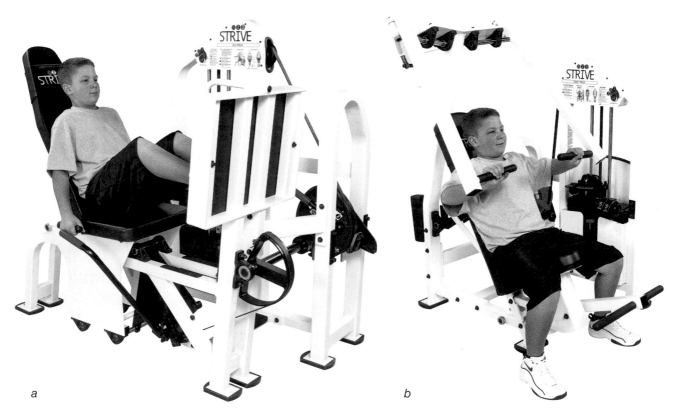

a   *b*

FIGURE 10.7 Some companies make resistance training machines designed to fit young children; they have small resistance increases to allow proper progression: *(a)* a leg press and *(b)* a chest press.

Courtesy of Strive Inc., McMurray, PA.

resisted exercises, fit is typically not a concern. With resistance training weight machines, however, fit can be critical. Although several companies now manufacture machines specifically for children, most resistance training machines are designed to fit adults (see figure 10.7). Most prepubescents lack the height and arm and leg length to properly fit many adult resistance training machines. If the machine does not fit the child properly, correct technique and full exercise range of motion are impossible. A critical danger of an ill-fitting machine is that a body part such as a foot or an arm may slip off its point of contact, resulting in injury.

Another common fit problem is a bench for machine or free weight exercises that is too wide to allow free movement of the shoulder during the exercise. When children perform exercises with inappropriate technique because of ill-fitting equipment, their joints and musculature can be exposed to undue stress, resulting in an injury.

Children should not use equipment that cannot be safely adapted to fit properly. Simple alterations of some machines, such as additional seat pads, can allow a trainee to use the machine safely. However, just adjusting the seat is often not enough. Although the seat adjustment may be appropriate, adjustments may also be needed to allow proper positioning of the arms or legs on the contact points of the machine. In addition, raising the seat may make it impossible for the child's feet to reach the floor, compromising balance. Placing blocks under the feet can help in such cases.

Altering a piece of equipment to fit one child does not guarantee that the equipment will fit another child. Proper fit must be checked before the equipment is used by each child. Care must be taken to ensure that additional padding or blocks do not slide during the exercise, which could result in injury. Sliding can be avoided in some alterations by attaching nonskid material to the top and bottom of blocks and the backs of additional pads. The safety of the lifter must always be the top priority when making any equipment adjustments.

Program Philosophy

Formal programs, such as those in schools and health clubs, should express their philosophies openly and clearly. Signs, wall charts, and handouts can reflect a positive attitude about weight training to prepubescents and adolescents. This is especially important when both adults and children are training in the same facility. The program philosophy can be promoted in the following ways:

- Posting age-related instructions for children next to the adult instructions. This can include both program and exercise instructions.
- Using posters and pictures that depict prepubescents and adolescents of both sexes using proper resistance training techniques.
- Using charts, contests, and awards to promote the principles on which prepubescents and adolescents need to concentrate (e.g., for training consistency, exercise technique, total conditioning and fitness, progress in other aspects of total fitness (i.e., flexibility, endurance), and preparation goals before and within a sports season)

The environment, exercise programs, and awards should all reflect the program philosophy. Because prepubescents and adolescents learn and retain information in different ways than adults do, the weight training program should communicate the expectations and philosophy in all forms of communication, including oral, written, audio, video, and pictorial media. All forms of communication need to be clear and appropriate for prepubescents and adolescents so that intimidation, confusion, or misunderstanding does not occur in any aspect of the program.

Summary

Resistance training for prepubescents and adolescents has gained acceptance and popularity because strength, power, and hypertrophy increases can occur, bone development may be enhanced, and injuries may be prevented in other sport activities with developmentally appropriate programs. Program designers should consider the developmental and physical differences among children, exercise tolerance, and safety issues to minimize acute and chronic injuries and maximize the benefits of participation.

SELECTED READINGS

Bass, S.L. 2000. The prepubertal years: A uniquely opportune stage of growth when the skeleton is most responsive to exercise? *Sports Medicine* 30: 73-70.

Canadian Society for Exercise Physiology. 2008. Position paper: Resistance training in children and adolescents. *Journal of Applied Physiology, Nutrition and Metabolism* 33: 547-561.

De Ste Croix, M.B.A., Deighan, M.A., and Armstrong, N. 2003. Assessment and interpretation of isokinetic muscle during growth and maturation. *Sports Medicine* 33: 727-743.

Falk, B, and Tenenbaum, G. 1996. The effectiveness of resistance training in children: A meta-analysis. *Sports Medicine* 22: 176-186.

Hass, C.J., Feigenbaum, M.S., and Franklin, B.A. 2001. Prescription of resistance training for healthy populations. *Sports Medicine* 31: 9539-9564.

Kraemer, W.J., and Fleck, S.J. 2005. *Strength training for young athletes,* 4th ed. Champaign, IL: Human Kinetics.

Malina, R. 2006. Weight training in youth—growth, maturation and safety: An evidence-based review. *Clinical Journal of Sports Medicine* 16: 478-487.

McGuigan, M.R., Tatasciore, M., Newton, R.U., and Pettigrew, S. 2009. Eight weeks of resistance training can significantly alter body composition in children who are overweight or obese. *Journal of Strength and Conditioning Research* 23: 80-85.

Miller, M.G., Cheathman, C.C., and Patel, N.D. 2010. Resistance training for adolescents. *Pediatric Clinics of North America* 57: 671-682.

National Strength and Conditioning Association. 2009. Youth resistance training: Updated position statement paper from the National Strength and Conditioning Association. *Journal of Strength and Conditioning Research* 23: S60-S79.

Naughton, G., Farpour-Lambert, N.J., Carlson, J., Bradney, M., and Van Praagh, E. 2000. Physiological issues surrounding the performance of adolescent athletes. *Sports Medicine* 30: 309-325.

Naylor, N.H., Watts, K., Sharpe, J.A., Jones, T.W., Davis, E.A., Thompson, A., George, K., Ramsay, J.M., O'Driscoll, G., and Green, D.J. 2008. Resistance training and diastolic myocardial tissue velocities in obese children. *Medicine & Science in Sports & Exercise* 40: 2027-2032.

Payne, V.G., Morrow, J.R., Jr., Johnson, L., and Dalton, S.N. 1997. Resistance training in children and youth: A meta-analysis. *Research Quarterly for Exercise and Sport* 68: 80-88.

Twisk, J.W.R. 2001. Physical activity guidelines for children and adolescents: A critical review. *Sports Medicine* 31: 617-627.

Resistance Training for Seniors

After studying this chapter, you should be able to

1. distinguish between modifiable and non-modifiable factors as they relate to the senior population,

2. describe the hormonal changes of aging men and women with respect to gonadopause and menopause and the overall implications relative to the senior population,

3. list the changes in body composition associated with aging and the individual, plus cumulative impacts,

4. explain the phenomenon of muscular strength and power loss seen, and the causes within the senior population,

5. list the key adaptations to resistance training for the senior population, and

6. identify the most important aspects of designing a resistance training program for seniors.

With increased age, seniors experience many changes in their bodies, including decreases in hormonal secretions, muscle atrophy, and decreases in bone density. The changes occurring with aging can have dramatic effects as a result of loss of function and independence. An optimal resistance training program can reduce physiological decrements, improve function, and enhance physical capabilities. For people of any age, the health of systems, tissues, and cells improves only when they are used. For skeletal muscle this means that training-related changes and adaptations occur in only those motor units that are used in an exercise. Interestingly, other systems also benefit from motor unit recruitment (e.g., reduced cardiovascular strain with increased peripheral strength). Seniors of all ages can benefit from and are capable of performing properly designed resistance training programs, including men and women of very advanced ages (see figure 11.1).

A person's age is just one factor within a larger context of variables, such as nutrition and level of physical activity, that can be modified to enhance physical capabilities. Although age, genotype, and sex are considered nonmodifiable factors, exercise is a key modifiable determinant of physiological function (Kraemer and Spiering 2006). Resistance training can influence physiological function, from the cells to whole-body physical performance, and therefore confers a remarkable number of benefits for seniors, even those with chronic illnesses. Ultimately, proper training can improve health, improve **functional abilities** (ability to perform tasks of daily living), and lead to a better quality of life. Improvement in the level of normal life or spontaneous physical activity may be one of the most important outcomes from resistance training. Resistance training is one of the most effective and least costly ways to preserve independent living in a wide segment of the population (Rogers and Evans 1993).

Those who design programs for senior populations need to understand the physiological changes that occur with age. Endocrine secretions of such hormones as testosterone, growth hormone, and estrogen decrease with age. We begin this

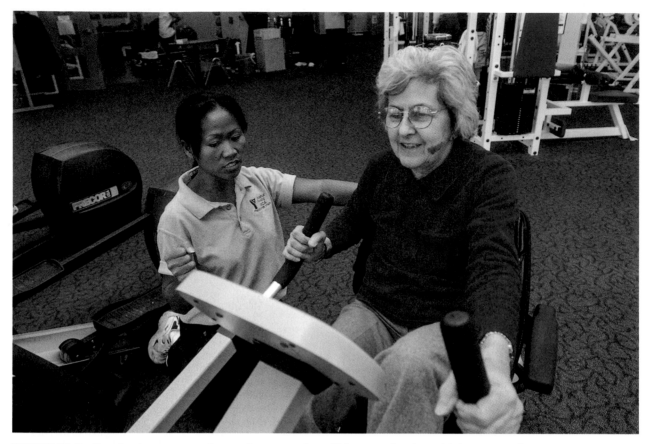

FIGURE 11.1 People at even very advanced ages can benefit from performing resistance exercises.

chapter by describing the hormonal changes with resistance exercise. The second section describes changes in body composition that tend to occur with age including increases in fat mass and decreases in the quality of muscle and connective tissues. All of these changes can influence physical performance with age. Next, we discuss age-related performance changes and how resistance training adaptations can enhance performance and body composition. Finally, we present some basic principles for resistance training program design in the senior population.

Hormonal Changes With Age and Resistance Training

It is well established that, with age, the endocrine glands' ability to secrete hormones decreases. Like any of the body's structures, endocrine glands also go through a cellular aging process. Resistance exercise and training may offset the magnitude

of decreases in the endocrine system's structure and function. This appears to be mediated by the stimulation of endocrine glands with resistance exercise, which results in their synthesizing and secreting the hormones needed for metabolic homeostasis (during exercise) and for anabolic signaling (during recovery).

Despite exercise training, as we age the endocrine system loses its ability to secrete hormones in response to exercise; however, without exercise training this process can be more dramatic as a result of disuse. Compromised glandular function results in reductions in resting concentrations of hormones, including anabolic hormones. The concept of a compromised endocrine system is supported by early studies of testosterone and growth hormone, in which a reduced responsiveness to resistance exercise stimuli in older adults was observed (Chakravati and Collins 1976; Häkkinen and Pakarinen 1993; Hammond et al. 1974; Vermeulen, Rubens, and Verdonck 1972). Figure 11.2 presents an overview of the hormonal changes

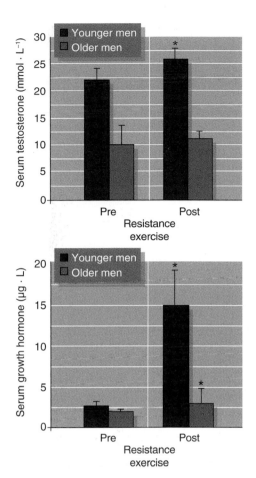

FIGURE 11.2 Hormonal alterations with aging.

* = significant difference from preexercise value.

Data courtesy of Dr. William J. Kraemer, Department of Kinesiology, University of Connecticut, Storrs, CT.

Testosterone

Testosterone is a key hormonal signal in both men and women for various physiological functions, cellular growth, and homeostasis (see chapter 3). Acute increases stimulate signals to a variety of target tissues, such as muscle and bone. The amount of testosterone, or any hormone, in the blood is related to the molar amounts that are released, degraded, or taken out of circulation by binding to target receptors. Binding proteins elongate the half-life of a hormone circulating in the blood. Circulatory changes are sensitive to each of these phenomena. Elevations in the blood mean that production has exceeded breakdown and the amount of target tissue binding that occurs, both of which lower the hormone's blood concentration. Increases in resting hormonal concentrations within the normal physiological ranges typically dictate small regulatory alterations in normal homeostatic function. As with any hormone, testosterone is a signal messenger to the nuclei of the cell to produce a specific genetic response. Therefore, changes in resting hormonal concentrations represent a partial regulation of the feedback systems for a given hormone. Most investigations examine hormones such as testosterone in the fasting state, and thus the interactions with nutrients at the level of the cell are missing. Therefore, the interpretation of testosterone responses and adaptations from most studies must be put into the context of a fasted state without the available influences of nutrients (e.g., amino acids) to modulate the hormonal response patterns and the amount of receptor binding (Vingren et al. 2010).

The resting concentrations of testosterone and the magnitude of its response to an acute bout of resistance exercise appear to diminish with age, especially in men. In general, it has been demonstrated that in older untrained men (62-70 years) the blood increase in both free and total testosterone concentration and the magnitude of increase are much lower than in younger men (≤32 years) in response to a resistance exercise stress, such as five or six sets of squats or leg presses with 10RM resistances with two to three minutes of rest between sets and exercises, or four sets of 10RM in a squat exercise with two minutes of rest between sets and exercises (Häkkinen and Pakarinen 1995; Häkkinen, Pakarinen et al. 2000; Kraemer, Häkkinen et al. 1998, 1999). However, with resistance training, enhancement of the magnitude of the

to resistance exercise with aging. In addition, increases in catabolic hormones and inflammatory cytokines can occur increasing the amount of protein breakdown and inflammation in the body with age (Roubenoff 2003). In combination, such changes are a concern for seniors because of the compromised ability to positively signal protein synthesis and fight inflammatory processes. A resistance training program can help to offset the magnitude of these changes with aging.

Anabolic hormones such as growth hormone can be stimulated to increase, both during and after resistance exercise, which helps to signal various physiological mechanisms and mediate muscle tissue remodeling and growth. This section addresses the changes in various hormones with age and how they interact with and can be modulated by resistance exercise.

exercise-induced response in older men has been shown, although not to the level of younger men. Also, with short-term training, resting concentrations are not affected (Izquierdo et al. 2001; Kraemer, Häkkinen et al. 1999). The lack of a change in resting concentrations is true regardless of whether cardiorespiratory exercise was also performed concurrently with the training program (Ahtiainen et al. 2009; Bell et al. 2000).

A hormone that is not bound to a binding protein, called a **free hormone**, can bind with a receptor. The amount of a free hormone is dictated by the total amount of hormone in circulation. In only 10 weeks of periodized training, resting free testosterone increases in 30-year-old men, but as discussed earlier, not in 62-year-old men (Kraemer, Häkkinen et al. 1999). After a six-month training program, during which both middle-aged (42 years) and older (70 years) men increased strength, no changes in exercise-induced or resting free testosterone were shown (Häkkinen, Pakarinen et al. 2000). Thus, whether training increases the acute response of testosterone in older men is unclear, but resting concentrations appear not to change with training.

Although increases in acute total testosterone have been repeatedly shown to occur in untrained younger men (~30 years) in response to exercise and training (Häkkinen and Pakarinen 1995), when this response capability might end as men age is unclear. Middle-aged men up to 50 years of age have shown an increase in total testosterone in response to an exercise challenge (Häkkinen and Pakarinen 1995). However, other studies have not observed any changes in resting or exercise-induced testosterone concentrations with up to six months of resistance training in middle-aged (~40 years) men despite increases in strength (Häkkinen, Pakarinen et al. 2000). In a case study, a 51-year-old male competitive lifter with 35 years of training experience had lower resting serum testosterone concentrations than young controls did, but a similar acute increase as a result of resistance exercise (Fry, Kraemer et al. 1995). Thus, the overwhelming amount of evidence indicates that testicular function diminishes with age compromising metabolic synthesis and testosterone release into the blood, yet at what age this so-called **gonadopause** (i.e., reduction in the production of the male hormone, testosterone) in men starts appears to be related to multiple factors including genetics, prior training history, and diet.

When gonadopause occurs needs further research.

It is well known that women have 20 to 40 times lower testosterone concentrations than men have. In women, testosterone secretions originate from the adrenal cortex and to a lesser extent from the ovaries. No increases have been demonstrated with acute resistance exercise in women 30 years of age and older. However, in younger women (~22 years) significant increases in total testosterone and free testosterone have been observed following a protocol of six sets of the squat at 10RM with two minutes of rest between sets, albeit at very low absolute concentrations compared to men, as noted earlier (Nindl, Kraemer, Gotshalk et al. 2001). Thus, younger women appear to have a greater acute testosterone response to resistance exercise than older women, and younger women with resistance exercise stimulate greater production of binding proteins (Vingren et al. 2010).

Recent evidence shows that trained women have a very rapid androgen receptor binding cycle for testosterone and can therefore rapidly use the testosterone produced (Vingren et al. 2009). As in men, age may be the predominant factor in women that determines whether they show an increase in resting testosterone with exercise training. No changes were observed after a six-month resistance training protocol during which both middle-aged (42 years) and older (70 years) women showed improvements in strength (Häkkinen, Pakarinen et al. 2000). As in men, this lack of change holds true regardless of whether cardiorespiratory exercise is performed concurrently with resistance exercise (Ahtiainen et al. 2009; Bell et al. 2000).

Such a lack of change in anabolic signaling by testosterone significantly diminishes the body's response in a variety of physiological targets (e.g., skeletal muscle, satellite cells, and motor neurons). Thus, aging can decrease concentrations of both resting and exercise-induced testosterone responses to a resistance exercise protocol. However, the small improvements in signaling seem to benefit the adaptational changes in tissues necessary to slow the aging process and the rate of decline with aging of cellular structure and function.

Cortisol

During the aging process complex interactions occur among inflammatory processes, the immune system, and the adrenal cortex. Exercise stress results in an acute inflammatory process related to the repair and remodeling of tissue, most prominently in skeletal muscle tissue. These inflammatory processes as one ages result in part from other cellular aging and immune function changes, which create a dramatic challenge to physiological well-being. Cortisol, a stress hormone, has multiple roles (see chapter 3) from acting as an anti-inflammatory agent to protecting glycogen stores in the body. Increased cortisol concentrations result in other changes that have earned it a reputation as a catabolic hormone, or a hormone involved in the degradation or breakdown of proteins. A wide array of catabolic influences are attributed to cortisol including inhibiting anabolic signals of testosterone at the gene level in the nuclei, inactivating the immune cells needed for the repair of damaged tissues, blocking downstream signaling systems for protein synthesis (e.g., mTOR), and promoting protein breakdown to spare the use of glycogen. Resistance training has been used to reduce the resting concentrations of cortisol and in some cases reduce the response to stressors such as exercise and environmental and psychological stress.

Obviously, with any intense exercise stressor, such as aerobic exercise greater than 70% of maximal oxygen consumption or a lifting protocol involving major muscle groups and multiple sets, cortisol increases in the blood. Several studies have shown some changes in blood cortisol response with resistance exercise training leading to an improvement in the so-called testosterone–cortisol ratio in older men but not in women (Häkkinen and Pakarinen 1994; Izquierdo et al. 2001). It has been shown that with short-term resistance exercise training, resting cortisol concentrations in the blood are reduced in older men (62 years). Also, although increases occur in response to resistance exercise stress, even after training, the magnitude of the response is diminished, meaning that the stress response has been reduced (Kraemer, Häkkinen et al. 1999). However, a great deal of study is needed to better understand the interactions of both testosterone and cortisol with the anabolic and catabolic signaling pathway responses that occur in the body especially with aging (Crewther et al. 2011).

Growth Hormones

Growth hormone has caught the aging public's eye because of the many extraordinary claims for its use in antiaging therapies. It was estimated in 2005 that the use of recombinant human growth hormone for antiaging therapy in America hovered around approximately 25,000 adults, and this may be even higher today (Perls, Reisman, and Olshansky 2005). Many of the purported benefits of growth hormone administration are speculative and have little support in the literature because increases in lean tissue in some cases may be the result of increased water retention alone (Kraemer et al. 2010). In fact, exogenous growth hormone administration has been shown not to cause any greater increase in muscle mass than resistance training in elderly subjects receiving no growth hormone (Thorner 2009). Given the risks and potentially limited benefits of exogenous growth hormone use, optimizing resistance training programs to make endocrine glands more effective in both the production and secretion of hormones may be the best treatment option to reduce the effects of aging (Thorner 2009).

As previously discussed, natural endogenous GH has over 100 variants apart from the classic 191 amino acid 22 kD monomer produced by the DNA machinery in the anterior pituitary (see chapter 3). It is thought that many of these variants, especially the higher-molecular-weight aggregates, have important anabolic functions because their concentrations are 10 to 100 times higher than those of the 22 kD form. To date, responses of bioactive growth hormone have not been investigated in seniors, but it is thought that even these higher-molecular-weight bioactive growth hormone variants are diminished by age (unpublished data from Dr. Kraemer's laboratory). The actions of growth hormone(s) are complex. Moreover, all of the data on growth hormone in older people have been studied examining only the 22 kD isoform that is measured by immunoassays (assays using antibodies) and not any of the bioactive isoforms measured by other biochemical assays (Kraemer et al. 2010). Thus, all of the growth hormone responses and adaptations discussed in this chapter are based on studies that have only been able to examine the response of this primary hormone that is produced by DNA machinery in the anterior pituitary somatrophs (i.e., classic 191 amino acid sequence) 22 kD isoform.

The acute responses of growth hormone to resistance exercise clearly differ with age. Growth hormone was shown to increase in response to acute 10RM resistance exercise in younger men, but not in older men or women (Häkkinen and

Pakarinen 1995). In a 10RM protocol with four sets, when older and younger men were matched for activity levels, both groups showed increased acute postexercise growth hormone levels, but these increases were significantly higher in the younger (30 years) group than in the older (62 years) group (Kraemer, Häkkinen et al. 1998, 1999). However, with 8 to 10 weeks of training, limited acute changes were observed in older men suggesting that longer-term training may be needed (e.g., over six months) for alterations to occur. In addition, other growth hormone variants could be changing on a much faster time line but not be represented by the adaptations seen in the 22 kD isoform. More research is needed to better understand the complexity of the anterior pituitary gland's responses. However, it does appear that if total work is increased, or if the glycolytic response is greater in a lifting protocol, a higher acute 22 kD growth hormone response will occur. Thus, the higher growth hormone values seen when comparing the younger and older men or women are typically due to higher work or metabolic capacity in the younger people. Even with isometric exercise, when comparing younger (26.5 years) and older (70 years) men, higher growth hormone responses are produced by the younger men because younger men can produce more force and greater amounts of total work (Häkkinen, Pakarinen et al. 1998).

In women, as in men, few changes occur in resting concentrations of growth hormone with training, and those that do occur are not as great in older women as they are in younger women (Häkkinen, Pakarinen 2000). However, the ability to increase growth hormone concentrations after a resistance exercise bout can be enhanced with training in older people, yet typically not to the extent that it can be in younger people (Häkkinen, Pakarinen 2001). Thus, it appears that the hypothalamic-pituitary-axis undergoes an aging process limiting its ability to produce growth hormone(s).

Insulin and Insulin-Like Growth Factor I

In both younger and older people, increases in body fat can compromise insulin sensitivity (Dela and Kjaer 2006). Resistance exercise improves insulin sensitivity in older people with diabetes or compromised insulin sensitivity (Strasser and Schobersberger 2011). Insulin in the fasted state displays an acute decrease with resistance exercise (Kraemer, Häkkinen et al. 1998). Six months of training has been shown to improve insulin sensitivity in older people (65-74 years) who are insulin resistant as a result of physical inactivity and obesity (Ryan et al. 2004). Resistance training in the 7- to 9RM zone over 26 weeks also decreased glycosylated hemoglobin (HbA1c) levels in 39- to 70-year-old diabetic men and women (Sigal et al. 2007). These benefits to **insulin resistance** and blood sugar control are especially important because most people with pathological conditions such as diabetes can perform resistance training.

With age, resting concentrations of insulin-like growth factor I (IGF-I) decrease. IGF-I was higher in younger men at all time points (pre- and post-training, acute and at rest) over the course of a 10-week training program. Additionally, only the younger men displayed an increase in IGF-I binding protein-3 after training (Kraemer, Häkkinen et al. 1999). Like younger people, frail elderly people show increases in IGF-I staining in muscle after chronic resistance training related to increased type II muscle hypertrophy (Singh et al. 1999). Older men (67-80 years) performing only two sets of 12RM and four sets of 5RM demonstrated increases in blood total and free IGF-I immediately after and six hours after a workout, yet no changes were observed in the binding proteins (Bermon et al. 1999). With training, resting IGF-I and binding proteins showed no significant changes, indicating that the acute response of IGF-I may be more important in the adaptations related to IGF-I and that acute signaling to nuclear DNA is the key to endocrine function.

Older women (~68 years) with low bone mineral density performed a resistance training program. Before training, concentrations of IGF-I, along with the binding proteins, were all significantly lower than those in an age-matched group of healthy women. Resistance training increased the resting IGF-I concentrations, but no changes took place in the binding proteins. The authors theorized that in women with low bone mineral density, the stimulation of IGF-I with training may contribute to improved physiological function (Parkhouse et al. 2000). It has also been shown that no change in resting IGF-I after 21 weeks of training in women 64 years of age occurs despite increased strength, power, and muscle size (Häkkinen, Pakarinen et al. 2001).

Estrogen

Just as testosterone production decreases in men with age, women undergo a decline in the sex hormone estrogen with age. This decrease in estrogen is characteristic of what is commonly referred to as **menopause**, a period that coincides with the ceasing of the menstrual cycle. This decrease in estrogen level contributes to the loss of strength, muscle mass, and bone mineral density associated with old age in women (Bemben et al. 2000; Leite et al. 2010). Resistance exercise, particularly of a high intensity (~80% of 1RM), has been shown to preserve bone mineral density in postmenopausal women (Bemben et al. 2000; Bocalini et al. 2009; Leite 2010). Additionally, resistance exercise has been shown to increase strength (Prestes, Shiguemoto et al. 2009) and muscle mass (Leite et al. 2010; Orsatti et al. 2008) in postmenopausal women. Resistance training that is periodized and uses heavier resistances seems to be important to optimize the end points of estrogen's target tissues in women.

Implications of Endocrine Changes With Age

Chronic performance of a resistance training program cannot maintain endocrine function, particularly resting endocrine concentrations, entirely. The acute responses to resistance exercise workouts may be lower in older men and women; however, both men and women typically display improved postexercise responses with training. The hormones of the body are important for muscle regeneration after mechanical damage in both younger and older people (Bamman et al. 2001). The changes in acute responses to resistance exercise facilitate endocrine secretions when they are most needed (directly after mechanical stimulus to muscle, tissue, and bone) and may therefore contribute to the strength and muscle fiber changes in seniors.

Again, it is important to remember that resistance training programs train not only skeletal muscle but also the other systems, tissues, and, specific to this section, endocrine glands. The structure and function of these glands can only be maintained in the fight against aging and disuse by challenging their functional abilities, just as skeletal muscle is challenged. The implementation and optimal design of a resistance training program

(i.e., individualized, periodized, and properly progressed) are vital for creating an effective exercise stimulus while limiting any potential for injury or such syndromes as overreaching and overtraining.

An appreciation of the acute hormonal responses to exercise helps in understanding the adaptations of muscle, bone, and other tissues. Understanding the hormonal responses to training in seniors also aids in understanding body composition changes, the topic of the next section.

Body Composition Changes in Seniors

Body composition describes the percentage of fat mass and various components of fat-free mass, including muscle, bone, tissue, and organs, of the body. With age, all components of body composition tend to change. This section is a review of the effects of body composition change on resting metabolic rate and includes a discussion of the changes in bone, tissue, and muscle with aging. Resistance training's effects on metabolic rate, muscle, bone, and tendon can help people maintain function during aging. The overall performance consequences and implications of age-related changes in muscle and body composition are addressed later in this chapter.

Decreased Metabolic Rate With Age and Resistance Exercise

One factor that may influence body composition in seniors is **resting metabolic rate (RMR)**, or the amount of energy expended during complete rest for vital physiological functions such as heart rate and breathing. Resting metabolic rates are lower in older (>60 years) men and women than in younger (20-35 years) men and women even when adjusting for fat-free mass, fat mass, and smoking history (Frisard et al. 2007; Krems et al. 2005; Woolf et al 2008). Interestingly, one investigation found that women who lived to at least 95 years of age had unexpectedly very low resting metabolic rates when compared to middle-aged women (Rizzo et al. 2005). This may have been less an indication of age and more an indication of the very old women's overall health. Resting metabolic rate in a longitudinal investigation decreased each decade by 5% in men and 4% in women (Luhrmann et al. 2009). Longitudinal data also show the decrease with age over the course of five years in those over 73 years of age (Rothenberg, Bosaeus, and Steen 2003); the decrease is more rapid in men between 70 and 80 years of age than in men between 40 and 50 years (Ruggiero et al. 2008).

One factor that appears to coincide with decreased metabolic rate is increased fat deposition. When tracking the same people over the course of eight years in a German population, height, waist-to-hip ratio, fat-free mass, and energy expenditure decreased while body mass index and fat mass increased (Luhrmann et al. 2009). As fewer calories are burned at rest as a result of the decrease in metabolic rate, aging may predispose people to increased fat mass (see box 11.1). As discussed later, resting metabolic rate is correlated to fat-free mass (Sparti et al. 1997), and resistance training can increase or slow the decrease in fat-free

mass. Thus, resistance training can be an important lifestyle intervention to offset some of the decrease in resting metabolic rate with aging.

One factor correlated to metabolic rate that resistance training can address is the amount of lean tissue mass. Resting metabolic rate is influenced by a number of factors, including muscle mass and lean tissue. Decreases in metabolic rate often coincide with decreased amounts of muscle tissue, which also influences the decreases in the mass of other tissues and organs and their specific metabolic rates (St-Onge and Gallagher 2010). By one estimate (Gallagher et al. 1998), skeletal muscle accounts for between 18 and 25% of resting energy expenditure. Although muscle mass may not account for all of the changes in energy expenditure, resistance training can help to optimize metabolic rate in the elderly.

 BOX 11.1 **RESEARCH**

Resistance Training and Age-Related Obesity

One might ask the question, Is obesity related only to age, and what might resistance training do to help? Obesity appears to increase with normal aging, from 18% in young adults to a peak of 31% in middle age. At the age range of 45 to 65 years, obesity affects 9% of Asian Americans, 30% of white Americans, 35% of Hispanic Americans, and 41% of black Americans. Although the increase in obesity up to age 65 appears to support an association between age and obesity, obesity actually falls to 24.7% after age 65 (Mendez 2010). The rationale for this is not entirely clear, but may be related to decreased life expectancy in those with obesity, resulting in a greater proportion of thinner people surviving long enough to be surveyed after age 65. In nonsmokers who are morbidly obese, life expectancy drops from 81 years to between 68 and 76 years in white men and from 75 years to between 59 and 74 years in black men (Finkelstein et al 2010). The decrease in obesity above 65 years could also be a function of malnutrition in seniors.

The prevalence of obesity at any age warrants action. In conjunction with nutritional interventions and cardiorespiratory exercise, resistance training may help to address the increase in body fat. Resistance training for 26 weeks increased total energy expenditure in older adults (61-77 years) and contributed to greater oxidation of lipids (Hunter et al. 2000). The increased total energy expenditure and spontaneous activity in seniors may have been related to increased aerobic ability caused by resistance training (Jubrias et al. 2001). With six months of resistance training, muscle oxidative ability increased 57%, muscle size increased 10%, and mitochondrial volume density increased 31%. Thus, along with other treatments, resistance training can help control total-body fat mass in seniors.

Finkelstein, E.A., Brown, D.S., Wrage, L.A., Allaire, B.T., and Thomas, J.H. 2010. Individual and aggregate years-of-life-lost associated with overweight and obesity. *Obesity* 18: 333-339.

Hunter, G.R., Wetzstein, C.J., Fields, D.A., Brown, A., and Bamman, M.M. 2000. Resistance training increases total energy expenditure and free-living physical activity in older adults. *Journal of Applied Physiology* 89: 977-984.

Jubrias, S.A., Esselman, P.C., Price, L.B., Cress, M.E., and Conley, K.E. 2001. Large energetic adaptations of elderly muscle to resistance and endurance training. *Journal of Applied Physiology* 90: 1663-1670.

Mendez, E. 2010. In U.S., obesity peaks in middle age. Gallup, Inc. www.gallup.com/poll/142736/obesity-peaks-middle-age.aspx.

Interestingly, resistance training for 24 weeks increased resting metabolic rate by 9% in both young and older men, although, surprisingly, this was not observed in younger or older women (Lemmer et al. 2001). Most likely the lack of metabolic response in women was due to the ineffectiveness of the training program used in the study to increase lean tissue mass. A low-volume training protocol was used (i.e., one set for the upper body and one or two sets for the lower body), and the subjects used self-selected resistances with pneumatic resistance training equipment. Although the program improved strength, apparently through neurological mechanisms, it did not stimulate enough muscle protein accretion to increase lean tissue significantly in women (see chapter 9).

Bone Density Changes With Age and Resistance Exercise

As previously described, the process of menopause is associated with decreases in bone density in women, although osteoporosis is a serious issue in both sexes. In addition to hip fractures, wrist and rib fractures are a major concern in the elderly. Only about half of seniors are able to regain independence following a hip fracture (Morrison, Chassin, and Siu 1998). Following hip fracture, one-year mortality rates are between 15 and 24% (LaVelle 2003; Wolinsky, Fitzgerald, and Stump 1997). Although hip fractures are often associated with a fall, surprisingly, the fracture is often the cause of the fall. In the elderly, about 90% of hip fracture falls occur from a simple standing position (Baumgaertner and Higgins 2002). Thus, proactive action must be taken to maintain healthy bone density before fracture occurs, which is often the first overt sign of osteoporosis. Fracture is not the only concern for joints in seniors, however (see box 11.2).

Resistance training increases bone density at a rate of 1 to 3% each year in seniors, whereas those who do not perform resistance exercise lose about 1 to 3% in bone density in the same time period (Frost 1997; Kohrt, Ehsani, and Birge 1997; Layne and Nelson 1999; Lohman 2004; Marcus 2002; Nelson 1994; Ryan et al. 2004; Smith et al. 1984; Vincent and Braith 2002; Warburton

BOX 11.2 RESEARCH

What Are the Benefits of Resistance Exercise for Joint Pain?

Osteoarthritis (OA) is one of the most common diseases of old age and is frequently encountered by practitioners who work with seniors. It is characterized by loss of cartilage at a joint and a subsequent overcompensation of bone growth to repair the damage. This growth exacerbates the cartilage loss issue, causing a painful, joint-wide problem (Fransen et al. 2009). OA is a very specific joint ailment with the effects specific to the joint affected (e.g., hip, knee, shoulder), the anatomical location within that joint (medial, lateral, anterior, posterior, combination), and the condition's grade of severity (grade 1 is the mildest; grade 4 is the most severe). Resistance exercise is beneficial for older people with OA because it results in increased strength, improved function, and decreased pain (Latham and Liu 2010).

Many people avoid exercise when joint pain is present, but exercise can improve clinical outcomes. A recent meta-analysis examined the effect of resistance training interventions on osteoarthritis, rheumatoid arthritis, and fibromyalgia in people with an average age of over 50 years (Kelley et al. 2011). The meta-analysis found significant improvements in pain and physical function with a low rate of adverse events across studies. The improvements were also clinically important, similar to those expected from analgesic agents such as acetaminophen and NSAIDS. Thus, resistance exercise interventions can be an important therapeutic aid for joint pain in seniors.

Fransen, M., McConnell, S., Hernandez-Molina, G., and Reichenbach, S. 2009. Exercise for osteoarthritis of the hip. *Cochrane Database of Systematic Reviews:* CD007912.

Latham, N., and Liu, C. J. 2010. Strength training in older adults: The benefits for osteoarthritis. *Clinics in Geriatric Medicine* 26: 445-459.

Kelley, G.A., Kelley, K.S., Hootman, J.M., and Jones, D.L. 2011. Effects of community deliverable exercise on pain and physical function in adults with arthritis and other rheumatic diseases: A meta-analysis. *Arthritis Care & Research* 63: 79-93.

and Bredin 2006). Resistance exercise increases markers of bone formation (Vincent and Braith 2002) and decreases markers of bone resorption (Whipple et al. 2004) resulting in increased bone formation. Although resistance training can benefit bone, appropriate resistance training prescription is important. Bone adapts and responds to the strain applied to it, including the strain that muscles place on bone during resistance exercise. This underlines the importance of using a resistance heavy enough to produce adaptations. An exercise must place strain on a particular bone to promote adaptations (Frost 1997; Winters-Stone and Snow 2006).

It is important to note that muscular strength and lean body mass are the best predictors of bone mineral density (Blain et al. 2001; Cussler et al. 2003; Egan, Reilly et al. 2006; Witzke and Snow 1999). Although runners engage in an activity that exerts a strain on the bones of the lower body, they tend to have lower bone density than those who are sedentary (Bilanin, Blanchard, and Russek-Cohen 1989; Hetland, Haarbo, and Christiansen 1993; Hind, Truscott, and Evans 2006; MacDougall 1992; MacKelvie et al. 2000), which can be addressed with resistance exercise (Smith et al. 1984; Hind, Truscott, and Evans 2006).

A resistance training program in older women (45-65 years) demonstrated no changes in bone density (dual-energy X-ray absorptiometry) after a linear periodized 24-week program despite increases in muscular strength. This indicates that a longer period of training may be necessary to affect bone density (Humphries et al. 2000). Although a linear periodization program of moderate to high intensity for 24 weeks produced similar changes in muscle strength in older men and women, men appeared to be capable of higher absolute training intensities and therefore stimulated increases in spinal bone density, whereas the older women saw no changes. This indicates that training intensity plays an important role in bone adaptations (Conroy and Earle 2000). Older women have shown significant increases in femoral and lumbar spine bone density when using higher-intensity resistance training programs (e.g., 80% of 1RM for 8-10 repetitions), but a year or more of training may be required to show bone density increases (Guadalupe-Grau et al. 2009). In addition, resistance training also resulted in an improvement in balance, total level of physical activity, and muscle mass. It has also been shown that one year of

jumping and bounding exercise performed two times per week increased proximal femur and tibial shaft bone mineral density in women from 50 to 57 years of age less than five years after the onset of menopause (Cheng et al. 2002). Thus, resistance training of the proper prescription over longer training periods does have a positive effect on bone density as well as most of the major risk factors for an osteoporotic fracture.

Tendon Changes With Age and Resistance Exercise

Tendons are the connective tissues that attach muscle to bone and are responsible for muscular force transmission to the skeleton. The muscle–tendon complex (MTC) (see chapter 4) describes the relationship between the muscle and tendon. Muscle–tendon stiffness is defined as the amount of force necessary to lengthen a tendon to a specific length. If a greater amount of force is needed to lengthen a tendon to a specific length, the MTC is stiffer. The interactions of changes in the muscle architecture and the tendon's mechanical properties change with age. Increases in muscle force production and the tendon's mechanical properties can occur as a result of several months of resistance training. A muscle fiber's fascicle length and tendon stiffness were shown to increase by 10 and 64%, respectively, with just 14 weeks of resistance training (Narici, Maffulli, and Maganaris 2008). However, resistance training had no effect on relative length–tension properties of the muscle suggesting that increased tendon stiffness and increased fascicle length neutralized each other's effects.

Because tendons are in a parallel series with muscle, their mechanical properties, such as stiffness, affect the efficiency of force transmission and the force-length-velocity relationship of the functional unit. The patella tendon in aged people (74.3 ± 3.5 years) increased in stiffness in response to 14 weeks of resistance training in comparison to sedentary controls (67.1 ± 2 years). The training routine consisted of leg press and leg extension exercises for two sets of 10 repetitions at 80% of 5RM, three times per week (Reeves, Maganaris, and Narici 2003). These authors concluded that increases in tendon stiffness may reduce tendon injury and increase functional task completion times. Although optimal training protocols for tendon strength and stiffness have not been completely elucidated, it appears that resistance training may reduce tendon injury, improve tendon stiffness, and thereby improve total force transfer in seniors.

Tendinopathy, the often asymptomatic degeneration of tendon, is best treated with an eccentric exercise program (Alfredson et al. 1998). For example, three sets of 10 repetitions of eccentric exercise have been employed at the Achilles (Ohberg, Lorentzen, and Alfredson 2004), patella (Jonsson et al. 2006), and rotator cuff tendons (Young et al. 2005); clinical success (e.g., no pain with activity and more normal tendon structure) was higher in young people. Although resistance exercise may help in the treatment of tendinopathy, the effect of eccentric training in elderly populations has not been examined. Additionally, the optimal eccentric program to affect tendons has not been elucidated.

Loss of Muscle With Age

It is well established that the properties of muscle change with increasing age. A plethora of investigations have shown a reduction in muscle mass as people age (Berger and Doherty 2010; Boirie 2009; Evans and Campbell 1993; Frontera et al. 1991; Häkkinen and Häkkinen 1991; Häkkinen, Kallinen, and Komi 1994; Janssen et al. 2000; Pillard et al 2011). This age-associated reduction in muscle mass historically had been termed **sarcopenia** (Berger and Doherty 2010; Evans and Campbell 1993), although as of today there is no real universal definition. It is generally considered to be related to a loss of muscle mass and low muscle strength or function. In addition, reduced tissue quality has also been considered a component of sarcopenia (e.g., fat replacing muscle fibers as in the white, marbled sections of red meat), as has fibrosis, increased inflammatory responses, obesity, reduced anabolic signaling, and degradation of the neuromuscular junction. Thus, many factors act in a type of constellation of catabolic influences in the aging of muscle. Loss of muscle mass, one component of that constellation, is a natural result of aging and muscle cell **apoptosis** (i.e., programmed cell death).

Using computerized EMG single motor unit analyses, Doherty and colleagues (1993) estimated a 47% reduction in the number of motor units in older people (60-81 years). For women in their 70s, the quadriceps cross-sectional area of muscle is 77% that of women in their 20s (Young, Stokes, and Crowe 1984). The decline in muscle mass appears to be due to the reduction in the cross-sectional area of the individual muscle fibers, the loss of individual muscle fibers, or both (Frontera et al. 1988; Larsson 1982; Lexell et al. 1983; Lexell, Taylor, and Sjostrom 1988). Although research on the phenomenon of sarcopenia continues, the aforementioned characteristics of sarcopenia are generally assumed.

Loss of muscle mass begins to be apparent by age 30 years but is most pronounced starting at age 50 (Faulkner et al. 2008; Janssen et al. 2000; Faulkner et al 2008). This effect on muscle mass is independent of muscle location (upper versus vs. lower extremities) and function (extension versus vs. flexion) (Frontera et al. 1991). However, greater decreases in lower-body compared to upper-body muscle mass have also been noted (Janssen et al. 2000). It is important to note that muscle fibers that are lost are subsequently replaced with fat or fibrous connective tissue (Taaffe et al. 2009). Not only is there a decrease in cross-sectional area of muscles, but there is also an increase of intramuscular fat, which is most pronounced in women (Imamura et al. 1983). Seniors have a twofold increase in non-contractile tissue in muscle compared to younger people (Kent-Braun, Ng, and Young 2000). Thus, in addition to muscle mass loss, other factors resulting in changes in muscle are also occurring.

In general, loss of motor units appears to affect fibers that have fallen into disuse. There appears to be a preferential loss of type II muscle fibers with aging, which would negatively affect power capabilities (Goodpaster et al. 2006; Korhonen et al 2006). The number of muscle fibers in the midsection of the vastus lateralis of autopsy specimens is lower by about 23% in elderly men (age 70-73) compared to young men (age 19-37) (Lexell et al. 1983). The decline is more marked in type II muscle fibers, which fall from an average of 60% in sedentary young men to below 30% of total fibers after the age of 80 (Larsson 1983). This preferential loss of type II muscle fibers causes a compression of the motor units and fibers, especially type II fibers, available to be recruited. The compression of motor units can have negative consequences on strength and power. Whether due to disuse or aging, the preferential loss of type II motor units and fibers may impair strength, power, speed, and functional abilities.

A host of potential mechanisms that may be involved in the loss of muscle fibers are still being uncovered as some begin to take a more global view of sarcopenia as a type of syndrome. The loss of muscle fibers with aging may be a result of muscle cell death, termed apoptosis, or a loss of contact with the nervous system, termed denervation (Häkkinen, Kallinen, and Komi 1994). In some cases, muscle fibers may regain contact with the nervous system, termed re-innervation, as a result of maintained or increased activity. Denervation of motor units occurs with age; therefore, the number of muscle fibers can be reduced by half in older age due to the death of alpha motor units and their associated muscle fibers (Doherty et al. 1993). The loss of muscle fibers compromises the individual motor unit's ability to produce force and affects the basic metabolic functions of the entire muscle, such as a reduced caloric resting metabolic rate due to reduced muscle mass. Figure 11.3 presents an overview of the basic muscle fiber changes with aging. Although hypertrophy of existing fibers is possible with resistance exercise, motor unit loss is irreversible.

Changes in Physical Performance With Age

The changes in body composition with age and the loss of skeletal muscle and especially type II motor units can have wide-ranging effects on strength and power performances. In this section, we will characterize the changes in performance that occur with age.

Patterns of Strength Loss With Age

A recent study of anthropometric predictors of physical performance in older men and women found that relative strength was the most important predictor of physical performance in men, but that body mass index (BMI) was a more important predictor for women (Fragala et al., 2012). Although loss of muscle strength may not always be the most substantial contributor to a reduction in physical performance, strength remains

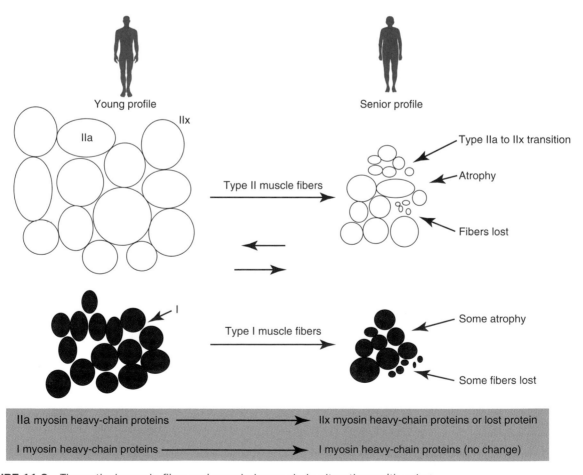

FIGURE 11.3 Theoretical muscle fiber and myosin heavy chain alterations with aging.

an important factor in maintaining functional abilities (Brill et al. 2000; Berger and Doherty 2010). Muscle weakness can advance to the stage at which an elderly person cannot perform common **activities of daily living**, such as getting out of a chair, sweeping the floor, lifting grocery bags, using the toilet, or taking out the trash. Reduced functional ability increases the chance of nursing home placement. Conversely, with greater muscle strength, increased levels of spontaneous activity have been seen in both healthy, free-living older people and very old, frail men and women. Strength training can enhance muscle strength in seniors (see figure 11.4)

Under normal conditions, strength appears to peak between the ages of 20 and 30, after which it remains relatively stable or slightly decreases over the next 20 years (Häkkinen, Kallinen, and Komi 1994; Faulkner et al 2008). In the sixth decade of life, a more dramatic decrease occurs in both men and women that is most dramatic after age 70, with this decrease perhaps more pronounced in women. More specifically, in subjects in the seventh and eighth decades of life, the average loss of strength due to age is between 20 and 40%, whereas reports of even greater strength losses (50% or more) have been made for those in the ninth decade of life and beyond (Berger and Doherty 2010).

Knee-extensor strength of a group of healthy 80-year-old men and women studied in the Copenhagen City Heart Study (Danneskoild-Samsoe et al. 1984) was found to be 30% lower than that reported in a previous population study (Aniansson and Gustavsson 1981) of 70-year-old men and women. In a comparison of middle-aged men (42 years) and older men (65 years), it has been demonstrated that the older men had a 14% reduction in 1RM squat, a 24% reduction in maximal isometric force, a 13% reduction in the quadriceps femoris muscle mass, and a lower concentration of free testosterone (Izquierdo et al. 2001). Cross-sectional as well as longitudinal data indicate that muscle strength declines by approximately 15% per decade in the sixth and seventh decades and about 30% thereafter (Danneskoild-Samsoe et al. 1984; Harries and Bassey

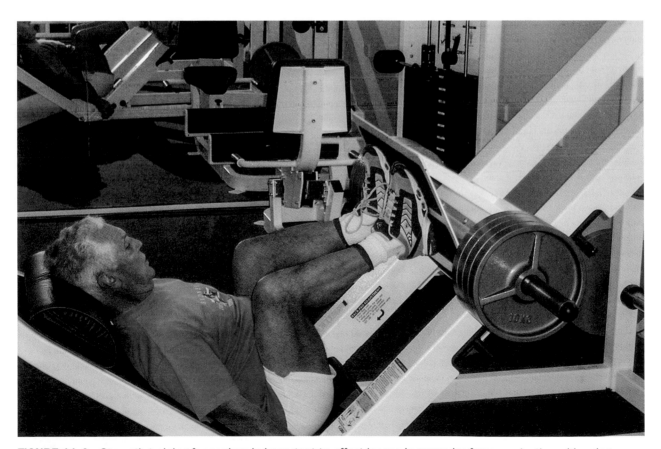

FIGURE 11.4   Strength training for seniors is important to offset losses in muscular force production with aging.
Photo courtesy of Dr. Robert Newton, Edith Cowan University, Perth, Australia.

1990; Larsson 1978; Murray et al. 1985). The loss of motor units appears to be most problematic for women as they pass the age of 60 years because their absolute starting point for muscle tissue mass is lower than that of men (Carmeli, Coleman, and Reznick 2002; Roubenoff 2001; Vandervoot and Symons 2001).

Conflicting reports concerning the magnitude of strength loss do exist. This may be due in part to the use of cross-sectional and longitudinal data. Cross-sectional studies may seriously underestimate the magnitude of strength loss with age (Bassey and Harries 1993). For example, the cross-sectional data (Bassey and Harries 1993) show a 2% loss of grip strength per year in the elderly. However, when people were followed longitudinally, the loss of hand grip strength was 3% per year for men and nearly 5% per year for women over a four-year period (Bassey and Harries 1993). Additionally, longitudinal rates of leg strength loss per decade are about 60% of estimates of strength loss from cross-sectional data (Hughes et al. 2001).

Long-term involvement with strength training appears to offset the magnitude of strength loss and enhances the actual absolute strength capabilities of an individual, but declines do occur even in competitive weightlifters (Faulkner et al. 2008; Kraemer 1992a; Meltzer 1994; Faulkner et al 2008). Interestingly, the aging curve of fitness parameters of "master athletes" indicates that the rate of decline of peak oxygen consumption with aging was not different from that of sedentary people, but that strength losses are not linear and exhibit plateaus at various ages (Wiswell et al. 2001). Master athletes involved in weight events and weightlifting for decades of their lives into their sixth and seventh decades of life had better strength and power performances than untrained men 10 to 20 years younger (Ojanen, Rauhala, and Häkkinen 2007). Thus, physiological age and chronological age may not be the same when training is performed throughout a lifetime. However, it is important to note that the maintenance of higher physiological and functional abilities appears to be mediated only with the maintenance of training, because strength and aerobic abilities will decline faster in untrained individuals or when people stop training or working out.

Figure 11.5 depicts a general theoretical aging curve for muscle strength in trained and untrained people. However, the magnitude of strength decrease varies by gender, sex, and individual

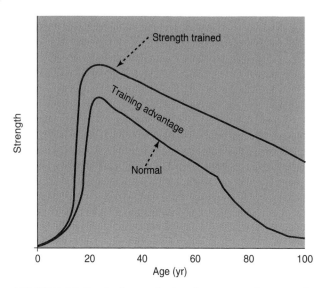

FIGURE 11.5 A theoretical aging curve for muscle strength. The magnitude of change will vary by muscle group and sex.

muscles and muscle groups. For example, the decline in the isokinetic strength of knee extensors and knee flexors averages about 14% and 16%, respectively, in both sexes (Hughes et al. 2001). However, women demonstrated slower rates of decline in elbow extensor and flexor strength (about 2% per decade) than men (about 12% per decade). The strength loss in the lower extremities has been shown to be greater than that of the upper extremities in both sexes (Häkkinen, Kallinen, and Komi 1994; Lynch et al. 1999). Concentric and eccentric peak torque per cross-sectional area of both the arm and leg musculature declines with age, but differences do exist between muscle groups and muscle action types (Lynch et al. 1999). Thus, strength will decrease with age, but the decrease is lessened with continued training and varies by muscle group and sex.

Causes of Decreased Strength With Age

The loss of motor units, even in healthy, active people, appears to be a primary factor underlying the age-associated reductions in strength (Doherty et al. 1993). In addition, a loss of force per cross-sectional area as a result of some unknown intrinsic factor in contractile proteins may occur with age (Frontera, Suh et al. 2000). The strength decline with aging may also be related to different factors in different various muscle groups. For example, it has been demonstrated that for leg tasks, factors other than lean tissue are involved in the force production loss, whereas in the arm flexors, the loss of lean tissue explains the functional decline in strength (Landers et al. 2001)

In effect, a number of factors potentially contribute to the loss of muscle strength and power. How these factors interact with each other and what exact mechanisms predominate under certain conditions or at certain ages remain speculative (see box 11.3). The following are some of the primary factors associated with muscle weakness with aging (Berger and Doherty 2010; Fiatarone and Evans 1993; Kraemer 1992b; Berger and Doherty 2010):

- Natural musculoskeletal changes that can come with aging
- Accumulation of chronic diseases
- Medications needed to treat diseases
- Disuse atrophy
- Undernourishment
- Reductions in hormonal secretions

 BOX 11.3 RESEARCH

Malnutrition in Seniors

While obesity receives significant attention, undernutrition also is a significant issue, particularly in seniors who are socially isolated, socioeconomically disadvantaged, or disabled (Lee and Berthelot 2010). In contrast to developing countries, where malnutrition is typically seen in infants (de Onis et al. 2004), in the United States between 2,000 and 3,000 American seniors die of malnutrition each year (Heron 2009). Food insecurity affects 11.4% of American seniors over age 60 years or approximately 5 million adults (Ziliak, Gundersen, and Haist et al. 2008), and with between 10 and 60% of older hospitalized adults suffering from malnutrition (Chen et al. 2007). The U.S. Centers for Disease Control in estimated that in the United States malnutrition affects about 1 person in every 100,000 Americans. By age 65, that number increases to about 1.4 people, then steadily increases in a highly variable manner due to inherent genetics to 20.9 people out of every 100,000 people at about 75 years of age. The causes for this undernutrition are not concrete completely understood at this time, but physiological (disease, decreased metabolism), psychological (depression and other cognitive disorders), social (no one to cook and eat with), economic, and behavioral (sedentary lifestyle) factors are potential contributors. A host of factors, endocrine changes, altered physical activity levels, changes in the nervous system, and muscle atrophy, result in decreased power and strength with age (Porter, Vandervoort, and Lexell 1995). However, malnutrition also appears to play an important role in this age-related loss of strength and power via the reduction in protein and total caloric intake needed for optimal maintenance of tissues.

Practitioners should consider working with dietetic staff to assess clients' nutrition. Additionally, reaching out to isolated (community dwelling or homebound), socioeconomically disadvantaged seniors may make the greatest difference. Practitioners can help by volunteering for senior care programs, meal delivery programs, charitable and religious organizations, and other services; starting senior health and fitness programs remembering that the problem is not always one of education but of means; and checking on neighbors, retired colleagues, relatives, and those in local or religious communities. In summary, although proper nutrition may appear to be the biggest concern, other social interventions may be the best approach for addressing malnutrition in the elderly.

Chen, C.C-H., Bai, Y.Y., Hang, G.H., Tang, S.T. 2007. Revisiting the concept of malnutrition in older people. *Journal of Clinical Nursing* 16: 2015-2026.

de Onis, M., Blössner, M., Borghi, E., Morris, R., Frongillo, E.A. 2004. Methodology for estimating regional and global trends of child malnutrition. *International Journal of Epidemiology* 33: 1260-70.

Heron, M., Hoyert, D., Murphy, S., Xu, J., Kochanek, K., and Tejada-Vera, B. 2009. Deaths: Final data for 2006. *National Vital Statistics Reports* 57: 33-37.

Porter, M.M., Vandervoort, A.A., Lexell, J. 1995. Aging of human muscle: Structure, function and adaptability. *Scandinavian Journal of Medicine and Science in Sports* 5: 129-42.

Ziliak, J.P., Gundersen, C., and Haist, M.P. 2008. The causes, consequences, and future of senior hunger in America. Meals on Wheels Association of America Foundation Technical Report.

- Nervous system changes
- Changes in bone density
- Loss of muscle fibers

Although it is unclear whether older people can activate their muscles maximally (i.e., recruit all muscle fibers maximally), twitch interpolation data indicate that both old and young people can do so (Korhonen et al. 2006; Phillips et al. 1992; Korhonen et al. 2006). However, it has also been concluded that older people are able to fully activate their muscles, but activation for dynamic activities may differ from activation for isometric muscle actions (Brown, McCartney, and Sale 1990). The extent to which central voluntary neural drive decreases with increasing age remains speculative. If aging does result in an inability to activate muscle, the factors primarily responsible may be peripheral neuromuscular mechanisms (e.g., neuromuscular junctions) (Häkkinen, Kallinen, and Komi 1994) rather than decreased neural ability to recruit motor units.

Patterns of Muscular Power Loss With Age

The decreased ability to produce force rapidly and relax rapidly, or decreased power production, may be one of the primary factors contributing to a loss of functional abilities and to injury from falls in older adults. Muscle power and its trainability in seniors have not received a great deal of study, but many everyday activities, such as walking, climbing stairs, and lifting objects, require rapid force development or a certain degree of power. Leg-extensor power in elderly men (88.5 ± 6 years) and women (86.5 ± 6 years) has been significantly correlated with chair-rising speed, stair-climbing speed and power, and walking speed (Bassey et al. 1992). Correlations between power and functional ability were greater in women than in men, but for both men and women power was important for the performance of daily activities. The ability of muscles to produce muscular force rapidly may also serve as a protective mechanism when falling, a major public health problem that is one of the top causes of injury in seniors and is associated with increased mortality risk (Wolinsky and Fitzgerald 1994).

Research also shows that muscle power is the major indicator of functional ability and disability for seniors (Keysor and Jette 2001; Latham et al. 2004). Furthermore, muscle power at ~40% of

1RM is more strongly related to functional performance than maximal strength (Doherty 1993).

Figures 11.6 and 11.7 depict the difference in rate of force development between older and younger people in bilateral (two limbs working together) and unilateral (single-limb) strength. Power production, especially in explosive movements, diminishes dramatically with age and to a greater extent than maximal strength does (Häkkinen, Kraemer, and Newton 1997; Paasuke et al. 2000). It has been estimated from cross-sectional studies that lower-limb power capabilities may be lost at a rate of 3.5% a year from the age of 65 to 84 years (Young and Skelton 1994). In women, cross-sectional data indicate a loss of maximal voluntary contraction and speed of contraction by the age of 40 years, while speed of relaxation is decreased by the age of 50 (Paasuke et al. 2000). The time needed to produce maximal isometric force early in the force–time curve (0 to 200 msec) was significantly longer in older women (70 years) than in middle-aged women (50 years) and younger women (30 years) (Häkkinen and Häkkinen 1991). Research has also shown that peak anaerobic power in master endurance and power athletes, when expressed in W · kg body mass^{-1}, decreased linearly as a function of age at a rate of about 1% a year (Grassi et al. 1991). This means that a 75-year-old has only 50% of the anaerobic power of a 20-year-old. For this reason, and because of the importance of power capabilities for health, improvement in muscular power should be a primary training goal in older populations.

Causes of Decreased Power With Age

Akin to strength losses, power losses may be related to muscle atrophy, muscle mass loss, loss of type II muscle fibers, and decreases in the rate of voluntary activation. However, other factors related to the quality of muscle may preferentially affect power. The contraction speed of the actin and myosin is reduced up to 25% in older adults (Hook, Sriramoju, and Larsson 2001; Larsson et al. 1997). Myosin heavy chains (MHC) shift to slower types with aging, which could affect the speed of myosin and actin cross-bridge cycling during muscle actions (Sugiura et al. 1992). This may be improved by weight training, because seniors (~65 years old) have a similar change in MHC transfor-

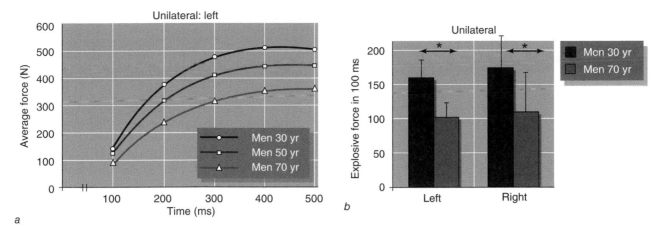

FIGURE 11.6 Unilateral force development in 100 ms for men 30 and 70 years old: (a) average force; (b) explosive force.

Figure 11.6a With kind permission from Springer Science+Business Media: *European Journal of Applied Physiology,* "Neuromuscular performance in voluntary bilateral and unilateral contraction and during electrical stimulation in men at different ages," 1995; 518-527, K. Häkkinen et al., figure 3b.

Figure 11.6b Adapted from *Electromyography Clinical Neurophysiology* Vol. 37: K. Häkkinen, W.J. Kraemer, and R. Newton, 1991, "Muscled activation and force production during bilateral and unilateral concentric and isometric contractions of the knee extensors in men and women at different ages," pgs. 131-142, copyright 1991, with permission from Elsevier.

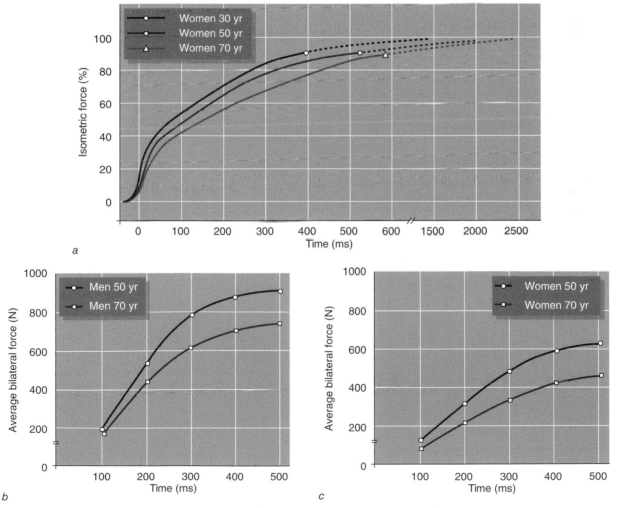

FIGURE 11.7 Bilateral force development curves for men and women at 50 and 70 years old.

Figure 11.7a With kind permission from Springer Science+Business Media: *European Journal of Applied Physiology,* "Muscle cross-sectional area, force production and relaxation characteristics in women at different ages," 1991, 62: 410-414, K. Häkkinen and A. Häkkinen, figure 6.

Figure 11.7b, c Adapted, by permission, from K. Häkkinen, W.J. Kraemer, and M. Kallinen et al., 1996, "Bilateral and unilateral neuromuscular function and muscle cross-sectional area in middle-aged and elderly men and women," *Journal of Gerontology and Biological Science* 51A: B21-B29. Copyright © The Gerontological Society of America.

mation (MHC IIb to MHC IIa) as younger people do with training (Sharman et al. 2001). The loss of type II muscle fibers with aging also means a loss of fast MHC proteins (Fry, Allemeier, and Staron 1994). Myosin ATPase activity also decreases with aging (Syrovy and Gutmann 1970). Thus, the loss of both the quantity and quality of proteins in the contractile units of muscle provides a structural biochemical basis for the loss of both strength and power with aging.

Another factor affecting power loss may involve the elastic property of connective tissue. When comparing the aging effects of people 18 to 73 years, Bosco and Komi (1980) noted a reduction in countermovement vertical jump heights with age (Bosco and Komi, 1980). Performing depth jumps from various heights so that the stretch-shortening cycle could be used resulted in greater decreases in vertical jump ability with aging. This indicates that the effects of aging on the elastic contractile components (e.g., non-contractile protein and connective tissue) in the muscle reduce inherent power.

Resistance Training Adaptations in Seniors

Because sarcopenia (and all of the factors associated with strength and power loss) is generally a universal characteristic of advancing age, strategies for preserving or increasing muscle mass in the elderly should be implemented. Considerations for training programs for seniors are discussed in the following sections.

Strength and Hypertrophy

Approaches to resistance exercise in seniors are often gentle and mild with the belief that seniors are frail or weak. While reasonable precautions and proper medical screening are important, seniors should not be approached in a paternalistic manner. Master male powerlifters over the age of 65 years weighing about 181 lb (82.1 kg) in drug-free competitions with no equipment aids (e.g., super suits) have squatted in excess of 330 lb (150 kg); and those over the age of 70 years have bench pressed over 250 lb (113.45 kg). Similarly, master female powerlifters who are women over the age of 50 years and in the 198 lb (90+ kg) weight class have benched in excess of 200 lbs (90.72 kg) and have squatted over 315 lbs (142.9 kg). These older

lifters demonstrate that seniors can maintain substantial strength with training, and this conclusion is supported by research.

Even in extremely old seniors, men and women (87-96 years) and women (mean age 92 years) who resistance trained for eight weeks showed training adaptations (Fiatarone et al. 1990; Serra-Rexach et al. 2011). These studies demonstrated that the capacity for muscle strength improvement and muscle size increases (determined by CAT scans) is preserved even in the very old. For example, very old women showed a 17% increase in 6-7RM leg press ability and a significant reduction in falls (Serra-Rexach et al. 2011). Substantial strength gains (up to a 200% increase in 1RM) and muscle hypertrophy (CAT scans and muscle biopsy) were also demonstrated in a group of sedentary older men (60-72 years) using a higher-intensity resistance training regimen (three sets of eight repetitions at 80% of 1RM, three days per week for 12 weeks) (Frontera et al. 1988). Increased strength and hypertrophy were again observed in 49- to 74-year-old women following a 21-week resistance training program with six to eight exercises at each biweekly session (Sallinen 2006).

Young men (30 years) and older men (62 years) trained for 10 weeks, three days per week, using a nonlinear periodization training protocol, and who were matched for similar activity profiles before training, had significant gains in muscular size and strength (Kraemer, Häkkinen, et al. 1999). In that study, increases in strength and MRI cross-sectional area of the thigh were observed, but the younger men demonstrated significantly higher absolute values both pre- and post-training. This indicated a more robust response to resistance training in the younger men most likely due to more dynamic physiological systems (e.g., endocrine system; see the preceding discussion).

In people over 70 years, six months of resistance exercise (three days per week) resulted in strength increases of 15% in the leg press, 25% in the bench press, and 30% in the bench pull, and, in a 6% increase in maximal workload (Strasser et al. 2009). In this study, subjects performed sets to volitional failure. However, this may not be advisable in older people because of increased joint stress and strain as well as higher cardiovascular pressure overloads as a result of Valsalva maneuvers at the end of each set. Nevertheless, both strength and hypertrophy can increase in seniors with heavy resistance exercise training.

In obtaining muscle biopsies, it has been shown that, in seniors, both type I and type II muscle fibers can increase in cross-sectional area, and total muscle size in seniors can increase in cross-sectional area with resistance training. Increases in fiber size with resistance training (biopsies and MRI analyses of individual muscles) in older men and women have been confirmed by a wide variety of studies from 12 to 36 weeks in length (Campbell et al. 1999; Charette et al. 1999; Häkkinen, Pakarinen et al. 2001; Hunter et al. 2001; Lemmer et al. 2001). Younger people compared to older individuals of similar training backgrounds typically have larger muscle fibers and intact muscles than the older people at the start of any resistance training program (Aagaard et al. 2010). Although there were obvious differences in the magnitude of increase in fiber size as a result of age, both men and women demonstrate increases in type II muscle fibers with heavy resistance training. The changes that occur with training depend on the program design. It appears that a key program design variable for producing hypertrophy of the entire muscle in older people is the intensity and volume of the resistance exercise protocols used (e.g., use of multiple sets at 70-80% of 1RM or use of 3- to 5RM zones as part of the periodized training program).

Analysis of muscle fiber types indicates that seniors maintain the ability to increase the size of type II muscle fibers if the intensity results in the recruitment of the motor units containing these fibers. It has been suggested that in men between 76 and 80 years of age who maintain physical activity, a compensatory hypertrophy of solely the type I muscle fibers is an adaptation for the inevitable age-related loss of motor units (Aniansson, Grimby, and Hedberg 1992). The percentages of type I and II muscle fibers do not change between the ages of 76 to 80, but there is a significant reduction of type IIx fibers. This could be interpreted as a loss of muscle fibers, but it is more likely a transition from type IIx to type IIa muscle fibers as a result of physical activity (Hikida et al. 2000). Following resistance training, the type I, type IIa, and type IIx fibers of seniors were all hypertrophied (Hikida et al. 2000). Yet the percentage of type IIx fibers are reduced as they transition to type IIa fibers because of the repeated recruitment with heavy resistance training exercise resulting in a shift to type IIa fiber type. Myosin heavy chains reflect this same transitional change with training

in the elderly as they do in younger people (see chapter 3). These observations have been supported by other studies (Häkkinen, Kraemer et al. 2001; Sharman et al. 2001). A statistical trend (p = .07) for the cytoplasm-to-myonucleus ratio to increase with resistance training has been shown in seniors (Hikida et al. 2000). As pointed out in chapter 3, the number of nuclei must increase as the muscle hypertrophies to maintain nuclear domains because this is a limiting factor in the size increases of muscle fibers and has been feared to be less in seniors.

Although many resistance training studies have examined short-term adaptations in seniors, only a few have examined strength and body composition changes during training periods of 52 weeks or more. A study of 39 healthy women (59 ± 0.9 years) who were randomized to either a control group or a progressive resistance training group (three sets of eight reps, 80% of 1RM, upper- and lower-body exercises) that trained twice weekly for 12 months demonstrated that strength continually improved in the training group, with no evidence of plateauing during the 12 months of training (Morganti et al. 1995). In the lat pull-down, knee extension, and leg press, the greatest changes in strength were observed in the first three months of the study. However, smaller but statistically significant increases were seen in the second six-month period of the study. This indicates that seniors may experience a reduction in the rate of strength gains over long-term training similar to that found in younger people.

In a group of older men (65-77 years) an initial 24 weeks of resistance training produced increases in strength and muscle fiber size, and with 12 weeks of detraining followed by 8 weeks of retraining, maximal strength was regained to post-24-week levels. However, muscle fiber size did not significantly change (Taaffe and Marcus 1997). The regaining of strength was attributed to neural mechanisms. For muscle fibers, a longer time course of retraining may well be needed to recover from a long detraining period. In this case, importantly, three months of detraining was too long to maintain the gains in myonuclei that should have occurred with the initial training period (Bruusgaard et al. 2010). Such maintenance of the number of myonuclei while the muscle fibers atrophy has been suggested as one important reason for the rapid retraining of muscle fiber size (see chapter 3).

Power and Training

Resistance exercise can help to develop muscular power in seniors and is recommended as a low-cost intervention that may reduce fall risk in the elderly (Caserotti, Aagaard, and Puggaard 2008). Power training is not only beneficial to elderly men and women but is also safe and well-tolerated (Caserotti et al 2008). High-velocity resistance training in the elderly (mean age of 77 years) significantly improved muscle power, particularly during the leg press exercise using a relatively high percentage of body mass (60-70%). The large power improvements were accompanied by a significant improvement in walking ability, but only small, non-significant improvements in chair rise time and balance (Earles, Judge, and Gunnarsson 2001). Thus, the success of translating a training program to functional movements may vary depending on the movements.

Twelve weeks of training at 80% of 1RM with two sets of eight repetitions and a third set to volitional fatigue did show power increases, but they were not specific to the 80% of 1RM resistance used in training (Campbell et al. 1999). Knee extension power significantly increased at 20%, 40%, and 60% of 1RM, but not at 80% of 1RM. While arm pull power increased significantly only at 20% of 1RM in older women (~64 years), a 21-week strength training program showed significant increases in maximal strength and rate of force development, showing that, with training, power capabilities are possible in elderly women (Häkkinen, Pakarinen et al. 2001). Older adults improved power over a 16-week training period because of improvements in both strength and concentric velocity, whereas young men and women saw improvements in power because of increased strength alone (Patrella et al. 2007). Thus, power increases in older people can occur, but they may be different from muscle group to muscle group and may not show specificity to the training load or velocity of movement.

Power development in seniors may depend upon the duration and type of resistance training program used. Ten weeks of using a nonlinear periodization training program resulted in significant improvements in 1RM strength in both older (61 ± 4 years) and younger (29 ± 5 years) men, but power did not improve in the older men (Häkkinen, Newton et al. 1998) despite similar percentage changes in thigh cross-sectional area and strength as in the younger men. Strength (1RM), jump performance, and walking speed increased in both older (63-78 years) and middle-aged (37-44 years) men and women when explosive power exercises were used in conjunction with biweekly resistance training over a training period of 24 weeks (Häkkinen and Alen 2003).

In a 12-week biweekly pneumatic resistance training program using 80% of 1RM as a resistance for three sets of five exercises, both older (56-66 years) and younger (21-30 years) men and women had similar increases in power at 40% and 60% of 1RM, respectively, but men responded with significantly greater absolute gains at these percentages (Jozsi et al. 1999). The increase in leg extensor power at 80% of the 1RM was similar in all groups. The men increased to a significantly greater extent than women in all exercises except for the two-legged leg press. However, pneumatic resistance was used in this study, which allowed high-velocity repetitions without any deceleration phase at the end of repetitions in all exercises thereby promoting power development (Jozsi et al. 1999).

Power training (i.e., training the velocity component of the power equation) is more effective than strength training (i.e., training the maximal force component of the power equation) at increasing power because of the specificity of training and thus may be more beneficial in enhancing physical function in older people (Caserotti et al 2008; Porter 2006, Caserotti et al. 2008). The use of high-velocity, low-intensity movements over an appropriate time period may improve power, thereby helping to enhance the function of the neuromuscular system and optimize functional abilities. It may also have secondary effects on other physiological systems, such as connective tissue. Table 11.1 presents an overview of some of the responses of older adults to resistance exercise training.

Neural Adaptations

Even in the elderly, the size principle of motor unit recruitment is maintained (Fling, Knight, and Kamen et al. 2009). For many years it has been known that neural adaptations with resistance training act as one of the primary mechanisms mediating improvements in strength over the first several weeks. This was demonstrated in very old, frail men and women who performed a high-intensity resistance training program (80% of 1RM for 10 weeks), resulting in significant

TABLE 11.1   **Basic Resistance Training Adaptations in Older Adults (60 years and older)**

Experimental variable	Response
Muscle strength (1RM)	Increased
Muscle power (W)	Increased
Muscle fiber size	Increased (both major types)
Isokinetic peak torque 60 deg · sec^{-1} 240 deg · s^{-1}	Increased Increased but less than 60 degrees
Isometric peak torque (Nm)	Increased
Local muscle endurance	Increased
Cross-sectional thigh muscle size	Increased
Regional bone mineral density	Increased
Total bone mineral density (men)	No change
Pain levels	Decreased
Intra-abdominal and subcutaneous fat	Decreased
Percent fat	Decreased
Daily tasks	Improved
Gastrointestinal motility	Improved
Flexibility	Increased
Resting metabolic rate	Increased
Balance	Increased
Walking ability	Increased
Functional performance rising from chair, stairs	Increased
Risk factors for falling	Reduced
Back strength	Increased
Peak oxygen consumption	Increased
Blood pressure/CV demand	Decreased
Capillary density	May increase
Blood lipid profiles	May improve
Insulin resistance	Reduced
Submaximal aerobic capacity	Increased
Psychological factors	Positive effects
Neural factors Integrated EMG Twitch half relaxation time Rate of force development	Enhanced Increased Increased No change or increased

increases in strength without any significant increases in muscle size. Additionally, the increase in strength was associated with an increase in gait speed, stair-climbing power, balance, and overall spontaneous activity (Fiatarone et al. 1994). In a classic study examining 72-year-old men using a training program consisting of two sets of 10 repetitions at 66% of the 1RM for maximal voluntary contractions of the elbow flexors, three days per week for eight weeks, increases were observed in strength but not in the size of the muscle (Moritani and DeVries 1980). Thus, longer training durations may be needed to elicit muscle size gains in seniors. The roles of intensity, volume, and duration of training for different various age groups of seniors needs further investigation. However, higher intensities, greater variations in training to allow recovery, and large muscle group exercises over longer training periods will most likely be needed to optimize muscle hypertrophy.

With short-term training and higher intensities, training may well be needed to see gains in both strength and muscle size, yet trying to realize the same magnitude of training adaptations as younger people appears improbable. Matching for activity levels and using the same relative intensity and varied resistance training program for 10 weeks (Häkkinen, Newton, et al. 1998), both younger and older men increased the average maximal integrated electromyography (IEMGs) of the vastus lateralis, and muscle size (MRI analysis) increased in both younger (~30 years) and older men (~62 years). However, isometric rate of force production was not changed in the older men, indicating challenges to power development with short-term training. Integrated EMG of the vastus lateralis has also been shown to increase dramatically over a six-month heavy resistance training period for middle-aged and older men and women (40 and 70 years), which mirrored increases in strength (Häkkinen, Pakarinen et al. 2000). Thus, as in younger people, neural factors appear to contribute considerably to the improvements in strength in the early phases of training in both middle-aged and older adults.

Protein Synthesis

Research efforts concerning protein synthesis and metabolism in seniors as a result of training and protein intake (see box 11.4) are ongoing. Nitrogen balance measured before and after 12 weeks of high-intensity resistance training (three sets of eight repetitions, 80% of 1RM, upper- and lower-body exercises) in a group of older men and women showed that resistance training increases nitrogen retention (Campbell et al. 1995). In addition, constant infusion of ^{13}C-leucine revealed that the training resulted in a significant increase in the rate of whole-body protein synthesis. In another study it was observed that older (63-66 years) people compared to younger (24 years) people had a lower rate of muscle protein synthesis as determined by measuring the *in vivo* incorporation rate of intravenously infused ^{13}C-leucine into mixed-muscle protein before and after a short-term two-week resistance training program (two to four sets of 4 to 10 repetitions at 60 to 90% of 1RM, five days per week). However, the resistance training resulted in a significant increase in muscle protein synthesis in both the younger and the older people (Yarasheski, Zachwieja, and Bier 1993). Thus, protein synthesis does increase with training in seniors.

Muscle Damage With Resistance Training

Muscle tissue damage and breakdown followed by repair and remodeling are part of the skeletal muscle tissue rebuilding process. In order to examine muscle fibers' ultrastructure damage, researchers had both young (20-30 years) and older (65-75 years) men participate in a pneumatic knee extensor training program three days a week for nine weeks (Roth et al. 1999). Only one limb was trained; the other acted as a control. Five sets of knee extensors of 5 to 20 repetitions for a total 55 repetitions were performed with each repetition requiring maximal effort. Biopsies were obtained from the thighs of both limbs, and muscle damage was quantified using electron microscopy to determine structural damage. Strength increased in both groups for the trained limb at about 27%. Before-training analysis of the muscle in both thighs demonstrated no more than 3% damage to the fibers in both younger and older men. After training, this doubled to about 6% to 7% in the trained thighs of the younger and older men, respectively. Using this type of pneumatic resistance training protocol, the myofibrillar damage was higher in the trained thigh than in the control thigh but showed no differences between the younger and older men. In contrast to the findings in men, results in a follow-up study with women, using a similar experimental approach, showed that older women exhibited higher levels of muscle damage than younger women did (Roth et al. 2000).

Markers of oxidative damage to DNA in younger and older men and women showed significantly greater oxidative damage in the older people

? BOX 11.4 PRACTICAL QUESTION

What Is the Minimal Amount of Protein Needed by Seniors?

Inadequate energy intake may reduce the body's ability to remodel tissues and is one of the major factors in the decrease of muscle mass with age. In addition a lack of sufficient protein inhibits the amount of protein accretion and muscle fiber hypertrophy that can occur with resistance training. Although many have voiced concerns that higher protein intake could have negative renal consequences, research has demonstrated that, with the exception of specific medical conditions, there are no contraindications for higher protein intake in seniors (Wolfe, Miller, and Miller et al. 2008). In fact, given their increased needs for immune function and healing, it appears normally active seniors require up to $1 \text{ g} \cdot \text{kg}^{-1} \cdot \text{day}^{-1}$ regardless of training status. With whole-body resistance training they may need even more protein to allow for adequate nitrogen availability for muscle fiber size increases with whole-body programs (Chernoff 2004; Evans 2001). Thus, when training and hypertrophy are factored in, adequate protein intake may exceed the recommended daily allowance of $0.8 \text{ g} \cdot \text{kg}^{-1} \cdot \text{day}^{-1}$ (Campbell and Evans 1996; Campbell et al. 2001).

Subjects who consumed a supplement containing protein, carbohydrate, vitamins, minerals, and fat (accounting for an additional 8 kilocalories and 0.33 grams of protein per kilogram of ideal body mass per day) during a 12-week resistance training study showed a greater increase in muscle tissue than those who did not receive supplementation (Meredith et al. 1992). It has also been shown that protein supplementation before and after a workout (nutrient timing) optimizes protein synthesis for both younger and older people (Esmarck et al. 2001). Whether through supplementation or diet, adequate protein intake is an important factor in health and for optimal adaptations of the neuromuscular system when seniors perform resistance training.

Campbell, W.W., and Evans, W.J. 1996. Protein requirements of elderly people. *European Journal of Clinical Nutrition* 50 (Suppl.): S180-S183.

Campbell, W.W., Trappe, T.A., Wolfe, R.R., and Evans, W.J. 2001. The recommended dietary allowance for protein may not be adequate for older people to maintain skeletal muscle. *Journal of Gerontology: Biological Medical Sciences* 56: M373-M380.

Campbell, W.W., and Evans, W.J. 1996. Protein requirements of elderly people. *European Journal of Clinical Nutrition* 50 (Suppl): S180-S183.

Chernoff, R. 2004. Protein and older adults. *Journal of the American College of Nutrition* 23: 627S-630S.

Evans, W.J. 2004. Protein nutrition, exercise and aging. *Journal of the American College of Nutrition* 23: 601S-609S.

Esmarck, B., Andersen, J.L., Olsen, S., Richter, E.A., Mizuno, M., and Kjaer M. 2001. Timing of postexercise protein intake is important for muscle hypertrophy with resistance training in elderly humans. *Journal of Physiology* 535 (Pt. 1): 301-311.

Meredith, C.N., Frontera, W.R., O'Reilly, K.P., and Evans, W.J. 1992. Body composition in elderly men: Effect of dietary modification during strength training. *Journal of the American Geriatric Society* 40: 155-162.

Wolfe, R.R., Miller, S.L., and Miller, K.B. 2008. Optimal protein intake in the elderly. *Clinical Nutrition* 27: 675-684.

following an eccentric work bout. Additionally, older men demonstrated higher levels of oxidative damage than older women (Fano et al. 2001). In older women, it was shown that that resistance training did provide some type of protective mechanism, reducing the amount of muscle damage from an eccentric work bout after training. Muscle tissue damage in older women after training showed no significant difference when compared to younger untrained women, indicating that training can offset the increased damage due to aging (Ploutz-Snyder, Giamis, and Rosenbaum 2001). Additionally, over the course of a six-month time period, resistance exercise between 50 and 80% of 1RM reduced exercise-induced oxidative stress and homocysteine concentrations in older adults who were overweight and obese (Vincent et al. 2006).

Resistance training does result in muscle damage in older people. However, the damage appears to be similar to that observed in younger people, and as in younger people, it may be needed for adaptation to occur. However, extreme damage and soreness are obviously counterproductive in allowing for normal recovery and repair. Training programs for seniors, like any training programs, should therefore be carefully monitored. Moreover, program designers should keep in mind that older muscle tissue still exhibits the development of protective mechanisms to combat damage due to physical activity, including heavy resistance training.

Developing a Resistance Training Program for Seniors

The fundamentals and principles of resistance training program design are the same no matter what the trainee's age (see chapter 5). Because of variations in the functional capacity of many older people, the best program is one that is individualized to meet the needs and medical concerns of each person. At present, periodized training has been used in several situations when training older adults (Hunter, Wetzstein et al. 2001; Newton et al. 1995). As with any untrained population, in the early phases of training, advanced program design is not required to produce positive results. When the older adult's long-term resistance training goal is progression toward higher levels of muscular strength and hypertrophy, evidence supports the use of variation in the resistance training program. It is important to emphasize that progression should be introduced at a gradual pace to avoid acute injury and to allow time for adaptation. The program design needs to consider the medical aspects of older adults, such as cardiovascular problems and arthritis. Some seniors may require a period of time for basic conditioning before they start to actually train with more intense programs.

Performance Evaluation

Prior to exercise prescription, to determine training progress and individualize the program of an older person, the trainer should evaluate strength (on the equipment used in training, if possible), body composition, functional ability (e.g., the person's ability to lift a chair, get out of chair, etc.), muscle size, nutrition, and pre-existing medical conditions. The American College of Sports Medicine (ASCM) recommends that when implementing a strength training program, trainers should consult a physician prior to strength training to determine if any other testing for people in category III is needed (see discussion in more detail later). Strength testing and resistance exercise workouts using as much as 75% of the 1RM have been shown to have resulted in fewer cardiopulmonary symptoms than graded treadmill exercise tests in cardiac patients with good left ventricular function

(Faigenbaum et al. 1990). In addition, 1RM testing has been shown to be a safe and effective means of evaluating the elderly provided they are adequately familiar with the protocol (Shaw, McCully, and Posner 1995). It is important to note that the resistance training injury risk in seniors is low; it is greatest during testing (particularly above 80% of 1RM) (Porter 2006). In some cases submaximal testing can be used in seniors to predict their 1RM for training monitoring purposes.

One important cautionary note concerning strength testing and study interpretation is that adequate familiarization with strength testing is necessary for gaining accurate information. Older (66 ± 5 years) and younger (23 ± 4 years) people were tested repetitively for knee extension 1RM strength (a relatively simple single-joint exercise). Older women required eight or nine sessions to gain a stable and reliable baseline strength measure compared to the three or four sessions required by the younger women despite both groups having had the same experience with lifting (Ploutz-Snyder and Giamis 2001). Thus, strength assessment does have a potential age-related need for greater numbers of familiarization sessions with maximal strength testing. Without adequate familiarization, some of the dramatically high percentage gains in strength in older individuals may be due to learning effects as to how to perform the exercise with heavier loads.

Proper exercise technique is vital to the safe implementation of a resistance training program. Many have the mistaken belief that machines are safer than free weights. However, with machines, people often push longer and strain harder with a repetition, even when technique fails, causing strains or pulls in muscles. However, this issue can be minimized with the use of most free weight exercises because of the need for balance and control in multiple planes of motion, which prevents continuation of an exercise if the proper technique is not used. Thus, technique training and supervision can be important in a resistance training program for both machines and free weights and are sometimes lost in the process of implementing a program for the elderly.

Needs Analysis

People respond differently to a given resistance training program based on their current training status, past training experience, and response to the training stress. The process of developing a strength training program in older adults consists of pretesting, setting individualized goals, designing a program, and developing evaluation methods. Competent supervision is also important for optimizing strength and conditioning programs (e.g., in the United States, the National Strength and Conditioning Association's [NSCA] Certified Strength and Conditioning Specialist [CSCS] certification) (see figure 11.8). There is now also a Special Population NSCA certification that includes the training of the elderly to the identification of minimal competence which is considered prudent for those working with this population. In older adults, resistance training should be part of a lifelong fitness lifestyle, so continual reevaluations of

program goals and program designs are necessary for optimal results and adherence.

The American College of Sports Medicine (ACSM 2001) has advised that people who start an exercise program be classified into one of three risk categories:

- Apparently healthy, less than one coronary risk factor (hypertension, smoking) or cardiopulmonary or metabolic disease.
- At higher risk, more than two coronary risk factors or cardiopulmonary or metabolic disease symptoms.
- Previously diagnosed with diseases such as cardiovascular, pulmonary, or metabolic disease.

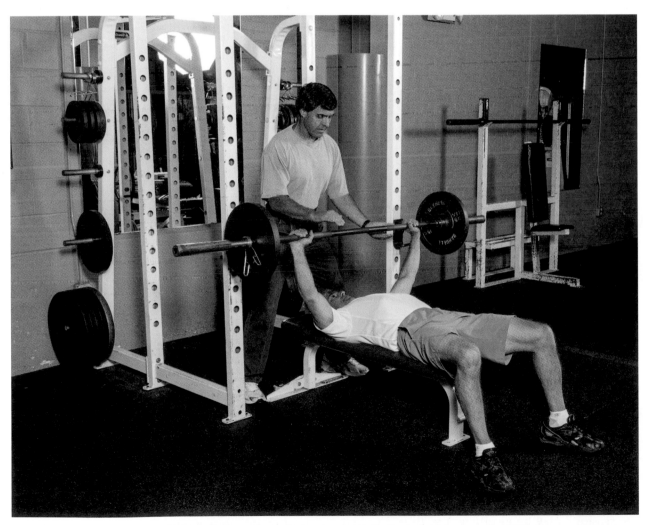

FIGURE 11.8 Proper supervision optimizes the safety and potentially the training outcomes of resistance training programs for seniors. Minimal competencies with proper certifications are helpful in determining effective personal trainers for the senior population.

As noted by the American College of Sports Medicine concerning coronary vascular disease (CVD) and coronary heart disease (CHD), as well as other risks, "Consultation with a medical professional and diagnostic exercise testing should be performed as medically indicated based on signs and symptoms of disease and according to clinical practice guidelines" (ACSM 2011, p. 1348). Also:

> Effective strategies to reduce the musculoskeletal and CVD risks of exercise include screening for and educating about prodromal signs and symptoms of cardiovascular disease in novice and habitual exercisers, consultation with a health professional and diagnostic exercise testing as medically indicated, and attention to several elements of the exercise prescription including warming up, cooling down, a gradual progression of exercise volume and intensity, and proper training technique. The supervision of an experienced fitness professional can enhance adherence to exercise and likely reduces the risk of exercise in those with elevated risk of adverse CHD events. Adults, especially novice exercisers and persons with health conditions or disabilities, likely can benefit from consultation with a well-trained fitness professional. (ACSM American College of Sports Medicine 2011, p. 1349)

Frequency

A major concern for older adults is proper progression to avoid injury or acute overuse. We might speculate that the muscles of older adults require longer periods of time to recover between exercise sessions. Therefore, workouts for seniors should be varied in intensity and volume to ensure recovery, especially after workouts in which significant muscle damage has occurred because of heavy resistances or high volumes. Care is needed not to "overshoot" the physiological ability to repair tissues after a workout. As in all age groups, proper nutritional intake and rest are needed for recovery.

Resistance training on two to three days per week has been recommended, yet three days a week offers a wider range of options for program design. If the number of sets is equated, two weekly training sessions may be as efficient as three in older people (Wieser and Haber 2007). Some research has shown resistance training program periodization to be beneficial for older adults (Hunter et al. 2001; Newton et al. 1995). The frequency at which each type of program emphasis is performed is also important. In a given week, at least one session that includes high resistance (80% of 1RM) (discussed later in the section on Resistance, or Load) should be used. Given the importance of power production to functional abilities, it is likely that high-speed power training should be performed a minimum of once each week, although many investigations have used power training twice per week. Training emphasizing hypertrophy, about 10- to 12RM, would be useful to incorporate about once per week to stimulate endocrine secretions for hypertrophy.

In addition to these primary modes of training, one systematic review suggests that balance training is best conducted frequently, or about three days a week for 10 minutes, although this was not examined in the elderly (DiStefano et al. 2009). This implies that balance training might be important to incorporate into each training session.

Choice of Exercise

With any type of equipment, care needs to be taken to help the person attain proper range of motion and safely control the resistance throughout the full range of motion. Older adults may need to supplement resistance exercise training with mobility training to achieve their full range of motion. In the absence of physical limitations, however, the exercise choice may not differ from that of any other person with the exception of decreased volume.

With the goal of maintaining appropriately low volume in seniors, it is important to focus primarily on all major muscle groups over the course of a given week. Depending upon familiarity and skill level, two to four compound, large-muscle-group exercises may be used: double-leg push (squat) or pull (deadlift); horizontal push (bench press) or pull (seated row); single-leg functional movements (stair climbing, step-ups with grocery bags); or power exercises (plyometrics) with two to four supplemental small-muscle-group exercises (abdominal, rotator cuff or scapula, balance). The squat, seated row, and similar multijoint or compound movements have all been used with success to increase bone mineral density in sedentary, post-menopausal women between 45 and 65 years of age (Houtkooper 2007). Therefore, inclusion of these exercises in programs for older women seems warranted.

As described earlier, upper-body exercise and exercises that stimulate muscles attached at primary bone sites of concern may be important for increasing spinal bone density and so should also be included in a program. As the program progresses, the progression of exercises should activate as much of the skeletal muscle mass as possible to facilitate adaptation. In addition, although heavy weight may not be appropriate for twisting and turning movements, exercises that incorporate these types of movements may help to develop functional abilities better than linear movements alone.

The exercise equipment used must fit the individual and her functional capacity; some machines are too large, have too much initial resistance, or have inappropriate load increments for some seniors. Free weights, isokinetic machines, pneumatic machines, and stack plate machines have all been commonly used. Isokinetics, pneumatics, or hydraulics may allow for easier initiations of the exercise movement and for a smoother resistance progression than normal machines. Programs have used all types of resistance tools: food cans of different sizes, rubber tubing, water-filled milk cartons, and more recently, functional devices such as medicine and stability balls. Although exercises with these devices may be novel and fun, it is important that they be used as part of a larger set of equipment, be properly tested with the person to ensure that they provide the adequate resistance to produce adaptations, and can be performed safely.

Functional resistance training, is a term often used, but it can be confusing as its origin came out of the occupational and physical therapy professions. It referred to the use of everyday activities, such as going up stairs and lifting groceries off the ground, helping to improve a senior's ability to perform activities of daily living while not using conventional resistance exercises in a weight room. However, weight training exercises do translate to improving such everyday functional task demands, and resistance exercises can be more carefully progressed and loaded than the everyday tasks. Research shows that stair-climbing ability at various speeds can improve with resistance exercise (Holsgqaard-Larsen et al. 2011) as can steadiness (which tends to decrease with age because of the increased coactivation of antagonistic muscles and increased variability in the discharge rate of motor units). Four weeks of weight training of the hand muscles (first dorsal interosseus) resulted

in improved steadiness of both concentric and eccentric actions, especially during eccentric actions (Laidlaw et al. 1999). Functional training should mimic functional abilities as closely as possible, such as performing stair-climbing exercises to improve stair-climbing ability, walking with loaded bags to simulate grocery carrying, or squat movements to aid in independence in rising from a seated position or the toilet.

The inclusion of balance training in resistance exercise protocols is an effective means of reducing falls in seniors (Granacher et al. 2011). It is important to note, however, that between 30 and 50% of falls in older community-dwelling individuals are caused by slips and trips (Gabell, Simons, and Nayak 1985; Lord et al. 1993; Gabell et al. 1985). Balancing on an unstable surface in a static standing posture has little functional carryover to most challenges encountered by seniors. Research indicates that rather than traditional techniques, it may be more beneficial to train seniors with challenges in equilibrium (**perturbation-based training**), such as a gentle push from behind by a practitioner (Granacher et al. 2011), particularly while seniors engage in simultaneous cognitive challenges.

In many cases, resistance exercise protocols used in balance comparison investigations do not include appropriate exercise selection. Dynamic balance tasks (step-ups, reverse or walking lunges, loaded or unloaded, with or without support), may be more appropriate in terms of both safety and functionality for seniors. In the absence of contraindications, properly selected free weight and power exercises can be used by seniors and are excellent for developing stability and balance, but more research that uses such movements is required. It is also important to remember that functional resistance training is an important adjunct to, and tool within, a broader practice of resistance exercise, but not a replacement for it.

Order of Exercise

In general, exercise order for seniors is the same as for any age. Following a warm-up, large-muscle-group exercises are typically placed at the beginning of the workout. This minimizes fatigue and enables people to use higher intensities or greater resistances in these exercises. Optimal stimulation of large-muscle groups in the lower extremities (e.g., with the leg press) and the upper body (e.g., with the bench press or seated row) should be a top priority in programs for older adults. Large-muscle-group exercises are followed by smaller-muscle-group exercises and cool-down activities. For total-body workouts, exercises may be rotated between the upper and lower body, and between opposing muscle groups.

Resistance, or Load

The most common percentage range examined is 50 to 85% of 1RM or a 6- to 12RM zone (12RM or heavier has been used in most effective investigations). Lighter resistances (30% and heavier) are recommended for high-velocity power movements. The starting level of strength fitness may be minimal in the frail elderly, with a maximal force capability of only a few pounds (~1.3 kg). In some cases, trainers and program designers should use care in choosing the proper equipment to allow manipulations of resistance in increments of less than 1 lb (0.5 kg). On the other hand, even frail men and women can safely perform and adapt to resistance exercise at 80% of 1RM (Fiatarone et al. 1994; Fiatarone and Evans 1993). It is important to note that, although low, the risk of injury is greater above 80% of 1RM relative to lower-intensity exercise (20% or 50% of 1RM) training in healthy older men and women (Porter 2006).

Loads closer to 80% are important for optimizing training adaptations, including bone adaptation. Using light elastic cords for training has been shown to be ineffective in achieving the same magnitude of adaptation as using free weights, in terms of muscle strength and muscle fiber training-related adaptations, even in younger men and women (Hostler, Schwirian et al. 2001). This is supported, in older people (68 years), who showed no beneficial effects in the measured training outcomes from using light hand weights (Engelles et al. 1998). In addition, older adults showed greater maintenance of hypertrophy gains during detraining when heavier resistances were used in training compared to lighter resistances (Bickel, Cross, and Bamman et al. 2011). Thus, heavier loading is important for optimal activation of muscle tissue and resulting adaptations to resistance exercise. However, this does not imply that moderate resistances do not result in significant fitness gains in middle-aged or elderly people, but the magnitude of adaptations are simply less. Significant increases in strength and muscle cross-sectional area in females 45 years old have been shown following training using three sets at approximately 50% of 1RM (Takarada and Ishii 2002).

Care must be taken not to overemphasize any one training zone (i.e., %RM or RM target zone) to the exclusion of others. Nevertheless, most investigations that have had unsuccessful outcomes in terms of bone density, strength, power, endocrine responses, and hypertrophy used loads heavier than 70% of the 1RM or less than 11RM (with the exception of power days). It is also important to remember, as discussed in the section that follows, that controlling volume is just as important for preventing injury as resistance.

Some data indicate that the application of the intensity must be carefully controlled so as not to initiate an overtraining syndrome in older adults. Heavy resistances need not be used in every training session because training three days per week with either 80% 1RM every session, or training with 80%, 65%, and 59% of 1RM one session per week, both resulted in significant and similar increases in strength and fat-free mass in senior (61-77 years old) men and women (Hunter et al. 2001). The group training with varied resistances showed a significant decrease in the difficulty of a carrying task compared to the group training with only 80% of 1RM. These results indicate that heavy resistances may only be necessary during one out of three training sessions per week to bring about optimal strength increases, and that varying resistance is effective with seniors. One investigation found that training with lighter resistances (50-60% of the 1RM) may result in greater increases in the 1RM in older women (Hunter and Treuth 1995). From these results, paired with the results of Hunter and colleagues (2001), one might conclude that a nonlinear periodized approach using both low and high resistances would be optimal for seniors.

Repetitions

At heavier loads, fewer repetitions can be performed. Improvements in local muscular endurance (which are enhanced by circuit weight training and high-repetition, short-rest, moderate-load programs in younger populations) may lead to an enhanced ability to perform submaximal work and recreational activities. Caution is important when such protocols are employed; although many fear high intensity with seniors, excessive repetition volume with lighter resistances can also cause problems as can inadequate rest between sets and exercises. No matter how many repetitions are performed, a set needs to end when there is a break in proper exercise technique.

Repetition number must also be carefully considered for safety reasons given the high prevalence of cardiovascular problems and risks in older adults. Performing a set to concentric failure results in higher blood pressures and heart rates compared to a set not performed to failure (see chapter 3). In addition, performing sets to concentric failure using resistances in the 70 to 90% of 1RM range results in blood pressures that are slightly higher than those resulting from sets to failure below and above this range. The highest blood pressures and heart rates normally occur in the last few repetitions of a set. Therefore, it is recommended that older adults should not perform sets to concentric failure, especially those with cardiovascular problems or risks and especially in the 70 to 90% of 1RM range. This recommendation is perhaps most important when beginning a program. Performance of a Valsalva maneuver (i.e., suppressing one's breath), which is typical in sets to failure, increases blood pressure and should also be discouraged in this population.

Lifting Velocity

Moderate, volitional lifting velocities have been recommended for strength and hypertrophy training. When power is a training goal, light loads with faster lifting velocities have been recommended. The use of proper equipment for power training (e.g., pneumatic resistance) and exercises (Olympic-style movements such as hang pulls and plyometric medicine ball exercises) is also vital for power development.

Number of Sets

The recommended minimal initial starting point consists of at least one set per exercise. Progression may ensue from one to three sets over time (depending on the number of exercises performed). It is important to note that tolerance of three sets has been shown by even the frail elderly. The number of sets is related to the exercise volume. Initially, some seniors can only tolerate a low exercise volume and single-set programs are the simplest starting point. Using the principle of progressive resistance training, the volume can be increased by increasing the number of sets or repetitions per set to help the person tolerate the use of a higher volume of exercise. Programs for older adults usually do not involve more than three sets of a given exercise. If the muscle group needs more stimulation, another exercise for that muscle group can be added to the program (e.g., seated rows or lat pull-downs). In addition, many programs for older adults should use a warm-up set at a much lighter resistance than the RM target zone or the resistance to be used for the working sets. This warm-up set allows the person to get a feel for the exercise movement and notice anything out of the ordinary (e.g., joint pain or muscle pain) before using the heavier training resistance.

Rest Between Sets and Exercises

The rest between sets and exercises dictates the metabolic intensity of a resistance training workout. In older people, tolerance of anaerobic acidic conditions (i.e., low pH) is less than in younger people (e.g., Wingate anaerobic testing) (see figure 11.9). Typically, rest periods of 2-3 minutes between sets and exercises can be used. The person should be carefully monitored for any symptoms (e.g., nausea, dizziness), and the program should be immediately changed if symptoms occur. Tolerance of the workout is paramount for optimal training. Rest periods that are too short can also produce a drastic reduction in the load used in successive sets if recovery is not sufficient before the next set or exercise is initiated. Short rest intervals are used to enhance local muscular endurance and improve acid-base status, which has been shown to be compromised with aging.

Because the activation of muscle tissue is related to the resistance and the total amount of work performed, rest period lengths should be consistent with the program goals. Shorter rest periods can be used with circuit programs. The rest periods should be longer if heavier resistances are being used and can be shortened as exercise tolerance increases. The amount of rest may also be dictated by the medical or physical condition of the individual. In some older adults (e.g., those with type 1 diabetes), gains in strength are the major goal, so care must be taken to properly control the length of rest between sets and exercises so as not to create severe or intolerable metabolic stress. Tolerance of the workout in the context of progression toward specific goals is the key to optimizing workout quality, and rest period length plays a crucial role in this program design process.

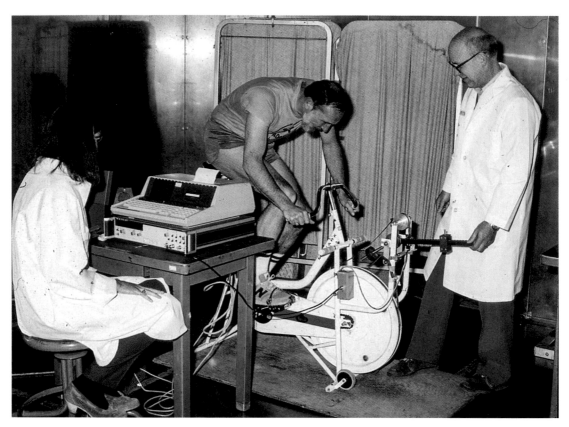

FIGURE 11.9 Anaerobic capacity, determined in tests like the Wingate cycling test, is diminished in seniors as a result of diminished tolerance of decreases in pH and increases in H^+ ions in the blood. Resistance training workouts using shorter rest period lengths must be carefully progressed, and symptoms should be monitored so as not to overshoot physiological buffering capacity.

Photo courtesy of Dr. Howard Knuttgen, one of the true pioneers in exercise physiology and the study of metabolism, shown here on the cycle ergometer.

Summary

Resistance training can be safely and successfully implemented in older populations. Even the frail and very sick elderly can gain benefits that will positively affect their quality of life. Muscle strength and power carries over into the enhancement of everyday activities and quality of life, positively affecting a long list of physiological characteristics, especially in muscle, bone, and connective tissue. Some of the findings in this chapter challenge common beliefs that power training and traditional resistance training are inappropriate for elderly people. Traditional resistance training and power training for this population are effective as long as the program is properly designed, properly supervised, and appropriately accounts for individual characteristics, such as clinical conditions and social, psychological, and economic considerations. Resistance training for seniors is well on its way to being an accepted modality for fighting the aging processes and improving physiological function and performance in this population.

SELECTED READINGS

Carmeli, E., Coleman, R., and Reznick, A.Z. 2002. The biochemistry of aging muscle. *Experimental Gerontology* 37: 477-489.

Doherty, T.J., Vandervoot, A.A., Taylor, A.W., and Brown, W.F. 1993. Effects of motor unit losses on strength in older men and women. *Journal of Applied Physiology* 74: 868-874.

Fiatarone, M.A., O'Neill, E.F., Ryan, N.D., Clements, K.M., Solares, G.R., Nelson, M.E., Roberts, S.B., Kehayias, J.J., Lipsitz, L.A., and Evans, W.J. 1994. Exercise training and nutritional supplementation for physical frailty in very elderly people. *The New England Journal of Medicine* 330: 1769-1775.

Gavrilov, L.A., and Gavrilova, N.S. 2001. The reliability theory of aging and longevity. *Journal of Theoretical Biology* 213: 527-545.

Hurley, B.F., Hanson, E.D., and Sheaff, A.K. 2011. Strength training as a countermeasure to aging muscle and chronic disease. *Sports Medicine* 41: 289-306.

Liu, C.K., and Fielding, R.A. 2011. Exercise as an intervention for frailty. *Clinical Geriatric Medicine* 27 (1): 101-110.

Meredith, C.N., Frontera, W.R., O'Reilly, K.P., and Evans, W.J. 1992. Body composition in elderly men: Effect of dietary modification during strength training. *Journal of the American Geriatric Society* 40: 155-162.

Nelson, M.E., Fiatarone, M.A., Morganti, C.M., Trice, I., Greenberg, R.A., and Evans, W.J. 1994. Effects of high-intensity strength training on multiple risk factors for osteoporotic fractures. *Journal of the American Medical Association* 272: 1909-1914.

Peterson, M.D., Rhea, M.R., Sen, A., and Gordon, P.M. 2010. Resistance exercise for muscular strength in older adults: A meta-analysis. *Ageing Research Review* 9: 226-237.

Peterson, M.D., Sen, A., and Gordon, P.M. 2011. Influence of resistance exercise on lean body mass in aging adults: A meta-analysis. *Medicine & Science in Sports & Exercise* 43: 249-258.

Roth, S.M., Martel G.F., Ivey, F.M., Lemmer, J.T., Tracy, B.L., Metter, E.J., Hurley, B.F., and Rogers, M.A. 2001. Skeletal muscle satellite cell characteristics in young and older men and women after heavy resistance strength training. *Journal of Gerontology: A Biological Sciences Medical Sciences* 56: B240-B247.

Strasser, B., Siebert, U., and Schobersberger, W. 2010. Resistance training in the treatment of the metabolic syndrome: A systematic review and meta-analysis of the effect of resistance training on metabolic clustering in patients with abnormal glucose metabolism. *Sports Medicine* 40: 397-415.

Sundell, J. 2011. Resistance training is an effective tool against metabolic and frailty syndromes. *Advances in Preventive Medicine* 2011:984683.

Tschopp, M., Sattelmayer, M.K., and Hilfiker, R. 2011. Is power training or conventional resistance training better for function in elderly persons? A meta-analysis. *Age Ageing* 40: 549-56.

GLOSSARY

absolute strength—The maximal amount of strength or force (i.e., 1RM) generated in a movement or exercise without adjusting for height, weight, or body composition.

accentuated eccentric training—Training that involves performing a complete repetition but with more resistance used in the eccentric phase than in the concentric phase. Also called *negative accentuated training*.

activities of daily living—Activities people can reasonably expect to encounter as part of daily life, such as getting out of a chair, sweeping the floor, using the toilet, or taking out the trash.

acute injury—An injury that is the result of a single trauma.

acute program variables—A group of variables that can be used to describe a resistance exercise session including the number of sets, number of repetitions per set, exercises, rest between sets, rest between exercises, and repetition speed.

aerobic—A term used for ATP production that requires oxygen.

aerobic conditioning—Exercise used to improve maximal or peak oxygen consumption and the associated cardiovascular functions that support endurance performances.

all or none law—The law that states that when a motor unit is activated by the nervous system, all of the associated muscle fibers contract.

alternating muscle group order—Performing exercises for the same muscle group in succession; a synonymous term is *stacking exercise order*.

anaerobic—A term used for ATP production that does not require oxygen.

apophyseal insertion—The place where a tendon attaches to bone.

apoptosis—An inherent program in every cell that involves a set of signal pathways leading to cell death; some call it the body's biological clock.

autocrine system—Referring to a hormone released from a cell to interact with the same cell.

avulsion fracture—The separation of a tendon from the bone; in many cases a small piece of bone is still attached to the tendon.

ballistic resistance training—Exercises in which a high rate of force development is needed and in which the mass being accelerated, such as body mass or external weight, can be projected into the air.

ballistic stretching—A fast dynamic movement through the entire range of motion that ends in a stretch.

bilateral deficit—The difference between the sum of the force developed by either the arms or legs independently and both limbs simultaneously.

bioenergetics—The study of the biochemistry that concerns energy flow through living systems.

body composition—The percentage of fat mass and various components of fat-free mass (including muscle, bone, tissue, and organs) in the body.

body-part exercise—Exercise that predominantly involves movement at one joint or muscle group; synonymous terms are *single-joint exercise* and *single-muscle-group exercise*.

bulked-up athlete—An athlete who, through resistance training and dietary practices, has gained substantial amounts of body weight during an athletic career.

cardiorespiratory endurance fitness—The ability of the heart, lungs, and blood vessels to deliver oxygen to exercising muscles and tissues, as well as the ability of those muscles and tissues to use that oxygen.

choice of exercise—One of the acute program variables; involves the choice of what exercises to perform.

chronic injury—An injury that is the result of repeated microtraumas.

classic strength and power periodization—Training that follows a general trend of decreasing volume and increasing intensity as training progresses; synonymous terms are *linear periodization* and *stepwise periodization*.

compatibility of exercise—Whether two types of exercise positively or negatively affect adaptations to either type.

compensatory acceleration—Lifting the resistance in an exercise as fast as possible throughout the range of motion to optimize force and power.

complex training—Performing a strength exercise, such as the squat, and then after a short rest period performing a power-type exercise, such as the vertical jump. The training goal is to increase maximal power output. A synonymous term is *contrast loading*.

concentric muscle action—The shortening of a muscle while it is generating force.

concurrent training—Performing two or more exercise types, such as strength and endurance, during a training cycle.

connective tissue sheath—Tissue that encloses a muscle fiber.

contraction specificity—The fact that strength and power increases due to training are greatest when determined using the type of muscle action performed during training.

contrast loading—Performing a strength exercise, such as the squat, and then after a short rest period performing a power-type exercise, such as the vertical jump. The training goal is to increase maximal power output. A synonymous term is *complex training*.

core musculature—The axial skeleton and all muscles, ligaments, and other soft tissues with an attachment originating on the axial skeleton whether or not this tissue terminates on the axial or appendicular (arm or leg) skeleton.

cortisol—A steroid hormone that is secreted from the adrenal cortex.

daily nonlinear periodization—Training in which intensity and volume are varied by using several RM or near-RM training zones that are changed in successive training sessions.

deceleration phase—Slowing in the last part of the concentric phase of a repetition even though there is an attempt to increase or maintain movement speed.

delayed-onset muscle soreness (DOMS)—Pain and discomfort after an exercise bout that is typically most severe approximately one to two days after the exercise bout.

detraining—A process that occurs when training is reduced or ceases completely; performance is affected because of diminished physiological capacity.

dynamic constant external resistance (DCER)—Exercise in which the weight or resistance used is held constant; a synonymous term is *isoinertial*.

dynamic stretching—Flexibility exercise involving motion during the stretch that results in movement through the entire range of motion of the joint(s) involved.

dysmenorrhea—Painful menstruation.

eccentric muscle action—The controlled lengthening of a muscle while it is generating force.

eccentric training—Training with only the eccentric, or muscle lengthening, phase of a repetition, or performing the eccentric phase with greater than the normal one-repetition maximum (1RM).

energy source specificity—The concept that physical training causes adaptations of the metabolic systems predominantly used to supply the energy needed by muscles to perform a given physical activity.

epiphyseal plates—Growth plates at the end of long bones.

epiphysis—Cartilage on the joint surface.

exercise specificity—The concept that adaptations are related to the specific demands imposed by the exercise protocol.

flexibility training—Exercise designed to improve absolute range of movement in a joint or series of joints.

flexible daily nonlinear periodization—A form of daily nonlinear periodization that involves changing the training zone based on the readiness of the trainee to perform in a specific training zone.

force–time curve—A curve that depicts the amount of force that can be produced in a given time period.

force–velocity curve—A curve that depicts maximal force capabilities with changes in velocity.

free hormone—A hormone not bound to a binding protein in the circulation.

full range of motion—The greatest range of motion possible dictated by the exercise position and the joints involved.

functional abilities—Abilities meant to replicate or closely simulate actual physical movements encountered as part of daily life, athletic competition, or occupation.

functional capacity—The maximal level of exercise intensity at which no abnormal symptoms or responses are present.

functional training—Training to increase performance in some type of functional task, such as activities of daily living or tests related to athletic performance.

Golgi tendon organ—A proprioceptive receptor found in tendons that monitors force development.

gonadopause—A reduction in the production of the male hormone testosterone that occurs with aging.

growth cartilage—A connective tissue located at the growth plate of bone, the epiphysis, or the apophyseal insertion.

growth hormone—A polypeptide hormone secreted from the anterior pituitary gland.

heart rate training zone—A quantified heart rate range used for determining the intensity of an exercise.

hormone—A molecule secreted from a gland into the blood, which transports it to a target cell where it binds to a receptor delivering a signal to the cell.

hyperplasia—An increase in cell number.

hypertrophy—An increase in cell size.

hysteresis—The amount of heat energy lost by the muscle–tendon complex during the recoil from a stretch.

implement training—Training using a variety of objects as the resistance to be lifted or moved, such as a weighted baseball bat, water-filled dumbbells, water-filled barrels, kettlebells, or a tire.

isoinertial—Exercise in which the weight or resistance used is held constant; a synonymous term is *dynamic constant external resistance*.

isokinetic—Exercise in which the velocity of movement is held constant.

isometric muscle action—A muscle action in which the muscle does not change in length while generating force.

isometric training—Training that involves muscle actions in which no change in muscle length occurs.

isotonic—Actions in which muscles exert a constant tension; do not typically occur because the force generated by a muscle changes throughout an exercise movement.

in-season detraining—Losses of performance or strength that occur when people stop completely or reduce resistance training volume while undertaking other sport-type training.

in-season program—Resistance training undertaken during the competitive portion of the year to further increase or at least maintain strength, power, and motor performance during the competitive season.

insulin—A peptide hormone secreted by the pancreas.

insulin-like growth factors—Peptide hormones that are released from various cells and tissues (e.g., muscle, liver).

insulin resistance—A diminished capability of cells (e.g., skeletal muscle) to respond to the action of insulin in transporting glucose from the bloodstream into cells.

intensity (of training)—A measure of training difficulty; for weight training, a percentage of the heaviest weight for one complete repetition (1RM) is used to determine intensity.

interval training—An exercise training protocol that involves alternating between exercise and rest phases of different durations or times, called an exercise(work)-to-rest ratio.

joint-angle specificity—The concept that strength gains made by training at a particular joint angle are greatest at that joint angle and decrease the farther from the training joint angle strength is measured.

length–tension (force) curve—The curve that depicts the relationship between the length of a muscle or sarcomere and force production capability.

linear periodization—Training that follows a general trend of decreasing volume and increasing intensity as training progresses; synonymous terms are *classic strength and power periodization* and *stepwise periodization.*

long detraining period—A period of detraining that lasts months or years.

long stretch-shortening cycle—A plyometric-type action in which the ground contact time is greater than 250 ms, such as a countermovement jump and a block jump in volleyball.

lordosis—An anterior bending of the spine, usually accompanied by flexion of the pelvis.

maximal strength—The maximal force possible in an exercise or generated by a muscle at a specific velocity of movement for an exercise. 1RM is often used as a measure of maximal strength.

maximal voluntary muscle action—Voluntarily developing the maximal force a muscle's present fatigue level will allow; thus, both lifting the maximal resistance possible for one repetition and the last repetition in a set to failure are maximal voluntary muscle actions even though the muscle can develop more force when not fatigued.

menopause—A stage in middle-aged women that coincides with the end of their reproductive ability; characterized by a decrease in estrogen and the ceasing of the menstrual cycle.

motor unit—The alpha motor neuron and its associated muscle fibers.

multijoint exercise—Exercise involving movement at more than one joint; synonymous terms are *structural exercise* and *multi-muscle-group exercise.*

multi-muscle-group exercise—Exercise involving the use of more than one muscle group; synonymous terms are *structural exercise* and *multijoint exercise.*

multiple-set system—A system in which trainees perform more than one set of the same exercise during a training session.

muscle action specificity—The concept that increases in muscle strength due to training are greatest when measured using the type of muscle action performed during training.

muscle biopsy—A medical procedure in which a needle is use to remove a small sample of skeletal muscle.

muscle group specificity—Increases in strength, hypertrophy, or local muscular endurance, or any other training outcome that occur only in the muscles undergoing training.

muscle spindle—A receptor found in the belly of the muscle that monitors the stretch and length of the muscle.

muscle–tendon complex—The interaction of the muscle and the tendon when activity is performed.

myonuclear domain—The area of a muscle fiber controlled by one nucleus.

myosin ATPase staining method—A histochemical assay used to characterize muscle fiber types.

needs analysis—An evaluation of the metabolic demands of a training program; the biomechanics of the movements needed to be successful in the program; and the injury profile of the trainee, sport, or activity.

negative accentuated training—See *accentuated eccentric training.*

negative training—Training that involves performing the eccentric portion of repetitions with more than the 1RM for a complete repetition.

neuromuscular junction—The interface between an alpha motor neuron and skeletal muscle.

nonlinear periodization—Training in which intensity and volume are varied by using several RM or near-RM training zones that are changed frequently (e.g., in successive training sessions or weekly).

oligomenorrhea—An irregular menstrual cycle (more than 36 days between menstrual flows) in women who previously had a normal menstrual pattern or cycle.

osteochondritis—Inflammation of growth cartilage.

osteochondritis dissecans—A condition in which a piece of bone or cartilage (or both) at a joint loses blood supply and dies.

paired set training—Training that involves performing sets of an exercise for an agonist immediately followed by sets of an exercise for an antagonist in an alternating fashion.

paracrine system—Referring to a hormone that is released from a cell and binds to the receptor of another cell.

pennation angle—The angle at which a muscle fiber attaches to its tendon in relation to the direction of pull of the tendon.

periodization—Planned variation in training with the goal of optimizing training outcomes and avoiding training plateaus.

perturbation-based training—A form of balance training that emphasizes perturbations to the trainee's center of mass that the trainee must respond to and try to maintain their balance.

plyometrics—Power-type training involving the stretch-shortening cycle and typically thought of as performing body weight jumping-type exercises and throwing medicine balls.

postactivation potentiation—The increased performance or power output shortly after performing a strength exercise; typically attributed to a neural accommodation resulting in an increased ability to recruit muscle fibers or the inhibition of neural protective mechanisms.

postexercise hypotension—The decrease in either systolic or diastolic blood pressure immediately after an exercise bout.

power—The rate of performing work calculated as force times distance divided by time.

pre-exhaustion—Performing a small-muscle-group exercise prior to performing a large-muscle-group exercise involving the muscle group used in the small-muscle-group exercise to cause fatigue in the muscle group used in both exercises.

prehabilitation—An exercise program intended to prevent injury.

primary exercises—Exercises that train the prime movers in a particular movement and usually involve major muscle group exercises.

program design—A systematic process that uses a sound understanding of the basic principles of resistance training to meet the needs of each trainee.

progression—The process of making changes in an exercise program over time to cause desired training outcomes.

progressive overload—Continually increasing the stress placed on the body as force, power, or endurance increases with training.

progressive resistance—Similar to progressive overload, except that it applies specifically to weight training; the most common method to increase the stress of training is to increase the resistance lifted for a specific number of repetitions.

proprioceptive neuromuscular facilitation (PNF)—A set of stretching techniques that uses various stretch-contract-relax protocols.

proprioceptors—Specialized receptors that sense the length, force, and movement of tendons and skeletal muscle.

pyramid system—A system that involves performing several sets of the same exercise beginning with light resistances and high numbers of repetitions per set and progressing toward several repetitions per set with heavy resistances followed by increasing numbers of repetitions per set with progressively lighter resistances; a synonymous term is *triangle system*.

Q-angle—The angle between a line connecting the anterior superior iliac crest and the midpoint of the patella and a line connecting the midpoint of the patella and the tibia tubercle.

rate of force development—The amount of change per unit of time in strength.

relative strength—Absolute strength divided by or expressed relative to total body weight or fat-free mass.

repetition—One complete motion of an exercise typically including both a concentric and an eccentric muscle action.

repetition maximum (RM)—The resistance that allows a specific number of repetitions but not more than that number of repetitions in an exercise.

repetition maximum target zone (RM target zone)—A resistance that typically allows a three-repetition range to be performed (3- to 5RM, 8- to 10RM).

repetition maximum training zone (RM training zone)—A training zone that results in momentary failure when the highest number of repetitions in a training zone per set of an exercise is performed, such as performing six repetitions per set at a 4- to 6RM training zone.

repetition speed—The velocity at which a movement occurs in an exercise.

resting metabolic rate (RMR)—The amount of energy expended at rest.

rest periods—Recovery time allowed between sets and exercises in a training session.

reverse linear periodization—Training that progresses from low volume and high intensity to high volume and low intensity, or in the opposite pattern to linear periodization.

sarcomere—The smallest contractile segment of a skeletal muscle.

sarcopenia—The age-associated reduction in muscle mass.

satellite cells—Small cells with no cytoplasm that are found in skeletal muscle between the basement membrane and the sarcolemma, or cell membrane, of the muscle fiber.

secondary amenorrhea—The absence of menstruation for 180 days or more in women who previously menstruated regularly.

set—A specific number of repetitions of an exercise performed in succession, typically with no rest between repetitions.

short stretch-shortening cycle—A plyometric-type action having a ground contact time of less than 250 ms (e.g., a drop jump in which an attempt is made to minimize ground contact time, and sprinting).

single-joint exercise—An exercise that involves movement at predominantly one joint; synonymous terms are *body-part exercise* and *single-muscle-group exercise*.

single-muscle-group exercise—An exercise that predominantly involves only one muscle group; synonymous terms are *single-joint exercise* and *body-part exercises*.

single-set system—A system that involves performing only one set of each exercise during a training session.

size principle—A principle that states that the recruitment of motor units is based on external force demands and size (e.g., number of fibers, size of muscle fibers); motor units are recruited from low-electrical-threshold-activated to high-electrical-threshold-activated motor units.

skeletal muscle fiber—The individual cells that make up an intact skeletal muscle.

sliding filament theory—The theory that muscle contraction results from actin filaments interacting and sliding over stationary myosin filaments to produce force.

slow-movement stretching—Dynamic movements of body parts in a slow and controlled manner (e.g., neck rotations).

specificity—The concept that training-related gains will be specific to the exact conditions used in the exercise program.

spotting—A safety measure performed by those other than the lifter to ensure the safety of the lifter.

stacking exercise order—Performing exercises for the same muscle group in succession; a synonymous term is *alternating muscle group order*.

static stretching—Flexibility exercise that requires the person to voluntarily relax the muscle while elongating it, and then holding the muscle in a stretched position at a point of slight muscular discomfort.

stepwise periodization—Training that follows a general trend of decreasing volume and increasing intensity as training progresses; synonymous terms are *classic strength and power periodization* and *linear periodization*.

stretch-shortening cycle—A sequence of muscle actions consisting of an eccentric action, a brief isometric action, and a concentric action performed in rapid succession.

structural exercise—Exercise that involves movement at multiple joints and involves multiple muscle groups; synonymous terms are *multijoint exercise* and *multi-muscle-group exercise*.

tendon hysteresis—See *hysteresis*.

tendon stiffness—The relationship between the forces applied to the muscle–tendon complex and the change in the length of the unit.

testing specificity—The concept that increases in muscle strength or power due to training are highest when tested using an exercise or muscle action performed during training.

testosterone—A steroid hormone released from the testes in men and at much lower concentration from the ovaries and adrenal cortex in women.

total conditioning program—A program that combines a variety of exercise protocols to improve physical or sport fitness or health (or both); typically addresses strength, power, local muscular endurance, cardiorespiratory endurance, and flexibility.

training volume—A measure of the total amount of work performed during training.

transfer specificity—The degree to which the exercise program results in changes in the performance of a specific activity or sport.

triangle system—A system that involves performing several sets of the same exercise beginning with light resistances and high numbers of repetitions per set and progressing toward only several repetitions per set with heavy resistances followed by increasing numbers of repetitions per set with progressively lighter resistances; a synonymous term is *pyramid system*.

type I (slow-twitch) muscle fibers—Muscle fibers that are characterized by higher levels of oxidative characteristics, or endurance capability, and lower force production capabilities; they are typically smaller than type II muscle fibers.

type II (fast-twitch) muscle fibers—Muscle fibers that are characterized by lower levels of oxidative characteristics, or endurance ability, and higher force production capabilities; they are typically larger than type I muscle fibers.

unstable surface training—Training that involves performing exercises on an unstable surface, such as a Swiss ball, inflatable disc, or wobble board.

Valsalva maneuver—Holding one's breath while attempting to exhale with a closed glottis.

variable resistance—Equipment having a lever arm, cam, or pulley arrangement that varies the resistance throughout the exercise's range of motion.

variable variable resistance—A type of variable resistance equipment allowing adjustments to or changes in the resistance curve of an exercise.

velocity specificity—The concept that strength or power gains are greatest when measured at or close to the velocity of movement used during training.

velocity spectrum training—Training that involves performing several sets of an exercise at several velocities; typically refers to isokinetic training.

vibration training—The application of vibration to a body part or the whole body while performing resistance training; the most popular type of whole-body vibration occurs while standing on an oscillating platform.

window of adaptation—The potential for improvement or positive changes in a given performance or physiological variable; the closer to the genetic potential a trainee is, the smaller the possibility of further gain will be.

REFERENCES

Aagaard, P., and Andersen, J.L. 2010. Effects of strength training on endurance capacity in top-level endurance athletes. *Scandinavian Journal of Medicine & Science in Sports* 20 (Suppl.) 2: 39-47.

Aagaard, P., Andersen, J.L., Bennekou, M., Larsson, B., Olsen, J.L., Crameri, R., Magnusson, S.P., and Kjaer, M. 2011. Effects of resistance training on endurance capacity and muscle fiber composition in young top-level cyclists. *Scandinavian Journal of Medicine & Science in Sports* 21: 298-307.

Aagaard, P., Andersen, J.L., Poulsen, P.D., Leffers, A.M., Wagner, A., Magnusson, S.P., Kristensen, J.H., and Simonsen, J. 2001. A mechanism for increased contractile strength of human pennate muscles in response to strength training: Changes in muscle architecture. *Journal of Physiology* 534: 613-623.

Abe, T., Bechue, W.F., Fujita, S., and Brown, J.R. 1998. Gender differences in FFM accumulation and architectural characteristics of muscle. *Medicine & Science in Sports & Exercise* 30: 1066-1070.

Abe, T., Brown, J.B., and Brechue, W.F. 1999. Architectural characteristics of skeletal muscle in black and white college football players. *Medicine & Science in Sports & Exercise* 31: 1448-1452.

Abe, T., Kearns, C., and Sato, Y. 2006. Muscle size and strength are increased following walk training with restricted venous blood flow from the leg muscle, kaatsu-walk training. *Journal of Applied Physiology* 100: 1460-1466.

Abernathy, P.J., Thayer, R., and Taylor, A.W. 1990. Acute and chronic responses of skeletal muscle to endurance and sprint exercise: A review. *Sports Medicine* 10: 365-389.

Abraham, S.F., Beumont, P.J., Fraser, I.S., and Llewellyn-Jones, D. 1982. Body weight, exercise and menstrual status among ballet dancers in training. *British Journal of Obstetrics and Gynecology* 89: 507-510.

Adams, G. 1998. Role of insulin-like growth factor-I in the regulation of skeletal muscle adaptation to increased loading. *Exercise and Sports Science Reviews* 26: 31-60.

Adams, G., Hather, B.M., Baldwin, K.M., and Dudley, G.A. 1993. Skeletal muscle myosin heavy chain composition and resistance training. *Journal of Applied Physiology* 74: 911-915.

Adams, G., and McCue, S. 1998. Localized infusion of IGF-I results in skeletal muscle hypertrophy in rats. *Journal of Applied Physiology* 84: 1716-1722.

Adams, J.B., Edwards, D., Servirettee, D., Bedient, A.M., Huntsman, E., Jacobs, K.A., Del Rossi, G., Roos, B.A., and Signorile, J.F. 2009. Optimal frequency, displacement, duration, and recovery patterns to maximize power output following acute whole-body vibration. *Journal of Strength and Conditioning Research* 3: 237-245.

Adams, K., O'Shea, J.P., O'Shea, K.L., and Climstein, M. 1992. The effect of six weeks of squat, plyometric and squat-plyometric training on power production. *Journal of Applied Sport Science Research* 6: 36-41.

Ades, P.A., Savage, P.D., Brochu, M., Tischler, M.D., Lee, N.M., and Poehlman, E.T. 2005. Resistance training increases total daily energy expenditure in disabled older women with coronary heart disease. *Journal of Applied Physiology* 98: 1280-1285.

Adler, Y., Fisman, E.Z., Koren-Morag, N., Tanne, D., Shemesh, J., Lasry, E. and Tenenbaum, A. 2008. Left ventricular diastolic function in trained male weight lifters at rest and during isometric exercise. *American Journal of Cardiology* 102: 97-101.

Aguilar, A.J., DiStefano, L.J., Brown, C.N., Herman, D.C., Guskiewicz, K.M., and Padua, D.A. 2012. A dynamic warm-up model increases quadriceps strength and hamstring flexibility. *Journal of Strength and Conditioning Research* 26: 1130-1141.

Ahtiainen, J.P., and Häkkinen, K. 2009. Strength athletes are capable to produce greater muscle activation and general fatigue during high-intensity resistance exercise than nonathletes. *Journal of Strength and Conditioning Research* 23: 1129-1134.

Ahtiainen, J.P., Hulmi, J.J., Kraemer, W.J., Lehti, M., Nyman, K., Selänne, H., Alen, M., Pakarinen, A.,

Komulainen, J., Kovanen, V., Mero, A.A., and Häkkinen, K. 2011. Heavy resistance exercise training and skeletal muscle androgen receptor expression in younger and older men. *Steroids* 76: 183-192.

Ahtiainen, J.P., Hulmi, J.J., Kraemer, W.J., Lehti, M., Pakarinen, A., Mero, A.A., Karavirta, L., Sillanpää, E., Selänne, H., Alen, M., Komulainen, J., Kovanen, V., Nyman, K., and Häkkinen, K. 2009. Strength, endurance or combined training elicit diverse skeletal muscle myosin heavy chain isoform proportion but unaltered androgen receptor concentration in older men. *International Journal of Sports Medicine* 30: 879-887.

Ahtiainen, J.P., Pakarinen, A., Alen, M., Kraemer, W.J., and Häkkinen, K. 2005. Short vs. long rest period between the sets in hypertrophic resistance training: Influence on muscle strength, size, and hormonal adaptations in trained men. *Journal of Strength and Conditioning Research* 19: 572-582.

Akima, H., Takahashi, H., Kuno, S., Masuda, K., Masuda, T., Shimojo, H., Anno, I., Ital, Y., and Katsuta, S. 1999. Early phase adaptations of muscle use and strength to isokinetic training. *Medicine & Science in Sports & Exercise* 31: 588-594.

Alcaraz, P.E., Sanchez-Lorente, J., and Blazevich, A.J. 2008. Physical performance and cardiovascular responses to an acute bout of heavy resistance circuit training versus traditional strength training. *Journal of Strength and Conditioning Research* 22: 667-671.

Alegre, L.M., Lara, A.J., Elvira J.L., and Aguado, X. 2009. Muscle morphology and jump performance: Gender and intermuscular variability. *Journal of Sports Medicine and Physical Fitness* 49: 320-360.

Alen, M., Pakarinen, A., Häkkinen, K., and Komi, P.B. 1988. Responses of serum androgenic-anabolic and catabolic hormones to prolonged strength training. *International Journal of Sports Medicine* 9: 229-233.

Alfredson, H., Pietila, T., Jonsson, P., and Lorentzon, R. 1998. Heavy-load eccentric calf muscle training for the treatment of chronic Achilles tendinosis. *American Journal of Sports Medicine* 26: 360-366.

Allen, T.E., Byrd, R.J., and Smith, D.P. 1976. Hemodynamic consequences of circuit weight training. *Research Quarterly* 47: 299-307.

Allsen, P.E., Parsons, P., and Bryce, G.R. 1977. Effect of menstrual cycle on maximum oxygen uptake. *The Physician and Sportsmedicine* 5: 52-55.

Aloia, J.F., Vaswani, A., Ma, R., and Flaster, E. 1995. To what extent is bone mass determined by fat-free for fat mass? *American Journal of Clinical Nutrition* 61: 1110-1114.

Alter, M.J. 1998. *Sports stretch*. Champaign, IL: Human Kinetics.

Alway, S.E. 1994. Characteristics of the elbow flexors in women bodybuilders using androgenic-anabolic steroids. *Journal of Strength and Conditioning Research* 8: 161-169.

Alway, S.E., Grumbt, W.H., Gonyea, W.J, and Stary-Gundersen, J. 1989. Contrast in muscle and myofibers of elite male and female bodybuilders. *Journal of Applied Physiology* 67: 24-31.

Alway, S.E., Grumbt, W.H., Stary-Gundersen, J., and Gonyea, W.J. 1992. Effects of resistance training on elbow flexors of highly competitive bodybuilders. *Journal of Applied Physiology* 72: 1512-1521.

Alway, S.E., MacDougall, J.D., and Sale, D.G. 1989. Contractile adaptations in the human triceps surae after isometric exercise. *Journal of Applied Physiology* 66: 2725-2732.

Alway, S.E., MacDougall, J.D., Sale, D.G., Sutton, J.R., and McComas, A.J. 1988. Functional and structural adaptations in skeletal muscle of trained athletes. *Journal of Applied Physiology* 64: 1114-1120.

Alway, S.E., Sale, D.G., and MacDougall, J.D. 1990. Twitch contractile adaptations are not dependent on the intensity of isometric exercise in the human triceps surae. *European Journal of Applied Physiology* 60: 346-352.

Alway, S.E., Winchester, P.K., Davies, M.E., and Gonyea, W.J. 1989. Regionalized adaptations and muscle fiber proliferation in stretch-induced enlargement. *Journal of Applied Physiology* 66: 771-781.

American Academy of Pediatrics. 2008. Strength training by children and adolescents. *Pediatrics* 121: 835-840.

American College of Sports Medicine. 1993. The prevention of sport injuries of children and adolescents. *Medicine & Science in Sports & Exercise* 25 (8 Suppl.): 1-7.

American College of Sports Medicine. 2001. Resource manual. *ACSM guidelines for exercise testing and prescription*, 4th ed. Baltimore: Lippincott Williams & Wilkins.

American College of Sports Medicine. 2002. Position stand. Progression models in resistance training for healthy adults. *Medicine & Science in Sports & Exercise* 34: 364-380.

American College of Sports Medicine. 2008. Selected issues for the adolescent athlete and team physician: Consensus statement. *Medicine & Science in Sports & Exercise* 40: 1997-2012.

American College of Sports Medicine. 2009. Progression models in resistance training for healthy adults. *Medicine & Science in Sports & Exercise* 41: 687-708.

American College of Sports Medicine. 2011. Quantity and quality of exercise for developing and maintaining cardiorespiratory, musculoskeletal, and neuromotor fitness in apparently healthy adults: Guidance for prescribing exercise. *Medicine & Science in Sports & Exercise* 43: 1334-1359.

American Orthopedic Society for Sports Medicine. 1988. *Proceedings of the conference on strength training and the prepubescent.* Chicago: American Orthopedic Society for Sports Medicine.

Amusa, L.O., and Obajuluwa, V.A. 1986. Static versus dynamic training programs for muscular strength using the knee-extensors in healthy young men. *Journal of Orthopaedic and Sports Physical Therapy* 8: 243-247.

Andersen, J.L., and Aagaard, P. 2000. Myosin heavy chain IIX overshoot in human skeletal muscle. *Muscle and Nerve* 23: 1095-1104.

Andersen, L.L., Andersen, J.L., Magnusson, S.P., and Aagaard, P. 2005. Neuromuscular adaptations to detraining following resistance training in previously untrained subjects. *European Journal of Applied Physiology* 93: 511-518.

Anderson, B. 2010. *Stretching.* Bolinas, CA: Shelter Publications.

Anderson, C.E., Sforzo, G.A., and Sigg, J.A. 2008. The effects of combining elastic and free weight resistance on strength and power in athletes. *Journal of Strength and Conditioning Research* 22: 567-574.

Anderson, T., and Kearney, J.T. 1982. Muscular strength and absolute and relative endurance. *Research Quarterly for Exercise and Sport* 53: 1-7.

Aniansson, A., Grimby, G., and Hedberg, M. 1992. Compensatory muscle fiber hypertrophy in elderly men. *Journal of Applied Physiology* 73: 812-816.

Aniansson, A., and Gustavsson, E. 1981. Physical training in elderly men with specific reference to quadriceps muscle strength and morphology. *Clinical Physiology* 1: 87-98.

Annino, G., Padua, E., Castagna, C., Di Salvo, V., Minichella, S., Tsarpela, O., Manzi, V., and D'Ottavio, S. 2007. Effect of whole body vibration training on lower limb performance in selected high-level ballet students. *Journal of Strength and Conditioning Research* 24: 1072-1076.

Antonio, J., and Gonyea, W.J. 1994. Muscle fiber splitting in stretch-enlarged avian muscle. *Medicine and Science in Sports and Exercise* 26: 973-977.

Ariel, G. 1977. Barbell vs. dynamic variable resistance. *U.S. Sports Association News* 1: 7.

Atha, J. 1981. Strengthening muscle. *Exercise and Sport Sciences Reviews* 9: 1-73.

Augustsson, J., Esko, A., Thomee, R., and Svantesson, U. 1998. Weight training of the thigh muscles using closed vs. open kinetic chain exercises: A comparison of performance enhancement. *Journal of Orthopedic and Sports Physical Therapy* 27: 3-8.

Augustsson, J., Thomeé, R., Hörnstedt, P., Lindblom, J., Karlsson J., and Grimby G. 2003. Effect of pre-exhaustion exercise on lower-extremity muscle activation during a leg press exercise. *Journal of Strength and Conditioning Research* 17: 411-416.

Aura, O., and Komi, P.V. 1986. The mechanical efficiency of locomotion in men and women with special emphasis on stretch-shortening exercises. *European Journal of Applied Physiology* 55: 37-43.

Australian Strength and Conditioning Association. 2007. Resistance training for children and youth: A position stand from the Australian Strength and Conditioning Association. Available at: www.strengthandconditioning.org.

Baar, K. 2006. Training for endurance and strength: Lessons from cell signaling. *Medicine & Science in Sports & Exercise* 38: 1939-1944.

Baar, K., and Esser K. 1999. Phosphorylation of p70S6k correlates with increased skeletal muscle mass following resistance exercise. *American Journal of Physiology (Cell Physiology)* 276: C120-C127.

Babault, N., Maffiuletti, N.A., and Pousson, M. 2008. Postactivation potentiation in human knee extensors during dynamic passive movements. *Medicine & Science in Sports & Exercise* 40: 735-743.

Baechle, T.R., Earle, R.W., and Wathen, D. 2000. Resistance training. In *Essentials of strength training and conditioning,* edited by T.R. Baechle and R.W. Earle, 2nd ed., 395-425. Champaign, IL: Human Kinetics.

Baker, D. 2001a. A series of studies on the training of high-intensity muscle power and rugby league football players. *Journal of Strength and Conditioning Research* 15: 198-209.

Baker, D. 2001b. Acute and long-term power responses to power training: Observations on the

413

training of an elite power athlete. *Strength and Conditioning Journal* 23: 47-56.

Baker, D. 2001c. Comparison of upper-body strength and power between professional and college-aged rugby league players. *Journal of Strength and Conditioning Research* 15: 30-35.

Baker, D., Nance, S., and Moore M. 2001a. The load that maximizes the average mechanical power output during explosive bench press throws in highly trained athletes. *Journal of Strength and Conditioning Research* 15: 20-24.

Baker, D., Nance, S., and Moore M. 2001b. The load that maximizes the average mechanical power output during jump squats in power-trained athletes. *Journal of Strength and Conditioning Research* 15: 92-97.

Baker, D.G., and Newton, R.U. 2005. Methods to increase the effectiveness of maximla power training for the upper body. *Strength and Conditioning Journal* 27: 24-32.

Baker, D.G., and Newton, R.U. 2009. Effect of kinetically altering a repetition via the use of chain resistance on velocity during the bench press. *Journal of Strength and Conditioning Research* 23: 1941-1946.

Baker, D., Wilson, G., and Carlyon, R. 1994a. Generality versus specificity: A comparison of dynamic and isometric measures of strength and speed-strength. *European Journal of Applied Physiology* 68: 350-355.

Baker, D., Wilson, G., and Carlyon, R. 1994b. Periodization: The effect on strength of manipulating volume and intensity. *Journal of Strength and Conditioning Research* 8: 235-242.

Bakhitary, A., Safavi-Farokhi, Z., and Aminian-Fra, A. 2006. Influence of vibration on delayed onset muscle soreness following eccentric exercise. *British Journal of Sports Medicine* 41: 145-148.

Ballor, D.L., Becque, M.D., and Katch, V.L. 1987. Metabolic responses during hydraulic resistance exercise. *Medicine & Science in Sports & Exercise* 19: 363-367.

Bamman, M.M., Hunger, G.R., Newton, L.E., Roney, R.K., and Khaled, M.A. 1993. Changes in body composition, diet, and strength of body builders during the 12 weeks prior to competition. *Journal of Sports Medicine and Physical Fitness* 33: 383-391.

Bamman, M.M., Shipp, J.R., Jiang, J., Gower, B.A., Hunter, G.R., Goodman, A., McLafferty, C.L., Jr., and Urban, R.J. 2001. Mechanical load increases muscle IGF-I and androgen receptor mRNA concentrations in humans. *American Journal of Physiology: Endocrinology and Metabolism* 280: E383-E390.

Barbosa, A.R., Santarem, J.M., Filho, W.J., Marucci, M.D.N. 2002. Effects of resistance training on the sit-and-reach test in elderly women. *Journal of Strength and Conditioning Research* 16: 14-18.

Barker, M., Wyatt, T.J., Johnson, R.L., Stone, M.H., O'Bryant, H.S., Poe, C., and Kent, M. 1993. Performance factors, psychological assessment, physical characteristics, and football playing ability. *Journal of Strength and Conditioning Research* 7: 224-233.

Barnekow-Bergkvist, M., Hedberg, G., Janlert, U., and Jansson, E. 1996. Physical activity pattern in men and women at the ages of 16 and 34 and development of physical activity from adolescence to adulthood. *Scandinavian Journal of Medicine & Science in Sports* 6: 359-370.

Barnett, L.S. 1985. Little league shoulder syndrome: Proximal humeral epiphyseolysis in adolescent baseball pictures. *Journal of Bone and Joint Surgery* 7A: 495-496.

Bartholomeu, S.A. 1985. Plyometrics and vertical jump training. Master's thesis, University of North Carolina, Chapel Hill.

Bass, A., Mackova, E., and Vitek, V. 1973. Activity of some enzymes of energy supplying metabolism in rat soleus after tenotomy of synergistic muscles and in contralateral control muscle. *Physiologica Bohemoslovaca* 22: 613-621.

Bass, S.L. 2000. The prepubertal years: A unique opportune stage of growth when the skeleton is most responsive to exercise? *Sports Medicine* 30: 73-70.

Bassey, E.J., Fiatarone, M.A., O'Neil, E.F., Kelly, M., Evans, W.J., and Lipsitz, L.A. 1992. Leg extensor power and functional performance in very old men and women. *Clinical Science* 82: 321-327.

Bassey, E.J., and Harries, U.J. 1993. Normal values for handgrip strength in 920 men and women aged over 65 years, and longitudinal changes over 4 years in 620 survivors. *Clinical Science* 84: 331-337.

Bastiaans, J.J., van Diemen, A.B., Veneberg, T., and Jeukendrup, A.E. 2001. The effects of replacing a portion of endurance training by explosive strength training on performance in trained cyclists. *European Journal of Applied Physiology* 86: 79-84.

Batista, M.A.B., Ugrinowitsch, C., Roschell, H., Lotufo, R., Ricard, M.D., and Tricoli, V.A.A. 2007.

Intermittent exercise as a conditioning activity to induce postactivation potentiation. *Journal of Strength and Conditioning Research* 21: 837-840.

Baty, J.J., Hwang, H., Ding, Z., Bernard, J.R., Wang, B., Kwon, B., and Ivy, J.L. 2007. The effect of a carbohydrate and protein supplement on resistance exercise performance, hormonal response, and muscle damage. *Journal of Strength and Conditioning Research*. 21: 321-329.

Bauer, J.A., Fry, A., and Carter, C. 1999. The use of lumbar-supporting weight belts while performing squats: Erector spinae electromyographic activity. *Journal of Strength Conditioning Research* 13: 384-388.

Bauer, T., Thayer, R.E., and Baras, G. 1990. Comparison of training modalities for power development in the lower extremity. *Journal of Applied Sport Science Research* 4: 115-121.

Baumann, G. 1991a. Growth hormone heterogeneity: Genes, isohormones, variants, and binding proteins. *Endocrine Reviews* 12: 424-443.

Baumann, G. 1991b. Metabolism of growth hormone (GH) and different molecular forms of GH in biological fluids. *Hormone Research Supplement* 36: 5-10.

Baumgaertner, M.R., and Higgins, T.F. 2002. Femoral neck fractures. In Rockwood and Green's Fractures in Adults, edited by R.W. Buchholz and J.D. Heckman, 5th ed. Philadelphia, PA: Lippincott Williams and Wilkins; 2001.

Baumgartner, T., and Wood, S. 1984. Development of shoulder-girdle strength-endurance in elementary children. *Research Quarterly for Exercise and Sport* 55: 169-171.

Bazett-Jones, D.M., Gibson, M.H., and McBride, J.M. 2008. Sprint and vertical jump performances are not affected by six weeks of static hamstring stretching. *Journal of Strength and Conditioning Research* 22: 25-31.

Beck, T.W., Housh, T.J., Johnson, G.O., Weir, J.P., Cramer, J.T., Coburn, J.W., Malek, M.H., and Mielke, M. 2007. Effects of two days of isokinetic training on strength electromyographic amplitude in the agonist and antagonist muscles. *Journal of Strength and Conditioning Research* 21: 757-762.

Beedle, B., Jesse, C., and Stone, M.H. 1991. Flexibility characteristics among athletes who weight train. *Journal of Applied Sport Science Research* 5: 150-154.

Behm, D.G., Button, D.C., and Butt, J.C. 2001. Factors affecting force loss with prolonged stretching. *Canadian Journal of Applied Physiology* 26: 261-272.

Behm, D.G., and Chaouachi, A. 2011. A review of the acute effects of static and dynamic stretching on performance. *European Journal of Applied Physiology* 111: 2633-2651.

Behm, D.G., Drinkwater, E.J., Willardson, J.M., and Cowley, P.M. 2010. Canadian Society for Exercise Physiology positions stand: The use of instability to train the core in athletic and nonathletic conditioning. *Applied Physiology, Nutrition and Metabolism* 35: 109-112.

Behm, D.G., and Sale, D.G. 1993. Velocity specificity of resistance training. *Sports Medicine* 15: 374-388.

Behm, D.G., Wahl, M.J., Button, D.C., Power, K.E., and Anderson, K.G. 2005. Relationship between hockey skating speed and select performance measures. *Journal of Strength and Conditioning Research* 19: 326-331.

Behringer, M., Heede, A., Yue, Z., and Mester, J. 2010. Effects of resistance training in children and adolescents: A meta-analysis. *Pediatrics* 125: 999-1000.

Belanger, A., and McComas, A.J. 1981. Extent of motor unit activation during effort. *Journal of Applied Physiology* 51: 1131-1135.

Bell, G.J., Petersen, S.R., Maclean I., Reid, D.C., and Quinney, H.A. 1992. Effect of high velocity resistance training on peak torque, cross sectional area and myofibrillar ATPase activity. *Journal of Sports Medicine and Physical Fitness* 32: 10-17.

Bell, G.J., Petersen, S.R., Wessel, J., Bagnall, K., and Quinney, H.A. 1991a. Adaptations to endurance and low velocity resistance training performed in a sequence. *Canadian Journal of Sport Science* 16: 186-192.

Bell, G.J., Petersen, S.R., Wessel, J., Bagnall, K., and Quinney, H.A. 1991b. Physiological adaptations to concurrent endurance training and low velocity resistance training. *International Journal of Sports Medicine* 12: 384-390.

Bell, G.J., Snydmiller, G.D., Neary, J.P., and Quinney, H.A. 1989. The effect of high and low velocity resistance training on anaerobic power output in cyclists. *Journal of Human Movement Studies* 16: 173-181.

Bell, G.J., Syrotuik, D.G., Attwood, K., and Quinney, H.A. 1993. Maintenance of strength gains while performing endurance training in oarswomen. *Journal of Applied Physiology* 18: 104-115.

Bell, G.J., Syrotuik, D., Martin, T.P., Burnham, R., and Quinney, H.A. 2000. Effect of concurrent strength and endurance training on skeletal muscle properties and hormone concentrations in humans. *European Journal of Applied Physiology* 81: 418-427.

Bell, G., Syrotuik, D., Socha, T., MacLean, I., and Quinney, H.A. 1997. Effects of strength training and concurrent strength and endurance training on strength, testosterone, and cortisol. *Journal of Strength and Conditioning Research* 11: 57-64.

Bellar, D.M., Muller, M.D., Barkley, J.E., Kim, C-H., Ida, K., Ryan, E.J., Bliss, M.V., and Glickman, E.L. 2011. The effects of combined elastic-and free-weight tension vs. free weight tension on one-repetition maximum strength in the bench press. *Journal of Strength and Conditioning Research* 25: 459-463.

Bemben, D.A., Fetters, N.L., Bemben, M.G., Nabavi, N., and Koh, E.T. 2000. Musculoskeletal responses to high-and low-intensity resistance training in early postmenopausal women. *Medicine & Science in Sports & Exercise* 32: 1949-1957.

Bender, J., and Kaplan, H. 1963. The multiple angle testing method for the evaluation of muscle strength. *Journal of Bone and Joint Surgery* 45A: 135-140.

Bennett, S. 2008. Using strongman exercises and training. *Strength and Conditioning Journal* 30 (3): 42-43.

Ben Sira, D., Amir, R., Amir, O., Yamin, C., Eynon, N., Meckel, Y., Sagiv, M., and Sagiv, M. 2010. Effect of different sprint training regimes on the oxygen delivery-extraction in elite sprinters. *Journal of Sports Medicine and Physical Fitness* 50: 121-125.

Benson, A.C., Torode, M.E., and Fiatarone-Singh, M.A. 2008. The effect of high-intensity progressive resistance training on adiposity in children: A randomized controlled trial. *International Journal of Obesity* 32: 1016-1027.

Benton, M.J., Kasper, M.J., Raab, S.A., Waggener, G.T., Swan, P.D. 2011. Short-term effects of resistance training frequency on body composition and strength in middle-aged women. *Journal of Strength and Conditioning Research* 25: 3142-3149.

Bera, S.G., Brown, L.E., Zinder, S.M., Noffal, G.J., Murray, D.P., and Garrett, N.M. 2007. The effects of velocity-spectrum training on the ability to rapidly step. *Journal of Strength and Conditioning Research* 21: 1101-1107.

Berger, M.J., and Doherty, T.J. 2010. Sarcopenia: Prevalence, mechanisms, and functional consequences. *Interdisciplinary Topics in Gerontology* 37: 94-114.

Berger, R.A. 1962a. Effect of varied weight training programs on strength. *Research Quarterly* 33: 168-181.

Berger, R.A. 1962b. Optimum repetitions for the development of strength. *Research Quarterly* 33: 334-338.

Berger, R.A. 1962c. Comparison of static and dynamic strength increases. *Research Quarterly* 33: 329-333.

Berger, R.A. 1963a. Comparative effects of three weight training programs. *Research Quarterly* 34: 396-398.

Berger, R.A. 1963b. Comparison between static training and various dynamic training programs. *Research Quarterly* 34: 131-135.

Berger, R.A. 1963c. Effects of dynamic and static training on vertical jump ability. *Research Quarterly* 34: 419-424.

Berger, R.A. 1963d. Comparison of the effect of various weight training loads on strength. *Research Quarterly* 36: 141-146.

Berger, R.A., and Hardage, B. 1967. Effect of maximum loads for each of ten repetitions on strength improvement. *Research Quarterly* 38: 715-718.

Bergeron, M.F., Nindl, B.C., Deuster, P.A., Baumgartner, N., Kane, S., Kraemer, W.J., Sexauer, L.R., Thompson, W.R., and O'Connor, F.G. 2011. Consortium for Health and Military Performance and American College of Sports Medicine consensus paper on extreme conditioning programs. *Current Sports Medicine Reports* 10: 383-389.

Bermon, S., Ferrari, P., Bernard, P., Altare, S., and Dolisi, C. 1999. Responses of total and free insulin-like growth factor-1 and insulin-like growth factor binding protein-3 after resistance exercise and training in elderly subjects. *Acta Physiologica Scandinavica* 165: 51-56.

Berning, J.M., Adams, K.J., DeBeliso, M., Sevene-Adams, P.G., Harris, C., and Stamford, B.A. 2010. Effect of functional isometric squats on vertical jump in trained and untrained men. *Journal of Strength and Conditioning Research* 24: 2285-2289.

Berning, J.M., Coker, C.A., and Briggs, D. 2008. The biomechanical and perceptual influence of chain resistance on the performance of the Olympic clean. *Journal of Strength and Conditioning Research* 22: 390-395.

Berryman, N., Maurel, D., and Bosquet, L. 2010. Effect of plyometric vs. dynamic weight training on the energy cost of running. *Journal of Strength and Conditioning Research* 24: 1818-1825.

Bickel, C.S., Cross, J.M., and Bamman, M.M. 2011. Exercise dosing to retain resistance training adaptations in young and older adults. *Medicine & Science in Sports & Exercise* 43: 1177-1187.

Biewener, A.A., and Roberts, T.J. 2000. Muscle and tendon contributions to force, work, and elastic energy savings: A comparative perspective. *Exercise and Sport Sciences Reviews* 28: 99-107.

Bilanin, J.E., Blanchard, M.S., and Russek-Cohen, E. 1989. Lower vertebral bone density in male long distance runners. *Medicine & Science in Sports & Exercise* 21: 66-70.

Billeter, R., Jostarndt-Fogen, K., Gunthor, W., and Hoppeler, H. 2003. Fiber type characteristics and myosin light chain expression in a world champion shot putter. *International Journal of Sports Medicine* 4: 203-207.

Biolo, G., Fleming, R.Y., Maggi, S.P., and Wolfe, R.R. 1995. Transmembrane transport and intracellular kinetics of amino acids in human skeletal muscle. *American Journal of Physiology* 268: E75-E84.

Biolo, G., Tipton, K.D., Klein, S., and Wolfe, R.R. 1997. An abundant supply of amino acids enhances the metabolic effect of exercise on muscle protein. *American Journal of Physiology* 36: E122-E129.

Biolo, G., Williams, B.D., Fleming, R.Y., and Wolfe, R.R. 1999. Insulin action on muscle protein kinetics and amino acid transport during recovery after resistance exercise. *Diabetes* 48: 949-957.

Bishop, D., Girard, O., and Mendez-Villanueva, A. 2011. Repeated-sprint ability-part II: Recommendations for training. *Sports Medicine* 41: 741-756.

Bishop, D.C., Smith, R.J., Smith, M.F., and Rigby, H.E. 2009. Effect of plyometric training on swimming block start performance in adolescents. *Journal of Strength and Conditioning Research* 23: 2137-2143.

Bishop, P., Cureton, K., and Collins, M. 1987. Sex difference in muscular strength in equally trained men and women. *Ergonomics* 30: 675-687.

Black, C.D., and McCully, K.K. 2008. Muscle injury after repeated bouts of voluntary and electrically stimulated exercise. *Medicine & Science in Sports & Exercise* 40: 1605-1615.

Blackey, J.B., and Southard, D. 1987. The combined effects of weight training and plyometrics on dynamic leg strength and leg power. *Journal of Applied Sport Science Research* 1: 14-16.

Blain, H., Vuillemin, A., Teissier, A., Hanesse, B., Guillemin, F., and Jeandel, C. 2001. Influence of muscle strength and body weight and composition on regional bone mineral density in healthy women aged 60 years and over. *Gerontology* 47: 207-212.

Bland, R. 2000. Steroid hormone receptor expression and action in bone. *Clinical Science* 98: 217-240.

Blattner, S.E., and Noble, L. 1979. Relative effects of isokinetic and plyometric training on vertical jumping performance. *Research Quarterly* 50: 583-588.

Blazevich, A.J. 2006. Effects of physical training and the training, mobilization, growth and aging on human fascicle geometry. *Sports Medicine* 36: 1003-1017.

Blazevich, A.J., Cannavan, D., Coleman, D.R., and Horne, S. 2007. Influence of concentric and eccentric resistance training on architectural adaptation in human quadriceps muscles. *Journal of Applied Physiology* 103: 1565-1575.

Blessing, D., Stone, M., Byrd, R., Wilson, D., Rozenek, R., Pushparani, D., and Lipner, H. 1987. Blood lipid and hormonal changes from jogging and weight training in middle-aged men. *Journal of Applied Sport Science Research* 1: 25-29.

Blimkie, C.J.R. 1992. Resistance training during pre- and early puberty: Efficacy, trainability, mechanisms, and persistence. *Canadian Journal of Sport Sciences* 17: 264-279.

Blimkie, C.J.R. 1993. Resistance training during pre-adolescence issues and controversies. *Sports Medicine* 15: 389-407.

Blimkie, C.J.R., Ramsay, J., Sale, D., MacDougall, D., Smith, K., and Garner, S. 1989. Effects of 10 weeks resistance training on strength development in pre-pubertal boys. In *Children and exercise XIII*, edited by S. Oseid and K.H. Carlsen, 183-197. Champaign, IL: Human Kinetics.

Blanksby, B., and Gregory, J. 1981. Anthropometric, strength, and physiological changes in male and female swimmers with progressive resistance training. *Australian Journal of Sport Science* 1: 3-6.

Blossner, M., and de Onis, M. 2005. Malnutrition: Quantifying the health impact at national and local levels. World Health Organization, *WHO Environmental Burdens of Disease Series*, No. 12. Geneva.

Bocalini, D.S., Serra, A.J., dos Santos, L., Murad, N., and Levy, R.F. 2009. Strength training preserves the bone mineral density of postmenopausal women without hormone replacement therapy. *Journal of Aging and Health* 21: 519-527.

Boirie, Y. 2009. Physiopathological mechanism of sarcopenia. *The Journal of Nutrition, Health & Aging* 13: 717-723.

Bond, V., Jr., Wang, P., Adams, R.G., Johnson, A.T., Vaccaro, P., Tearney, R.J., Millis, R.M., Franks, B.D., and Bassett, D.R. Jr. 1996. Lower leg high-intensity resistance training and peripheral hemodynamic adaptations. *Canadian Journal of Physiology* 21: 209-217.

Bonde-Peterson, F. 1960. Muscle training by static, concentric and eccentric contractions. *Acta Physiologica Scandinavica* 48: 406-416.

Bonde-Peterson, F., and Knuttgen, H.G. 1971. Effect of training with eccentric muscle contractions on human skeletal muscle metabolites. *Acta Physiologica Scandinavica* 80: 16A-17A.

Bonde-Peterson, F., Knuttgen, H.G., and Henriksson, J. 1972. Muscle metabolism during exercise with concentric and eccentric contractions. *Journal of Applied Physiology* 33: 792-795.

Bonde-Peterson, F., Mork, A.L., and Nielsen, E. 1975. Local muscle blood flow and sustained contractions of human arms and back muscles. *European Journal of Applied Physiology and Occupational Physiology* 34: 43-50.

Borst, S.E., De Hoyos, D.V., Garzarella, L., Vincent, K., Pollock, B.H., Lowenthal, D.T., and Pollock, M.L. 2001. Effects of resistance training on insulin-like growth factor-I and IGF binding proteins. *Medicine and Science in Sports and Exercise* 33: 648-653.

Bosco, C., Colli, R., Bonomi, R., von Duvillard, S.P., and Viru, A. 2000. Monitoring strength training: Neuromuscular and hormonal profile. *Medicine & Science in Sports & Exercise* 32: 202-208.

Bosco, C., and Komi, P.V. 1980. Influence of aging on the mechanical behavior of leg extensor muscles. *European Journal of Applied Physiology* 45: 209-219.

Bosco, C., Montanari, G., Ribacchi, R., Giovenali, P., Latteri, F., Iachelli, G., Faina, M., Coli, R., Dal Monte, A., La Rosa, M., Cortili, G., and Saibene, F. 1987. Relationship between the efficiency of muscular work during jumping and the energetics of running. *European Journal of Applied Physiology* 56: 138-143.

Bosco, C., and Pittera, C. 1982. Zur trainings Wirkung neuentwicker Sprungubungen auf die Explosivkraft. *Leistungssport* 12: 36-39.

Bosco, C., Tarkka, I., and Komi, P.V. 1982. Effects of elastic energy and myoelectrical potentiation of triceps surae during stretch-shortening cycle exercises. *Sports Medicine* 3: 137-140.

Boyer, B.T. 1990. A comparison of the effects of three strength training programs on women. *Journal of Applied Sport Science Research* 4: 88-94.

Brady, T., Cahill, B., and Bodnar, L. 1982. Weight training related injuries in the high school athlete. *American Journal of Sports Medicine* 10: 1-5.

Braith, R.W., Graves, J.E., Leggett, S.H., and Pollock, M.L. 1993. Effect of training on the relationship between maximal and submaximal strength. *Medicine & Science in Sports & Exercise* 25: 132-138.

Braith, R.W., and Stewart, K.J. 2006. Resistance exercise training: Its role in the prevention of cardiovascular disease. *Circulation* 113: 2642-2650.

Brandenburg, J.P. 2005. Acute effects of prior dynamic resistance exercise using different loads on subsequent upper-body explosive performance in resistance-trained men. *Journal of Strength and Conditioning Research* 19: 427-432.

Brandenburg, J.P., and Docherty, D. 2002. The effects of accentuated eccentric loading on strength, muscle hypertrophy, and neural adaptations in trained individuals. *Journal of Strength and Conditioning Research* 16: 25-32.

Brandy, W.D., Irion, J.M., and Briggler, M. 1997. The effect of time and frequency of static stretching on flexibility of the hamstring muscles. *Physical Therapy* 77: 1090-1096.

Brandy, W.D., Irion, J.M., and Briggler, M. 1998. The effect of static stretch and dynamic range of motion training on the flexibility of the hamstring muscles. *Journal of Orthopedic Sports Physical Therapy* 27: 295-300.

Brazell-Roberts, J.V., and Thomas, L.E. 1989. Effects of weight training frequency on the self-concept of college females. *Journal of Applied Sports Science Research* 3: 40-43.

Brechue, W.F., and Abe, T. 2002. The role of FFM accumulation and skeletal muscle architecture in powerlifting performance. *European Journal of Applied Physiology* 84 (4): 327-336.

Brechue, W.F., and Mayhew, J.L. 2009. Upper-body work capacity and 1 RM prediction are unaltered by increasing muscular strength in college football players. *Journal of Strength and Conditioning Research* 23: 2477-2486.

Brechue, W.F., and Mayhew, J.L. 2012. Lower-body work capacity and one-repetition maximum squat prediction in college football players. *Journal of Strength and Conditioning Research* 26: 364-372.

Brennecke, A., Gumarães, T.M., Leone, R., Cadarci, M., Mochizuki, L., Simao, R., Amadio, A.C., and Serrato, J.C. 2009. Neuromuscular activity during bench press exercise performed with and without the preexhaustion method. *Journal of Strength and Conditioning Research* 23: 1933-1940.

Brentano, M.A., Cadore, E.L., Da Silva, E.M., Ambrosini, A.B., Coertjens, M., Petkowicz, R., Viero, I., and Kruel, L.F. 2008. Physiological adaptations to strength and circuit training in postmenopausal women with bone loss. *Journal of Strength and Conditioning Research* 22: 1816-1825.

Bricourt, V.A., Germain, P.S., Serrurier, B.D., and Guezeennec, C.Y. 1994. Changes in testosterone muscle receptors: Effects of an androgen treatment on physically trained rats. *Cellular and Molecular Biology* 40: 291-294.

Brill, P.A., Macera, C.A., Davis, D.R., Blair, S.N., and Gordon, N. 2000. Muscular strength and physical function. *Medicine & Science in Sports & Exercise* 32: 412-416.

British Association of Exercise and Sport Sciences. 2004. BASES position statement on guidelines for resistance training and young people. *Journal of Sport Sciences* 22: 283-390.

Brockett, C.L., Morgan, D.L., and Proske, U. 2001. Human hamstring muscles adapt to eccentric exercise by changing optimal length. *Medicine & Science in Sports & Exercise* 33: 783-790.

Brooks, G.A. 2010. What does glycolysis make and why is it important? *Journal of Applied Physiology* 108: 1450-1451.

Brooks, G.A., Butterfield, G.E., Wolfe, R.R., Groves, B.M., Mazzeo, R.S., Sutton, J.R., Wolfel, E.E., and Reeves, J.T. 1991. Decreased reliance on lactate during exercise after acclimatization to 4,300 m. *Journal of Applied Physiology* 71: 333-341.

Brooks, G.A., and Fahey, T.D. 1984. *Exercise physiology: Human bioenergetics and its applications.* New York: Wiley & Son.

Brooks, N., Layne, J.E., Gordon, P.L., Roubenoff, R., Nelson, M.E., and Castaneda-Sceppa, C. 2007. Strength training improves muscle quality and insulin sensitivity in Hispanic older adults with type 2 diabetes. *International Journal of Medical Sciences*, 4: 19-27.

Brooks-Gunn, J., and Rubb, D.N. 1983. The experience of menarche from a developmental perspective. In *Girls at puberty: Biological and psychosocial perspectives,* edited by J. Brooks-Gunn and A.C. Peterson, 155-177. New York: Plenum Press.

Brown, A.B., McCartney, N., and Sale, D.G. 1990. Positive adaptations to weight-lifting training in the elderly. *Journal of Applied Physiology* 69: 1725-1733.

Brown, B.S., Gorman, D.R., DiBrezzom, R., and Fort, I. 1988. Anaerobic power changes following short term, task specific, dynamic and static overload training. *Journal of Applied Sport Science Research* 2: 35-38.

Brown, C.H., and Wilmore, J.H. 1974. The effects of maximal resistance training on the strength and body composition of women athletes. *Medicine and Science in Sports & Exercise* 6: 174-177.

Brown, L.E., Whitehurst, M., Findley, B.W., Gilbert, R., Groo, D.R., and Jimenez, J.A. 1998. Effect of repetitions and gender on acceleration range of motion during knee extension on an isokinetic device. *Journal of Strength and Conditioning Research* 12: 222-225.

Brown, S., Byrd, R., Jayasinghe, M.D., and Jones, D. 1983. Echocardiographic characteristics of competitive and recreational weight lifters. *Journal of Cardiovascular Ultrasonography* 2: 163-165.

Brughelli, M., and Cronin, J. 2007. Altering the length-tension relationship with eccentric exercise implications for performance and injury. *Sports Medicine* 37: 807-826.

Bruusgaard, J.C., Johansen, I.B., Egner, I.M., Rana, Z.A., and Gundersen, K. 2010. Myonuclei acquired by overload exercise precede hypertrophy and are not lost on detraining. *Proceedings of the National Academy of Sciences* 107: 15111-15116.

Buchanan, P.A., and Vardaxis, V.G. 2009. Lower-extremity strength profiles and gender-based classification of basketball players ages 9-22 years. *Journal of Strength and Conditioning Research* 23: 406-419.

Buford, T.W., Rossi, S.J., Smith, D.B., and Warren, A.J. 2007. A comparison of periodization models during nine weeks of equated volume and intensity for strength. *Journal of Strength and Conditioning Research* 21: 1245-1250.

Bullock, N., Martin, D.T., Ross, A., Rosemond, C.D., Jordan, M.J., and Marino, F.E. 2008. Acute effect of whole-body vibration on sprint and jumping performance in elite skeleton athletes. *Journal of Strength and Conditioning Research* 22: 1371-1374.

Burgess, K.E., Connick, M.J., Graham-Smith, P., and Pearson, S.J. 2007. Plyometric vs. isometric training influences on tendon properties and muscle output. *Journal of Strength and Conditioning Research* 21: 986-989.

Burgess, K.E., Pearson, S.J., and Onambélé, G.L. 2010. Patellar tendon properties with fluctuating menstrual cycle hormones. *Journal of Strength and Conditioning Research* 24: 2088-2095.

Burgomaster, K.A., Moore, D.R., Schofield, L.M., Phillips, S.M., Sale, D.G., and Gibala, M.J. 2003. Resistance training with vascular occlusion: Metabolic adaptations in human muscle. *Medicine and Science and Sports and Exercise* 35: 1203-1208.

Burke, R.E., Levine, D.N., Salcman, M., and Tsairis, P. 1974. Motor units in cat soleus muscle: Physiological, histochemical and morphological characteristics. *Journal of Applied Physiology* 238: 503-514.

Bush, J.A., Kraemer, W.J., Mastro, A.M., Triplett-McBride, N.T., Volek, J.S., Putukian, M., Sebastianelli, W.J., and Knuttgen, H.G. 1999. Exercise and recovery responses of adrenal medullary neurohormones to heavy resistance exercise. *Medicine & Science in Sports & Exercise* 31: 554-559.

Butts, N.K., and Price, S. 1994. Effects of a 12-week weight training program on the body composition of women over 30 years of age. *Journal of Strength and Conditioning Research* 8: 265-269.

Byrd, S.K. 1992. Alterations in the sarcoplasmic reticulum: A possible link to exercise-induced muscle damage. *Medicine & Science in Sports & Exercise* 24: 531-536.

Byrne, C., Twist, C., and Eston, R. 2004. Neuromuscular function after exercise-induced muscle damage: Theoretical and practical implications. *Sports Medicine* 34: 149-169.

Byrne, H.K., and Wilmore, J.H. 2000. The effects of resistance training on resting blood pressure in women. *Journal of Strength and Conditioning Research* 14: 411-418.

Byrne, S., and McLean, N. 2002. Elite athletes: Effects of the pressure to be thin. *Journal of Science and Medicine in Sport* 5: 80-94.

Cabell, L., and Zebras, C.J. 1999. Resistive torque validation of the Nautilus multi-biceps machine. *Journal of Strength and Conditioning Research* 13: 20-23.

Cacchio, A., Don, R., Ranavolo, A., Guerra, E., McCaw, S.T., Procaccianti, R., Camerota, F., Frascarell, M., and Santilli, V. 2008. Effects of 8-week strength training with two models of chest press machines on muscular activity pattern and strength. *Electromyography and Kinesiology* 18: 618-627.

Cadore, E.L., Pinto, R.S., Lhullier, F.L., Correa, C.S., Alberton, C.L., Pinto, S.S., Almeida, A.P., Tartaruga, M.P., Silva, E.M., and Kruel, L.F. 2010. Physiological effects of concurrent training in elderly men. *International Journal of Sports Medicine* 31: 689-697.

Cadore, E.L., Pinto, R.S., Pinto, S.S., Alberton, C.L., Correa, C.S., Tartaruga, M.P., Silva, E.M., Almeida, A.P., Trindade, G.T., and Kruel, L.F. 2011. Effects of strength, endurance, and concurrent training on aerobic power and dynamic neuromuscular economy in elderly men. *Journal of Strength and Conditioning Research* 25: 758-766.

Caine, D., DiFiori, J., and Maffulli, N. 2006. Physeal injuries and children's and youth sports: Reasons for concern? *British Journal of Sports Medicine* 40: 749-760.

Caiozzo, V.J., Laird, T., Chow, K., Prietto, C.A., and McMaster, W.C. 1983. The use of precontractions to enhance the in-vivo force velocity relationship. *Medicine & Science in Sports & Exercise* 14: 162.

Caiozzo, V.J., Perrine, J.J., and Edgerton, V.R. 1981. Training-induced alterations of the in vivo force-velocity relationship of human muscle. *Journal of Applied Physiology: Respiratory, Environmental and Exercise Physiology* 51: 750-754.

Calder, A.W., Chilibeck, P.D., Webber, C.E., and Sale, D.G. 1994. Comparison of whole and split weight training routines in young women. *Canadian Journal of Applied Physiology* 19: 185-199.

Callister, R., Shealy, M.J., Fleck, S.J., and Dudley, G.A. 1988. Performance adaptations to sprint, endurance and both modes of training. *Journal of Applied Physiology* 2: 46-51.

Camargo, M.D., Stein, R., Ribeiro, J.P., Schvartzman, P.R., Rizzatti, M.O., and Schaan, B.D. 2008. Circuit weight training and cardiac morphology: A trial with magnetic resonance imaging. *British Journal of Sports Medicine* 42: 141-145.

Cameron, K.R., Wark, J.D., and Telford, R.D. 1992. Stress fractures and bone loss: The skeletal cost of intense athleticism. *Excel* 8: 39-55.

Campbell, R.C. 1962. Effects of supplemental weight training on the physical fitness of athletic squads. *Research Quarterly* 33: 343-348.

Campbell, W.W., Crim, M.C., Young, V.R., Joseph, L.J., and Evans, W.J. 1995. Effects of resistance training and dietary protein intake on protein metabolism in older adults. *American Journal of Applied Physiology* 268: E1143-E1153.

Campbell, W.W., and Evans, W.J. 1996. Protein requirements of elderly people. *European Journal of Clinical Nutrition* 50 (Suppl.): S180-S183.

Campbell, W.W., Joseph, L.J.O., Davey, S.L., Cyr-Campbell, D., Anderson, R.A., and Evans, W.J. 1999. Effects of resistance training and chromium picolinate on body composition and skeletal muscle in older men. *Journal of Applied Physiology* 86: 29-39.

Campbell, W.W., Trappe, T.A., Wolfe, R.R., and Evans, W.J. 2001. The recommended dietary allowance for protein may not be adequate for older people to maintain skeletal muscle. *Journal of Gerontology: Biological Medical Sciences* 56: M373-M380.

Campos, G.E.R., Luecke, T.J., Wendeln, H.K., Toma, K., Hagerman, F.C., Murray, T.F., Ragg, K.E., Ratamess, N.A., Kraemer, W.J., and Staron, R.S. 2002. Muscular adaptations in response to three different resistance-training regimens: Specificity of repetition maximum training zones. *European Journal of Applied Physiology* 88: 50-60.

Canadian Society for Exercise Physiology. 2008. Position paper: Resistance training in children and adolescents. *Journal of Applied Physiology, Nutrition and Metabolism* 33: 547-561.

Candow, D.G., and Burke, D.G. 2007. Effect of short-term equal-volume resistance training with different workout frequency on muscle mass and strength in untrained men and women. *Journal of Strength and Conditioning Research* 21: 204-207.

Cann, C.E., Martin, M.C., Genant, H.K., and Jaffe, R. 1984. Decreased spinal mineral content in amenorrheic females. *Journal of the American Medical Association* 251: 626-629.

Cannon, R., and Cafarelli, E. 1987. Neuromuscular adaptations to training. *Journal of Applied Physiology* 63: 2396-2402.

Capen, E.K. 1950. The effect of systematic weight training on power, strength and endurance. *Research Quarterly* 21: 83-93.

Capen, E.K., Bright, J.A., and Line, P.Q. 1961. The effects of weight training on strength, power, muscular endurance and anthropometric measurements on a select group of college women. *Journal of the Association for Physical and Mental Rehabilitation* 15: 169-173.

Carmeli, E., Coleman, R., and Reznick, A.Z. 2002. The biochemistry of aging muscle. *Experimental Gerontology* 37: 477-489.

Carolyn, B., and Cafarelli, E. 1992. Adaptations in coactivation after isometric resistance training. *Journal of Applied Physiology* 73: 911-917.

Carpinelli, R.N., and Gutin, B. 1991. Effects of miometric and pliometric muscle actions on delayed muscle soreness. *Journal of Applied Sport Science Research* 5: 66-70.

Carroll, T.J., Riek, S., and Carson, R.G. 2001. Neural adaptations to resistance training implications for movement control. *Sports Medicine* 31: 829-840.

Carroll, T.J., Selvanayagam, V.S., Riek, S., and Semmler, J.G. 2011. Neural adaptations to strength training: Moving beyond transcranial magnetic stimulation and reflex studies. *Acta Physiologica* (Oxford) 202: 119-140.

Caruso, J.F., Coday, M.A., Ramsey, C.A., Griswold, S.H., Polanski, D.W., Drumond, J.L., and Walker, R.H. 2008. Leg and calf press training modes and their impact on jump performance adaptations. *Journal of Strength and Conditioning Research* 22: 766-772.

Caruso, J.F., Signorile, J.F., Perry, A.C., Clark, M., and Bamman, M.M. 1997. Time course changes in contractile strength resulting from isokinetic exercise and b2 agonist administration. *Journal of Strength and Conditioning Research* 11: 8-13.

Casa, D.J., Guskiewicz, K.M., Anderson, S.A., Courson, R.W., Heck, J.F., Jimenez, C.C., McDermott, B.P., Miller, M.G., Stearns, R.L., Swartz, E., and Walsh, K.M. 2012. National Athletic Trainers' Association position statement: Preventing sudden death in sports. *Journal of Athletic Training* 47: 96-118.

Caserotti, P., Aagaard, P., Larsen, J.B., and Puggaard, L. 2008. Explosive heavy-resistance training in old and very old adults: Changes in rapid muscle force, strength and power. *Scandinavian Journal of Medicine & Science in Sports* 18: 773-782.

Caserotti, P., Aagaard, P., and Puggaard, L. 2008. Changes in power and force generation during coupled eccentric-concentric versus concentric muscle contraction with training and aging. *European Journal of Applied Physiology* 103: 151-161.

Castro, M.J., McCann, D.J., Shaffrath, J.D., and Adams, W.C. 1995. Peak torque per unit cross-sectional area differs between strength-trained and untrained young adults. *Medicine & Science in Sports & Exercise* 27: 397-403.

Chakravati, S., and Collins, W. 1976. Hormonal profiles after menopause. *British Medical Journal* 2: 782-787.

Chapman, D.W., Newton, M.J., McGuigan, M.R., and Nosaka, K. 2011. Effect of slow-velocity lengthening contractions on muscle damage induced by fast-velocity lengthening contractions. *Journal of Strength and Conditioning Research* 25: 211-219.

Chalmers, G.R. 2008. Can fast-twitch muscle fibres be selectively recruited during lengthening contractions? Review and applications to sport movements. *Sports Biomechanics.* 7: 137-157.

Chandler, R.M., Byrne, H.K., Patterson, J.G., and Ivy, J.L. 1994. Dietary supplements affect the anabolic hormones after weight-training exercise. *Journal of Applied Physiology* 76: 839-845.

Chang, D.E., Buschbacker, L.P., and Edlich, R.F. 1988. Limited mobility in power lifters. *The American Journal of Sports Medicine* 16: 280-284.

Channell, B.T., and Barfield, J.P. 2008. Effect of Olympic and traditional resistance training on vertical jump improvement in high school boys. *Journal of Strength and Conditioning Research* 22: 1522-1527.

Charette, S.L., McEvoy, L., Pyka, G., Snow-Harter, C., Guido, D., Wiswell, R.A., and Marcus, R. 1991. Muscle hypertrophy response to resistance training in older women. *Journal of Applied Physiology* 70: 1912-1916.

Chatzinikolaou, A., Fatouros, I.G., Gourgoulis, V., Avloniti, A., Jamurtas, A.Z., Nikolaidis, M.G., Douroudos, I., Michailidis, Y., Beneka, A., Malliou, P., Tofas, T., Georgiadis, I., Mandalidis, D., and Taxildaris, K. 2010. Time course of changes in performance and inflammatory responses after acute plyometric exercise. *Journal of Strength and Conditioning Research* 24: 1389-1398.

Chen, C.C.-H., Bai, Y.-Y., Huang, G.-H., and Tang, S.T. 2007. Revisiting the concept of malnutrition in older people. *Journal of Clinical Nursing* 16: 2015-2026.

Chen, H.L., Nosaka, K., and Chen, T.C. 2012. Muscle damage protection by low-intensity eccentric contractions remains for 2 weeks but not 3 weeks. *European Journal of Applied Physiology* 112: 555-565.

Chen, T.C., Chen, H.-L., Lin, C.-J., Wu, C.-J., and Nosaka, K. 2010. Potent protective effect conferred by four bouts of low-intensity eccentric exercise. *Medicine & Science in Sports & Exercise* 42: 1004-1012.

Chen, T.C., and Nosaka, K. 2006. Response of elbow flexors to two strenuously eccentric exercise bouts separated by three days. *Journal of Strength and Conditioning Research* 20: 108-116.

Cheng, S., Sipilä, S., Taaffe, D.R., Puolakka, J., and Suominen, H. 2002. Change in bone mass distribution induced by hormone replacement therapy and high-impact physical exercise in post-menopausal women. *Bone* 31: 126-135.

Chernoff, R. 2004. Protein and older adults. *Journal of the American College of Nutrition* 23: 627S-630S.

Chesley, A., MacDougall, J.D., Tarnopolsky, M.A., Atkinson, S.A., and Smith, K. 1992. Changes in human muscle protein synthesis after resistance exercise. *Journal of Applied Physiology* 73: 1383-1388.

Cheung, K., Hume, P.A., and Maxwell, L. 2003. Delayed onset muscle soreness treatment strategies and performance factors. *Sports Medicine* 33: 145-164.

Chevan, J. 2008. Demographic determinants of participation in strength training activities among U.S. adults. *Journal of Strength and Conditioning Research* 22: 553-558.

Chilibeck, P.D., Calder, A.W., Sale, D.G., and Webber, C.E. 1998. A comparison of strength and muscle mass increases during resistance training in young women. *European Journal of Applied Physiology* 77: 170-175.

Chilibeck, P.D., Sale, D.G., and Webber, C.E. 1995. Exercise and bone mineral density. *Sports Medicine* 19: 103-122.

Chilibeck, P.D., Syrotuik, D.G., and Bell, G.J. 1999. The effect of strength training on estimates of mitochondrial density and distribution throughout muscle fibers. *European Journal of Applied Physiology* 80: 604-609.

Chilibeck, P.D., Syrotuik, D.G., and Bell, G.J. 2002. The effect of concurrent endurance and strength training on quantitative estimates of subsarcolemmal and intermyofibrillar mitochondria. *International Journal of Sports Medicine* 23: 33-39.

Chow, J.W.M. 2000. Role of nitrate oxide and prostaglandins in the bone formation response to mechanical loading. *Exercise and Sport Sciences Reviews* 28: 185-188.

Chow, R.S., Medri, M.K., Martin, D.C., Leekam, R.N., Agur, A.M., and McKee, N.H. 2000. Sonographic studies of human soleus and gastrocnemius muscle architecture: Gender variability. *European Journal of Applied Physiology* 82: 236-244.

Christou, M., Smilios, I., Sotiropoulos, K., Volakis, K., Pilianidis, T., and Tokmakidis, S.P. 2006. Effects of resistance training on the physical capacities of adolescent soccer players. *Journal of Strength and Conditioning Research* 20: 783-791.

Chromiak, J.A., and Mulvaney, D.R. 1990. A review: The effects of combined strength and endurance training on strength development. *Journal of Applied Sport Science Research* 4: 55-60.

Chu, E. 1950. The effect of systematic weight training on athletic power. *Research Quarterly* 21: 188-194.

Church, J.B., Wiggins, M.S., Moode, F.M., and Crist, R. 2001. Effect of warm-up and flexibility treatments on vertical jump performance. *Journal of Strength and Conditioning Research* 15: 332-336.

Cirello, V.M., Holden, W.C., and Evans, W.J. 1983. The effects of two isokinetic training regimens on muscle strength and fiber composition. In *Biochemistry of exercise*, edited by H.G. Knuttgen, J.A. Vogel, and S. Poortmans, 787-793. Champaign, IL: Human Kinetics.

Claassen, H., Gerber, C., Hoppeler, H., Luthi, J.M., and Vock, P. 1989. Muscle filament spacing and short-term heavy-resistance exercise in humans. *Journal of Physiology* 409: 491-495.

Claflin, D.R., Larkin, L.M., Cederna, P.S., Horowitz, J.F., Alexander, N.B., Cole, N.M., Galecki, A.T., Chen, S., Nyquist, L.V., Carlson, B.M., Faulkner, J.A., and Ashton-Miller, J.A. 2011. Effects of high- and low-velocity resistance training on the contractile properties of skeletal muscle fibers from young and older humans. *Journal of Applied Physiology* 111: 1021-1030.

Clarke, D.H. 1973. Adaptations in strength and muscular endurance resulting from exercise. *Exercise and Sport Sciences Reviews* 1: 73-102.

Clarkson, P. 2006. Case report of exertional rhabdomyolysis in a 12-year-old boy. *Medicine & Science in Sports & Exercise* 38: 197-200.

Clarkson, P.M., Devaney, J.M., Gordish-Dressman, H., Thompson, P.D., Hubal, M.J., Urso, M., Price, T.B., Angelopoulos, T.J., Gordon, P.M., Moyna, N.M., Pescatello, L.S., Visich, P.S., Zoeller, R.F., Seip, R.L., and Hoffman, E.P. 2005. ACTN3 genotype is associated with increases in muscle strength in response to resistance training in women. Journal of Applied Physiology 99: 154-163.

Clarkson, P.M., Nosaka, K., and Braun, B. 1992. Muscle function after exercise-induced muscle damage and rapid adaptation. *Medicine & Science in Sports & Exercise* 24: 512-520.

Clarkson, P.M., and Tremblay, I. 1988. Exercise-induced muscle damage, repair and adaptation in humans. *Journal of Applied Physiology* 65: 1-6.

Clutch, D., Wilson, C., McGown, C., and Bryce, G.R. 1983. The effect of depth jumps and weight training on leg strength and vertical jump. *Research Quarterly* 54: 5-10.

Coburn, J.W., Housh, T.J., Malek, M.H., Weir, J.P., Cramer, J.T., Beck, T.W., and Johnson, G.O. 2006. Neuromuscular responses to three days of velocity-specific isokinetic training. *Journal of Strength and Conditioning Research* 20: 892-890.

Cochrane, D.J., and Hawke, E.J. 2007. Effects of acute upper-body vibration on strength and power variables in climbers. *Journal of Strength and Conditioning Research* 21: 527-531.

Cochrane, D.J., and Stannard, S.R. 2005. Acute whole body vibration training increases vertical jump and flexibility performance in elite field hockey players. *British Journal Sports Medicine* 39: 860-865.

Coker, C.A., Berning, J.M., and Briggs, D.L. 2006. A preliminary investigation of the biomechanical and perceptual influence of chain resistance on the performance of the snatch. *Journal of Strength and Conditioning Research* 20: 887-891.

Colan, S., Sanders, S.P., and Borrow, K.M. 1987. Physiologic hypertrophy: Effects on left ventricular systolic mechanisms in athletes. *Journal of the American College of Cardiology* 9: 776-783.

Colan, S., Sanders, S.P., McPherson, D., and Borrow, K.M. 1985. Left ventricular diastolic function in elite athletes with physiologic cardiac hypertrophy. *Journal of the American College of Cardiology* 6: 545-549.

Colduck, C.T., and Abernathy, P.J. 1997. Changes and surface EMG of biceps brachii with increasing velocity of eccentric contraction in women. *Journal of Strength and Conditioning Research* 11: 50-56.

Coleman, A.E. 1977. Nautilus vs. Universal gym strength training in adult males. *American Corrective Therapy Journal* 31: 103-107.

Collett-Solberg, P.F., and Cohen, P. 1996. The role of the insulin-like growth factor binding proteins and the IGFBP proteases in modulating IGF action. *Endocrinology and Metabolism Clinics of North America* 25: 591-614.

Colliander, E.B., and Tesch, P. 1988. Blood pressure in resistance-trained athletes. *Canadian Journal of Sports Science* 13: 31-34.

Colliander, E.B., and Tesch, P.A. 1989. Bilateral eccentric and concentric torque of quadriceps and hamstring in females and males. *European Journal of Applied Physiology* 59: 227-232.

Colliander, E.B., and Tesch, P.A. 1990a. Effects of eccentric and concentric muscle actions in resistance training. *Acta Physiologica Scandinavica* 140: 31-39.

Colliander, E.B., and Tesch, P.A. 1990b. Responses to eccentric and concentric resistance training in females and males. *Acta Physiologica Scandinavica* 141: 149-156.

Comfort, P., Haigh, A., and Matthews, M.J. 2012. Are changes in maximal squat strength during preseason training reflected in changes in sprint performance in rugby athletes? *Journal of Strength and Conditioning* 26: 772-776.

Comyns, T.M., Harrison, A.J., Hennessy, L.K., and Jensen, R.L. 2006. The optimal complex training rest interval for athletes from anaerobic sports. *Journal of Strength and Conditioning Research* 20: 471-476.

Conale, S.T., and Belding, R.H. 1980. Osteochondral lesions of the talus. *Journal of Bone and Joint Surgery* 62A: 97-102.

Conley, M.S., Stone, M.H., Nimmons, M., and Dudley, G.A. 1997. Resistance training and human cervical muscle recruitment plasticity. *Journal of Applied Physiology* 83: 2105-2111.

Conroy, B., and Earle, R.W. 2000. Bone, muscle, and connective tissue adaptations to physical activity. In *Essentials of strength training and conditioning*, edited by T. Baechle and R.W. Earle, 2nd ed. Champaign, IL: Human Kinetics.

Conroy, B.P., Kraemer, W.J., Maresh, C.M., and Dalsky, G.P. 1992. Adaptive responses of bone to physical activity. *Medicine, Exercise, Nutrition, and Health* 1: 64-74.

Conroy, B.P., Kraemer, W.J., Maresh, C.M., Dalsky, G.P., Fleck, S.J., Stone, M.H., Miller, P., and Fry, A.C. 1993. Bone mineral density in elite junior weightlifters. *Medicine & Science in Sports & Exercise* 25: 1103-1109.

Consitt, L.A., Copeland, J.L., and Tremblay, M.S. 2001. Hormone responses to resistance vs. endurance exercise in premenopausal females. *Canadian Journal of Applied Physiology* 26: 574-587.

Constantini, N.W. 1994. Clinical consequences of athletic amenorrheic. *Sports Medicine* 17: 213-223.

Cook, G., Burton, L., and Hoogenboom, B. 2006. The use of fundamental movements as an assessment of function—part 1. *North American Journal of Physical Therapy* 1: 62-72.

Cook, G., Burton, L., and Hoogenboom, B. 2006. The use of fundamental movements as an assessment of function—part 2. *North American Journal of Physical Therapy* 1: 132-139.

Corder, K.P., Potteiger, J.A., Nau, K.L., Feigoni, S.E., and Hershberger, S.L. 2000. Effects of active and passive recovery conditions on blood lactate, rating of perceived exertion, and performance during resistance exercise. *Journal of Strength and Conditioning Research* 14: 151-156.

Cordova, M.L., Ingersoll, C.D., Kovaleski, J.E., and Knight, K.L. 1995. A comparison of isokinetic and isotonic predictions of a functional task. *Journal of Athletic Training* 30: 319-322.

Cormie, P., Deane, R.S., Triplett, N.T., and McBride, J.M. 2006. Acute effects of whole-body vibration on muscle activity, strength, and power. *Journal of Strength and Conditioning Research* 20: 257-261.

Cormie, P., McGuigan, M.R., and Newton, R.U. 2010a. Influence of strength and magnitude and mechanisms of adaptation to power training. *Medicine & Science in Sports & Exercise* 42: 1566-1581.

Cormie, P., McGuigan, M.R., and Newton, R.U. 2010b. Adaptations in athletic performance after ballistic power versus strength training. *Medicine & Science in Sports & Exercise* 42: 1582-1598.

Cornelissen, V.A., and Fagard, R.H. 2005. Effect of resistance training on resting blood pressure: A meta-analysis of randomized controlled trials. *Journal of Hypertension* 23: 251-259.

Cornu, C., Almeida Silveira, M.I., and Goubel, F. 1997. Influence of plyometric training on the mechanical impedance of the human ankle joint. *European Journal of Applied Physiology* 76: 282-288.

Costill, D.L., Coyle, E.F., Fink, W.F., Lesmes, G.R., and Witzmann, F.A. 1979. Adaptations in skeletal muscle following strength training. *Journal of Applied Physiology: Respiratory, Environmental and Exercise Physiology* 46: 96-99.

Cote, C., Simoneau, J.A., Lagasse, P., Boulay, M., Thibault, M.C., Marcotte, M., and Bouchard, C. 1988. Isokinetic strength training protocols: Do they induce skeletal muscle fiber hypertrophy? *Archives of Physical Medicine and Rehabilitation* 69: 281-285.

Coutts, A.J., Murphy, A.J., and Dascombe, B.J. 2004. Effect of direct supervision of a strength coach on measures of muscular strength and power in young rugby league players. *Journal of Strength and Conditioning Research* 18: 316-323.

Coviello, A.D., Zhuang, W.V., Lunetta, K.L., Bhasin, S., Ulloor, J., Zhang, A., Karasik, D., Kiel, D.P., Vasan, R.S., and Murabito, J.M. 2011. Circulating testosterone and SHBG concentrations are heritable in women: The Framingham Heart Study. *Journal of Clinical Endocrinology and Metabolism* 96: E1491-1495.

Coyle, E.F., Feiring, D.C., Rotkis, T.C., Cote, R.W., Roby, F.B., Lee, W., and Wilmore, J.H. 1981. Specificity of power improvements through slow and fast isokinetic training. *Journal of Applied Physiology* 51: 1437-1442.

Craig, B.W., and Kang, H. 1994. Growth hormone release following single versus multiple sets of back squats: Total work versus power. *Journal of Strength and Conditioning Research* 8: 270-275.

Cramer, J.T., Housh, T.J., Coburn, J.W., Beck, T.W., and Johnson, G.O. 2006. Acute effects of static stretching on maximal eccentric torque production in women. *Journal of Strength and Conditioning Research* 20: 354-358

Cramer, J.T., Stout, J.R., Culbertson, J.Y., and Egan, A.D. 2007. Effects of creatine supplementation and three days of resistance training on muscle strength, power output, and neuromuscular function. *Journal of Strength and Conditioning Research* 21: 668-677.

Cressey, E.M., West, C.A., Tiberio, D.P., Kraemer, W.J., and Maresh, C.M. 2007. The effects of ten weeks of lower-body unstable surface training on markers of athletic performance. *Journal of Strength and Conditioning Research* 21: 561-567.

Crewther, B.T., and Christian, C. 2010. Relationships between salivary testosterone and cortisol concentrations and training performance in Olympic weightlifters. *Journal of Sports Medicine and Physical Fitness* 50: 371-375.

Crewther, B.T., Cook, C., Cardinale, M., Weatherby, R.P, and Lowe, T. 2011 Two emerging concepts for elite athletes: The short-term effects of testosterone and cortisol on the neuromuscular system and the dose-response training role of these endogenous hormones *Sports Medicine* 41: 103-123.

Crewther, B., Cronin, J., and Keogh, J. 2005. Possible stimuli for strength and power adaptation acute mechanical responses. *Sports Medicine* 35: 967-989.

Crist, D.M., Peake, G.T., Egan, P.A., and Waters, D.L. 1988. Body composition responses to exogenous GH during training in highly conditioned adults. *Journal of Applied Physiology* 65: 579-584.

Cronin, J., and Sleivert, G. 2005. Challenges in understanding the influence of maximal power training on improving athletic performance. *Sports Medicine* 35: 213-234.

Crowley, M.A., and Matt, K.S. 1996. Hormonal regulation of skeletal muscle hypertrophy in rats: The testosterone to cortisol ratio. *European Journal of Applied Physiology* 73: 66-72.

Cumming, D.C., Wall, S.R., Galbraith, M.A., and Belcastro, A.N. 1987 Reproductive hormone responses to resistance exercise. *Medicine and Science in Sports and Exercise* 19:234-238.

Cuneo, R.C., Salomon, F., Wiles, C.M., Hesp, R., and Sonksen, P.H. 1991. Growth hormone treatment in growth hormone-deficient adults. I. Effects on muscle mass and strength. *Journal of Applied Physiology* 70: 688-694.

Cureton, K.J., Collins, M.A., Hill, D.W., and McElhannon, F.M. 1988. Muscle hypertrophy in men and women. *Medicine & Science in Sports & Exercise* 20: 338-344.

Cussler, E.C., Lohman, T.G., Going, S.B., Houtkooper, L.B., Metcalfe, L.L., Flint-Wagner, H.G., Harris, R.B., and Teixeira, P.J. 2003. Weight lifted in strength training predicts bone change in postmenopausal women. *Medicine & Science in Sports & Exercise* 35: 10-17.

Dale, E., Gerlach, D., and Wilhite, A. 1979. Menstrual dysfunction in distance runners. *Obstetrics and Gynecology* 54: 47-53.

Dalsky, G.P., Stocke, K.S., Ehasani, A.A., Slatpolsky, E., Lee, W.C., and Birge, S. 1988. Weight-bearing exercise training and lumbar bone mineral content in post menopausal female. *Annuals of Internal Medicine* 108: 824-828.

Dalton, S.E. 1992. Overuse injuries and adolescent athletes. *Sports Medicine* 13: 58-70.

D'Andrea, A., Cocchia, R., Riegler, L., Scarafile, R., Salerno, G., Gravino, R., Golia, E., Pezzullo, E., Citro, R., Limongelli, G., Pacilco, G., Cuomo, S., Caso, P., Giovana, M., Bossone, E., and Calabrò, R. 2010. Left ventricular myocardial velocities and deformation indexes in top-level athletes. *Journal of the American Society of Echocardiography* 23: 1281-1288.

D'Andrea, A., Riegler, L., Cocchia, R., Scarafile, R., Salerno, G., Gravino, R., Golia, E., Vriz, O., Citro, R., Limongelli, G., Calabro, P., Di Salvo, G., Caso, P., Russo, M.G., Bossone, E., and Calabro, R.. 2010. Left atrial volume index in highly trained athletes. *American Heart Journal* 159: 1155-1161.

Dannelly, B.D., Othey, S.C., Croy, T., Harrison, B., Rynders, C.A., Hertel, J.N., and Weltman, A. 2011.

The effectiveness of traditional and sling exercise strength training in women. *Journal of Strength and Conditioning Research* 25: 464-471.

Danneskoild-Samsoe, B., Kofod, V., Munter, J., Grimby, G., and Schnohr, P. 1984. Muscle strength and functional capacity in 77-81-year-old men and women. *European Journal of Applied Physiology* 52: 123-135.

Darden, E. 1973. Weight training systems in the U.S.A. *Journal of Physical Education* 44: 72-80.

DaSilva-Grigoletto, M.E., Vaamonde, D.M., Castillo, E., Poblador, M.S., Gracia-Manso, J.M., and Lancho, J.L. 2009. Acute and cumulative effects of different times of recovery from whole body vibration exposure on muscle performance. *Journal of Strength and Conditioning Research* 23: 2073-2082.

Davies, A.H. 1977. Chronic effects of isokinetic and allokinetic training on muscle force, endurance, and muscular hypertrophy. *Dissertation Abstracts International* 38: 153A.

Davies, B.N., Greenwood, E.J., and Jones, S.R. 1988. Gender differences in the relationship of performance in the handgrip and standing long jump tests to lean limb volume in young adults. *European Journal of Applied Physiology* 58: 315-320.

Davies, C.T.M., and Young, K. 1983. Effects of training at 30 and 100% maximal isometric force on the contractile properties of the triceps surae of man. *Journal of Physiology* 36: 22-23.

Davies, J., Parker, D.F., Rutherford, O.M., and Jones, D.A. 1988. Changes in strength and cross sectional area of the elbow flexors as a result of isometric strength training. *European Journal of Applied Physiology* 57: 667-670.

Davis, W.J., Wood, D.T., Andrews, RG., Elkind, L.M., and Davis, W.B. 2008. Concurrent training enhances athletes' strength, muscle endurance, and other measures. *Journal of Strength and Conditioning Research* 22: 1487-1502.

Dawood, M.Y. 1983. Dysmenorrhea. *Clinical Obstetrics and Gynecology* 26: 719-727.

Dawson, B., Goodman, C., Lawrence, S., Preen, D., Polglaze, T., Fitzsimons, M., and Fourier, P. 1997. Muscle phosphocreatine repletion following single and repeated short sprint efforts. *Scandinavian Journal of Medicine & Science in Sports* 7: 206-213.

Deane, R.S., Chow, J.W., Tillman, M.D., and Fournier, K.A. 2005. Effects of hip flexor training on sprint, shuttle run, and vertical jump performance. *Journal of Strength and Conditioning Research* 19: 615-621.

DeBeliso, M., Harris, C., Spitzer-Gibson, T., and Adams, K.J. 2005. A comparison of periodized and fixed repetition training protocol on strength in older adults. *Journal of Science and Medicine in Sport* 8: 190-199.

Decoster, L.C., Cleland, J., Altieri, C., and Russell, P. 2005. The effects of hamstring stretching on range of motion: A systematic review of the literature. *Journal of Orthopedic and Sports Physical Therapy* 35: 377-387.

DeCree, C., Vermeulen, A., and Ostyn, M. 1991. Are high-performance young women athletes doomed to become low-performance old wives? A reconsideration of the increased risk of osteoporosis in amenorrheic women. *Journal of Sports Medicine and Physical Fitness* 31: 108-114.

DeKoning, F.L., Binkhorst, R.A., Vissers, A.C.A., and Vos, J.A. 1982. Influence of static strength training on the force-velocity relationship of the arm flexors. *International Journal of Sports Medicine* 3: 25-28.

Dela, F., and Kjaer, M. 2006. Resistance training, insulin sensitivity and muscle function in the elderly. *Essays in Biochemistry* 42: 75-88.

Deligiannis, A., Zahopoulou, E., and Mandroukas, K. 1988. Echocardiographic study of cardiac dimensions and function in weight lifters and body builders. *International Journal of Sports Cardiology* 5: 24-32.

Delecluse, C., Coppenolle, H.V., Willems, E., Van Leemputte, M., Diles, R., and Goris, M. 1995. Influence of high-resistance and high velocity training on sprint performance. *Medicine & Science in Sports & Exercise* 27: 1203-1209.

Delorme, T.L., Ferris, B.G., and Gallagher, J.R. 1952. Effect of progressive exercise on muscular contraction time. *Archives of Physical Medicine* 33: 86-97.

Delorme, T.L., and Watkins, A.L. 1948. Techniques of progressive resistance exercise. *Archives of Physical Medicine* 29: 263-273.

DeLuca, C.J., Lefever, R.S., McCue, M.P., and Xenakis, A.P. 1982. Behavior of human motor units in different muscles during linearly varying contractions. *Journal of Physiology* 329: 113-128.

DeMeyts, P., Wallach, B., Christoffersen, C.T., Ursø, B., Grønskov, K., Latus, L.J., Yakushiji, F., Ilondo, M.M., and Shym-ko, R.M. 1994. The insulin-like growth factor-I receptor. *Hormone Research* 42: 152-169.

DeMichele, P.D., Pollock, M.L., Graves, J.E., Foster, D.N., Carpenter, D., Garzarella, L., Brehue, W., and Fulton, M. 1997. Isometric dorsal rotations strength: Effective training frequency on its development.

Archives of Physiology and Medical Rehabilitation 78: 64-69.

Deminice, R., Sicchieri, T., Mialich, M., Milani, F., Ovidio, P., and Jordao, A.A. 2011. Acute session of hypertrophy-resistance traditional interval training and circuit training. *Journal of Strength and Conditioning Research* 25: 798-804.

de Onis, M., Blössner, M., Borghi, E., Morris, R., and Frongillo, E.A. 2004. Methodology for estimating regional and global trends of child malnutrition. *International Journal of Epidemiology* 33: 1260-1270.

Depino, G.M., Webright, W.G., and Arnold, B.L. 2000. Duration of maintained hamstring flexibility after cessation of an acute static stretching protocol. *Journal of Athletic Training* 35: 56-59.

DeRenne, C., Hetzler, R.K., Buxton, B.P., and Ho, K.W. 1996. Effects of training frequency on strength maintenance in pubescent baseball players. *Journal of Strength and Conditioning Research* 10: 8-14.

de Salles, B.F., Maior, A.S., Polito, M., Alexander, J., Rhea, M., and Simão, R. 2010. Influence of rest interval lengths on hypotensive response after strength training sessions performed by older men. *Journal of Strength and Conditioning Research* 24: 3049-3054.

de Salles, B.F., Simão, R., Miranda, F., Novaes Jda, S., Lemos, A., and Willardson, J.M. 2009. Rest interval between sets in strength training. *Sports Medicine* 39: 765-777.

Deschenes, M.R., Judelson, D.A., Kraemer, W.J., Meskaitis, V.J., Volek, J.S., Nindl, B.C., Harman, F.S., and Deaver, D.R. 2000. Effects of resistance training on neuromuscular junction morphology. *Muscle Nerve* 10: 1576-1581.

Deschenes, M.R., Maresh, C.M., Armstrong, L.E., Covault, J., Kraemer, W.J., and Crivello J.F. 1994. Endurance and resistance exercise induce muscle fiber type specific responses in androgen binding capacity. *Journal of Steroid Biochemistry and Molecular Biology* 50: 175-179.

Deschenes, M.R., Maresh, C.M., Crivello, J.F., Armstrong, L.E., Kraemer, W.J., and Covault, J. 1993. The effects of exercise training of different intensities on neuromuscular junction morphology. *Journal of Neurocytology* 22: 603-615.

Deschenes, M.R., Roby, M.A., and Glass, E.K. 2011. Aging influences adaptations of the neuromuscular junction to endurance training. *Neuroscience* 190: 56-66.

Deschenes, M.R., Tenny, K., Eason, M.K., and Gordon, S.E. 2007. Moderate aging does not modulate mor-phological responsiveness of the neuromuscular system to chronic overload in Fischer 344 rats. *Neuroscience* 148: 970-977.

Desmedt, J.E. 1981. The size principle of motor-neuron recruitment in ballistic or ramp-voluntary contractions in man. In *Progress in clinical neuro-physiology*, vol. 9, *Motor unit types, recruitment and plasticity in health and disease*, edited by J.E. Desmedt, 250-304. Basel: Karger.

Desmedt, J.E., and Godaux, E. 1977. Ballistic contractions in man: Characteristic recruitment pattern of single motor units of the tibialis muscle. *Journal of Physiology* 264: 673-694.

DeSouza, M.J., Hontscharuk, R., Olmsted, M., Kerr, G., and Williams, N.I. 2007. Drive for thinness score is a proxy indicator of energy deficiency in exercising women. *Appetite* 48: 359-367.

DeSouza, M.J., and Metzger, D.A. 1991. Reproductive dysfunction in amenorrheic athletes and anorexia patients: A review. *Medicine & Science in Sports & Exercise* 23: 995-1007.

DeSouza, M.J., Miller, B.E., Loucks, A.B., Luciano, A.A., Pescatello, L.S., Campbell, C.G., and Lasley, B.L. 1998. High frequency of luteal phase deficiency and anovulation in recreational women runners: Blunted elevation in follicle-stimulating hormone observed during luteal-follicular transition. *Journal of Clinical Endocrinology and Metabolism* 83: 4220-4232.

De Ste Croix, M.B.A., Deighan, M.A., and Armstrong, N. 2003. Assessment and interpretation of isoki-netic muscle during growth and maturation. *Sports Medicine* 33: 727-743.

De Van, A.E., Anton, M.M., Cook, J.N., Neidre, D.B., Cortez-Cooper, M.Y., and Tanaka, H. 2005. Acute effects of resistance exercise on arterial compliance. *Journal of Applied Physiology* 98: 2287-2291.

Diallo, O., Dore, E., Duche, P., and Van Praagh, E. 2001. Effects of plyometric training followed by a reduced training programme on physical per-formance in prepubescent soccer players. *Journal of Sports Medicine and Physical Fitness* 41: 342-348.

Dickerman, R.D., Pertusi, R., and Smith, G.H. 2000. The upper range of lumbar spine bench bone min-eral density? An examination of the current world record holder in the squat lift. *International Journal of Sports Medicine* 21: 469-470.

Dickhuth, H.H., Simon, G., Kindermann, W., Wild-berg, A., and Keul, J. 1979. Echocardiographic stud-ies on athletes of various sport-types and non-ath-letic persons. *Zeitschrift für Kardiologie* 68: 449-453.

DiPrampero, P.E., and Margaria, R. 1978. Relationship between O_2 consumption, high energy phosphates and the kinetics of the O_2 debt in exercise. *Pflugers Archives* 304: 11-19.

DiStefano, L.J., Clark, M.A., and Padua, D.A. 2009. Evidence supporting balance training in healthy individuals: A systematic review. *Journal of Strength and Conditioning Research* 23: 2718- 2731.

DiStefano, L.J., Padua, D.A., Blackburn, J.T., Garrett, W.E., Guskiewicz, K.M., and Marshall, S.W. 2010. Integrated injury prevention program improves balance and vertical jump height and children. *Journal of Strength and Conditioning Research* 24: 332-342.

DiStefano, L.J., Padua, D.A., DiStefano, M.J., and Marshall, S.W. 2009. Influence of age, sex, technique, and exercise program on movement patterns after an anterior cruciate ligament injury prevention program in youth soccer players. *American Journal of Sports Medicine* 37: 495-505.

Dixon, P.G., Kraemer, W.J., Volek, J.S., Howard, R.L., Gomez, A.L., Comstock, B.A., Dunn-Lewis, C., Fragala, M.S., Hooper, D.R., Häkkinen, K., and Maresh, C.M. 2010. The impact of cold-water immersion on power production in the vertical jump and the benefits of a dynamic exercise warm-up. *Journal of Strength and Conditioning Research* 24: 3313-3317.

Doan, B.K., Newton, R.U., Marsit, J.L., Triplett-McBride, N.T., Kozaris, L.P., Fry, A.C., and Kraemer, W.J. 2002. The effects of increased eccentric loading on bench press. *Journal of Strength and Conditioning Research* 16: 9-13.

Docherty, D., Wenger, H.A., Collis, M.L., and Quinney, H.A. 1987. The effects of variable speed resistance training on strength development in prepubertal boys. *Journal of Human Movement Studies* 13: 377-382.

Dodd, D.J., and Alvar, B.A. 2007. Analysis of acute explosive training modalities to improve lower-body power in baseball players. *Journal of Strength and Conditioning Research* 21: 1177-1182.

Doherty, T.J., Vandervoort, A.A., Taylor, A.W., and Brown, W.F. 1993. Effects of motor unit losses on strength in older men and women. *Journal of Applied Physiology* 74: 868-874.

Dohm, G.L., Williams, R.T., Kasperek, G.J., and Van, R.J. 1982. Increased excretion of urea and N tan-methylhistidine by rats and humans after a bout of exercise. *Journal of Applied Physiology* 64: 350-353.

Donnelly, A.E., Clarkson, P.M., and Maughan, R.J. 1992. Exercise-induced muscle damage: Effects of light exercise on damaged muscle. *European Journal of Applied Physiology* 64: 350-353.

Doolittle, R.L., and Engebretsen, J. 1972. Performance variations during the menstrual cycle. *Journal of Sports Medicine and Physical Fitness* 12: 54-58.

Dornemann, T.M., McMurray, R.G., Renner, J.B., and Anderson, J.J.B. 1997. Effects of high-intensity resistance exercise on bone mineral density and muscle strength of 40 to 50-year-old women. *Journal of Sports Medicine and Physical Fitness* 37: 246-251.

Drinkwater, B.L. 1984. Women and exercise: Physiological aspects. In *Exercise and sport science reviews*, edited by R.L. Terjung, 21-52. Lexington, KY: MAL Callamore Press.

Drinkwater, B.L., Bruemmer, B., and Chestnut, C.H. III. 1990. Menstrual history as determinant of current bone density in young athletes. *Journal of the American Medical Association* 263: 545-548.

Drinkwater, E.J., Lawton, T.W., McKenna, M.J., Lindsell, R.P., Hunt, P.H., and Pyne, D.B. 2007. Increased number of forced repetitions does not enhance strength development with resistance training. *Journal of Strength and Conditioning Research* 21: 841-847.

Duchateau J., and Enoka, R.M. 2011. Human motor unit recordings: Origins and insight into the integrated motor system. *Brain Research* 1409: 42-61.

Duchateau, J., and Hainaut, K. 1984. Isometric and dynamic training: Differential effects on mechanical properties of a human muscle. *Journal of Applied Physiology* 56: 296-301.

Duchateau, J., Semmler, J.G., and Enoka, R.M. 2006. Training adaptations in the behavior of human motor units. *Journal of Applied Physiology* 101: 1766-1775.

Ducher, G., Turner, A.I., Kukuljan, S., Pantano, K.J., Carlson, J.L., Williams, N.I., and De Souza, M.J. 2011. Obstacles in the optimization of bone health outcomes in the female athlete triad. *Sports Medicine* 41: 587-607.

Dudley, G.A., and Djamil, R. 1985. Incompatibility of endurance and strength training modes of exercise. *Journal of Applied Physiology* 59: 1446-1451.

Dudley, G.A., and Fleck, S.J. 1987. Strength and endurance training: Are they mutually exclusive? *Sports Medicine* 4: 79-85.

Dudley, G.A., Harris, R.T., Duvoisin, M.R., Hather, B.M., and Buchanan, P. 1990. Effect of voluntary vs. artificial activation on the relationship of muscle torque to speed. *Journal of Applied Physiology* 69: 2215-2221.

Dudley, G.A., Tesch, P.A., Miller, B.J., and Buchannan, P. 1991. Importance of eccentric actions in performance adaptations to resistance training. *Aviation, Space, and Environmental Medicine* 62: 543-550.

Duehring, M.D., Feldmann, C.R., and Ebben, W.P. 2009. Strength and conditioning practices of United States high school strength and conditioning coaches. *Journal of Strength and Conditioning Research* 23: 2188-2203.

Duffey, M.J., and Challis, J.H. 2007. The key effects on bar kinematics during the benchpress. *Journal of Strength and Conditioning Research* 21: 556-560.

Earles, D.R., Judge, J.O., and Gunnarsson, O.T. 2001. Velocity training induces power-specific adaptations in highly functioning older adults. *Archives of Physical Medicine and Rehabilitation* 82: 872-878.

Ebbeling, C.B., and Clarkson, P.M. 1989. Exercise-induced muscle damage and adaptation. *Sports Medicine* 7: 207-234.

Ebbeling, C.B., and Clarkson, P.M. 1990. Muscle adaptation prior to recovery following eccentric exercise. *European Journal of Applied Physiology* 60: 26-31.

Ebben, W.P. 2006. A brief review of concurrent activation potentiation: Theoretical and practical constructs. *Journal of Strength and Conditioning Research* 20: 985-991.

Ebben, W.P., and Blackard, D.O. 2001. Strength and conditioning practices of national football league strength and conditioning coaches. *Journal of Strength and Conditioning Research* 15: 48-58.

Ebben, W.P., Feldman, C.R., VanderZanden, T.L., Fauth, M.L., and Petushek, E.J. 2010. Periodized plyometric training is effective for women, and performance is not influenced by the length of post-training recovery. *Journal of Strength and Conditioning Research* 24: 1-7.

Ebben, W.P., Hintz, M.J., and Simenz, C.J. 2005. Strength and conditioning practices of major league baseball strength and conditioning coaches. *Journal of Strength and Conditioning Research* 19: 538-546.

Ebben, W.P., and Jensen, R.L. 2002. Electromyographic and kinetic analysis of traditional, chain, and elastic band squats. *Journal of Strength and Conditioning Research* 16: 547-550.

Ebben, W.P., Kindler, A.G., Chirdon, K.A., Jenkins, N.C., Polichnowski, A.J., and Ng, A.V. 2004. The effect of high-low vs high-repetition training on endurance performance. *Journal of Strength and Conditioning Research* 18: 513-517.

Edgerton, V.R. 1978. Mammalian muscle fiber types and their adaptability. *American Physiology* 60: 26-31.

Edwards, R.H.T., Hill, D.K., and McDonnell, M.N. 1972. Monothermal and intramuscular pressure measurements during isometric contractions of the human quadriceps muscle. *Journal of Physiology* 224: 58-59.

Effron, M.B. 1989. Effects of resistance training on left ventricular function. *Medicine & Science in Sports & Exercise* 21: 694-697.

Egan, A.D., Cramer, J.T., Massey, L.L., and Marek, S.M. 2006. Acute effects of static stretching on peak torque and mean power output in National Collegiate Athletic Association Division I women's basketball players. *Journal of Strength and Conditioning Research.* 20: 778-782.

Egan, E., Reilly, T., Giacomoni, M., Redmond, L., and Turner, C. 2006. Bone mineral density among female sports participants. *Bone* 38: 227-233.

Ellenbecker, T.S., Davies, G.J., and Rowinski, M.J. 1988. Concentric versus eccentric isokinetic strengthening of the rotator cuff. *The American Journal of Sports Medicine* 16: 64-69.

Ellias, B.A., Berg, K.E., Latin, R.W., Mellion, M.B., and Hofschire, P.J. 1991. Cardiac structure and function in weight trainers, runners, and runner/weight trainers. *Research Quarterly for Exercise and Sport* 62: 326-332.

Elliot, B.C., Wilson, G.J., and Kerr, G.K. 1989. A biomechanical analysis of the sticking region in the bench press. *Medicine & Science in Sports & Exercise* 21: 450-462.

Elliot, D.L., and Goldberg, L. 1983. Weight lifting and amenorrhea. *Journal of the American Medical Association* 249: 354.

Elliott, K.J., Sale, C., and Cable, N.T. 2002. Effects of resistance training and detraining on muscle strength and blood lipid profiles in postmenopausal women. *British Journal of Sport Medicine* 36: 340-345.

Eloranta, V., and Komi, P.V. 1980. Function of the quadriceps femoris muscle under maximal concentric and eccentric contraction. *EMG and Clinical Neurophysiology* 20: 159-174.

Emeterio, C.A., Antuñano, N.P., López-Sobaler, A.M., and González-Badillo, J.J. 2011. Effect of strength training and the practice of alpine skiing on bone mass density, growth, body composition, and the strength and power of the legs of adolescent skiers. *Journal of Strength and Conditioning Research* 25: 2879-2890.

Enea, C., Boisseau, N., Ottavy, M., Mulliez, J., Millet, C., Ingrand, I., Diaz, V., and Dugué, B. 2009. Effects of menstrual cycle, oral contraception, and training on exercise-induced changes in circulating DHEA-sulphate and testosterone in young women. *European Journal of Applied Physiology* 106: 365-373.

Engels, H.J., Drouin, J., Zhu, W., and Kazmierski, J.F. 1998. Effects of low-impact, moderate-intensity exercise training with and without wrist weights on functional capacities and mood states in older adults. *Gerontology* 44: 239-244.

Epley, B. 1985. *Dynamic strength training for athletes.* Lincoln, NE: William C. Brown.

Erskine, R.M., Jones, D.A., Maffulli, N., Williams, A.G., Stewart, C.E., and Degens, H. 2011. What causes in vivo muscle specific tension to increase following resistance training? *Experimental Physiology* 96: 145-155.

Erskine, R.M., Jones, D.A., Williams, A.G., Stewart, C.E., and Degens, H. 2010. Resistance training increases in vivo quadriceps femoris muscle specific tension in young men. *Acta Physiologica* (Oxford) 199: 83-89.

Escamilla, R.F., Fleisig, G.S., Zheng, N., Lander, J.E., Barrentine, S.W., Andrews, J.R., Bergemann, B.W., and Moorman, C.T. III. 2001. Effects of technique variations on knee biomechanics during the squat and leg press. *Medicine & Science in Sports & Exercise* 33: 1552-1566.

Esformes, J.I., Keenan, M., Moody, J., and Bampouras, T.M. 2011. Effect of different types of conditioning contraction on upper body post-activation potentiation. *Journal of Strength and Conditioning Research* 25: 143-148.

Esmarck, B., Andersen, J.L., Olsen, S., Richter, E.A., Mizuno, M., and Kjaer, M. 2001. Timing of postexercise protein intake is important for muscle hypertrophy with resistance exercise in elderly humans. *Journal of Physiology* 535: 301-311.

Essen, B., Jansson, E., Henriksson, J., Taylor, A.W., and Saltin, B. 1975. Metabolic characteristics of fiber types in human skeletal muscle. *Acta Physiologica Scandinavica* 95: 153-165.

Evans, W.J. 2004. Protein nutrition, exercise and aging. *Journal of the American College of Nutrition* 23: 601S-609S.

Evans, W.J., and Campbell, W.W. 1993. Sarcopenia and age-related changes in body composition and functional capacity. In: Symposium: Aging and body composition: Technological advances and physiological interrelationships. *Journal of Nutrition* 123: 465-468.

Ewing, J.L., Wolfe, D.R., Rogers, M.A., Amundson, M.L., and Stull, G.A. 1990. Effects of velocity of isokinetic training on strength, power, and quadriceps muscle fibre characteristics. *European Journal of Applied Physiology* 61: 159-162.

Exner, G.U., Staudte, H.W., and Pette, D. 1973. Isometric training of rats: Effects upon fats and slow muscle and modification by an anabolic hormone in female rats. *Pflugers Archives* 345: 1-4.

Fagard, R. 2006. Exercise is good for your blood pressure: Effects of endurance training in resistance training. *Clinical and Experimental Pharmacology and Physiology* 33: 853-856.

Fagard, R.H. 1996. Athlete's heart: A meta-analysis of the echocardiographic experience. *International Journal of Sports Medicine* 17 Suppl 3:S140-S144.

Fahey, T.D., Akka, L., and Rolph, R. 1975. Body composition and $\dot{V}O_2$ max of exceptional weight trained athletes. *Journal of Applied Physiology* 39: 559-561.

Fahey, T.D., and Brown, H. 1973. The effects of an anabolic steroid on the strength, body composition, and endurance of college males when accompanied by a weight training program. *Medicine and Science in Sports* 5: 272-276.

Fahey, T.D., Rolph, R., Moungmee, P., Nagel, J., and Mortara, S. 1976. Serum testosterone, body composition and strength of young adults. *Medicine and Science in Sports* 8: 31-34.

Faigenbaum, A.D., Larosa Loud, R., O'Connell, J., Glover, S., O'Connell, J., and Westscott, W.L. 2001. Effects of different resistance training protocols on upper-body strength and endurance development in children. *Journal of Strength and Conditioning Research* 15: 459-465.

Faigenbaum, A.D., McFarland, J.E., Buchanan, E., Ratamess, N.A., Kang, J., and Hoffman, J.R. 2010. After-school fitness performance is not altered after physical education lessons in adolescent athletes. *Journal of Strength and Conditioning Research* 24: 765-770.

Faigenbaum, A.D., McFarland, J.E., Johnson, L., Kang, J., Bloom, J., Ratamess, N.A., and Hoffman, J.R. 2007. Preliminary evaluation of an after school resistance training program for improving physical fitness in middle school age boys. *Perceptual Motor Skills* 104: 407-415.

Faigenbaum, A.D., Milliken, L.A., Loud, R.L., Burak, B.T., Doherty, C.L., and Westcott, W.L. 2002. Comparison of 1 and 2 days per week of strength training in children. *Research Quarterly for Exercise and Sport* 73: 416-424.

Faigenbaum, A.D., Skrinar, G.S., Cesare, W.F., Kraemer, W.J., and Thomas, H.E. 1990. Physiologic and symptomatic responses of cardiac patients to resistance exercise. *Archives of Physical Medicine and Rehabilitation* 71: 395-398.

Faigenbaum, A.D., Westcott, W.L., La-Rosa Loud, R., and Long, C. 1999. The effects of different resistance training protocols on muscular strength and endurance development in children. *Pediatrics* 104: 1-7.

Faigenbaum, A.D., Westcott, W.L., Micheli, L.J., Outerbridge, A.R., Long, C.J., La-Rosa Loud, R., and Zaichkowsky, L.D. 1996. The effects of strength training and detraining on children. *Journal of Strength and Conditioning Research* 10: 109-114.

Faigenbaum, A.D., Zaichkowsky, L., Westcott, W., Micheli, L., and Fehandt, A. 1993. The effects of a twice per week strength training program on children. *Pediatrics Exercise Science* 5: 339-346.

Faigenbaum, M.S., and Pollock, M.L. 1997. Strength training: Rationale for current guidelines for adult fitness programs. *Physician and Sportsmedicine* 25: 44-64.

Falk, B., and Mor, G. 1996. The effects of resistance and martial arts training in total 6- to 8-year-old boys. *Pediatrics Exercise Science* 8: 48-56.

Falk, B., and Tenenbaum, G. 1996. The effectiveness of resistance training in children: A meta-analysis. *Sports Medicine* 22: 176-186.

Falkel, J.E., Fleck, S.J., and Murray, T.F. 1992. Comparison of central hemodynamics between powerlifters and body builders during exercise. *Journal of Applied Sport Science Research* 6: 24-35.

Fano, G., Mecocci, P., Vecchiet, J., Belia, S., Fulle, S., Polidori, M.C., Felzani, G., Senin, U., Vecchiet, L., and Beal, M.F. 2001. Age and sex influence on oxidative damage and functional status in human skeletal muscle. *Journal of Muscle Research Cell Motility* 22: 345-351.

Fardy, P.S., Maresh, C.M., Abbott, R., and Kristiansen, T. 1976. An assessment of the influence of habitual physical activity, prior sport participation, smoking habits and aging upon indices of cardiovascular fitness: Preliminary report of a cross-section and retrospective study. *Journal of Sports Medicine and Physical Fitness* 16: 77-90.

Farley, C.T., Blickhan, R., Saito, J., and Taylor, C.R. 1991. Hopping frequency in humans: A test of how springs set stride frequency in bouncing gaits. *Journal of Applied Physiology* 71: 2127-2132.

Farrell, P.A., Hernandez, J.M., Fedele, M.J., Vary, T.C., Kimball, S.R., and Jefferson, L.S. 2000. Eukaryotic initiation factors and protein synthesis after resistance exercise in rats. *Journal of Applied Physiology* 88: 1036-1042.

Farthing, J.P., and Chilibeck, P.D. 2003. The effects of eccentric and concentric training at different velocities on muscle hypertrophy. *European Journal of Applied Physiology* 89: 578-586.

Fath, F., Blazevich, A.J., Waugh, C.M., Miller, S.C., and Korff, T. 2010. Direct comparison of in vivo Achilles tendon moment arms obtained from ultrasound and MR scans. *Journal of Applied Physiology* 109: 1644-1652.

Fatouros, I.G., Jamurtas, A.Z., Leontsini, D., Taxildaris, K., Kostopoulos, N., and Buckenmeyer, P. 2000. Evaluation of plyometric exercise training, weight training, and their combination on vertical jump in performance and leg strength. *Journal of Strength and Conditioning Research* 14: 470-476.

Fatouros, I.G., Kambas, A., Katrabasas, I., Leontsini, D., Chatzinikolaou, A., Jamurta, A.Z., Douroudos, I., Aggelousis, N., and Taxildaris, K. 2006. Resistance training and detraining effects on flexibility performance in the elderly are intensity-dependent. *Journal of Strength and Conditioning Research* 20: 634-642.

Fatouros, I.G., Taxildaris, K., Tokmakidis, S.P., Kalapotharakos, V., Aggelousis, N., Athanasopoulos, S., Zeeris, I., and Katrabasas, I. 2002. The effects of strength training, cardiovascular training and their combination on flexibility of inactive older adults. *International Journal of Sports Medicine* 23: 112-119.

Faulkner, J.A., Davis, C.S., Mendias, C.L., and Brooks, S.V. 2008. The aging of elite male athletes: Age-related changes in performance and skeletal muscle structure and function. *Clinical Journal of Sport Medicine* 18: 501-507.

Felici, F., Rosponi, A., Sbriccoli, P., Filligoi, G.C., Fattorini, L., and Marchetti, M. 2001. Linear and non-linear analysis of surface electromyograms in weightlifters. *European Journal of Applied Physiology* 84: 337-342.

Fernandez-Rio, J., Terrados, N., Fernandez-Garcia, B., and Suman, O.E. 2010. Effects of vibration training on force production in female basketball players. *Journal of Strength and Conditioning Research* 24: 1373-1380.

Fiatarone, M.A., and Evans, W.J. 1993. The etiology and reversibility of muscle function in the aged. *Journal of Gerontology* 48: 77-83.

Fiatarone, M.A., Marks, E.C., Ryan, N.D., Meredith, C.N., Lipsitz, L.A., and Evans, W.J. 1990. High-intensity strength training in nonagenarians. Effects on skeletal muscle. *Journal of the American Medical Association* 263: 3029-3034.

Fiatarone, M.A., O'Neill, E.F., Ryan, N.D., Clements, K.M., Solares, G.R., Nelson, M.E., Roberts, S.B., Kehayias, J.J., Lipsitz, L.A., and Evans, W.J. 1994. Exercise training and nutritional supplementation for physical frailty in very elderly people. *The New England Journal of Medicine* 330: 1769-1775.

Finkelstein, E.A., Brown, D.S., Wrage, L.A., Allaire, B.T., and Thomas, J.H. 2010. Individual and aggregate years-of-life-lost associated with overweight and obesity. *Obesity* 18: 333-339.

Finni, T. 2006. Structural and functional features of human muscle-tendon unit. *Scandinavian Journal of Medicine & Science in Sports* 16: 147-158.

Finni, T., Ikegawa, S., and Komi, P.V. 2001. Concentric force enhancement during human movement. *Acta Physiologica Scandinavica* 173: 369-377.

Finnie, S.B., Wheeldon, T.J., Hensrud, D.D., Dahm, D.L., and Smith, J. 2003. Weight lifting belt use patterns among a population of health club members. *Journal of Strength and Conditioning Research* 17: 498-502.

Fitts, R. 1996. Cellular, molecular, and metabolic basis of muscle fatigue. In *Handbook of physiology exercise: Regulation and integration of multiple systems,* 1151-1183. Besthesda, MD: American Physiological Society.

Fleck, S.J. 1983. Bridging the gap: Interval training physiological basis. *NSCA Journal* 5: 40, 57-62.

Fleck, S.J. 1988. Cardiovascular adaptations to resistance training. *Medicine & Science in Sports & Exercise* 20: S146-S151.

Fleck, S.J. 1998. *Successful long-term weight training.* Chicago: NTP/Contemporary Publishing Group.

Fleck, S.J. 1999. Periodized strength training: A critical review. *Journal of Strength and Conditioning Research* 13: 82-89.

Fleck, S.J. 2002. Cardiovascular responses to strength training. In *Strength and power in sport,* edited by P.V. Komi, 387-406. Oxford: Blackwell Science.

Fleck, S.J., Bartels, R., Fox, E.L., and Kraemer, W. 1982. Isokinetic total work increases and peak force training cut-off points. *National Strength and Conditioning Association Journal* 4 (2): 20-21.

Fleck, S.J., Bennett, J.B. III, Kraemer, W.J., and Baechle, T.R. 1989. Left ventricular hypertrophy in highly strength trained males. *Sports Cardiology 2nd International Conference Volume Two,* pp. 303-311.

Fleck, S.J., and Dean, L.S. 1987. Previous resistance-training experience and the pressor response during resistance exercise. *Journal of Applied Physiology* 63: 116-120.

Fleck, S.J., Henke, C., and Wilson, W. 1989. Cardiac MRI of elite junior Olympic weight lifters. *International Journal of Sports Medicine* 10: 329-333.

Fleck, S.J., and Kontor, K. 1986. Complex training. *National Strength and Conditioning Association Journal* 8: 66-69.

Fleck, S.J., Mattie, C., and Martensen H.C. III. 2006. Effect of resistance and aerobic training on regional body composition in previously recreationally trained middle-aged women. *Applied Physiology, Nutrition and Metabolism* 31: 261-270.

Fleck, S.J., and Schutt, R.C. 1985. Types of strength training. *Clinics in Sports Medicine* 4: 159-169.

Fling, B.W., Knight, C.A., and Kamen, G. 2009. Relationships between motor unit size and recruitment threshold in older adults: Implications for size principle. *Experimental Brain Research,* 197: 125-133.

Florini, J.R. 1987. Hormonal control of muscle growth. *Muscle and Nerve* 10: 577-598.

Florini, J.R., Ewton, D.Z., and Coolican, S.A. 1996. Growth hormone and the insulin-like growth factor system in myogenesis. *Endocrine Reviews* 17: 481-517.

Florini, J.R., Samuel, D.S., Ewton, D.Z., Kirk, C., and Sklar, R.M. 1996. Stimulation of myogenic differentiation by a neuregulin, glial growth factor 2. Are neuregulins the long-sought muscle trophic factors secreted by nerves? Journal of Biological Chemistry 27: 12699-12702.

Focht, B.C., and Koltyn, K.F. 1998. Influence of resistance exercise of different intensities on state anxiety and blood pressure. *Medicine & Science in Sports & Exercise* 31: 456-463.

Fogelholm, M., Kaprio, J., and Sarna, S. 1994. Healthy lifestyles of former Finnish world class athletes.

Medicine & Science in Sports & Exercise 26: 224-229.

Folland, J.P., Hawker, K., Leach, B., Little, T., and Jones, D.A. 2005. Strength training: Isometric training at a range of joint angles versus dynamic training. *Journal Sports Science* 23: 817-824.

Folland, J., and Morris, B. 2008. Variable-cam resistance training machines: Do they match the angle-torque relationship in humans? *Journal of Sports Science* 26: 163-169.

Folland, J.P., and Williams, A.G. 2007. The adaptations to strength training: Morphological and neurological contributions to increased strength *Sports Medicine* 37: 145-168.

Ford, H.T., Puckett, J.R., Drummond, J.P., Sawyer, K., Gantt, K., and Fussell, C. 1983. Effects of three combinations of plyometric and weight training programs on selected physical fitness test items. *Perceptual and Motor Skills* 56: 919-922.

Foschini, D., Araujo, R.C., Bacurau, R.F.B., De Piano, A., De Almeida, S.S., Carnier, J., Rosa, T.D.S., Tufik, S., and Damaso, A.R. 2010. Treatment of obese adolescents: The influence of periodization models and ace genotype. *Obesity* 18: 766-772.

Fowles, J.R., MacDougall, J.D., Tarnopolsky, M.A., Sale, D.G., Roy, B.D., and Yarasheski, K.E. 2000. The effects of acute passive stretch on muscle protein synthesis in humans. *Canadian Journal of Applied Physiology* 25: 165-180.

Fox, E.L. 1979. *Sports physiology*. Philadelphia: Saunders.

Fradkin, A.J., Zazryn, T.R., and Smoliga, J.M. 2010. Effects of warming-up on physical performance: A systematic review with meta-analysis. *Journal of Strength and Conditioning Research* 24: 140-148.

Fragala, M.S., Clark, M.H., Walsh, S.J., Kleppinger, A., Judge, J.O., Kuchel, G.A., and Kenny, A.M. 2012. Gender differences in anthropometric predictors of physical performance in older adults. *Gender Medicine* 9: 445-56.

Fragala, M.S., Kraemer, W.J., Denegar, C.R., Maresh, C.M., Mastro, A.M., and Volek, J.S. 2011a. Neuro-endocrine-immune interactions and responses to exercise. *Sports Medicine* 41: 621-639.

Fragala, M.S., Kraemer, W.J., Mastro, A.M., Denegar, C.R., Volek, J.S., Häkkinen, K., Anderson, J.M., Lee, E.C., and Maresh, C.M. 2011b. Leukocyte β2-adrenergic receptor expression in response to resistance exercise. *Medicine & Science in Sports & Exercise* 43: 1422-1432.

Fragala, M.S., Kraemer, W.J., Mastro, A.M., Denegar, C.R., Volek, J.S., Kupchak, B.R., Häkkinen, K., Anderson, J.M., and Maresh, C.M. 2011c. Glucocorticoid receptor expression on human B cells in response to acute heavy resistance exercise. *Neuroimmunomodulation* 18: 156-164.

Freedson, P.S., Micheuic, P.M., Loucks, A.B., and Birandola, R.M. 1983. Physique, body composition, and psychological characteristics of competitive female body builders. *Physician and Sportsmedicine* 11: 85-93.

Frisard, M.I., Broussard, A., Davies, S.S., Roberts, L.J., Rood, J., de Jonge, L., Fang, X., Jazwinski, S.M., Deutsch, W.A., and Ravussin, E. 2007. Aging, resting metabolic rate, and oxidative damage: Results from the Louisiana Healthy Aging Study. *Journals of Gerontology Series A: Biological Sciences and Medical Sciences* 62: 752-759.

Frisch, R.E., and McArthur, J.W. 1974. Menstrual cycles: Fatness as a determinant of minimum weight and height necessary for their onset. *Science* 185: 949-951.

Frontera, W.R., Hughes, V.A., Fielding, R.A., Fiatarone, M.A., Evans, W.J., and Roubenoff, R. 2000. Aging of skeletal muscle: A 12-yr longitudinal study. *Journal of Applied Physiology* 88: 1321-1326.

Frontera, W.R., Hughes, V.A., Lutz, K.J., and Evans, W.J. 1991. A cross-sectional study of muscle strength and mass in 45- to 78-year-old men and women. *Journal of Applied Physiology* 71: 644-650.

Frontera, W.R., Meredith, C.N., O'Reilly, K.P., Knuttgen, H.G., and Evans, W.J. 1988. Strength conditioning in older men: Skeletal muscle hypertrophy and improved function. *Journal of Applied Physiology* 64: 1038-1044.

Frontera, W.R., Suh, D., Krivickas, L.S., Hughes, V.A., Goldstein, R., and Roubenoff, R. 2000. Skeletal muscle fiber quality in older men and women. *American Journal Physiology Cell Physiology* 279: C611-C618.

Frost, H.M. 1997. Why do marathon runners have less bone than weight lifters? A vital-biomechanical view and explanation. *Bone* 20: 183-189.

Frost, R.A., and Lang, C.H. 1999. Differential effects of insulin-like growth factor I (IGF-I) and IGF-binding protein-1 on protein metabolism in human skeletal muscle cells. *Endocrinology* 140: 3962-3970.

Fry, A.C. 2004. The role of resistance exercise intensity on muscle fibre adaptations. *Sports Medicine* 34: 663-679.

Fry, A.C., Allemeier, C.A., and Staron, R.S. 1994. Correlation between percentage of fiber type area and myosin heavy chain content in human skeletal muscle. *European Journal of Applied Physiology and Occupational Physiology* 68: 246-251.

Fry, A.C., Ciroslan, D., Fry, M.D., LeRoux, C.D., Schilling, B.K., and Chiu, L.Z. 2006. Anthropometric and performance variables discriminating elite American junior men weightlifters. *Journal of Strength and Conditioning Research* 20: 861-866.

Fry, A.C., and Kraemer, W.J. 1991. Physical performance characteristics of American collegiate football players. *Journal of Applied Sport Science Research* 5: 126-138.

Fry, A.C., and Kraemer, W.J. 1997. Resistance exercise overtraining and overreaching. Neuroendocrine responses. *Sports Medicine* 23: 106-129.

Fry, A.C., Kraemer, W.J., Stone, M.H., Warren, B.J., Fleck, S.J., Kearney, J.T., and Gordon, S.E. 1994. Endocrine responses to overreaching before and after 1 year of weightlifting. *Canadian Journal of Applied Physiology* 19: 400-410.

Fry, A.C., Kraemer, W.J., Stone, M.J., Fleck, S.J., Kearney, J.T., Triplett, N.T., and Gordon, S.E. 1995. Acute endocrine responses with long-term weightlifting in a 51-year old male weightlifter. *Journal of Strength and Conditioning Research* 9: 193 (abstract).

Fry, A.C., Kraemer, W.J., van Borselen, F., Lynch, J.M., Marsit, J.L, Roy, E.P., Triplett, N.T., and Knuttgen, H.G. 1994. Performance decrements with high-intensity resistance exercise overtraining. *Medicine & Science in Sports & Exercise* 26: 1165-1173.

Fry, A.C., Stone, M.H., Thrush, J.T., and Fleck, S.J. 1995. Precompetition training sessions enhance competitive performance of high anxiety junior weightlifters. *Journal of Strength and Conditioning Research* 9: 37-42.

Fryburg, D.A. 1994. Insulin-like growth factor I exerts growth hormone- and insulin-like actions on human muscle protein metabolism. *American Journal of Physiology* 267: E331-E336.

Fryburg, D.A. 1996. NG-monomethyl-L-arginine inhibits the blood flow but not the insulin-like response of forearm muscle to IGF-I: Possible role of nitric oxide in muscle protein synthesis. *Journal of Clinical Investigation* 97: 1319-1328.

Fryburg, D.A., and Barrett, E.J. 1995. Insulin, growth hormone and IGF-I regulation of protein metabolism. *Diabetes Reviews* 3: 93-112.

Fryburg, D.A., Jahn, L.A., Hill, S.A., Oliveras, D.M., and Barrett, E.J. 1995. Insulin and insulin-like growth factor-I enhance human skeletal muscle protein anabolism during hyperaminoacidemia by different mechanisms. *Journal of Clinical Investigation* 96: 722-729.

Fukashiro, S., Hay, D.C., and Nagano, A. 2006. Biomechanical behavior of muscle-tendon complex during dynamic human movements. *Journal of Applied Biomechanics* 22: 131-147.

Fukunaga, T., Funato, K., and Ikegawa, S. 1992. The effects of resistance training on muscle area and strength in prepubescent age. *Annals of Physiology and Anthropology* 11: 357-364.

Fulco, C.S., Rock, P.B., Muza, S.R., Lammi, E., Cymerman, A., Butterfield, G., Moore, L.G., Braun, B., and Lewis, S.F. 1999. Slower fatigue and faster recovery of the adductor pollicis muscle in women matched for strength with men. Acta Physiologica Scandinavica 167: 233-239.

Gabbett, T.J., Johns, J., and Riemann, M. 2008. Performance changes following training in junior rugby league players. *Journal of Strength and Conditioning Research* 22: 910-917.

Gabell, A., Simons, M.A., and Nayak, U.S. 1985. Falls in the healthy elderly: Predisposing causes. *Ergonomics* 28: 965-975.

Gaja, B. 1965. The new revolutionary phase or sequence system of training. *Iron Man* 26: 14-17.

Gallagher, D., Belmonte, D., Deurenberg, P., Wang, Z., Krasnow, N., Pi-Sunyer, F.X., and Heymsfield, S.B. 1998. Organ-tissue mass measurement allows modeling of REE and metabolically active tissue mass. *American Journal of Physiology—Endocrinology and Metabolism* 275: E249-258.

Galvao, D.A., and Taaffe, D.R. 2005. Resistance exercise dosage in older adults: Single- versus multiset effects on physical performance and body composition. *Journal of American Geriatrics Society* 53: 2090-2097.

Garber, C.E., Blissmer, B., Deschenes, M.R., Franklin, B.A., Lamonte, M.J., Lee, I.M., Nieman, D.C., and Swain, D.P. 2011. Quantity and quality of exercise for developing and maintaining cardiorespiratory, musculoskeletal, and neuromotor fitness in apparently healthy adults: Guidance for prescribing exercise. *Medicine & Science in Sports & Exercise* 43: 1334-1359.

García-Pallarés, J., and Izquierdo, M. 2011. Strategies to optimize concurrent training of strength and aerobic fitness for rowing and canoeing. *Sports Medicine* 41: 329-343.

Gardner, G. 1963. Specificity of strength changes of the exercised and nonexercised limb following isometric training. *Research Quarterly* 34: 98-101.

Garfinkel, S., and Cafarelli, E. 1992. Relative changes in maximal force, EMG, and muscle cross-sectional area after isometric training. *Medicine & Science in Sports & Exercise* 24: 1220-1227.

Garhammer, J., and Takano, B. 1992. Training for weightlifting. *Strength and Power in Sports* 5: 357-381.

Gasier, H.G., Fluckey, J.D., Preivs, S.F., Wiggs, M.P., and Riechman, S.E. 2012. Acute resistance exercise augments integrative myofibrillar protein synthesis. *Metabolism* 61: 153-156.

Gehri, D.J., Ricard, M.D., Kleiner, D.M., and Kirkendall, D.T. 1998. A comparison of plyometric training techniques for improving vertical jump ability and energy production. *Journal of Strength and Conditioning Research* 12: 85-89.

Gellish, R.I., Goslin, B.R., Olson, R.E., McDonald, A., Russi, G.D., and Moudgil, V.K. 2007. Longitudinal modeling of the relationship between age and maximal heart rate. *Medicine & Science in Sports & Exercise* 39: 822-829.

Gentil, P., and Bottaro, M. 2010. Influence of supervision ratio on muscle adaptations to resistance training in nontrained subjects. *Journal of Strength and Conditioning Research* 24: 639-643.

George, K.P., Wolfe, L.A., Burggraf, G.W., and Norman, R. 1995. Electrocardiographic and echocardiographic characteristics of female athletes. *Medicine & Science in Sports & Exercise* 27: 1362-1370.

Gergley, J.C. 2009. Comparison of two lower-body modes of endurance training on lower-body strength development while concurrently training. *Journal of Strength and Conditioning Research* 23: 979-987.

Gettman, L.R., and Ayers, J.J. 1978. Aerobic changes through 10 weeks of slow and fast speed isokinetic training. *Medicine and Science in Sports* 10: 47.

Gettman, L.R., Ayres, J.J., Pollock, M.L., Durstine, J.C., and Grantham, W. 1979. Physiological effects on adult men of circuit strength training and jogging. *Archives of Physical Medicine and Rehabilitation* 60: 115-120.

Gettman, L.R., Ayres, J.J., Pollock, M.L., and Jackson, A. 1978. The effect of circuit weight training on strength, cardiorespiratory function and body composition of adult men. *Medicine and Science in Sports* 10: 171-176.

Gettman, L.R., Culter, L.A., and Strathman, T. 1980. Physiological changes after 20 weeks of isotonic vs. isokinetic circuit training. *Journal of Sports Medicine and Physical Fitness* 20: 265-274.

Gettman, L.R., and Pollock, M.L. 1981. Circuit weight training: A critical review of its physiological benefits. *The Physician and Sportsmedicine* 9: 44-60.

Ghigiarelli, J.J., Nagle, E.F., Gross, F.L., Robertson, R.J., Irrgang, J.J., and Myslinski, T. 2009. The effects of a 7-week heavy elastic band and weight chain program on upper-body strength and upper-body power and a sample of division 1-AA football players. *Journal of Strength and Conditioning Research* 23: 756-764.

Gibala, M.J., Interisano, S.A., Tarnopolsky, M.A., Roy, B.D., MacDonald, J.R., Yarasheski, K.E., and MacDougall, J.D. 2000. Myofibrillar disruption following acute concentric and eccentric resistance exercise in strength-trained men. *Canadian Journal of Physiology and Pharmacology* 78: 656-661.

Gillam, G.M. 1981. Effects of frequency of weight training on muscle strength enhancement. *Journal of Sports Medicine* 21: 432-436.

Gillies, E.M., Putman, C.T., and Bell, G.J. 2006. The effect of varying the time of concentric and eccentric muscle actions during resistance training on skeletal muscle adaptations in women. *European Journal of Applied Physiology* 97: 443-453.

Giorgi, A., Wilson, G.J., Weatherby, R.P., and Murphy, A. 1998. Functional isometric weight training: Its effects on the development of muscular function and the endocrine system over an 8-week training period. *Journal of Strength and Conditioning Research* 12: 18-25.

Girouard, C.K., and Hurley, B.F. 1995. Does strength training inhibit gains in range of motion from flexibility training in older adults? *Medicine & Science in Sports & Exercise* 27: 1444-1449.

Gjøvaag, T.P., and Dahl, H.A. 2009. Effect of training and detraining with different mechanical loadings on MyHC and GLUT4 changes. *Medicine & Science in Sports & Exercise* 41: 129-136.

Gladden, L.B., and Colacino, D. 1978. Characteristics of volleyball players and success in a national tournament. *Journal of Sports Medicine and Physical Fitness* 18: 57-64.

Glowacki, S.P., Martin, S.E., Maurer, A., Baek, W., Green, J.S., and Crouse, S.F. 2004. Effects of resistance, endurance, and concurrent exercise on training outcomes in men. *Medicine & Science in Sports & Exercise* 36: 2119-2127.

Godard, M.P., Wygand, J.W., Carpinelli, R.N., Catalano, S., and Otto, R.M. 1998. Effects of accentuated eccentric resistance training on concentric knee extensor strength. *Journal of Strength and Conditioning Research* 12: 26-29.

Goldberg, L., Elliot, D.L., and Kuehl, K.S. 1994. A comparison of the cardiovascular effects of running and weight training. *Journal of Strength and Conditioning Research* 8: 219-224.

Goldberg, L., Elliot, D.L., and Kuehl, K.S. 1988. Assessment of exercise intensity formulas by use of ventilatory threshold. *Chest* 94: 95-98.

Golden, C.L., and Dudley, G.A. 1992. Strength after bouts of eccentric or concentric actions. *Medicine & Science in Sports & Exercise* 24: 926-933.

Goldspink, G. 1992. Cellular and molecular aspects of adaptation in skeletal muscle. In *Strength and power in sport*, edited by P.V. Komi, 211-229. Oxford: Blackwell Scientific.

Goldspink, G. 1998. Cellular and molecular aspects of muscle growth, adaptation and aging. *Gerontology* 15: 35-43.

Goldspink, G. 1999. Changes in muscle mass and phenotype and the expression of autocrine and systemic growth factors by muscle in response to stretch and overload. *Journal of Anatomy* 194: 323-334.

Goldspink, G., Wessner, B., and Bachl, N. 2008. Growth factors, muscle function, and doping. *Current Opinions in Pharmacology* 8: 352-357.

Goldspink, G., and Yang, S.Y. 2001. Effects of activity on growth factor expression. *International Journal of Sport Nutrition and Exercise Metabolism* 11: S21-S27.

Gollhofer, A. 1987. Innervation characteristics of m. gastrocnemius during landing on different surfaces. In *Biomechanics X-B*, edited by B. Johnson, 701-706. Champaign, IL: Human Kinetics.

Gollnick, P.D., Timson, B.F., Moore, R.L., and Riedy, M. 1981. Muscular enlargement and number of fibers in skeletal muscles of rats. *Journal of Applied Physiology: Respiratory, Environmental and Exercise Physiology* 50: 936-943.

Gomides, R.S., Costa, L.A.R., Souza, D.R., Queiroz, A.C.C., Fernandes, J.R.C., Ortega, K.C., Junior, D.M.,

Tinucci, T., and Forjaz, C.L.M. 2010. Atenolol blunts blood pressure increase during dynamic resistance exercise in hypertensives. *British Journal of Clinical Pharmacology* 70: 664-673.

Gomides, R.S., Dias, R.M., Souza, D.R., Costa, L.A., Ortega, K.C., Mion, D., Jr., Tinucci, T., de Moraes, and Forjaz, C.L. 2010. Finger blood pressure during leg resistance exercise. *International Journal of Sports Medicine* 31: 590-595.

Gonyea, W.J. 1980. Role of exercise in inducing increases in skeletal muscle fiber number. *Journal of Applied Physiology: Respiratory, Environmental and Exercise Physiology* 48: 421-426.

Gonyea, W.J., and Sale, D. 1982. Physiology of weight-lifting exercise. *Archives of Physical Medicine and Rehabilitation* 63: 235-237.

Gonyea, W.J., Sale, D., Gonyea, F., and Mikesky, A. 1986. Exercise induced increases in muscle fiber number. *European Journal of Applied Physiology* 55: 137-141.

Gonzalez-Camarena, R., Carrasco-Sosa, S., Roman-Ramos, R., Gaitan-Gonzalez, M.J., Medina-Banuelos, V., and Azpiroz-Leehan, J. 2000. Effect of static and dynamic exercise on heart rate and blood pressure variabilities. *Medicine & Science in Sports & Exercise* 32: 1719-1728.

Goodman, C.A., Pearce, A.J., Nicholes, C.J., Gatt, B.M., and Fairweather, I.H. 2008. No difference in 1 RM strength and muscle activation during the barbell chest press on a stable and unstable surface. *Journal of Strength and Conditioning Research* 22: 288-294.

Goodpaster, B.H., Park, S.W., Harris, T.B., Kritchevsky, S.B., Nevitt, M., Schwartz, A.V., Simonsick, E.M., Tylavsky, F.A., Visser, M., and Newman, A.B. 2006. The loss of skeletal muscle strength, mass, and quality in older adults: The health, aging and body composition study. *Journal of Gerontology A Biological Science Medical Science* 61: 1059-64.

Gordon, S.E., Kraemer, W.J., and Pedro, J.G. 1991. Increased acid-base buffering capacity via dietary supplementation: Anaerobic exercise implications. *Journal of Applied Nutrition* 43: 40-48.

Gordon, S.E., Kraemer, W.J., Vos, N.H., Lynch, J.M., and Knuttgen, H.G. 1994. Effect of acid base balance on the growth hormone response to acute, high-intensity cycle exercise. *Journal of Applied Physiology* 76: 821-829.

Gordon, S.E., Lake, J.A., Westerkamp, C.M., and Thomson, D.M. 2008. Does AMP-activated protein kinase negatively mediate aged fast-twitch skeletal muscle mass? *Exercise and Sport Science Reviews* 36: 179-186.

Gotshalk, L.A., Loebel, C.C., Nindl, B.C., Putukian, M., Sebastianelli, W.J., Newton, R.U., Häkkinen, K., and Kraemer, W.J. 1997. Hormonal responses to multiset versus single-set heavy-resistance exercise protocols. *Canadian Journal of Applied Physiology* 22: 244-255.

Gotshall, R.W., Gootman, J., Byrnes, W.C., Fleck, S.J., and Volovich, T.C. 1999. Noninvasive characterization of the blood pressure response to the double-leg press exercise. *Journal of Exercise Physiology online* 2, www.css.edu/users/tboone2.

Granacher, U., Muehlbauer T., Zahner, L., Gollhofer, A., and Kressig, R. 2011. Comparison of traditional and recent approaches in the promotion of balance and strength in older adults. *Sports Medicine* 41: 377-400.

Grassi, B., Cerretelli, P., Narici, M.V., and Marconi, C. 1991. Peak anaerobic power in master athletes. *European Journal of Applied Physiology* 62: 394-399.

Gravelle, B.L. and Blessing, D.L. 2000. Physiological adaptation in women concurrently training for strength and endurance. *Journal of Strength and Conditioning Research* 14: 5-13.

Graves, J.E., and James, R.J. 1990. Concurrent augmented feedback and isometric force generation during familiar and unfamiliar muscle movements. *Research Quarterly for Exercise and Sport* 61: 75-79.

Graves, J.E., Pollock, M.L., Foster, D.N., Leggett, S.H., Carpenter, D.M., Vuoso, R., and Jones, A. 1990. Effects of training frequency and specificity on isometric lumbar extension strength. *Spine* 15: 504-509.

Graves, J.E., Pollock, M.L., Jones, A.E., Colvin, A.B., and Leggett, S.H. 1989. Specificity of limited range of motion variable resistance training. *Medicine & Science in Sports & Exercise* 21: 84-89.

Graves, J.E., Pollock, M.L., Leggett, S.H., Braith, R.W., Carpenter, D.M., and Bishop, L.E. 1988. Effect of reduced frequency on muscular strength. *International Journal of Sports Medicine* 9: 316-319.

Graves, J.E., Pollock, M.I., Leggett, S.H., Carpenter, D.M., Fix, C.R., and Fulton, M.N. 1992. Limited range-of-motion lumbar extension strength training. *Medicine & Science in Sports & Exercise* 24: 128-133.

Gray, D.P., and Dale, E. 1984. Variables associated with secondary amenorrhea in women runners. *Journal of Sports Sciences* 1: 55-67.

Green, H., Dahly, A., Shoemaker, K., Goreham, C., Bombardier, E., and Ball-Burnett, M. 1999. Serial effects of high-resistance and prolonged endurance training on Na+-K+ pump concentration and enzymatic activities in human vastus lateralis. *Acta Physiologica Scandinavica* 165: 177-184.

Green, H., Goreham, C., Ouyang, J., Ball-Burnett, M., and Ranney, D. 1998. Regulation of fiber size, oxidative potential, and capillarization in human muscle by resistance exercise. *American Journal of Physiology* 276: R591-R596.

Green, H., Grange, F., Chin, C., Goreham, C., and Ranney, D. 1998. Exercise-induced decreases in sarcoplasmic reticulum Ca2+-ATPase activity attenuated by high-resistance training. *Acta Physiologica Scandinavica* 164: 141-146.

Greenspan, F.S. 1994. The thyroid gland. In *Basic and clinical endocrinology,* edited by F.S. Greenspan, and J.D. Baxter, 4th ed., 160-226. Norwalk, CT: Appleton and Lange.

Griffin, J., Tooms, R., Vander Zwaag, R., Bertorini, T., and O'Toole, M. 1993. Eccentric muscle performance of elbow and knee muscle groups and untrained men and women. *Medicine & Science in Sports & Exercise* 25: 936-944.

Grimby, G., Bjorntorp, P., Fahlen, M., Hoskins, T.A., Hook, O., Oxhof, H., and Saltin, B. 1973. Metabolic effects of isometric training. *Scandinavian Journal of Chemical Laboratory Investigation* 31: 301-305.

Grimby, G., and Hannerz, J. 1977. Firing rate and recruitment order of toe extensor motor units in different modes of voluntary contraction. *Journal of Physiology (London)* 264: 867-879.

Grimby, G., Hannerz, J., and Hedman, B. 1981. The fatigue and voluntary discharge properties of single motor units in man. *Journal of Physiology* 36: 545-554.

Guezennec, Y., Leger., L., Lhoste, F., Aymonod, M., and Pesquies, P.C. 1986. Hormone and metabolite response to weight-training sessions. *International Journal of Sports Medicine* 7: 100-105.

Guggenheimer, J.D., Dickin, D.C., Reyes, G.F., and Dolny, D.G. 2009. The effects of specific preconditioning activities on acute sprint performance. *Journal of Strength and Conditioning Research* 23: 1135-1139.

Guglielmo, L.G., Greco, C.C., and Denadai, B.S. 2009. Effects of strength training on running economy. *International Journal of Sports Medicine* 30: 27-32.

Gundersen, K. 2011. Excitation-transcription coupling in skeletal muscle: The molecular pathways of exercise. *Biological Reviews of the Cambridge Philosophical Society* (London) 86: 564-600.

Gur, H., Cakfin, N., Akova, B., Okay, E., and Kuchkoglu, S. 2002. Concentric versus combined concentric-eccentric isokinetic training: Effects on functional capacity and syndromes in patients with osteoarthritis of the knee. *Archives of Physical Medicine and Rehabilitation* 83: 308-316.

Guyton, A.C. 1991. *Textbook of medical physiology*, 8th ed. Philadelphia: W.B. Saunders.

Haennel, R., Teo, K.K., Quinney, A., and Kappagoda, T. 1989. Effects of hydraulic circuit training on cardiovascular function. *Medicine & Science in Sports & Exercise* 21: 605-612.

Haggmark, T., Jansson, E., and Eriksson, E. 1982. Fiber type area and metabolic potential of the thigh muscle in man after knee surgery and immobilization. *International Journal of Sports Medicine* 2: 12-17.

Haggmark, T., Jansson, E., and Svane, B. 1978. Cross-sectional area of the thigh muscle in man measured by computed tomography. *Scandinavian Journal of Clinical and Laboratory Investigation* 38: 354-360.

Häkkinen, K. 1985. Factors influencing trainability of muscular strength during short term and prolonged training. *National Strength and Conditioning Association Journal* 7: 32-37.

Häkkinen, K. 1987. Force production characteristics of leg extensor, trunk flexor and extensor muscles in male and female basketball players. *Journal of Sports Medicine and Physical Fitness* 31: 325-331.

Häkkinen, K. 1989. Neuromuscular and hormonal adaptations during strength and power training. *Journal of Sports Medicine* 29: 9-26.

Häkkinen, K. 1992. Neuromuscular responses in male and female athletes to two successive strength training sessions in one day. *Journal of Sports Medicine and Physical Fitness* 32: 234-242.

Häkkinen, K. 1993. Changes in physical fitness profile in female basketball players during the competitive season including explosive strength training. *Journal of Sports Medicine and Physical Fitness* 33: 19-26.

Häkkinen, K., Alen, M., Kallinen, M., Newton, R.U., and Kraemer, W.J. 2002. Neuromuscular adaptation during prolonged strength training, detraining and re-strength training in middle aged and elderly people. *European Journal of Applied Physiology* 83: 51-62.

Häkkinen, K., Alen, M., Kraemer, W.J., Gorostiaga, E., Izquierdo, M., Rusko, H., Mikkola, J., Häkkinen, A., Valkeinen, H., Kaarakainen, E., Romu, S., Erola, V., Ahtiainen, J., and Paavolainen, L. 2003. Neuromuscular adaptations during concurrent strength and endurance training versus strength training. *European Journal of Applied Physiology* 89: 42-52.

Häkkinen, K., Alen, M., and Komi, P.V. 1985. Changes in isometric force- and relaxation-time, electromyographic and muscle fibre characteristics of human skeletal muscle during strength training and detraining. *Acta Physiologica Scandinavica* 125: 573-585.

Häkkinen, K., and Häkkinen, A. 1991. Muscle cross-sectional area, force production and relaxation characteristics in women at different ages. *European Journal of Applied Physiology* 62: 410-414.

Häkkinen, K., and Kallinen, M. 1994. Distribution of strength training volume into one or two daily sessions on muscular adaptations in female athletes. *Electromyography and Clinical Neurophysiology* 34: 117-124.

Häkkinen, K., Kallinen, M., and Komi, P.V. 1994. Neuromuscular adaptations in strength athletes during strength training distributed into one or two daily sessions. *European Journal of Applied Physiology* 68: 269-270.

Häkkinen, K., and Komi, P. 1981. Effect of different combined concentric and eccentric muscle work on maximal strength development. *Journal of Human Movement Studies* 7: 33-44.

Häkkinen, K., and Komi, P.V. 1983. Changes in neuromuscular performance in voluntary and reflex contraction during strength training in man. *International Journal of Sports Medicine* 4: 282-288.

Häkkinen, K., and Komi, P.V. 1985a. Changes in electrical and mechanical behavior of leg extensor muscles during heavy resistance strength training. *Scandinavian Journal of Sports Science* 7: 55-64.

Häkkinen, K., and Komi, P.V. 1985b. Effect of explosive type strength training on electromyographic and force production characteristics of leg extensor muscles during concentric and various stretch-shortening cycle exercises. *Scandinavian Journal of Sports Science* 7: 65-76.

Häkkinen, K., and Komi, P.V. 1985c. Changes in electrical and mechanical behavior of leg extensor muscles during heavy resistance strength training. *Scandinavian Journal of Sports Science* 7: 55-64.

Häkkinen, K., and Komi, P.V. 1986. Effects of fatigue and recovery on electromyographic and isometric force- and relaxation-time characteristics of human skeletal muscle. *European Journal of Applied Physiology* 55: 588-596.

Häkkinen, K., Komi, P.V., and Alen, M. 1985. Effect of explosive type strength training on isometric force- and relaxation-time, electromyographic and muscle fibre characteristics of leg extensor muscles. *Acta Physiologica Scandinavica* 125: 587-600.

Häkkinen, K., Komi, P.V., Alen, M., and Kauhanen, H. 1987. EMG, muscle fibre and force production characteristics during a 1 year training period in elite weightlifters. *European Journal of Applied Physiology* 56: 419-427.

Häkkinen, K., Komi, P.V., and Tesch, P.A. 1981. Effect of combined concentric and eccentric strength training and detraining on force-time, muscle fiber and metabolic characteristics of leg extensor muscles. *Scandinavian Journal of Sports Science* 3: 50-58.

Häkkinen, K., Kraemer, W.J., and Newton, R. 1997. Muscle activation and force production during bilateral and unilateral concentric and isometric contractions of the knee extensors in men and women at different ages. *Electromyography Clinical Neurophysiology* 37: 131-142.

Häkkinen, K., Kraemer, W.J., Newton, R.U., and Alen, M. 2001. Changes in electromyographic activity, muscle fibre and force production characteristics during heavy resistance/power strength training in middle-aged and older men and women. *Acta Physiologica Scandinavica* 141: 51-62.

Häkkinen, K., Newton, R.U., Gordon, S.E., McCormick, M., Volek, J.S., Nindl, B.C., Gotshalk, L.A., Campbell, W.W., Evans, W.J., Häkkinen, A., Humphries, B., and Kraemer, W.J. 1998. Changes in muscle morphology, electromyographic activity, and force production characteristics during progressive strength training in young and older men. *Journal of Gerontology: Biological Medical Sciences* 53: 415-423.

Häkkinen, K., and Pakarinen, A. 1991. Serum hormones in male strength athletes during intensive short term strength training. *European Journal of Applied Physiology* 63: 194-199.

Häkkinen, K., and Pakarinen, A. 1993. Muscle strength and serum testosterone, cortisol and SHBG concentrations in middle-aged and elderly men and women. *Acta Physiologica Scandinavica* 148:199-207.

Häkkinen, K., and Pakarinen, A. 1994 Serum hormones and strength development during strength training in middle-aged and elderly males and females. *Acta Physiologica Scandinavia* 150: 211-219.

Häkkinen, K., and Pakarinen, A. 1995. Acute hormonal responses to heavy resistance exercise in men and women at different ages. *International Journal of Sports Medicine* 16: 507-513.

Häkkinen, K., Pakarinen, A., Alen, M., Kauhanen, H., and Komi, P.V. 1987. Relationships between training volume, physical performance capacity, and serum hormone concentration during prolonged training in elite weight lifters. *International Journal of Sports Medicine* 8: 61-65.

Häkkinen, K., Pakarinen, A., Alen, M., Kauhanen, H., and Komi, P.V. 1988a. Neuromuscular and hormonal responses in elite athletes to two successive strength training sessions in one day. *European Journal of Applied Physiology* 57: 133-139.

Häkkinen, K., Pakarinen, A., Alen, M., Kauhanen, H., and Komi, P.V. 1988b. Daily hormonal and neuromuscular responses to intensive strength training in 1 week. *International Journal of Sports Medicine* 9: 422-428.

Häkkinen, K., Pakarinen, A., Alen, M., Kauhanen, H., and Komi, P.V. 1988c. Neuromuscular and hormonal adaptations in athletes to strength training in two years. *Journal of Applied Physiology* 65: 2406-2412.

Häkkinen, K., Pakarinen, A., Alen, M., and Komi, P.V. 1985. Serum hormones during prolonged training of neuromuscular performance. *European Journal of Applied Physiology* 53: 287-293.

Häkkinen, K., Pakarinen, A., and Kallinen, M. 1992. Neuromuscular adaptations and serum hormones in women during short-term intensive strength training. *European Journal of Applied Physiology* 64: 106-111.

Häkkinen, K., Pakarinen, A., Komi, P.V., Ryushi, T., and Kauhanen, H. 1989. Neuromuscular adaptations and hormone balance in strength athletes, physically active males, and females during intensive strength training. In *Proceedings of the XII International Congress of Biomechanics*, no. 8, edited by R.J. Gregor, R.F. Zernicke, and W.C. Whiting, 889-894. Champaign, IL: Human Kinetics.

Häkkinen, K., Pakarinen, A., Kraemer, W.J., Häkkinen, A., Valkeinen, H., and Alen, M. 2001. Selective muscle hypertrophy, changes in EMG and force, and serum hormones during strength training in older women. *Journal of Applied Physiology* 91: 569-580.

Häkkinen, K., Pakarinen, A., Kraemer, W.J., Newton, R.U., and Alen, M. 2000. Basal concentrations and acute responses of serum hormones and strength development during heavy resistance training in middle-aged and elderly men and women. *Journal of Gerontology: Biological Sciences, Medical Sciences* 55: B95-B105.

Häkkinen, K., Pakarinen, A., Kyrolainen, H., Cheng, S., Kim, D.H., and Komi, P.V. 1990. Neuromuscular adaptations and serum hormones in females during prolonged power training. *International Journal of Sports Medicine* 11: 91-98.

Häkkinen, K., Pakarinen, A., Newton, R.U., and Kraemer, W.J. 1998. Acute hormone responses to heavy resistance lower and upper extremity exercise in young versus old men. *European Journal of Applied Physiology* 77: 312-319.

Hall, Z.W., and Ralston, E. 1989. Nuclear domains in muscle cells. *Cell* 59: 771-772.

Hamada, T., Sale, D.G., MacDougall, J.D., and Tarnopolsky, M.A. 2000. Postactivation potentiation, fiber type, and twitch contraction time in human knee extensor muscles. *Journal of Applied Physiology* 88: 2131-2137.

Hamil, B.P. 1994. Relative safety of weightlifting and weight training. *Journal of Strength and Conditioning Research* 8: 53-57.

Hamilton, W.F., Woodbury, R.A., and Harper, H.T. 1943. Arterial, cerebrospinal, and venous pressures in man during cough and strain. *American Journal of Physiology* 141: 42-50.

Hamlin, M.J., and Quigley, B.M. 2001. Quadriceps concentric and eccentric exercise 2: Differences in muscle strength, fatigue and EMG activity in eccentrically-exercised sore and non-sore muscles. *Journal of Science and Medicine in Sport* 4: 104-115.

Hammond, G.L., Kontturi, M., Vihko, P., and Vihko, R. 1974. Serum steroids in normal males and patients with prostatic diseases. *Clinical Endocrinology* 9: 113-121.

Hansen, K.T., Cronin, J.B., and Newton, M.J. 2011. The effect of cluster loading of force, velocity, and power during ballistic jump squat training. *International Journal of Sports Physiology and Performance* 6: 455-468.

Hansen, K.T., Cronin, J.B., Pickering, S.L., and Newton, M.J. 2011. Does cluster loading enhance lower body power development in preseason preparation of elite rugby union players? *Journal of Strength and Conditioning Research* 25: 2118-2126.

Hanson, E.D., Leigh, S., and Mynark, R.G. 2007. Acute effects of heavy-and light-load squat exercise on the kinetic measures of vertical jumping. *Journal of Strength and Conditioning Research* 21: 1012-1017.

Hardee, J.P., Triplett, N.T., Utter, A.C., Zwetsloot, K.A., and McBride, J.M. 2012. Effect of interpretation rest on power output in the power clean. *Journal of Strength and Conditioning Research* 26: 883-889.

Hardy, D.O., and Tucker, L.A. 1998. The effects of a single bout of strength training on ambulatory blood pressure levels in 24 mildly hypertensive men. *American Journal of Health Promotion* 13: 69-72.

Harman, E. 1983. Resistive torque analysis of 5 Nautilus exercise machines. *Medicine & Science in Sports & Exercise* 15: 113.

Harman, E.A., Rosenstein, R., Frykman, P., and Nigro, G. 1989. Effects of a belt on intra-abdominal pressure during weight lifting. *Medicine & Science in Sports & Exercise* 21: 186-190.

Harries, U.J., and Bassey, E.J. 1990. Torque-velocity relationships for the knee extensors in women in their 3rd and 7th decades. *European Journal of Applied Physiology* 60: 87-190.

Harris, N.K., Cronn, J.B., Hopkins, W.G., and Hansen, K.T. 2008. Squat jump training at maximal power low versus heavy loads: Effect on sprint ability. *Journal of Strength and Conditioning Research* 22: 1742-1749.

Harr Romey, B.M., Denier Van Der Gon, J.J., and Gielen, C.C. 1982. Changes in recruitment order of motor units in the human biceps muscle. *Experimental Neurology* 78: 360-368.

Hartmann, H., Bob, A., Wirth, K., and Schmidtbleicher, D. 2009. Effects of different periodization models on rate of force development and power ability of the upper extremity. *Journal of Strength and Conditioning Research* 23: 1921-1932.

Hass, C.J., Feigenbaum, M.S., and Franklin, B.A. 2001. Prescription of resistance training for healthy populations. *Sports Medicine* 31: 953-964.

Hass, C.J., Garzarella, L., de Hoyos, D., and Pollock, M.L. 2000. Single versus multiple sets in long-term recreational weightlifters. *Medicine & Science in Sports & Exercise* 32: 235-242.

Hatfield, D.L., Kraemer, W.J., Spiering, B.A. Häkkinen, K., Volek, J.S., Shimano, T., Spreuwenberg, L.P.B., Silvestre, R., Vingren, J.L., Fragala, M.S., Gómez, A.L., Fleck, S.J., Newton, R.U., and Maresh, C.M. 2006. The impact of velocity of movement on performance factors in resistance exercise. *Journal of Strength and Conditioning Research* 20: 760-766.

Hatfield, F.C. 1989. *Power: A scientific approach.* Chicago: Contemporary Books.

Hatfield, F.C., and Krotee, M.L. 1978. *Personalized weight training for fitness and athletics from theory and practice.* Dubuque, IA: Kendall/Hunt.

Hather, B.M., Mason, C.E., and Dudley, G.A. 1991. Histochemical demonstration of skeletal muscle fiber types and capillaries on the same transverse section. *Clinical Physiology* (Oxford) 11: 127-134.

Hather, B.M., Tesch, P.A., Buchanan, P., and Dudley, G.A. 1991. Influence of eccentric actions on skeletal muscle adaptations to resistance training. *Acta Physiologica Scandinavica* 143: 177-185.

Hatta, H., Atomi, Y., Yamamoto, Y., Shinohara, S., and Yamada, S. 1989. Incorporation of blood lactate and glucose into tissues in rats after short-duration strenuous exercise. *International Journal of Sports Medicine* 10: 272-278.

Hawke, T.J., and Garry, D.J. 2001. Myogenic satellite cells: Physiology to molecular biology. *Journal of Applied Physiology* 91: 534-551.

Hawkins, S.A., Schroeder, E.T., Wiswell, R.A., Jaque, S.V., Marcell, T.J., and Costa, K. 1999. Eccentric muscle action increases site-specific osteogenic response. *Medicine & Science in Sports & Exercise* 31: 1287-1292.

Hawkins, S.B., Doyle, T.L.A., and McGuigan, M.R. 2009. The effect of different training programs on eccentric energy utilization and college-aged males. *Journal of Strength and Conditioning Research* 23: 1996-2002.

Haykowsky, M.J., Quinney, H.A., Gillis, R., and Thompson, C.R. 2000. Left ventricular morphology in junior and master resistance trained athletes. *Medicine & Science in Sports & Exercise* 32: 349-352.

Hedrick, A. 2003. Using uncommon implements in the training of athletes. *Strength and Conditioning Journal* 25 (4): 18-24.

Heidt, R.S. Jr., Sweeterman, L.M., Carlonas, R.L., Traub, J.A., and Tekulve, F.X. 2000. Avoidance of soccer injuries with preseason conditioning. *American Journal of Sports Medicine* 28: 659-662.

Heinonen, A., Sievanen, H., Kannus, P., Oja, P., and Vuori, I. 1996. Effects of unilateral strength training and detraining on bone mineral mass and estimated mechanical characteristics of upper limb bones in young women. *Journal of Bone Mineral Research* 11: 490-501.

Hejna, W.F., Rosenberg, A., Buturusis, D.J., and Krieger, A. 1982. The prevention of sports injuries in high school students through strength training. *National Strength and Conditioning Association Journal* 4: 28-31.

Helgerud, J., Rodas, G., Kemi, O.J., and Hoff, J. 2011. Strength and endurance in elite football players. *International Journal of Sports Medicine* 32: 677-682.

Helzberg, J.H., Camilo, J., Waeckerle, J.F., and O'Keefe, J.H. 2010. Review of cardiometabolic risk factors among current professional football and professional baseball players. *Physician and Sportsmedicine.* 38: 77-83.

Henneman, E., Somjen, G., and Carpenter, D.O. 1985. Functional significance of cell size in spinal motorneurons. *Journal of Neurophysiology* 28: 560-580.

Hennessy, L., and Kilty, J. 2001. Relationship of the stretch-shortening cycle to sprint performance and trained female athletes. *Journal of Strength and Conditioning Research* 15: 326-331.

Hennessy, L.C., and Watson, A.W.S. 1994. The interference effects of training for strength and endurance simultaneously. *Journal of Strength and Conditioning Research* 8: 12-19.

Henriksson-Larsen, K. 1985. Distribution, number, and size of different types of fibers in whole cross-sections of female m. tibialis anterior. An enzyme histochemical study. *Acta Physiologica Scandinavica* 123: 229-235.

Henwood, T.R., Riek, S., and Taaffe, D.R. 2008. Strength versus muscle power-specific resistance training in community-dwelling older adults. *Journal of Gerontology: Medical Sciences* 63A: 83-91.

Herbert, R.D., de Noronha, M., and Kamper, S.J. 2011. Stretching to prevent or reduce muscle soreness after exercise. *Cochrane Database Systematic Reviews* 6: CD004577.

Herman, J.R. 2009. Muscular adaptations to slow-speed versus traditional resistance training protocols. PhD dissertation, Ohio University.

Herman, K., Barton, C., Malliaras, P., and Morrissey, D. 2012. The effectiveness of neuromuscular warm-up strategies that require no additional equipment, for preventing lower limb injuries during sports participation: A systematic review. *BMC Medicine* 1075. doi: 10.1186/1741-7015-10-75.

Hermansen, L., Machlum, S., Pruett, E.R., Vaage, O., Waldrum, H., and Wessel-Aas, T. 1976. Lactate removal at rest and during exercise. In *Metabolic adaptation to prolonged physical exercise*, edited by H. Howard and J.R. Pootsmans, 101-105. Basel: Birhauser Verlag.

Heron, M., Hoyert, D., Murphy, S., Xu, J., Kochanek, K., and Tejada-Vera, B. 2009. Deaths: Final data for 2006. *National Vital Statistics Reports* 57: 33-37.

Herrero, A.J., Martin, J., Abadla, O., Fernandez, B., and Garcia-Lopez, D. 2010a. Short-term effect of strength training with and without superimposed electrical stimulation on muscle strength and anaerobic performance. A randomized controlled trial. Part I. *Journal of Strength and Conditioning Research* 24: 1609-1615.

Herrero, A.J., Martin, J., Abadla, O., Fernandez, B., and Garcia-Lopez, D. 2010b. Short-term effect of plyometrics and strength training with and without superimposed electrical stimulation on muscle strength and anaerobic performance: A randomized controlled trial. Part II. *Journal of Strength and Conditioning Research* 24: 1616-1622.

Herrick, A.B., and Stone, W.J. 1996. The effects of periodization versus progressive resistance exercise on upper and lower body strength in women. *Journal of Strength and Conditioning Research* 10: 72-76.

Hetland, M.L., Haarbo, J., and Christiansen, C.1993. Low bone mass and high bone turnover in male long distance runners. *Journal of Clinical Endocrinology and Metabolism* 77: 770-775.

Hettinger, R. 1961. *Physiology of strength*. Springfield, IL: Charles C. Thomas.

Hettinger, R., and Muller, E. 1953. Muskelleistung und muskeltraining. *Arbeits Physiology* 15: 111-126.

Hetzler, R.K., Schroeder, B.L., Wages, J.J, Stickley, C.D., and Kimura, I.F. 2010. Anthropometry increases 1 repetition maximum predictive ability of NFL-225 test for Division IA college football players. *Journal of Strength and Conditioning Research* 24: 1429-39.

Hewett, T.E. 2000. Neuromuscular and hormonal factors associated with knee injuries in female athletes' strategies for intervention. *Sports Medicine* 29: 313-327.

Hewett, T.E., Lindenfeld, T.N., Riccobene, J.V., and Noyes, F.R. 1999. The effect of neuromuscular training on the incidence of knee injury in female athletes: A prospective study. *American Journal of Sports Medicine* 27: 699-706.

Heyward, V.H., and Wagner, D.R. 2004. *Applied body composition assessment*, 2nd ed. Champaign, IL: Human Kinetics.

Hibbs, A.E., Thompson, K.G., French, D., Wrigley, A., and Spears, I. 2008. Optimizing performance by improving core stability and core strength. *Sports Medicine* 38: 1995-2008.

Hickson, R.C. 1980. Interference of strength development by simultaneously training for strength and endurance. *European Journal of Applied Physiology* 45: 255-269.

Hickson, R.C., Dvorak, B.A., Gorostiaga, E.M., Kurowski, T.T., and Foster, C. 1988. Potential for strength and endurance training to amplify endurance performance. *Journal of Applied Physiology* 65: 2285-2290.

Hickson, R.C., Hidaka, K., and Foster, C. 1994. Skeletal muscle fiber type, resistance training, and strength-related performance. *Medicine & Science in Sports & Exercise* 26: 593-598.

Hickson, R.C., Hidaka, K., Foster, C., Falduto, M.T., and Chatterton, R.T. 1994. Successive time courses of strength development and steroid hormone responses to heavy-resistance training. *Journal of Applied Physiology* 76: 663-670.

Hickson, R.C., and Marone, J.R. 1993. Exercise and inhibition of glucocorticoid-induced muscle atrophy. *Exercise and Sports Sciences Reviews* 21: 135-167.

Hickson, R.C., Rosenkoetter, M.A., and Brown, M.M. 1980. Strength training effects on aerobic power and short-term endurance. *Medicine & Science in Sports & Exercise* 12: 336-339.

Higbie, E.J., Cureton, K.J., Warren, G.I., and Prior, B.M. 1996. Effects of concentric and eccentric training on muscle strength, cross-sectional area, and neural activation. *Journal of Applied Physiology* 81: 2173-2181.

Higgs, F., and Winter, S.L. 2009. The effect of a four-week proprioceptive neuromuscular facilitation stretching program on isokinetic torque production. *Journal of Strength and Conditioning Research* 23: 1442-1447.

Hikida, R.S., Staron, R.S., Hagerman, F.C., Walsh, S., Kaiser, E., Shell, S., and Hervey, S. 2000. Effects of high-intensity resistance training on untrained older men. II. Muscle fiber characteristics and nucleo-cytoplasmic relationships. *Journal of Gerontology: A Biological Sciences Medical Sciences* 55: B347-B354.

Hikida, R.S., Van Nostran, S., Murray, J.D., Staron, R.S., Gordon, S.E., and Kraemer, W.J. 1997. Myonuclear loss in atrophied soleus muscle fibers. *Anatomical Record* 247: 350-354.

Hildebrandt, W., Schutze, H., and Stegemann, J. 1992. Cardiovascular limitations of active recovery from strenuous exercise. *European Journal of Applied Physiology and Occupational Physiology* 64: 250-257.

Hill-Hass, S., Bishop, D., Dawson, B., Goodman, C., and Edge, J. 2007. Effects of rest interval during high-repetition resistance training on strength, aerobic fitness, and repeated sprint ability. *Journal of Sports Sciences* 25: 619-628.

Hill, D.W., and Butler, S.D. 1991. Hemodynamic responses to weightlifting exercise. *Sports Medicine* 12: 1-7.

Hind, K., Truscott, J.G., and Evans, J.A. 2006. Low lumbar spine bone mineral density in both male and female endurance runners. *Bone* 39: 880-885.

Ho, K.W., Roy, R.R., Tweedle, C.D., Heusner, W.W., Van Huss, W.D., and Carrow, R. 1980. Skeletal muscle fiber splitting with weight-lifting exercise in rats. *American Journal of Anatomy* 157: 433-440.

Ho, R.C., Alcazar, O., and Goodyear, L.J. 2005. Exercise regulation of insulin action in skeletal muscle. In: *The endocrine system in sports and exercise*, edited by W.J. Kraemer and A.D. Rogol, 388-407. Oxford, UK: Blackwell.

Hodson-Tole, E.F., and Wakeling, J.M. 2009. Motor unit recruitment for dynamic tasks: Current understanding and future directions. *Journal of Comparative Physiology B: Biochemical, Systemic, and Environmental Physiology* 179: 57-66.

Hoeger, W.W.K., Barette, S.L., Hale, D.F., and Hopkins, D.R. 1987. Relationship between repetitions and selected percentages of one repetition maximum. *Journal of Applied Sport Science Research* 1: 11-13.

Hoeger, W.W.K., Hopkins, D.R., Barette, S.L. and Hale, D.F. 1990. Relationship between repetitions and selected percentages of one repetition maximum: A comparison between untrained and trained males and females. *Journal of Applied Sport Science Research* 4: 47-54.

Hoffman, J.R., Fry, A.C., Howard, R., Maresh, C.M., and Kraemer, W.J. 1991. Strength, speed and endurance changes during the course of a division I basketball season. *Journal of Applied Sport Science Research* 3: 144-149.

Hoffman, J.R., and Kalfeld, S. 1998. The effect of resistance training on injury rate and performance in a self-defense instructors course for women. *Journal of Strength and Conditioning Research* 12: 52-56.

Hoffman, J.R., Kraemer, W.J., Fry, A.C., Deschenes, M., Kemp, M. 1990. The effects of self-selection for frequency of training in a winter conditioning program for football. *Journal of Applied Sport Science Research* 4: 76-82.

Hoffman, J.R., Ratamess, N.A., Klatt, M., Faigenbaum, A.D., Ross, R.E., Tranchina, N.M., McCurry, R.C., Kang, J., and Kraemer, W.J. 2009. Comparison between different off-season resistance training programs in division III American college football players. *Journal of Strength and Conditioning Research* 23: 11-19.

Hoffman, T., Stauffer, R.W., and Jackson, A.S. 1979. Sex difference in strength. *American Journal of Sports Medicine* 7: 265-267.

Hogan, M.C., Gladden, L.B., Kurdak, S.S., and Poole, D.C. 1995. Increased (lactate) in working dog muscle reduces tension development independent of pH. *Medicine & Science in Sports & Exercise* 27: 371-377.

Hoge, K.M., Ryan, E.D., Costa, P.B., Herda, T.J., Walter, A.A., Stout, J.R., and Cramer, J.T. 2010. Gender differences in musculotendinous stiffness and range of motion after an acute bout of stretching. *Journal of Strength and Conditioning Research* 24: 2618-2626.

Holcomb, W.R., Rubley, M.D., Lee, H.J., and Guadagnoli, M.A. 2007. Effect of hamstring-emphasized resistance training on hamstrings: Quadriceps strength ratios. *Journal of Strength and Conditioning Research* 21: 41-47.

Hollander, D.B., Kraemer, R.R., Kilpatrick, M.W., Ramadan, Z.G., Reeves, G.V., Francois, M.F., Hebert, E.P., and Tryniecki, J.L. 2007. Maximal eccentric and concentric strength discrepancies between young men and women for dynamic resistance exercise. *Journal of Strength and Conditioning Research* 21: 34-40.

Holmdahl, D.C., and Ingelmark, R.E. 1948. Der Bau des Gelenknorpels unter verschiedenen funktionellen Verhältnissen. *Acta Anatomica* 6: 113-116.

Holsgaard-Larsen, A., Caserotti, P., Puggaard, L., and Aagaard, P. 2011. Stair-ascent performance in elderly women: Effect of explosive strength training. *Journal of Aging and Physical Activity* 19: 117-136.

Hook, P., Sriramoju, V., and Larsson, L. 2001. Effects of aging on actin sliding speed on myosin from single skeletal muscle cells of mice, rats, and humans. *American Journal of Cell Physiology* 280: C782-C788.

Hopkins, T., Pak, J.O., Robertshaw, A.E., Feland, J.B., Hunter, I., and Gage, M. 2008. Whole body vibration and dynamic restraint. *International Journal of Sports Medicine* 29: 424-428.

Hori, N., Newton, R.U., Kawamori, N., McGuigan, M.R., Andrews, W.A., Chapman, D.W., and Nosaka, K. 2008. Comparison of weighted jump squat training with and without eccentric braking. *Journal of Strength and Conditioning Research* 22: 54-65.

Hortobagyi, T., Devita, P., Money, J., and Barrier, J. 2001. Effects of standard and eccentric overload strength training in young women. *Medicine & Science in Sports & Exercise* 33: 1206-1212.

Hortobagyi, T., Hill, J.P., Houmard, J.A., Fraser, D.D., Lambert, N.J., and Israel, R.G. 1996. Adaptive responses to muscle lengthening and shortening in humans. *Journal of Applied Physiology* 80: 765-772.

Hortobagyi, T., Houmard, J.A., Stevenson, J.R., Fraser, D.D., Johns, R.A., and Israel, R.G. 1993. The effects of detraining on power athletes. *Medicine & Science in Sports & Exercise* 25: 929-935.

Hortobagyi, T., Katch, F.I., and LaChance, P.F. 1991. Effects of simultaneous training for strength and endurance on upper and lower body strength and running performance. *Journal of Sports Medicine and Physical Fitness* 31: 20-30.

Hostler, D., Crill, M.T., Hagerman, F.C., and Staron, R.S. 2001. The effectiveness of 0.5-lb. increments in progressive resistance exercise. *Journal of Strength and Conditioning Research* 15: 86-91.

Hostler, D., Schwirian, C.I., Campos, G., Toma, K., Crill, M.T., Hagerman, G.R., Hagerman, F.C., and Staron, R.S. 2001. Skeletal muscle adaptations in elastic resistance-trained young men and women. *European Journal of Applied Physiology* 86: 112-118.

Housh, D.J., Housh, T.J., Johnson, G.O., and Chu, W.K. 1992. Hypertrophic response to unilateral concentric isokinetic training. *Journal of Applied Physiology* 73: 65-70.

Housh, D.J., Housh, T.J., Weir, J.P., Weir, L.L., Evetovich, T.K., and Dolin, P.E. 1998. Effects of unilateral eccentric-only dynamic constant external resistance training on quadriceps femoris cross-sectional area. *Journal of Strength and Conditioning Research* 12: 192-198.

Houston, M.E., Froese, E.A., Valeriote, S.P., Green, H.J., and Ramey, D.A. 1983. Muscle performance, morphology and metabolic capacity during strength training and detraining: A one leg model. *European Journal of Applied Physiology and Occupational Physiology* 51: 25-35.

Houston, M.E., Norman, R.W., and Froese, E.A. 1988. Mechanical measures during maximal velocity knee extension exercise and their relation to fiber composition of the human vastus lateralis muscle. *European Journal of Applied Physiology* 58: 1-7.

Houtkooper, L.B., Stanford, V.A., Metcalfe, L.L., Lohman, T.G., and Going, S.B. 2007. Preventing osteoporosis the Bone Estrogen Strength Training way. *ACSM's Health & Fitness Journal* 11: 21-27.

Howatson, G., and van Someren, K.A. 2008. The prevention and treatment of exercise-induced muscle damage. *Sports Medicine* 38: 483-503.

Howe, T.E., Shea, B., Dawson, L.J., Downie, F., Murray, A., Ross, C., Harbour, R.T., Caldwell, L.M., and Creed, G. 2011. Exercise for preventing and treating osteoporosis in postmenopausal women. *Cochrane Database of Systematic Reviews* 6: CD000333.

Howald, H. 1982. Training induced morphological and functional changes in skeletal muscle. *International Journal of Sports Medicine* 3: 1-12.

Hrysomallis, C. 2011. Balance ability and athletic performance. *Sports Medicine* 41: 221-232.

Huang, J.S., Pietrosimone, B.G., Ingersoll, C.D., Weltman, A.L., and Saliba, S.A. 2011. Sling exercise in traditional warm-up have similar effects on the velocity and accuracy of throwing. *Journal of Strength and Conditioning Research* 25: 1673-1679.

Hubal, M.J., Rubinstein, S.R., and Clarkson, P.M. 2007. Mechanisms of variability in strength loss after muscle-lengthening actions. *Medicine & Science in Sports & Exercise* 39: 461-468.

Hubal, M.J., Rubinstein, S.R., and Clarkson, P.M. 2008. Muscle function in men and women during maximal eccentric exercise. *Journal of Strength and Conditioning Research* 22: 1332-1338.

Hughes, V.A., Frontera, W.R., Dallal, G.E., Lutz, K.J., Fisher, E.C., and Evans, W.J. 1995. Muscle strength and body composition: Associations with bone density in older subjects. *Medicine & Science in Sports & Exercise* 27: 967-974.

Hughes, V.A., Frontera, W.R., Weed, M., Evans, W.J., Dallal, G.E., Roubenoff, R., and Fiatarone, M.A. 2001. Longitudinal muscle strength changes in older adults: Influence of muscle mass, physical activity, and health. *Journal of Gerontology: Biological Sciences, Medical Sciences* 56: B209-B217.

Hulmi, J.J., Lockwood, C.M., and Stout, J.R. 2010. Effect of protein/essential amino acids and resistance training on skeletal muscle hypertrophy: A case for whey protein. *Nutrition and Metabolism (London)* 17: 7-15.

Hulsey, C.R., Soto, D.T., Koch, A.J., and Mayhew, J.L. 2012. Comparison of kettlebell swings and treadmill running equivalent rating of perceived exertion values. *Journal of Strength and Conditioning Research* 26: 1203-1207.

Hultman, E., Bergstrom, J., and Anderson, N.M. 1967. Breakdown and resynthesis of phosphorylcreatine and adenosine triphosphate in connection with muscular work in man. *Scandinavian Journal of Clinical Investigation* 19: 56-66.

Humburg, H., Baas, H., Schroder, J., Reer, R., and Braumann, K-M. 2007. 1-set vs. 3-set resistance training: A crossover study. *Journal of Strength and Conditioning Research* 21: 578-582.

Humphries, B., Newton, R.U., Bronks, R., Marshall, S., McBride, J., Triplett-McBride, T., Häkkinen, K., Kraemer, W.J., and Humphries, N. 2000. Effect of exercise intensity on bone density, strength, and calcium turnover in older women. *Medicine & Science in Sports & Exercise* 32: 1043-1050.

Hunter, G.R. 1985. Changes in body composition, body build and performance associated with different weight training frequencies in males and females. *National Strength and Conditioning Association Journal* 7: 26-28.

Hunter, G.R., and Culpepper, M.I. 1995. Joint angle specificity of fixed mass versus hydraulic resistance knee flexion training. *Journal of Strength and Conditioning Research* 9: 13-16.

Hunter, G.R., Demment, R., and Miller, D. 1987. Development of strength and maximum oxygen uptake during simultaneous training for strength and endurance. *Journal of Sports Medicine and Physical Fitness* 27: 269-275.

Hunter, G.R., McGuirk, J., Mitrano, N., Pearman, P., Thomas, B., and Arrington, R. 1989. The effects of a weight training belt on blood pressure during exercise. *Journal of Applied Strength and Conditioning Research* 3: 13-18.

Hunter, G.R., Seelhorst, D., and Snyder, S. 2003. Comparison of metabolic and heart rate responses to super slow versus traditional resistance training. *Journal of Strength and Conditioning Research* 17: 76-81.

Hunter, G.R., and Treuth, M.S. 1995. Relative training intensity and increases in strength in older women. *Journal of Strength and Conditioning Research* 9: 188-191.

Hunter, G.R., Wetzstein, C.J., Fields, D.A., Brown, A., and Bamman, M.M. 2000. Resistance training increases total energy expenditure and free-living physical activity in older adults. *Journal of Applied Physiology* 89: 977-984.

Hunter, G.R., Wetzstein, C.J., McLafferty, C.L., Jr., Zuckerman, P.A., Landers, K.A., and Bamman, M.M. 2001. High-resistance versus variable-resistance training in older adults. *Medicine & Science in Sports & Exercise* 33: 1759-1764.

Hunter, J.P., and Marshall, R.N. 2002. Effects of power and flexibility training on vertical jump technique. *Medicine & Science in Sports & Exercise* 34: 470-486.

Hunter, S.K., Thompson, M.W., Ruell, P.A., Harmer, A.R., Thom, J.M., Gwinn, T.H., and Adams, R.D. 1999. Human skeletal sarcoplasmic reticulum Ca2+ uptake and muscle function with aging and strength training. *Journal of Applied Physiology* 86: 1858-1865.

Hurley, B.F. 1989. Effects of resistance training on lipoprotein-lipid profiles: A comparison to aerobic exercise training. *Medicine & Science in Sports & Exercise* 21: 689-693.

Hurley, B.F., Hagberg, J.M., Seals, D.R., Ehsani, A.A., Goldberg, A.P., and Holloszy, J.O. 1987. Glucose tolerance and lipid-lipoprotein levels in middle-age powerlifters. *Clinical Physiology* 7: 11-19.

Hurley, B.F., Seals, D.R., Ehsani, A.A., Cartier, L.J., Dalsky, G.P., Hagberg, J.M., and Holloszy, J.O. 1984. Effects of high-intensity strength training on cardiovascular function. *Medicine & Science in Sports & Exercise* 16: 483-488.

Hurley, B.F., Seals, D.R., Hagberg, J.M., Goldberg, A.C., Ostrove, S.M., Holloszy, J.O., Wiest, W.G., and Goldberg, A.P. 1984. High-density-lipoprotein cholesterol in bodybuilders vs. powerlifters. *Journal of the American Medical Association* 252: 507-513.

Huston, L.J., and Wojtys, E.M. 1996. Neuromuscular performance characteristics in elite female athletes. *American Journal of Sports Medicine* 24: 427-436.

Hutton, R.S., and Atwater, S.W. 1992. Acute and chronic adaptations of muscle proprioceptors in response to increased use. *Sports Medicine* 14: 406-421.

Huxley A.F. 2000. Cross-bridge action: Present views, prospects, and unknowns. *Journal of Biomechanics* 33: 1189-1195.

Huxley, A.F., and Niedergerke, R. 1954. Structural changes in muscle during contraction. *Nature* 173: 971-972.

Huxley, H.E., and Hanson, E.J. 1954. Changes in cross-striations of muscle during contraction and stretch and their structural interpretation. *Nature* 173: 973-976.

Hyatt, J.-P.K., and Clarkson, P.M. 1998. Creatine kinase release and clearance using mm variants following repeated bouts of eccentric exercise. *Medicine & Science in Sports & Exercise* 30: 1059-1065.

Hymer, W.C., Kirshnan, K., Kraemer, W.J., Welsch, J., and Lanham, W. 2000. Mammalian pituitary growth hormone: Applications of free flow electrophoresis. *Electrophoresis* 21: 311-317.

Hymer, W.C., Kraemer, W.J., Nindl, B.C., Marx, J.O., Benson, D.E., Welsch, J.R., Mazzetti, S.A., Volek, J.S., and Deaver, D.R. 2001. Characteristics of circulating growth hormone in women following acute heavy resistance exercise. *American Journal of Physiology: Endocrinology and Metabolism* 281: E878-E887.

Ibañez, J., Izquierdo, M., Argüelles, I., Forga, L., Larrión, J.L., García-Unciti, M., Idoate, F., and Gorostiaga, E.M. 2005. Twice-weekly progressive resistance training decreases abdominal fat and improves insulin sensitivity in older men with type 2 diabetes. *Diabetes Care* 28: 662-667.

Ichinose, Y., Kanehisa, H., Ito, M., Kawakami, Y., and Fukunaga, T. 1998. Relationship between muscle fiber pennation and force capability in Olympic athletes. *International Journal of Sports Medicine* 19: 541-546.

Iellamo, F., Legramante, J.M., Raimondi, G., Castrucci, F., Damiani, C., Foti, C., Peruzzi, G., and Caruso, I. 1997. Effects of isokinetic, isotonic and isometric submaximal exercise on heart rate and blood pressure. *European Journal of Applied Physiology* 75: 89-96.

Ikai, M., and Fukunaga, T. 1970. A study on training effect on strength per unit cross-sectional area of muscle by means of ultrasonic measurement. *European Journal of Applied Physiology* 28: 173-180.

Ikai, M., and Steinhaus, A.H. 1961. Some factors modifying the expression of human strength. *Journal of Applied Physiology* 16: 157-163.

Ikegawa, S., Funato, K., Tsunoda, N., Kanehisa, H., Fukunaga, T., and Kawakami, Y. 2008. Muscle force per cross-sectional area is inversely related with pennation angle in strength trained athletes. *Journal of Strength and Conditioning Research* 22: 128-131.

Imamura, K., Ashida, H., Ishikawa, T., and Fujii, M. 1983. Human major psoas muscle and sacrospinalis muscle in relation to age: A study by computed tomography. *Journal of Gerontology* 38: 678-681.

Ingelmark, B.E., and Elsholm, R. 1948. A study on variations in the thickness of the articular cartilage in association with rest and periodical load. *Uppsala Lakaretorenings Foxhandlinger* 53: 61-64.

Ingjer, F. 1969. Effects of endurance training on muscle fiber ATPase activity, capillary supply and mitochondrial content in man. *Journal of Physiology* 294: 419-432.

Ingle, L., Sleap, M., and Tolfrey, K. 2006. The effects of a complex training and detraining programme on selected strength and power variables in early pubertal boys. *Journal of Sports Sciences* 24: 987-997.

International Federation of Sports Medicine (FIMIS). 1998. Resistance training for children and adolescents. In *Sports and Children*, edited by K. Chan and L. Micheli, 265-270. Hong Kong: Lippincott Williams & Wilkins.

International Olympic Committee. 2008. Consensus statement. Training the elite young athlete. *Clinical Journal of Sport Medicine* 18: 122-123.

Ishida, K., Moritani, T., and Itoh, K. 1990. Changes in voluntary and electrically induced contractions during strength training and detraining. *European Journal of Applied Physiology* 60: 244-248.

Ivey, F.M., Tracy, B.L., Lemmer, J.T., NessAiver, M., Metter, E.J., Fozard, J.L., and Hurley, B.F. 2000. Effects of strength training and detraining on muscle quality: Age and gender comparisons. *Journal of Gerontology. Series A Biological Science Medicine Science* 55: B152-B157.

Izquierdo, M., Häkkinen, K., Ibanez, J., Garrues, M., Anton, A., Zuniga, A., Larrión, J.L., and Gorostiaga, E.M. 2001. Effects of strength training on muscle power and serum hormones in middle aged and older men. *Journal of Applied Physiology* 90: 1497-1507.

Izquierdo, M., Häkkinen, K., Ibanez, J., Kraemer, W.J., and Gorostiage, E.M. 2005. Effects of combined resistance and cardiovascular training on strength, power, muscle cross-sectional area, and endurance markers in middle-aged men. *European Journal of Applied Physiology* 94: 70-75.

Izquierdo, M., Ibanez, J., Gonzalez-Badillo, J.J., Häkkinen, K., Ratamess, N.A., Kraemer, W.J., French, D.N., Eslava, J., Altadill, A., Asiain, X., and Gorostiaga, E.M. 2006. Different effects of strength training leading to failure versus not to failure of hormonal responses, strength, and muscle power games. *Journal of Applied Physiology* 100: 1647-1656.

Izquierdo, M., Ibanez, J., Gonzalez-Badillo, J.J., Ratamess, N.A., Kraemer, W.J., Häkkinen, K., Granados, C., French, D.N., and Gorostilaga, E.M. 2007. Detraining and tapering effects of hormonal responses and strength performance. *Journal of Strength and Conditioning Research* 1: 768-775.

Izquierdo, M., Ibañez, J., Häkkinen, K., Kraemer, W.J., Larrión, J.L., and Gorostiaga, E.M. 2004. Once weekly combined resistance and cardiovascular training in healthy older men. *Medicine & Science in Sports & Exercise* 36: 435-443.

Izquierdo-Gabarren, M., Gonzalez De Txabarri Exposito, R., Gracia-Pallares, J., Sanchez-Medina, L., De Villarreal, G., and Izquierdo, M. 2010. Concurrent endurance and strength training not to failure optimizes performance gains. *Medicine & Science in Sports & Exercise* 42: 1191-1199.

Jackson, A., Jackson, T., Hnatek, J., and West, J. 1985. Strength development: Using functional isometric in isotonic strength training program. *Research Quarterly for Exercise and Sport* 56: 324-337.

Jacobson, B.H. 1986. A comparison of two progressive weight training techniques on knee extensor strength. *Athletic Training* 21: 315-318, 390.

Jacobson, P.C., Bever, W., Brubb, S.A., Taft, T.N., and Talmage, R.V. 1984. Bone density in female: College athletes and older athletic female. *Journal of Orthopaedic Research* 2: 328-332.

Jakobi, J.M., and Chilibeck, P.D. 2001. Bilateral and unilateral contractions: Possible differences in maximal voluntary force. *Canadian Journal of Applied Physiology* 26: 12-33.

Janssen, I., Heymsfield, S.B., Wang, Z., and Ross, R. 2000. Skeletal muscle mass and distribution in 468 men and women aged 18-80 yr. *Journal of Applied Physiology* 89: 81-88.

Jefferson, L.S., and Kimball, S.R. 2001. Translational control of protein synthesis: Implications for understanding changes in skeletal muscle mass. *International Journal of Sport Nutrition and Exercise Metabolism* 11: S143-S149.

Jenkins, W.L., Thackaberry, M., and Killian, C. 1984. Speed-specific isokinetic training. *Journal of Orthopaedic and Sports Physical Therapy* 6: 181-183.

Jensen, C., and Fisher, G. 1979. *Scientific basis of athletic conditioning*. Philadelphia: Lea and Febiger.

Johnson, B.A., Salzberg, C.L., and Stevenson, D.A. 2012. Effects of a plyometric training program for 3 children with neurofibromatosis type 1. *Pediatric Physical Therapy* 24: 199-208.

Johnson, B.L., Adamczy, K.J.W., Tennoe, K.O., and Stromme, S.B. 1976. A comparison of concentric and eccentric muscle training. *Medicine & Science in Sports & Exercise* 8: 35-38.

Johnson, C.C., Stone, M.H., Lopez, S.A., Hebert, J.A., Kilgore, L.T., and Byrd, R.J. 1982. Diet and exercise in middle-age men. *Journal of the American Dietetic Association* 81: 695-701.

Johnson, J.H., Colodny, S., and Jackson, D. 1990. Human torque capability versus machine resistive torque for four eagle resistance machines. *Journal of Applied Sport Science Research* 4: 83-87.

Jones, A. 1973. The best kind of exercise. *Ironman* 32: 36-38.

Jones, D.A., and Rutherford, O.M. 1987. Human muscle strength training: The effects of three different regimes and the nature of the resultant changes. *Journal of Physiology* 391: 1-11.

Jones, K., Hunter, G., Fleisig, G., Escamilla, R., and Lemak, L. 1999. The effects of compensatory acceleration on upper-body strength and power in collegiate football players. *Journal of Strength and Conditioning Research* 13: 99-105.

Jonsson, P., Wahlström, P., Ohberg, L., and Alfredson, H. 2006. Eccentric training in chronic painful impingement syndrome of the shoulder: Results of a pilot study. *Knee Survey Sports Traumatology Arthroscopy* 14: 76-81.

Joseph, M.F., Lillie, K.R., Bergeron, D.J., and Denegar, C.R. 2012. Measuring Achilles tendon mechanical properties: A reliable, noninvasive method. *Journal of Strength and Conditioning Research* 26: 2017-2020.

Jozsi, A.C., Campbell, W.W., Joseph, L., Davey, S.L., and Evans, W.J. 1999. Changes in power with resistance training in older and younger men and women. *Journal of Gerontology: Biological Sciences* 54: M591-M596.

Jubrias, S.A., Esselman, P.C., Price, L.B., Cress, M.E., and Conley, K.E. 2001. Large energetic adaptations of elderly muscle to resistance and endurance training. *Journal of Applied Physiology* 90: 1663-1670.

Kadi F., Bonnerud, P., Eriksson, A., and Thornell, L.E. 2000. The expression of androgen receptors in human neck and limb muscles: Effects of training and self-administration of androgenic-anabolic steroids. *Histochemistry and Cell Biology* 113: 25-29.

Kadi, F., Charifi, N., Denis, C., Lexell, J., Andersen, J.L., Schjerling, P., Olsen, S., and Kjaer, M. 2005. The behaviour of satellite cells in response to exercise: What have we learned from human studies? *Pflugers Archive* 451: 319-327.

Kadi, F., Eriksson, A., Holmner, S., Butler-Browne, G.S., and Thornell, L.E. 1999. Cellular adaptation of the trapezius muscle in strength-trained athletes. *Histochemistry and Cell Biology* 111: 189-195.

Kadi, F., Schjerling, P., Andersen, L.L., Charifi, N., Madsen, J.L., Christensen, L.R., and Andersen, J.L. 2004. The effects of heavy resistance training and detraining on satellite cells in human skeletal muscles. *Journal of Physiology* 558: 1005-1012.

Kadi, F., and Thornell, L.E. 2000. Concomitant increases in myonuclear and satellite cell content in female trapezius muscle following strength training. *Histochemistry and Cell Biology* 113: 99-103.

Kahn, J.F., Kapitaniak, B., and Monod, H. 1985. Comparisons of two modalities when exerting isometric contractions. *European Journal of Applied Physiology* 54: 331-335.

Kalapotharakos, V., Smilios, I., Parlavatzas, A., and Tokmakidis, S.P. 2007. The effect of moderate resistance srength training and detraining on muscle strength and power in older men. *Journal of Geriatric Physical Therapy* 30: 109-113.

Kale, M., Asci, A., Bayrak, C., and Acikada, C. 2009. Relationships among jumping performance and sprint parameters during maximum speed phase in sprinters. *Journal of Strength and Conditioning Research* 23: 2272-2279.

Kalra, P.S., Sahu, A., and Kalra, S.P. 1990. Interleukin-1 inhibits the ovarian steroid-induced luteinizing hormone surge and release of hypothalamic luteinizing hormone-releasing hormone in rats. *Endocrinology* 126: 2145-2152.

Kamen, G., Kroll, W., and Ziagon, S.T. 1984. Exercise effects upon reflex time components in weight lifters and distance runners. *Medicine & Science in Sports & Exercise* 13: 198-204.

Kamen, G., and Roy A. 2000. Motor unit synchronization in young and elderly adults. *European Journal of Applied Physiology* 81: 403-410.

Kanakis, C., and Hickson, C. 1980. Left ventricular responses to a program of lower-limb strength training. *Chest* 78: 618-621.

Kanehisa, H., Ikegawa, S., and Fukunaga, T. 1998. Body composition and cross-sectional areas of limb lean tissues in Olympic weight lifters. *Scandinavian Journal of Medicine & Science in Sports* 8: 271-278.

Kanehisa, H., Ikegawa, S., Tsunoda, N., and Fukunaga, T. 1994. Strength and cross-sectional area of knee extension muscles in children. *European Journal of Applied Physiology* 68: 402-405.

Kanehisa, H., and Miyashita, M. 1983a. Effect of isometric and isokinetic muscle training on static strength and dynamic power. *European Journal of Applied Physiology* 50: 365-371.

Kanehisa, H., and Miyashita, M. 1983b. Specificity of velocity in strength training. *European Journal of Applied Physiology* 52: 104-106.

Kanehisa, H., Nagareda, H., Kawakami, Y., Akima, H., Masani, K., Kouzaki, M., and Fukanaga, T. 2002. Effects of equivolume isometric training programs comprising medium or high resistance on muscle size and strength. *European Journal of Applied Physiology* 87: 112-119.

Kanehisa, H., Okuyama, H., Ikegawa, S., and Fukunga, T. 1996. Sex difference in force generation capacity during repeated maximal knee extensions. *European Journal of Applied Physiology* 73: 557-562.

Kaneko, M., Fuchimoto, T., Toji, H., and Suei, K. 1983. Training effect of different loads on the force-velocity relationship and mechanical power output in human muscle. *Scandinavian Journal of Sports Science* 5: 50-55.

Kang, J., Hoffman, J.R., Im, J., Spiering, B.A., Ratamess, N.A., Rundell, K.W., Nioka, S., Cooper, J., and Chance, B. 2005. Evaluation of physiological responses during recovery following three resistance exercise programs. *Journal of Strength and Conditioning Research* 19: 305-309.

Karavirta, L., Tulppo, M.P., Laaksonen, D.E., Nyman, K., Laukkanen, R.T., Kinnunen, H., Häkkinen, A., and Häkkinen, K. 2009. Heart rate dynamics after combined endurance and strength training in older men. *Medicine & Science in Sports & Exercise* 41: 1436-1443.

Karlsson, J., Bonde-Petersen, F., Henriksson, J., and Knuttgen, H.G. 1975. Effects of previous exercise with arms or legs on metabolism and performance in exhaustive exercise. *Journal of Applied Physiology* 38: 208-211.

Karp, J.R. 2000. Interval training for the fitness professional. *Journal of Strength and Conditioning Research* 22: 64-69.

Katch, U.L., Katch, F.I., Moffatt, R., and Gittleson, M. 1980. Muscular development and lean body weight in body builders and weight lifters. *Medicine & Science in Sports & Exercise* 12: 340-344.

Katz, B. 1939. The relationship between force and speed in muscular contraction. *Journal of Physiology* 96: 45-64.

Kauhanen, H., and Häkkinen, K. 1989. Short term effects of voluminous heavy resistance training and recovery on the snatch technique in weightlifting. In *Proceedings of the XII International Congress of*

Biomechanics, edited by R.J. Gregor, R.F. Zernicke, and W.C. Whitting. Abstract, 31.

Kawakami, Y., Abe T., and Fukunaga T. 1993. Muscle-fiber pennation angles are greater in hypertrophied than in normal muscles. *Journal of Applied Physiology* 74: 2740-2744.

Kawakami, Y., Abe, T., Kuno, S., and Fukunaga, T. 1995. Training induced changes in muscle architecture and specific tension. *European Journal of Applied Physiology* 72: 37-43.

Kawamori, N., Rossi, S.J., Justice, B.D., Haff, E.E., Pistili, E.E., O'Bryant, H.S., Stone, M.H., and Haff, G.G. 2006. Peak force and rate of force development during isometric and dynamic mid-thigh clean pulls performed at various intensities. *Journal of Strength and Conditioning Research* 20: 483-491.

Kawano, H., Tanaka, H., and Miyachi, M. 2006. Resistance training and arterial compliance: Keeping the benefits while minimizing the stiffness. *Journal of Hypertension* 24: 1753-1759.

Kearns, C.F., Abe, T., and Brechue, W.F. 2000. Muscle enlargement in sumo wrestlers includes increased muscle fascicle length. *European Journal of Applied Physiology* 83: 289-296.

Keeler, L.K., Finkelstein, L.H., Miller, W., and Fernhall, B. 2001. Early-phase adaptations of traditional speed vs. superslow resistance training on strength and aerobic capacity in sedentary individuals. *Journal of Strength and Conditioning Research* 15: 309-314.

Kell, R.T. 2011. The influence of periodized resistance training on strength changes in men and women. *Journal of Strength and Conditioning Research* 25: 735-744.

Kelleher, A.R., Hackney, K.J., Keslacy, S., and Ploutz-Snyder, L.L. 2010. The metabolic costs of reciprocal supersets vs. traditional resistance exercise in young recreational active adults. *Journal of Strength and Conditioning Research* 24: 1043-1049.

Kelley, G. 1997. Dynamic resistance exercise and resting blood pressure in adults: A meta-analysis. *Journal of Applied Physiology* 82: 1559-1565.

Kelley, G.A., and Kelley, K.S. 2000. Progressive resistance exercise and resting blood pressure: A meta-analysis of randomized controlled trials. *Hypertension* 35: 838-843.

Kelley, G.A. and Kelley, K.S. 2009a. Impact of progressive resistance training on lipids and lipoproteins in adults: A meta-analysis of randomized controlled trials. *Preventative Medicine* 48: 9-19.

Kelley, G.A., and Kelley, K.S. 2009b. Impact of progressive resistance training on lipids and lipoproteins in adults: Another look at a meta-analysis using prediction intervals. *Preventative Medicine* 49: 473-475.

Kelley, G.A., Kelley, K.S., Hootman, J.M., and Jones, D.L. 2011. Effects of community-deliverable exercise on pain and physical function in adults with arthritis and other rheumatic diseases: A meta-analysis. *Arthritis Care & Research* 63: 79-93.

Kelley, G.A., Kelley, K.S., and Tran, Z.V. 2000. Exercise and bone mineral density in men: A meta-analysis. *Journal of Applied Physiology* 88: 1730-1736.

Kelley G.A., Kelley, K.S., and Tran, Z.V. 2001. Resistance training and bone mineral density in women: A meta-analysis of controlled trials. *American Journal of Physical Medicine and Rehabilitation* 80: 65-77.

Kellis, E., and Baltzopoulos, V. 1995. Isokinetic eccentric exercise. *Sports Medicine* 19: 202-222.

Kelly, S.B., Brown, L.E., Coburn, J.W., Zinder, S.M., Gardner, L.M., and Nguyen, D. 2007. The effect of single versus multiple sets on strength. *Journal of Strength and Conditioning Research* 21: 1003-1006.

Kemertzis, M.A., Lythgo, N.D., Morgan, D.L., and Galea, M.P. 2008. Ankle flexors produce peak torque at longer muscle lengths after whole-body vibration. *Medicine & Science in Sports & Exercise* 40: 1977-1983.

Kemmler, W.K., Lauber, D., Engelke, K., and Weineck, J. 2004. Effects of single- vs. multiple-set resistance training on maximum strength and body composition in trained postmenopausal women. *Journal of Strength and Conditioning Research* 18: 689-694.

Kent-Braun, J.A., Ng, A.V., and Young, K. 2000. Skeletal muscle contractile and noncontractile components in young and older women and men. *Journal of Applied Physiology* 88: 662-668.

Keogh, J.W.L., Payne, A.L., Anderson, B.B., and Atkins, P.J. 2010. A brief description of the biomechanics and physiology of a strongman event: The tire flip. *Journal of Strength and Conditioning Research* 24: 1223-1228.

Keogh, J.W.L., Wilson, G.J., and Weatherby, R.P. 1999. A cross-sectional comparison of different resistance training techniques in the bench press. *Journal of Strength and Conditioning Research* 13: 247-258.

Kerksick, C.M., Wilborn, C.D., Campbell, B.I., Roberts, M.D., Rasmussen, C.J., Greenwood, M., and Kreider, R.B. 2009. Early-phase adaptations to a split-body, linear periodization resistance training program in college-aged in middle-aged men. *Journal of Strength and Conditioning Research* 23: 962-1971..

Kerr, D., Ackland, T., Maslen, B., Morton, A., and Prince, R. 2001. Resistance training over 2 years increases bone mass in postmenopausal women. *Journal of Bone and Mineral Research* 16: 175-181.

Kesidis, N., Metaxas, T.I., Vrabas, I.S., Stefanidis, P., Vamvakoudis, E., Christoulas, K., Mandroukas, A., Balasas, D., and Mandroukas, K. 2008. Myosin heavy chain isoform distribution in single fibres of bodybuilders. *European Journal of Applied Physiology* 10: 579-583.

Keul, J., Haralambei, G., Bruder, M., and Gottstein, H.J. 1978. The effect of weight lifting exercise on heart rate and metabolism in experienced lifters. *Medicine & Science in Sports & Exercise* 10: 13-15.

Keysor, J.J., and Jette, A.M. 2001. Have we oversold the benefits of late-life exercise? *Journal of Gerontology* 56: M412-423.

Khamoui, A.V., Brown, L.E., Nguyen, D., Uribe, B.P., Coburn, J.W., Noffal, G.J., and Tran, T. 2011. Relationship between force-time and velocity-time characteristics of dynamic isometric muscle actions. *Journal of Strength and Conditioning Research* 25: 198-204.

Khan, K., McKay, H.A., Haapassalo, H., Bennell, K.L., Forwood, M.R., Kannus, P., and Wark, J.D. 2000. Does childhood and adolescence provide a unique opportunity for exercise to strengthen the skeleton? *Journal of Science and Medicine in Sport* 3: 150-164.

Kilduff, L.P., Bevan, H.R., Kingsley, M.I.C., Owen, N.J., Bennett, M.A., Bunce, P.J., Hore, A.M., Maw, J.R., and Cunningham, D.J. 2007. Postactivation potentiation in professional rugby players: Optimal recovery. *Journal of Strength and Conditioning Research* 21: 1134-1138.

Kilinc, F. 2008. An intensive combined training program modulates physical, physiological, biomotoric, and technical parameters in women basketball players. *Journal of Strength and Conditioning Research* 22: 1769-1778.

Kim, E., Dear, A., Ferguson, S.L., Seo, D., and Bemben, M.G. 2011. Effects of 4 weeks of traditional resistance training vs. superslow strength training on early phase adaptations in strength, flexibility, and aerobic capacity in college-aged women. *Journal of Strength and Conditioning Research* 25: 3006-3013.

Kimball, S.R. 2006. Interaction between the AMP-activated protein kinase and mTOR signaling pathways. *Medicine & Science in Sports & Exercise* 38: 1958-1964.

Kin-Isler, A., Acikada, C., and Artian, S. 2006. Effects of vibration on maximal isometric muscle contraction at different joint angles. *Isokinetics and Exercise Science* 14: 213-220.

Kinser, A.M., Ramsey, M.W., O'Bryant, H.S., Ayres, C.A., Sands, W.A., and Stone, M.H. 2008. Vibration and stretching effects on flexibility and explosive strength in young gymnasts. *Medicine & Science in Sports & Exercise* 40: 133-140.

Kistler B.M., Walsh, M.S., Horn, T.S., and Cox, R.H. 2010. The acute effects of static stretching on the sprint performance of collegiate men in the 60- and 100-m dash after a dynamic warm-up. *Journal of Strength and Conditioning Research* 24: 2280-2284.

Kitai, T.A., and Sale, D.G. 1989. Specificity of joint angle in isometric training. *European Journal of Applied Physiology* 58: 744-748.

Kjaer, M., and Secher, N.H. 1992. Neural influences on cardiovascular and endocrine responses to static exercise in humans. *Sports Medicine* 13: 303-319.

Kleiner, D.M., Blessing, D.L., Davis, W.R., and Mitchell, J.W. 1996. Acute cardiovascular responses to various forms of resistance exercise. *Journal of Strength and Conditioning Research* 10: 56-61.

Kleiner, D.M., Blessing, D.L., Mitchell, J.W., and Davis, W.R. 1999. A description of the acute cardiovascular responses to isokinetic resistance at three different speeds. *Journal of Strength and Conditioning Research* 13: 360-366.

Kleiner, S.M., Bazzarre, T.L., and Ainsworth, B.E. 1994. Nutritional status of nationally ranked elite bodybuilders. *International Journal of Sports Medicine* 4: 54-69.

Klitgaard, H., Ausoni, S., and Damiani, E. 1989. Sarcoplasmic reticulum of human skeletal muscle: Age-related changes and effect of training. *Acta Physiologica Scandinavica* 137: 23-31.

Klitgaard, H., Mantoni, M., Schiaffino, S., Ausoni, S., Gorza, L., Laurent-Winter, C., Schnohr, P., and Saltin, B. 1990. Function, morphology and protein expression of ageing skeletal muscle: A cross-sectional study of elderly men with different training backgrounds. *Acta Physiologica Scandinavica* 140: 41-54.

Knapik, J.J., Mawdsley, R.H., and Ramos, M.U. 1983. Angular specificity and test mode specificity of isometric and isokinetic strength training. *Journal of Orthopedic Sports Physical Therapy* 5: 58-65.

Knapik, J.J., Wright, J.E., Kowal, D.M., and Vogel, J.A. 1980. The influence of U.S. Army basic initial entry training on the muscular strength of men and women. *Aviation, Space and Environmental Medicine* 51: 1086-1090.

Knuttgen, H.G., and Kraemer, W.J. 1987. Terminology and measurement in exercise performance. *Journal of Applied Sport Science Research* 1: 1-10.

Kohler, J.M., Flanagan, S.P., and Whitting, W.C. 2010. Muscle activation patterns while lifting stable and unstable loads on unstable and unstable surfaces. *Journal of Strength and Conditioning Research* 24: 313-321.

Kohrt, W.M., Ehsani, A.A., and Birge, S.J. 1997. Effects of exercise involving predominately either joint-reaction or ground-reaction forces on bone mineral density in older women. *Journal of Bone and Mineral Research* 12: 1253-1261.

Kok, L.-Y., Hamer, P.W., and Bishop, D.J. 2009. Enhancing muscular qualities in untrained women: Linear versus undulating periodization. *Medicine & Science in Sports & Exercise* 41: 1797-1807.

Kokkonen, J., Bangerter, B., Roundy, E., and Nelson, A. 1988. Improved performance through digit strength gains. *Research Quarterly for Exercise and Sport* 59: 57-63.

Kokkonen, J., Nelson, A.G., Eldredge, C., and Winchester, J.B. 2007. Chronic static stretching improves exercise performance. *Medicine & Science in Sports & Exercise* 39: 1825-1831.

Kolber, M.J., Beekhuizen, K.S., Cheng, M.S., and Hellman, M.A. 2010. Shoulder injuries attributed to resistance training: A brief review. *Journal of Strength and Conditioning Research* 24: 1696-1704.

Komi, P.V. 1979. Neuromuscular performance: Factors influencing force and speed production. *Scandinavian Journal of Sports Sciences* 1: 2-15.

Komi, P.V., and Buskirk, E.R. 1972. Effect of eccentric and concentric muscle conditioning on tension and electrical activity of human muscle. *Ergonomics* 15: 417-434.

Komi, P.V., and Häkkinen, K. 1988. Strength and power. In *The Olympic book of sports medicine*, edited by A. Dirix, H.G. Knuttgen, and K. Tittel, 183. Boston: Blackwell Scientific.

Komi, P.V., Kaneko, M., and Aura, O. 1987. EMG activity of the leg extensor muscles with special reference to mechanical efficiency in concentric and eccentric exercise. *International Journal of Sports Medicine* 8: 22-29.

Komi, P.V., and Karlsson, J. 1978. Skeletal muscle fiber types, enzyme activities and physical performance in young males and females. *Acta Physiologica Scandinavica* 103: 210-218.

Komi, P.V., Linnamo, V., Ventoinen, P., and Sillanpaa, M. 2000. Force and EMG power spectrum during eccentric and concentric actions. *Medicine & Science in Sports & Exercise* 32: 1757-1762.

Komi, P.V., Suominen, H., Heikkinen, E., Karlsson, J., and Tesch, P. 1982. Effects of heavy resistance and explosive-type strength training methods on mechanical, functional, and metabolic aspects of performance. In *Exercise and sport biology,* edited by P.V. Komi, 90-102. Champaign, IL: Human Kinetics.

Kongsgaard, M., Reitelseder, S., Pedersen, T.G., Holm, L., Aagaard, P., Kjaer, M., and Magnusson, S.P. 2007. Region specific patellar tendon hypertrophy in humans following resistance training. Acta Physiologica (Oxford) 191: 111-1121.

Kopp-Woodroffe, S.A., Manore, M.M., Dueck, C.A., Skinner, J.S., and Matt, K.S. 1999. Energy and nutrient status of amenorrheic athletes participating in a diet and exercise training intervention program. *International Journal of Sport Nutrition* 9: 70-88.

Korhonen, M.T., Cristea, A., Alen, M., Häkkinen, K., Sipila, S., Mero, A., Viitasalo, J.T., Larsson, L., and Suominen, H. 2006. Aging, muscle fiber type, and contractile function in sprint-trained athletes. *Journal of Applied Physiology* 101: 906-917.

Kosek, D.J., and Bamman, M.M. 2008. Modulation of the dystrophin-associated protein complex in response to resistance training in young and older men. *Journal of Applied Physiology* 104: 1476-1484.

Kotzamanidis, C. 2006. Effect of plyometric training on running performance and vertical jumping in prepubertal boys. *Journal of Strength and Conditioning Research* 20: 441-445.

Koutedakis, Y., Boreham, C., Kabitsis, C., and Sharp, N.C.C. 1992. Seasonal deterioration of selected physiological variables in elite male skiers. *International Journal of Sports Medicine* 13: 548-551.

Kovaleski, J.E., and Heitman, R.J. 1993a. Effects of isokinetic velocity spectrum exercise on torque production. *Sports Medicine, Training and Rehabilitation* 4: 67-71.

Kovaleski, J.E., and Heitman, R.J. 1993b. Interaction of velocity and progression order during isokinetic velocity spectrum exercise. *Isokinetics and Exercise Science* 3: 118-122.

Kovaleski, J.E., Heitman, R.J., Scaffidi, F.M., and Fondren, F.B. 1992. Effects of isokinetic velocity spectrum exercise on average power and total work. *Journal of Athletic Training* 27: 54-56.

Kovaleski, J.E., Heitman, R.H., Trundle, T.L., and Gilley, W.F. 1995. Isotonic preload versus isokinetic knee extension resistance training. *Medicine & Science in Sports & Exercise* 27: 895-899.

Kowalchuk, J.M., Heigenhauser, F.J.F., Lininger, M.I., Obminski, G., Sutton, J.R., and Jones, N.L. 1988. Role of lungs and inactive muscle in acid-base control after maximal exercise. *Journal of Applied Physiology* 65: 2090-2096.

Koziris, L.P., Hickson, R.C., Chatterton, R.T., Groseth, R.T., Christie, J.M., Goldflies, D.G., and Unterman, T.G. 1999. Serum levels of total and free IGF-1 and IGFBP-3 are increased and maintained in long-term training. *Journal of Applied Physiology* 86: 1436-1442.

Koziris, L.P., Kraemer, W.J., Patton, J.F., Triplett, N.T., Fry, A.C., Gordon, S.E., and Knuttgen, H.G. 1996. Relationship of aerobic power to anaerobic performance indices. *Journal of Strength and Conditioning Research* 10: 35-39.

Kraemer, W.J. 1983a. Detraining the "bulked-up" athlete: Prospects for lifetime health and fitness. *National Strength and Conditioning Association Journal* 5: 10-12.

Kraemer, W.J. 1983b. Exercise prescription in weight training: A needs analysis. *National Strength and Conditioning Association Journal* 5: 64-65.

Kraemer, W.J. 1983c. Exercise prescription in weight training: Manipulating program variables. *National Strength and Conditioning Association Journal* 5: 58-59.

Kraemer, W.J. 1988. Endocrine responses to resistance exercise. *Medicine & Science in Sports & Exercise* 20 (Suppl.): S152-S157.

Kraemer, W.J. 1992a. Endocrine responses and adaptations to strength training. In *Strength and power in sports,* edited by P.V. Komi, 291-304. Boston: Blackwell Scientific.

Kraemer, W.J. 1992b. Hormonal mechanisms related to the expression of muscular strength and power. In *Strength and power in sports,* edited by P.V. Komi, 64-76. Boston: Blackwell Scientific.

Kraemer, W.J. 1994. Neuroendocrine responses to resistance exercise. In *Essentials of strength and conditioning,* edited by T.R. Baechle, 86-107. Champaign, IL: Human Kinetics.

Kraemer, W.J. 1997. A series of studies: The physiological basis for strength training in American football: Fact over philosophy. *Journal of Strength and Conditioning Research* 11: 131-142.

Kraemer, W.J., Aguilera, B.A., Terada, M., Newton, R.U., Lynch, J.M., Rosendaal, G., McBride, J.M., Gordon, S.E., and Häkkinen, K. 1995. Responses of IGF-I to endogenous increases in growth hormone after heavy-resistance exercise. *Journal of Applied Physiology* 77: 206-211.

Kraemer, W.J., Clemson, A., Triplett, N.T., Bush, J.A., Newton, R.U., and Lynch, J.M. 1996. The effects of plasma cortisol evaluation on total and differential leukocyte counts in response to heavy-resistance exercise. *European Journal of Applied Physiology* 73 (1-2): 93-97.

Kraemer, W.J., Deschenes, M.R., and Fleck, S.J. 1988. Physiological adaptations to resistance exercise implications for athletic conditioning. *Sports Medicine* 6: 246-256.

Kraemer, W.J., Dudley, G.A., Tesch, P.A., Gordon, S.E., Hather, B.M., Volek, J.S., and Ratamess, N.A. 2001. The influence of muscle action on the acute growth hormone response to resistance exercise and short-term detraining. *Growth Hormone and IGF Research* 11: 75-83.

Kraemer, W.J., Dunn-Lewis, C., Comstock, B.A., Thomas, G.A., Clark, J.E., and Nindl, B.C. 2010. Growth hormone, exercise, and athletic performance: A continued evolution of complexity. *Current Sports Medicine Reports* 9: 242-252.

Kraemer, W.J., Dziados, J.E., Marchitelli, L.J., Gordon, S.E., Harman, E.A., Mello, R., Fleck, S.J., Frykman, P.N., and Triplett, N.T. 1993. Effects of different heavy-resistance exercise protocols on plasma B-endorphin concentrations. *Journal of Applied Physiology* 74: 450-459.

Kraemer, W.J., and Fleck, S.J. 2007. *Optimizing strength training designing nonlinear periodization workouts,* Human Kinetics.

Kraemer, W.J., and Fleck S.J. 2005. *Strength training for young athletes,* 2nd ed. Champaign, IL: Human Kinetics.

Kraemer, W.J., Fleck, S.J., and Deschenes, M. 2012. *Exercise physiology integrating theory and application.* Lippincott, Williams and Wilkins, Baltmore, Maryland.

Kraemer, W.J., Fleck, S.J., Dziados, J.E., Harman, E., Marchitelli, L.J., Gordon, S.E., Mello, R., Frykman, P.N., Koziris, L.P., and Triplett, N.T. 1993. Changes in hormonal concentrations following different heavy resistance exercise protocols in women. *Journal of Applied Physiology* 75: 594-604.

Kraemer, W.J., Fleck, S.J., and Evans, W.J. 1996. Strength and power training: Physiological mechanisms of adaptation. In *Exercise and sport sciences reviews*, edited by J.O. Holoszy, 363-398. Baltimore: Williams & Wilkins.

Kraemer, W.J., Fleck, S.J., Maresh, C.M., Ratamess, N.A., Gordon, S.E., Goetz, K.L., Harman, E.A., Frykman, P.N., Volek, J., Mazzetti, S.A., Fry, A.C., Marchitelli, L.J., and Patton, J.F. 1999. Acute hormonal responses to a single bout of heavy resistance exercise in trained power lifters and untrained men. *Canadian Journal of Applied Physiology* 24: 524-537.

Kraemer, W.J., and Fry, A.C. 1995. Strength testing: Development and evaluation of methodology. In *Physiological assessment of human fitness*, edited by P. Maud and C. Foster. Champaign, IL: Human Kinetics.

Kraemer, W.J., Fry, A.C., Rubin, M.R., Triplett-McBride, T., Gordon, S.E., Koziris, L.P., Lynch, J.M., Volek, J.S., Meuffels, D.E., Newton, R.U., and Fleck, S.J. 2001. Physiological and performance responses to tournament wrestling. *Medicine & Science in Sports & Exercise* 33: 1367-1378.

Kraemer, W.J., Fry, A.C., Warren, B.J., Stone, M.H., Fleck, S.J., Kearney, J.T., Conroy, B.P., Maresh, C.M., Weseman, C.A., Triplett, N.T., and Gordon, S.E. 1992. Acute hormonal responses of elite junior weightlifters. *International Journal of Sports Medicine* 12: 228-235.

Kraemer, W.J., Gordon, S.E., Fleck, S.J., Marchitelli, L.J., Mello, R., Dziados, J.E., Friedl, K., Harman, E., Maresh, C., and Fry, A.C. 1991. Endogenous anabolic hormonal and growth factor responses to heavy resistance exercise in males and females. *International Journal of Sports Medicine* 12: 228-235.

Kraemer, W.J., and Gotshalk, L.A. 2000. Physiology of American football. In *Exercise and sport science*, edited by W.E. Garrett and D.T. Kirkendall, 798-813. Philadelphia: Lippincott Williams & Wilkins.

Kraemer, W.J., Häkkinen, K., Newton, R.U., McCormick, M., Nindl, B.C., Volek, J.S., Gotshalk, L.A., Fleck, S.J., Campbell, W.W., Gordon, S.E., Farrell, P.A., and Evans, W.J. 1998. Acute hormonal responses to heavy resistance exercise in younger and older men. *European Journal of Applied Physiology* 77: 206-211.

Kraemer, W.J., Häkkinen, K., Newton, R.U., Nindl, B.C., Volek, J.S., McCormick, M., Gotshalk, L.A., Gordon, S.E., Fleck, S.J., Campbell, W.W., Putukian, M., and Evans, W.J. 1999. Effects of heavy-resistance training on hormonal response patterns in younger vs. older men. *Journal of Applied Physiology* 87: 982-992.

Kraemer, W.J., Häkkinen, K., Triplett-McBride, N.T., Fry, A.C., Koziris, L.P., Ratamess, N.A., Bauer, J.E., Volek, J.S., McConnell, T., Newton, R.U., Gordon, S.E., Cummings, D., Hauth, J., Pullo, F., Lynch, J.M., Fleck, S.J., Mazzetti, S.A., and Knuttgen, H.G. 2003. Physiological changes with periodized resistance training in women tennis players. *Medicine & Science in Sports & Exercise* 35: 157-168.

Kraemer, W.J., Hatfield, D.L., Volek, J.S., Fragala, M.S., Vingren, J.L., Anderson, J.M., Spiering, B.A., Thomas, G.A., Ho, J.Y., Quann, E.E., Izquierdo, M., Häkkinen, K., and Maresh, C.M. 2009. Effects of amino acids supplement on physiological adaptations to resistance training. *Medicine & Science in Sports & Exercise* 41: 1111-1121.

Kraemer, R.R., Heleniak, R.J, Tryniecki, J.L, Kraemer, G.R, Okazaki, N.J., and Castracane, V.D. 1995. Follicular and luteal phase hormonal responses to low-volume resistive exercise. *Medicine & Science in Sports & Exercise* 27: 809-817.

Kraemer, W.J., Keuning, M., Ratamess, N.A., Volek, J.S., McCormick, M., Bush, J.A., Nindl, B.C., Gordon, S.E., Mazzetti, S.A., Newton, R.U., Gomez, A.L., Wickham, R.B., Rubin, M.R., and Häkkinen, K. 2001. Resistance training combined with bench-stepping enhances women's health profile. *Medicine & Science in Sports & Exercise* 33: 259-269.

Kraemer, W.J., and Koziris, L.P. 1992. Muscle strength training: Techniques and considerations. *Physical Therapy Practice* 2: 54-68.

Kraemer, W.J. and Koziris, L.P. 1994. Olympic weightlifting and power lifting. In *Physiology and Nutrition for Competitive Sport*, edited by D.R. Lamb, H.G. Knuttgen, and R. Murray 1-54. Cooper Publishing Group, Carmel, IN.

Kraemer, W.J., Koziris, L.P., Ratamess, N.A., Häkkinen, K., Triplett-McBride, N.T., Fry, A.C., Gordon, S.E., Volek, J.S., French, D.N., Rubin, M.R., Gomez, A.L., Sharman, M.J., Lynch, J.M., Izquierdo, M., and Fleck, S.J. 2002. Detraining produces minimal changes in physical performance and hormonal variables in recreationally strength-trained men. *Journal of Strength and Conditioning Research* 16: 373-382.

Kraemer, W.J., Loebel, C.C., Volek, J.S., Ratamess, N.A., Newton, R.U., Wickham, R.B., Gotshalk, L.A., Duncan, N.D., Mazzetti, S.A., Gomez, A.L., Rubin,

M.R., Nindl, B.C., and Häkkinen, K. 2001. The effect of heavy resistance exercise on the circadian rhythm of salivary testosterone in men. *European Journal of Applied Physiology* 84: 13-18.

Kraemer, W.J., Marchitelli, L., McCurry, D., Mello, R., Dziados, J.E., Harman, E., Frykman, P., Gordon, S.E., and Fleck, S.J. 1990. Hormonal and growth factor responses to heavy resistance exercise. *Journal of Applied Physiology* 69: 1442-1450.

Kraemer, W.J., Mazzetti, S.A., Nindl, B.C., Gotshalk, L.A., Volek, J.S., Bush, J.A., Marx, J.O., Dohi, K., Gomez, A.L., Miles, M., Fleck, S.J., Newton, R.U., and Häkkinen, K. 2001. Effect of resistance training on women's strength/power and occupational performances. *Medicine & Science in Sports & Exercise* 33: 1011-1025.

Kraemer, W.J., and Newton, R.U. 2000. Training for muscular power. *Physical and Medical Rehabilitation Clinics of North America* 11: 341-368.

Kraemer, W.J., Nindl, B.C., Marx, J.O., Gotshalk, L.A., Bush, J.A., Welsch, J.R., Volek, J.S., Spiering, B.A., Maresh, C.M., Mastro, A.M., and Hymer, W.C. 2006. Chronic resistance training in women potentiates growth hormone in vivo bioactivity: Characterization of molecular mass variants. *American Journal of Physiology: Endocrinology and Metabolism* 291: E1177-E1187.

Kraemer, W.J., Nindl, B.C., Ratamess, N.A., Gotshalk, L.A., Volek, J.S., Fleck, S.J., Newton, R.U., and Häkkinen, K. 2004. Changes in muscle hypertrophy in women with periodized resistance training. *Medicine & Science in Sports & Exercise* 36: 697-708.

Kraemer, W.J., Noble, B., Culver, B., and Lewis, R.V. 1985. Changes in plasma proenkephalin peptide F and catecholamine levels during graded exercise in men. *Proceedings of the National Academy of Sciences U S A.* 82: 6349-6351.

Kraemer, W.J., Noble, B.J., Culver, B.W., and Clark, M.J. 1987. Physiologic responses to heavy-resistance exercise with very short rest periods. *International Journal of Sports Medicine* 8: 247-252.

Kraemer, W.J., Patton, J., Gordon, S.E., Harman, E.A., Deschenes, M.R., Reynolds, K., Newton, R.U., Triplett, N.T., and Dziados, J.E. 1995. Compatibility of high intensity strength and endurance training on hormonal and skeletal muscle adaptations. *Journal of Applied Physiology* 78: 976-989.

Kraemer, W.J., and Ratamess, N.A. 2000. Physiology of resistance training: Current issues. In *Orthopaedic physical therapy clinics of North America: Exercise technologies* 9: 467-513. Philadelphia: W.B. Saunders.

Kraemer, W.J., and Ratamess, N.A. 2005. Hormonal responses and adaptations resistance exercise and training. *Sports Medicine* 35: 540-561.

Kraemer, W.J., and Ratamess, N.A. 2004. Fundamentals of resistance training: Progression and exercise prescription. *Medicine & Science in Sports & Exercise* 36: 674-678.

Kraemer, W.J., and Ratamess, N.A. 2005. Hormonal responses and adaptations to resistance exercise and training. *Sports Medicine* 35: 339-361.

Kraemer, W.J., Ratamess, N.A., Fry, A.C., and French, D.N. 2006. Strength training: Development and evaluation of methodology. In *Physiological assessment of human fitness,* edited by P.J. Maud and C. Foster, 119-150. Champaign, IL: Human Kinetics.

Kraemer, W.J., Ratamess, N., Fry, A.C., Triplett-McBride, T., Koziris, L.P., Bauer, J.A., Lynch, J.M., and Fleck, S.J. 2000. Influence of resistance training volume and periodization on physiological and performance adaptations in collegiate women tennis players. *American Journal of Sports Medicine* 28: 626-633.

Kraemer, W.J., Rubin, M.R., Häkkinen, K., Nindl, B.C., Marx, J.O., Volek, J.S., French, D.N., Gómez, A.L., Sharman, M.J., Scheett, T., Ratamess, N.A., Miles, M.P., Mastro, A., VanHeest, J., Maresh, C.M., Welsch, J.R., and Hymer, W.C. 2003. Influence of muscle strength and total work on exercise-induced plasma growth hormone isoforms in women. *Journal of Science and Medicine in Sport* 6: 295-306.

Kraemer, W.J., and Spiering, B.A. 2006. Skeletal muscle physiology: Plasticity and responses to exercise. *Hormone Research* 66: 2-16.

Kraemer, W.J., Spiering, B.A., Volek, J.S., Ratamess, N.A., Sharman, M.J., Rubin, M.R., French, D.N., Silvestre, R., Hatfield, D.L., Van Heest, J.L., Vingren, J.L., Judelson, D.A., Deschenes, M.R., and Maresh, C.M. 2006. Androgenic responses to resistance exercise: Effects of feeding and L-carnitine. *Medicine & Science in Sports & Exercise* 38: 1288-1296.

Kraemer, W.J., Staron, R.S., Hagerman, F.C., Hikida, R.S., Fry, A.C., Gordon, S.E., Nindl, B.C., Gotshalk, L.A., Volek, J.S., Marx, J.O., Newton, R.U., and Häkkinen, K. 1998. The effects of short-term resistance training on endocrine function in men and women. *European Journal of Applied Physiology* 78: 69-76.

Kraemer, W.J., Vingren, J.L., Schuenke, M.D., Kopchick, J.J., Volek, J.S., Fragala, M.S., Häkkinen, K.,

Jen-Ho, Thomas, G.A., and Staron, R.S. 2009. Effect of circulating growth hormone on muscle IGF-I protein concentration in female mice with growth hormone receptor gene disruption. *Growth Hormone and IGF Research* 19: 242-244.

Kraemer, W.J., Vogel, J.A., Patton, J.F., Dziados, J.E., and Reynolds, K.L. 1987. The effects of various physical training programs on short duration high intensity load bearing performance and the Army physical fitness test. *USARIEM Technical Report,* 30/87 August.

Kraemer, W.J., Volek, J.S., Bush, J.A., Putukian, M., and Sebastianelli, W.J. 1998. Hormonal responses to consecutive days of heavy-resistance exercise with or without nutritional supplementation. *Journal of Applied Physiology* 85: 1544-1555.

Kramer, J.B., Stone, M.H., O'Bryant, H.S., Conley, M.S., Johnson, R.L., Nieman, D.C., Honeycutt, D.R., and Hoke, T.P. 1997. Effects of single vs. multiple sets of weight training: Impact of volume, intensity, and variation. *Journal of Strength and Conditioning Research* 11: 143-147.

Krems, C., Luhrmann, P.M., Strassburg, A., Hartmann, B., and Neuhauser-Berthold, M. 2005. Lower resting metabolic rate in the elderly may not be entirely due to changes in body composition. *European Journal of Clinical Nutrition* 59: 255-262.

Krieger, J.W. 2009. Single versus multiple sets of resistance exercise: A meta-regression. *Journal of Strength and Conditioning Research* 23: 1890-1901.

Krieger, J.W. 2010. Single vs. multiple sets of resistance exercise for muscle hypertrophy: A meta-analysis. *Journal of Strength and Conditioning Research* 24: 1150-1159.

Kubiak, E.N., Klugman, J.A., and Bosco, J.A. 2006. Hand injuries in rock climbers. *Bulletin of the NYU Hospital for Joint Diseases* 64: 172-177.

Kubo, K., Ikebukuro, T., Maki, A., Yata, H., and Tsunoda, N. 2012. Time course of changes in the human Achilles tendon properties and metabolism during training and detraining in vivo. *European Journal of Applied Physiology* 12: 2679-2691.

Kubo, K., Ikebukro, I., Yata, H., Tsnoda, N., and Kanehisa, H. 2010. Time course of changes in muscle properties during strength training and detraining. *Journal of Strength and Conditioning Research* 24: 322-331.

Kubo, K., Kanehisa, H., Azuma, K., Ishizu, M., Kuno, S.Y., Okada, M., and Fukunaga, T. 2003. Muscle architectural characteristics in young and elderly men and women. *International Journal of Sports Medicine* 24: 125-130.

Kubo, K., Kanehisa, H., Ito, M., and Fukunaga, T. 2001. Effects of isometric training on the elasticity of human tendon structures in vivo. *Journal of Applied Physiology* 91: 26-32.

Kubo, K., Kanehisa, H., and Fukunaga, T. 2002. Effects of resistance and stretching training programmes on the viscoelastic properties of human tendon structures *in vivo. Journal of Physiology* 538: 219-226.

Kujala, U.M., Sarna, S., Kaprio, J., Tikkanen, H.O., and Koskenvuo, M. 2000. Natural selection to sports, later physical activity habits, and coronary heart disease. *British Journal of Sports Medicine* 34: 445-449.

Kumagai, K., Abe, T., Brechue, W.F., Ryushi, T., Takano, S., and Mizuno, M. 2000. Sprint performance is related to muscle fascicle length in male 100-m sprinters. *Journal of Applied Physiology* 88: 811-816.

Kusintz, I., and Kenney, C. 1958. Effects of progressive weight training on health and physical fitness of adolescent boys. *Research Quarterly* 29: 295-301.

Kvorning, T., Andersen, M., Brixen, K., and Madsen, K. 2006. Suppression of endogenous testosterone production attenuates the response to strength training: A randomized, placebo-controlled, and blinded intervention study. *American Journal of Physiology: Endocrinology and Metabolism* 291: E1325-E1332.

Kvorning, T., Andersen, M., Brixen, K., Schjerlin, P., Suetta, C., and Madsen, K. 2007. Suppression of testosterone does not blunt mRNA expression of myoD, myogenin, IGF, myostatin or androgen receptor post strength training in humans. *Journal of Physiology* 578: 579-593.

Kvorning, T., Bagger, M., Caserotti, P., and Madsen, K. 2006. Effects of vibration and resistance training on neural muscular and hormonal measures. *European Journal of Applied Physiology* 96: 615-625.

Lacerte, M., deLateur, B.J., Alquist, A.D., and Questad, K.A. 1992. Concentric versus combined concentric-eccentric isokinetic training programs: Effect on peak torque of human quadriceps femoris muscle. *Archives of Physical Medicine and Rehabilitation* 73: 1059-1062.

LaChance, P.F., and Hortobagyi, T. 1994. Influence of cadence on muscular performance during push-up and pull-up exercises. *Journal of Strength and Conditioning Research* 8: 76-79.

Laidlaw, D.H., Kornatz, K.W., Keen, D.A., Suzuki, S., and Enoka, R.M. 1999. Strength training improves the steadiness of slow lengthening contractions performed by old adults. *Journal of Applied Physiology* 87: 1786-1795.

Lamont, H.S., Cramer, J.T., Bemben, D.A., Shehab, R.L., Anderson, M.A., and Bemben, M.G. 2008. Effects of 6 weeks of periodized squat training with or without whole-body vibration on short-term adaptations in job performance within recreationally resistance trained men. *Journal of Strength and Conditioning Research* 22: 1882-1893.

Lamont, H.S., Cramer, J.T., Bemben, D.A., Shehab, R.L., Anderson, M.A., and Bemben, M.G. 2009. Effects of a 6-week periodized squat training program with or without whole-body vibration on jump height and power output following acute vibration exposure. *Journal of Strength and Conditioning Research* 23: 2317-2325.

Lamont, H.S., Cramer, J.T., Bemben, D.A., Shehab, R.L., Anderson, M.A., and Bemben, M.G. 2010. Effects of adding whole body vibration to squat training isometric force/time characteristics. *Journal of Strength and Conditioning Research* 24: 171-183.

Lander, J.E., Bates, B.T., Sawhill, J.A., and Hamill, J.A. 1985. Comparison between free-weight and isokinetic bench pressing. *Medicine & Science in Sports & Exercise* 17: 344-353.

Lander, J.E., Hundley, J.R., and Simonton, R.L. 1992. The effectiveness of weight-belts during multiple repetitions of the squat exercise. *Medicine & Science in Sports & Exercise* 24: 603-609.

Lander, J.E., Simonton, R., and Giacobbe, J. 1990. The effectiveness of weight-belts during the squat exercise. *Medicine & Science in Sports & Exercise* 22: 117-126.

Landers, K.A., Hunter, G.R., Wetzstein, C.J., Bamman, M.M., and Weisier, R.L. 2001. The interrelationship among muscle mass, strength, and the ability to perform physical tasks of daily living in younger and older women. *Journal of Gerontology: Biological Sciences, Medical Sciences* 56: B443-B448.

LaRoche, D.P., Lussier, M.V., and Roy, S.J. 2008. Chronic stretching and voluntary muscle force. *Journal of Strength and Conditioning Research* 22: 589-596.

Larsson, L. 1978. Morphological and functional characteristics of the aging skeletal muscle in man. *Acta Physiological Scandinavica* 457 (Suppl.): 1-36.

Larsson, L. 1982. Physical training effects on muscle morphology in sedentary males at different ages. *Medicine & Science in Sports & Exercise* 14: 203-206.

Larsson, L. 1983. Histochemical characteristics of human skeletal muscle during aging. *Acta Physiologica Scandinavica* 117: 469-471.

Larsson, L., Li, X., Yu, F., and Degens, H. 1997. Age-related changes in contractile properties and expression of myosin isoforms in single skeletal muscle cells. *Muscle Nerve* (Suppl.) 5: S74-S78.

Latham, N., Bennett, D., Stretton, C., and Anderson, C.S. 2004. Systematic review of progressive resistance strength training in older adults. *Journal of Gerontology* 59: M48-61.

Latham, N., and Liu, C.J. 2010. Strength training in older adults: The benefits for osteoarthritis. *Clinics in Geriatric Medicine* 26: 445-459.

Lathinghouse, L.H., and Trimble, M.H. 2000. Effects of isometric quadriceps activation on the q-angle in women before and after quadriceps exercise. *Journal of Orthopaedic and Sports Physical Therapy* 30: 211-216.

Laubach, L.L. 1976. Comparative muscular strength of men and women: A review of the literature. *Aviation, Space and Environmental Medicine* 47: 534-542.

Laurent, D., Reutenauer, H., Payen, J.F., Favre-Javin, A., Eterradossi, J., Lekas, J.F., and Rossi, A. 1992. Muscle bioenergetics in skiers: Studies using NMR. *International Journal of Sports Medicine* 13 (Suppl. 1): S150-S152.

Laurent, G.J., Sparrow, M.P., Bates, P.C., and Millward, D.J. 1978. Collagen content and turnover in cardiac and skeletal muscles of the adult fowl and the changes during stretch induced growth. *Biochemistry Journal* 176: 419-427.

Laurentino, G., Ugrinowitsch, C., Aihara, A.Y., Fernandes, A.R., Parcell, A.C., Ricard, M., and Tricoli, V. 2008. Effects of strength training and vascular occlusion. *International Journal of Sports Medicine* 29: 664-667.

Laurentino, G.C., Ugrinowitsch, C., Roschel, H., Aoki, M.S., Soares, A.G., Neves, M., Aihara, A.Y., Da Rocha Correa Fernandes, A., and Tricoli, V. 2012. Strength training with blood flow restriction diminishes myostatin gene expression. *Medicine & Science in Sports & Exercise* 44: 406-412.

Laursen, P.B., and Jenkins, D.G. 2002. The scientific basis for high-intensity interval training: Optimizing training programs and maximizing performance in highly trained endurance athletes. *Sports Medicine* 32: 53-73.

LaVelle, D.G. 2003. Fractures of hip. In *Campbell's operative orthopaedics*, edited by S.T. Canale, 10th ed., 2873. Philadelphia: Mosby.

Lawton, T.W., Cronin, J.B., Drinkwater, E., Lindsell, R., and Pyne, D. 2004. The effect of continuous repetition training and intra-set rest training on bench press strength and power. *Journal of Sports Medicine and Physical Fitness* 44: 361-367.

Lawton, T.W., Cronin, J.B., and Lindsell, R.P. 2006. Effect of interrepetition rest period on weight training repetition power output. *Journal of Strength and Conditioning Research* 20: 172-176.

Laycoe, R.R., and Marteniuk, R.G. 1971. Leaning and tension as factors in strength gains produced by static and eccentric training. *Research Quarterly* 42: 299-305.

Layne, J.E., and Nelson, M.E. 1999. The effects of progressive resistance training on bone density: A review. *Medicine & Science in Sports & Exercise* 31: 25-30.

Lebenstedt, M., Platte, P., and Pirke, K.M. 1999. Reduced resting metabolic rate in athletes with menstrual disorders. *Medicine & Science in Sports & Exercise* 31: 1250-1256.

LeBrasseur, N.K., Walsh, K., and Arany, Z. 2011. Metabolic benefits of resistance training and fast glycolytic skeletal muscle. *American Journal of Physiology, Endocrinology and Metabolism* 300: E3-E10.

Lebrun, C.M. 1994. The effect of the phase of the menstrual cycle and the birth control pill on athletic performance. *Clinics in Sports Medicine* 13: 419-441.

Lee, A., Craig, B.W., Lucas, J., Pohlman, R., and Stelling, H. 1990. The effect of endurance training, weight training and a combination of endurance and weight training on blood lipid profile of young males subjects. *Journal of Applied Sport Science Research* 4: 68-75.

Lee, M.R., and Berthelot, E.R. 2010. Community covariates of malnutrition based mortality among older adults. *Annals of Epidemiology* 20: 371-379.

Legwold, G. 1982. Does lifting weights harm a prepubescent athlete? *Physician and Sportsmedicine* 10: 141-144.

Leiger, A.B., and Milner, T.E. 2001. Muscle function at the wrist after eccentric exercise. *Medicine & Science in Sports & Exercise* 33: 612-620.

Leighton, J. 1955. Instrument and technique for measurement of range of joint motion. *Archives of Physical Medicine and Rehabilitation* 38: 24-28.

Leighton, J. 1957. Flexibility characteristics of three specialized skill groups of champion athletes. *Archives of Physical Medicine and Rehabilitation* 38: 580-583.

Leighton, J.R., Holmes, D., Benson, J., Wooten, B., and Schmerer, R. 1967. A study of the effectiveness of ten different methods of progressive resistance exercise on the development of strength, flexibility, girth and body weight. *Journal of the Association of Physical and Mental Rehabilitation* 21: 78-81.

Leite, R.D., Prestes, J., Pereira, G.B., Shiguemoto, G.E., and Perez, S.E. 2010. Menopause: Highlighting the effects of resistance training. *International Journal of Sports Medicine* 31: 761-767.

Lemmer, J.T., Hurlbut, D.E., Martel, G.F., Tracy, B.L., Ivey, F.M., Metter, E.J., Fozard, J.L., Fleg, J.L., and Hurley, B.F. 2000. Age and gender responses to strength training and detraining. *Medicine & Science in Sports & Exercise* 32: 1505-1512.

Lemmer, J.T., Ivey, F.M., Ryan, A.S., Martel, G.F., Hurlbut, D.E., Metter, J.E., Fozard, J.L., Fleg, J.L., and Hurley, B.F. 2001. Effect of strength training on resting metabolic rate and physical activity: Age and gender comparisons. *Medicine & Science in Sports & Exercise* 33: 532-541.

Lemmer, J.T., Martel, G.F., Hurlbut, D.E., and Hurley, B.F. 2007. Age and sex differentially affect regional changes in one repetition maximum strength. *Journal of Strength and Conditioning Research* 21: 731-737.

Lemon, P.W., and Mullin, J.P. 1980. Effect of initial muscle glycogen levels on protein catabolism during exercise. *Journal of Applied Physiology: Respiratory, Environmental and Exercise Physiology* 48: 624-629.

LeMura, L.M., von Duvillard, S.P., Andreacci, J., Klebez, J.M., Chelland, S.A., and Russo, J. 2000. Lipid and lipoprotein profiles, cardiovascular fitness, body composition, and diet during and after resistance, aerobic and combination training in young women. *European Journal of Applied Physiology* 82: 451-458.

Lepley, A.S., Gribble, P.A., and Pietrosimone, B.G. 2011. Effects of electromyographic biofeedback on quadriceps strength: A systematic review. *Journal of Strength and Conditioning* 26: 873-882.

Lesmes, G.R., Costill, D.L., Coyle, E.F., and Fink, W.J. 1978. Muscle strength and power changes during maximal isokinetic training. *Medicine & Science in Sports & Exercise* 4: 266-269.

Levin, G.T., McGuigan, M.R., and Laursen, P.B. 2009. Effect of concurrent resistance and endurance training on physiologic and performance parameters of well-trained endurance cyclists. *Journal of Strength and Conditioning Research* 23: 2280-2286.

Lewis, S., Nygaard, E., Sanchez, J., Egelbald, H., and Saltin, B. 1984. Static contraction of the quadriceps muscle in man: Cardiovascular control and responses to one-legged strength training. *Acta Physiologica Scandinavica* 122: 341-353.

Lexell, J., Hendriksson-Larsen, K., Winblad, B., and Sjostrom, M. 1983. Distribution of different fiber types in human skeletal muscles: Effects of aging studied in whole muscle cross section. *Muscle Nerve* 6: 588-595.

Lexell, J., Taylor, C.C., and Sjostrom, M. 1988. What is the cause of the ageing atrophy? Total number, size and proportion of different fiber types studied in whole vastus lateralis muscle from 15- to 83-year-old men. *Journal of Neurological Sciences* 84: 275-294.

Liederman, E. 1925. *Secrets of strength*. New York: Earle Liederman.

Li, R.C., Maffulli, N., Hsu, T.C., and Chan, K.M. 1996. Isokinetic strength of the quadriceps and hamstrings and functional ability of anterior cruciate deficient knees in recreation athletes. *British Journal of Sports Medicine* 30: 161-164.

Lind, A.R., and Petrofsky, J.S. 1978. Isometric tension from rotary stimulation of fast and slow cat muscles. *Muscle and Nerve* 1: 213-218.

Lindh, M. 1979. Increase of muscle strength from isometric quadriceps exercises at different knee angles. *Scandinavian Journal of Rehabilitation Medicine* 11: 33-36.

Linnamo, V., Pakarinen, A., Komi, P.V., Kraemer, W.J., and Häkkinen, K. 2005. Acute hormonal responses to submaximal and maximal heavy resistance and explosive exercises in men and women. *Journal of Strength and Conditioning Research* 19: 566-571.

Linsenbardt, S.T., Thomas, T.R., and Madsen, R.W. 1992. Effect of breathing technique on blood pressure response to resistance exercise. *British Journal of Sports Medicine* 26: 97-100.

Lithinghouse, L.H., and Trimble, M.H. 2000. Effects of isometric quadriceps activation on the q-angle in women before and after quadriceps exercise. *Journal of Orthopedic and Sports Physical Therapy* 20: 211-230.

Liu, H., Liu, P., and Qin, X. 1987. *Investigation of menstrual cycle and female weightlifters*. Beijing: Department of Exercise Physiology, National Institute of Sports Science.

Lo, M.S., Lin, L.L.C., Yao, W-J., and Ma, M-C. 2011 Training and detraining effects of the resistance vs. endurance program on body composition, body size, and physical performance in young men. *Journal of Strength and Conditioning Research* 25: 2246-2254.

Lockie, R.G., Murphy, A.J., Schultz, A.B., Knight, T.J., and Janse de Jonge, X.A.K. 2012. The effects of different speed training protocols on sprint acceleration kinematics and muscle strength and power in feel sport athletes. *Journal of Strength and Conditioning Research* 26: 1539-1550.

Loenneke, J.P., Wilson, J.M., Wilson, G.J., Pujol, T.J., and Bemben, M.G. 2011. Potential safety issues with blood flow restriction training. *Scandinavian Journal of Medicine & Science in Sports* 21: 510-518.

Lohman, T. 2004. The BEST exercise program for osteoporosis prevention. DSW Fitness. www.dswfitness.com.

Lloyd, T., Buchanan, J.R., Bitzer, S., Waldman, C.J., Myers, C., and Ford, B.G. 1987. Interrelationship of diet, athletic activity, menstrual status and bone density in collegiate women. *American Journal of Clinical Nutrition* 46: 681-684.

Lombardi, V.P., and Troxel, R.K. 1999. Weight training injuries and deaths in the U.S. *Medicine & Science in Sports & Exercise* 31: S93.

Lord, S.R., Ward, J.A., Williams, P., and Anstey, K.J. 1993. An epidemiological study of falls in older community-dwelling women: The Randwick falls and fractures study. *Australian and New Zealand Journal of Public Health* 17: 240-245.

Losnegard, T., Mikkelsen, K., Rønnestad, B.R., Hallén, J., Rud, B., and Raastad, T. 2011. The effect of heavy strength training on muscle mass and physical performance in elite cross country skiers. *Scandinavian Journal of Medicine & Science in Sports* 21: 389-401.

Loucks, A.B., and Horvath, S.M. 1985. Athletic amenorrhea: A review. *Medicine & Science in Sports & Exercise* 17: 56-72.

Loucks, A.B., Kiens, B., and Wright, H.H. 2011. Energy availability in athletes. *Journal of Sports Science* 29: S7-15.

Ludbrook, J., Faris, I.B., Iannos, J., Jamieson, G.G., and Russel, W.J. 1978. Lack of effect of isometric handgrip exercise on the responses of the carotid sinus baroreceptor reflex in man. *Clinical Science and Molecular Medicine* 55: 189-194.

Luhrmann, P.M., Bender, R., Edelmann-Schafer, B., and Neuhauser-Berthold, M. 2009. Longitudinal changes in energy expenditure in an elderly German population: A 12-year follow-up. *European Journal of Clinical Nutrition* 63: 986-992.

Lund, H., Vestergaard-Poulsen, P., Kanstrup, I.-L., and Sejr-sen, P. 1998. The effect of passive stretching on delayed onset muscle soreness, and other detrimental effects following eccentric exercise. *Scandinavian Journal of Medicine & Science in Sports* 8: 216-221.

Lundberg, T.R., Fernandez-Gonzalo, R., Gustafsson, T., and Tesch, P.A. 2012. Aerobic exercise alters skeletal muscle molecular responses to resistance exercise. *Medicine & Science in Sports & Exercise* 44:1680-1688.

Lusiani, L., Ronsisvalle, G., Bonanome, A., Castellani, V., Macchia, C., and Pagan, A. 1986. Echocardiographic evaluation of the dimensions and systolic properties of the left ventricle in freshman athletes during physical training. *European Heart Journal* 7: 196-203.

Lusk, S.J., Hale, B.D., and Russell, D.M. 2010. Grip width and forearm orientation effects on muscle activity during the lat pull-down. *Journal of Strength and Conditioning Research*. 16: 539-546.

Luthi, J.M., Howald, H., Claassen, H., Rosler, K., Vock, P., and Hoppler, H. 1986. Structural changes in skeletal muscle tissue with heavy-resistance exercise. *International Journal of Sports Medicine* 7: 123-127.

Lyle, N., and Rutherford, O.M. 1998. A comparison of voluntary versus stimulated strength training of the human abductor pollicis muscle. *Journal Sports Sciences* 16: 267-270.

Lyman, S., Fleisig, G.S., Waterbor, J.W., Funkhouser, E.M., Pulley, L., Andrews, J.R., Osiniki, E.D., and Roseman, J.M. 2001. Longitudinal study of elbow and shoulder pain in youth baseball pitchers. *Medicine & Science in Sports & Exercise* 33: 1803-1810.

Lynch, N.A., Metter, E.J., Lindle, R.S., Fozard, J.L., Tobin, J.D., Roy, T.A., Fleg, J.L., and Hurley, B.F. 1999. Muscle quality. I. Age associated differences between arm and leg muscle groups. *Journal of Applied Physiology* 86: 188-194.

Macaluso, A., De Vitto, G., Felici, F., and Nimmo, M.A. 2000. Electromyogram changes during sustained contraction after resistance training in women in their 3rd and 8th decades. *European Journal of Applied Physiology* 82: 418-424.

MacDonald, C.J., Lamont, H.S., and Garner, J.C. 2012. A comparison of the effects of 6 weeks of traditional resistance training, biometric training, and complex training on measures of strength and anthropometrics. *Journal of Strength and Conditioning Research* 26: 422-431.

MacDonald, J.R. 2002. Potential causes, mechanisms, and implications of post exercise hypotension. *Journal of Human Hypertension* 16: 225-236.

MacDougall, J.D. 1986. Adaptability of muscle to strength training—A cellular approach. In *Biochemistry of exercise* 6th ed. 501-513. Champaign, IL: Human Kinetics.

MacDougall, J.D. 1992. Hypertrophy or hyperplasia. In *Strength and power in sport*, edited by P.V. Komi, 230-238. Oxford: Blackwell Scientific.

MacDougall, J.D., Gibala, M.J., Tarnopolsky, M.A., MacDonald, J.R., Interisano, S.A., and Yarasheski, K.E. 1995. The time course for elevated muscle protein synthesis following heavy resistance exercise. *Canadian Journal of Applied Physiology* 20: 480-486.

MacDougall, J.D., Sale, D.G., Alway, S.E., and Sutton, J.R. 1984. Muscle fiber number in biceps brachii in bodybuilders and control subjects. *Journal of Applied Physiology* 57: 1399-1403.

MacDougall, J.D., Sale, D.G., Elder, G.C.B., and Sutton, J.R. 1982. Muscle ultrastructural characteristics of elite powerlifters and bodybuilders. *European Journal of Applied Physiology* 48: 117-126.

MacDougall, J.D., Sale, D.G., Moroz, J.R., Elder, G.C.B., Sutton, J.R., and Howald, H. 1979. Mitochondrial volume density in human skeletal muscle following heavy resistance training. *Medicine & Science in Sports & Exercise* 11: 164-166.

MacDougall, J.D., Tarnopolsky, M.A., Chesley, A., and Atkinson, S.A. 1992. Changes in muscle protein synthesis following heavy resistance exercise in humans: A pilot study. *Acta Physiologica Scandinavica* 146: 403-404.

MacDougall, J.D., Tuxen, D., Sale, D.G., Moroz, J.R., and Sutton, J.R. 1985. Arterial blood pressure response to heavy resistance exercise. *Journal of Applied Physiology* 58: 785-790.

MacDougall, J.D., Ward, G.R., Sale, D.G., and Sutton, J.R. 1977. Biochemical adaptations of human skeletal muscle to heavy resistance training and immobilization. *Journal of Applied Physiology* 43: 700-703.

MacKelvie, K.J., Taunton, J.E., McKay, H.A., and Khan, K.M. 2000. Bone mineral density and serum testosterone in chronically trained, high mileage 40-55-year-old male runners. *British Journal of Sports Medicine* 34: 273-278.

Madsen, N., and McLaughlin, T. 1984. Kinematic factors influencing performance and injury risk in the bench press exercise. *Medicine & Science in Sports & Exercise* 16: 429-437.

Maestu, J., Eliakim, A., Jurima, J., Valter, I., and Jurima, T. 2010. Anabolic and catabolic hormones and energy balance of the male bodybuilders during the preparation for competition. *Journal of Strength and Conditioning Research* 24: 1074-1081.

Maffiuletti, N.A., and Martin, A. 2001. Progressive versus rapid rate of contraction during 7 wk of isometric resistance training. *Medicine & Science in Sports & Exercise* 33: 1220-1227.

Magnusson, S.P. 1998. Passive properties of human skeletal muscle during stretch maneuvers: A review. *Scandinavian Journal of Medicine & Science in Sports* 8: 65-77.

Magnusson, S.P., Aagaard, P., and Nielson, J.J. 2000. Passive energy return after repeated stretches on the hamstring muscle-tendon unit. *Medicine & Science in Sports & Exercise* 32: 1160-1164.

Magnusson, S.P., Hansen, M., Langberg, H., Miller, B., Haraldsson, B., Westh, E.K., Koskinen, S., Aagaard, P., and Kjaer, M. 2007. The adaptability of tendon to loading differs in men and women. *International Journal of Experimental Pathology* 88: 237-240.

Magnusson, S.P., Narici, M.V., Maganaris, C.N., and Kjaer, M. 2008. Human tendon behaviour and adaptation, in vivo. *Journal of Physiology* 586: 71-81.

Maguire, M.S., Gabaree, C.L., and Hoffman, J.R. 1992. Oxygen consumption following exercise of moderate intensity and duration. *European Journal of Applied Physiology* 65: 421-426.

Mahieu, N.N., McNair, P., De Muynck, M., Stevens, V., Blanckaert, I., Smits, N., and Witvrouw, E. 2007. Effect of static and ballistic stretching on the muscle-tendon tissue properties. *Medicine & Science in Sports & Exercise* 39: 494-501.

Mair, J., Mayr, M., Muller, E., Koller, A., Haid, C., Artner-Dworzak, E., Calzolari, C., Larue, C., and Pushchendorf, B. 1995. Rapid adaptation to eccentric exercise-induced muscle damage. *International Journal of Sports Medicine* 16: 352-356.

Malina, R. 2006. Weight training in youth—growth, maturation and safety: An evidence-based review. *Clinical Journal of Sports Medicine* 16: 478-487.

Manal, K., Roberts, D.P., and Buchanan, T.S. 2008. Can pennation angles be predicted from EMGs for the primary ankle plantar and dorsi flexors during isometric contractions? *Journal of Biomechanics* 41: 2492-2497.

Mangine, G.T., Ratamess, N.A., Hoffman, J.R., Faigenbaum, A.D., Kang, J., and Chilakos, A. 2008. The effects of combined ballistic and heavy resistance training on maximal lower- and upper-body strength in recreationally trained men. *Journal of Strength and Conditioning Research* 22: 132-139.

Mangus, B.C., Takahashi, M., Mercer, J.A., Holcomb, W.R., McWhorter, J.W., and Sanchez, R. 2006. Investigation of vertical jump performance after completing heavy squat exercises. *Journal of Strength and Conditioning Research* 20: 597-600.

Manni, T.M., and Clark, B.C. 2009. Blood flow restricted exercise and skeletal muscle health. *Exercise and Sport Sciences Reviews* 37: 78-85.

Manning, R.J., Graves, J.E., Carpenter, D.M., Leggett, S.H., and Pollock, M.L. 1990. Constant vs. variable resistance knee extension training. *Medicine & Science in Sports & Exercise* 22: 397-401.

Mannion, A.F., Jakeman, P.M., and Willan, P.L.T. 1992. Effect of isokinetic training of the knee extensors on isokinetic strength and peak power output during cycling. *European Journal of Applied Physiology* 65: 370-375.

Manore, M.M., Thompson, J., and Russo, M. 1993. Diet and exercise strategies of a world-class bodybuilder. *International Journal of Sports Medicine* 3: 76-86.

Marcinek, D.J., Kushmerick, M.J., and Conley, K.E. 2010. Lactic acidosis in vivo: Testing the link between lactate generation and H+ accumulation in ischemic mouse muscle. *Journal of Applied Physiology* 108: 1479-1486.

Marcinik, E.J., Potts, J., Schlabach, G., Will, S., Dawson, P., and Hurley, B.F. 1991. Effects of strength training on lactate threshold and endurance performance. *Medicine & Science in Sports & Exercise* 23: 739-743.

Marcus, R. 2002. Mechanisms of exercise effects on bone. In *Principles of bone biology*, edited by J.P. Bilezikian et al., 2nd ed., 1477-1488. San Diego, CA: Academic Press.

Markovic, G. 2007. Does plyometric training improve vertical jump height? A meta-analytical review. *British Journal of Sports Medicine* 41: 349-355.

Maresh, C.M., Abraham, A., DeSouza, M.J., Deschenes, M.R., Kraemer, W.J., Armstrong, L.E., Maresh, C.M., Allison, T.G., Noble, B.J., Drash, A., and Kraemer,

W.J. 1989. Substrate and endocrine responses to race-intensity exercise following a marathon run. *International Journal of Sports Medicine* 10: 101-106.

Marin, P.J., and Rhea, M.R. 2010. Effects of vibration training on muscle strength: A meta-analysis. *Journal of Strength and Conditioning Research* 24: 548-556.

Markiewitz, A.D., and Andrish, J.T. 1992. Hand and wrist injuries in the preadolescent athlete. *Clinics in Sports Medicine* 11: 203-225.

Markovic, G., Simek, S., and Bradic, A. 2008. Are acute effects of maximal dynamic contractions on upper-body ballistic performance load specific? *Journal of Strength and Conditioning Research* 22: 1811-1815.

Marques, M.C., and Gonzalez-Badillo, J.J. 2006. In-season resistance training and detraining in professional team handball players. *Journal of Strength and Conditioning Research* 20: 563-571.

Marshall, P.W.M., and Desai, I. 2010. Electromyographic analysis of upper body, lower body, and abdominal muscles during advanced Swiss ball exercises. *Journal of Strength and Conditioning Research* 24: 1537-1545.

Marshall, P.W., McEwen, M., and Robbins, D.W. 2011. Strength and neuromuscular adaptation following one, four, and eight sets of high intensity resistance exercise in trained males. *European Journal of Applied Physiology* 111: 3007-3016.

Marshall, P.W.M., and Murphy, B.A. 2006. Increased deltoid and abdominal muscle activity during Swiss ball bench press. *Journal of Strength and Conditioning Research* 20: 745-750.

Martin, A., Martin, I., and Morlon, B. 1995. Changes induced by eccentric training on force-velocity relationships of the elbow flexor muscles. *European Journal of Applied Physiology* 72: 183-185.

Martyn-St. James, M., and Carroll, S. 2010. Effects of different impact exercise modalities on bone mineral density in premenopausal women: A meta-analysis. *Journal of Bone Mineral Metabolism* 28: 251-267.

Marx, J.O., Ratamess, N.A., Nindl, B.C., Gotshalk, L.A., Volek, J.S., Dohi, K., Bush, J.A., Gomez, A.L., Mazzetti, S.A., Fleck, S.J., Häkkinen, K., Newton, R.U., and Kraemer, W.J. 2001. Low-volume circuit versus high-volume periodized resistance training in women. *Medicine & Science in Sports & Exercise* 33: 635-643.

Massey, B.H., and Chaudet, N.L. 1956. Effects of heavy resistance exercise on range of joint movement in young male adults. *Research Quarterly* 27: 41-51.

Massey, C.D., Vincent, J., Maneval, M., Moore, M., and Johnson, J.T. 2004. An analysis of full range of motion vs. partial range of motion training into development of strength in untrained men. *Journal of Strength and Conditioning Research* 18: 518-521.

Massey, C.D., Vincent, J., Maneval, M., Moore, M., and Johnson, J.T. 2005. Influence of range of motion in resistance training in women: Early phase adaptations. *Journal of Strength and Conditioning Research* 19: 409-411.

Masterson, G. 1999. The impact of menstrual phases on anaerobic power performance in collegiate women. *Journal of Strength and Conditioning Research* 13: 325-329.

Masterson, G.L., and Brown, S.P. 1993. Effects of weighted rope jump training on power performance tests in collegians. *Journal of Strength and Conditioning Research* 7: 108-114.

Masuda, K., Choi, J.Y., Shimojo, H., and Katsuta, S. 1999. Maintenance of myoglobin concentration in human skeletal muscle after heavy resistance training. *European Journal of Applied Physiology* 79: 347-352.

Matavulj, D., Kukolj, M., Ugarkovic, D., Tihanyi, J., and Jaric, S. 2001. Effects of plyometric training on jumping performance in junior basketball players. *Journal of Sports Medicine and Physical Fitness* 41: 159-164.

Matheny, R.W., Jr., Nindl, B.C., and Adamo, M.L. 2010. Minireview: Mechano-growth factor: A putative product of IGF-I gene expression involved in tissue repair and regeneration. *Endocrinology* 151: 865-875.

Matheson, J.W., Kernozek, T.W., Fater, D.C., and Davies, G.J. 2001. Electromyographic activity and applied load during seated quadriceps exercises. *Medicine & Science in Sports & Exercise* 33: 1713-1725.

Matsakas, A., and Patel, K. 2009. Intracellular signaling pathways regulating the adaptation of skeletal muscle to exercise and nutritional changes. *Histology and Histopathology* 24: 209-222.

Maud, R.J., and Shultz, B.B. 1986. Gender comparisons and anaerobic power and anaerobic capacity tests. *British Journal of Sports Medicine* 20: 51-54.

Maughan, R.J., Harmon, M., Leiper, J.B., Sale, D., and Delman, A. 1986. Endurance capacity of untrained males and females in isometric and dynamic muscular contractions. *European Journal of Applied Physiology* 55: 395-400.

Mayhew, J.L., Ball, T.E., and Bowen, J.C. 1992. Prediction of bench press ability from submaximal repetitions before and after training. *Sports Medicine Training and Rehabilitation* 3: 195-201.

Mayhew, J., Bemben, M., Rohrs, D., et al. 1994. Specificity among anaerobic power tests in college female athletes. *Journal of Strength and Conditioning Research* 8: 43-47.

Mayhew, J.L., and Gross, P.M. 1974. Body composition changes in young women with high intensity weight training. *Research Quarterly* 45: 433-440.

Mayhew, J.L., and Salm, P.C. 1990. Gender differences and anaerobic power tests. *European Journal of Applied Physiology* 60: 133-138.

Maynard, J., and Ebben, W.P. 2003. The effects of antagonist prefatigue on agonist torque and electromyography. *Journal of Strength and Conditioning Research* 17: 469-474.

Mazzetti, S.A., Kraemer, W.J., Volek, J.S., Duncan, N.D., Ratamess, N.A., Gómez, A.L., Newton, R.U., Häkkinen, K., and Fleck, S.J. 2000. The influence of direct supervision of resistance training on strength performance. *Medicine & Science in Sports & Exercise* 32: 1043-1050.

Mazzetti, S.A., Ratamess, N.A., and Kraemer, W.J. 2000. Pumping down: After years of bulking up, when they graduate, strength-trained athletes must be shown how to safely detrain. *Training and Conditioning* 10: 10-13.

McBride, J.M., Larkin, T.R., Dayne, A.M., Haines, T.L., and Kirby, T.J. 2010. Effect of absolute and relative loading on muscle activity during stable and unstable squatting. *International Journal Sports Physiology and Performance* 5: 177-183.

McBride, J.M., Nuzzo, J.L., Dayne, A.M., Israetel, M.A., Nieman, D.C., and Triplett, N.T. 2010. Effect of an acute bout of whole body vibration exercise on muscle force output and motor neuron excitability. *Journal of Strength and Conditioning Research* 24:184-189.

McBride, J.M., Triplett-McBride, T., Davie, A., and Newton, R.U. 1999. A comparison of strength and power characteristics between power lifters, Olympic lifters, and sprinters. *Journal of Strength and Conditioning Research* 13: 58-66.

McBride, J.M., Triplett-McBride, T., Davie, A., and Newton, R.U. 2002. The effect of heavy- vs light-load jump squats on the development of strength, power, and speed. *Journal of Strength and Conditioning Research* 16: 75-82.

McCall, G.E., Byrnes, W.C., Dickinson, A., Pattany, P.M., and Fleck, S.J. 1996. Muscle fiber hypertrophy, hyperplasia, and capillary density in college men after resistance training. *Journal of Applied Physiology* 81: 2004-2012.

McCall, G.E., Byrnes, W.C., Fleck, S.J., Dickinson, A., and Kraemer, W.J. 1999. Acute and chronic hormonal responses to resistance training designed to promote muscle hypertrophy. *Canadian Journal of Applied Physiology* 24: 96-107.

McCall, G.E., Grindeland, R.E., Roy, R.R., and Edgerton, V.R. 2000. Muscle afferent activity modulates bioassayable growth hormone in human plasma. *Journal of Applied Physiology* 89: 1137-1141.

McCann, M.R., and Flanagan, S.P. 2010. The effects of exercise selection and rest interval on postactivation potentiation of vertical jump performance. *Journal of Strength and Conditioning Research* 25: 1285-1291.

McCarrick, M.J., and Kemp, J.G. 2000. The effect of strength training and reduced training on rotator cuff musculature. *Clinical Biomechanics* 15 (Suppl. 1): S42-S45.

McCarthy, J.P., Agre, J.C., Graf, B.K., Poziniak, M.A., and Vailas, A.C. 1995. Compatibility of adaptive responses with combining strength and endurance training. *Medicine & Science in Sports & Exercise* 27: 429-436.

McCartney, N., McKelvie, R.S., Martin, J., Sale, D.G., and MacDougall, J.D. 1993. Weight-training induced attenuation of the circulatory response of older males to weight lifting. *Journal of Applied Physiology* 74: 1056-1060.

McCurdy, K., Langford, G., Jenkerson, D., and Doscher, M. 2008. The validity and reliability of the one RM bench press using chain-loaded resistance. *Journal of Strength and Conditioning Research* 22: 678-683.

McDonagh, M.J.N., and Davies, C.T.M. 1984. Adaptive response of mammalian skeletal muscle to exercise with high loads. *European Journal of Applied Physiology* 52: 139-155.

McDonagh, M.J.N., Hayward, C.M., and Davies, C.T.M. 1983. Isometric training in human elbow flexor muscles. *Journal of Bone and Joint Surgery* 65: 355-358.

McDowell, M.A., Fryar, C.D., Ogden, C.L., and Flegal, K.M. 2008. Anthropometric reference data for children and adults: United States, 2003-2006. *National Health Statistics Reports* 10: 1-44.

McGee, D., Jessee, T.C., Stone, M.H., and Blessing, D. 1992. Leg and hip endurance adaptations to three weight-training programs. *Journal of Applied Sports Science Research* 6: 92-95.

McGuigan, M.R., Tatasciore, M., Newton, R.U., and Pettigrew, S. 2009. Eight weeks of resistance training can significantly alter body composition in children who are overweight or obese. *Journal of Strength and Conditioning Research* 23: 80-85.

McHugh, M.P., and Cosgrave, C.H. 2010. To stretch or not to stretch: The role of stretching in injury prevention and performance. *Scandinavian Journal of Medicine & Science in Sports* 20: 169-181.

McHugh, M.P., Tyler, T.F., Greenberg, S.C., and Gleim, G. 2002. Differences in activation patterns between eccentric and concentric quadriceps contractions. *Journal of Sports Sciences* 20: 83-91.

McKenna, M.J., Harmer, A.R., Fraser, S.F., and Li, J.L. 1996. Effects of training on potassium, calcium and hydrogen ion regulation in skeletal muscle and blood during exercise. *Acta Physiologica Scandinavica* 156: 335-346.

McLellan, C.P., Lovell, D.I., and Gass, G.C., 2011. Markers of postmatch fatigue in professional Rugby League players. *Journal of Strength and Conditioning Research* 25: 1030-1039.

McLoughlin, P., McCaffrey, N., and Moynihan, J.B. 1991. Gentle exercise with previously inactive muscle group hastens the decline of blood lactate concentration after strenuous exercise. *European Journal of Applied Physiology* 62: 274-278.

McLaughlin, T.M., Dillman, C.J., and Lardner, T.J. 1977. A kinematic model of performance of the parallel squat. *Medicine and Science in Sports* 9: 128-133.

McLester, J.R., Bishop, P., and Guilliams, M.E. 2000. Comparison of 1 day and 3 days per week of equal volume resistance training in experienced subjects. *Journal of Strength and Conditioning Research* 14: 273-281.

McMorris, R.O., and Elkins, E.C. 1954. A study of production and evaluation of muscular hypertrophy. *Archives of Physical Medicine and Revocation* 35: 420-426.

McNair, P.J., Dombroski, E.W., Hewson, D.J., and Stanley, S.N. 2001. Stretching at the ankle joint: Viscoelastic response to holds and continuous passive motion. *Medicine & Science in Sports & Exercise* 33: 354-358.

McNamara, J.M., and Stearne, D.J. 2010. Flexible nonlinear periodization and beginner college weight training class. *Journal of Strength and Conditioning Research* 24: 17-22.

Melo, C.M., Alencar-Filho, A.C., Tinucci, T., Mion, J.D., and Forjaz, C.L.M. 2006. Postexercise hypotension induced by low-intensity resistance exercise in hypertensive women receiving captopril. *Blood Pressure Monitoring* 11: 183-189.

Meltzer, D.E. 1994. Age dependence of Olympic weightlifting ability. *Medicine & Science in Sports & Exercise* 26: 1053-1067.

Mendelsohn, F.A., and Warren, M.P. 2010. Anorexia, bulimia, and the female athlete triad: Evaluation and management. *Endocrinology & Metabolism Clinics of North America* 39: 155-167.

Mendez, E. 2010, December 6. In U.S., obesity peaks in middle age. Gallup, Inc. www.gallup.com/poll/142736/obesity-peaks-middle-age.aspx.

Meredith, C.N., Frontera, W.R., O'Reilly, K.P., and Evans, W.J. 1992. Body composition in elderly men: Effect of dietary modification during strength training. *Journal of the American Geriatric Society* 40: 155-162.

Mero, A. 1988. Blood lactate production and recovery from anaerobic exercise in trained and untrained boys. *European Journal of Applied Physiology* 57: 660-666.

Mero, A., Luhtanen, P., Vitasalo, J.T., and Komi, P.V. 1981. Relationship between maximal running velocity, muscle fiber characteristics, force production and force relaxation of sprinters. *Scandinavian Journal of Sport Science* 3: 16-22.

Messier, S.P., and Dill, M.E. 1985. Alterations in strength and maximal oxygen uptake consequent to Nautilus circuit weight training. *Research Quarterly in Exercise and Sport* 56: 345-351.

Metcalf, B.S., Voss, L.D., Hosking, J., Jeffery, A.N., and Wilkin, T.J. 2008. Physical activity at the government-recommended level and obesity-related health outcomes: A longitudinal study (Early Bird 37). *Archives of Disease in Childhood* 93: 772-777.

Meyer, G.D., Quatman, C.E., Khoury, J., Wall, E.J., and Hewett, T.E. 2009. Youth versus adult "weightlifting" injuries presenting to United States emergency rooms: Accidental versus non-accidental injury mechanisms. *Journal of Strength and Conditioning Research* 3: 2054-2060.

Meyer, R.A., and Terjung, R.L. 1979. Differences in ammonia and adenylate metabolism in contracting fast and slow muscle. *American Journal of Physiology* 237: C11-C18.

Meyers, C.R. 1967. Effect of two isometric routines on strength, size and endurance in exercised and non-exercised arms. *Research Quarterly* 38: 430-440.

Meylan, C., and Malatesta, D. 2009. Effects in-season plyometric training within soccer practice on explosive actions of young players. *Journal of Strength and Conditioning Research* 23: 2605-2613.

Micheli, L.J. 1983. Overuse injuries and children's sports: The growth factor. *Orthopedic Clinics of North America* 14: 337-360.

Micheli, L.J., and Wood, R. 1995. Back pain in young athletes: Significant differences from adults in causes and patterns. *Archives of Pediatric and Adolescent Medicine* 149: 15-18.

Migiano, M.J., Vingren, J.L., Volek, J.S., Maresh, C.M., Fragala, M.S., Ho, J-Y., Thomas, G.A., Hatfield, D.L., Häkkinen, K., Ahtiainen, J., Earp, J.E., and Kraemer, W.J. 2010. Endocrine responses patterns to acute unilateral and bilateral resistance exercise in men. *Journal of Strength and Conditioning Research* 24: 128-134.

Mihalik, J.P., Libby, J.J., Battaglini, C.L., and McMurray, R.G. 2008. Comparing short-term complex and compound training programs on vertical jump height and power output. *Journal of Strength and Conditioning Research* 22: 47-53.

Mikkola, J., Rusko, H., Izquierdo, M., Gorostiaga, E.M., and Häkkinen, K. 2012. Neuromuscular and cardiovascular adaptations during concurrent strength and endurance training in untrained men. *International Journal of Sports Medicine* 33: 702-709.

Mikkola, J., Rusko, H., Nummela, A., Pollari, T., and Häkkinen, K. 2007. Concurrent endurance and explosive type strength training improves neuromuscular and anaerobic characteristics in young distance runners. *International Journal of Sports Medicine* 28: 602-611.

Miles, D.S., Owens, J.J., Golden, J.C., and Gotshall, R.W. 1987. Central and peripheral hemodynamics during maximal leg extension exercise. *European Journal of Applied Physiology* 56: 12-17.

Mileva, K.N., Naleem, A.A., Biswas, S.K., Marwood, S., and Bowtell, J.L. 2006. Acute effects of a vibra-

tion-like stimulus during extension exercise. *Medicine & Science in Sports & Exercise* 38: 1317-1328.

Miller, A.E.J., MacDougall, J.D., Tarnopolsky, M.A., and Sale, D.G. 1992. Gender differences in strength and muscle fiber characteristics. *European Journal of Applied Physiology* 66: 254-262.

Miller, B.P. 1982. The effects of plyometric training on the vertical jump performance of adult female subjects. *British Journal of Sports Medicine* 16: 113-115.

Miller, L.E., Pierson, L.M., Nickols-Richardson, S.M., Wooten, D.F., Selmon, S.S., Ramp, W.K., and Herbert, W.G. 2006. Knee extensor and flexor torque development with concentric and eccentric isokinetic training. *Research Quarterly for Exercise and Sport* 77: 158-163.

Miller, M.G., Cheathman, C.C., and Patel, N.D. 2010. Resistance training for adolescents. *Pediatric Clinics of North America* 57: 671-682.

Miller, T.A., White, E.D., Kinley, K.A., Congleton, J.J., and Clark, M.J. 2002. The effects of training history, player position, and body composition on exercise performance in collegiate football players. *Journal of Strength and Conditioning Association* 16: 44-49.

Miller, W.J., Sherman, W.M., and Ivy, J.L. 1984. Effect of strength training on glucose tolerance and post-glucose insulin response. *Medicine & Science in Sports & Exercise* 16: 539-543.

Millet, G.P., Jaouen, B., Borrani, F., and Candau, R. 2002. Effects of concurrent endurance and strength training on running economy and $\dot{V}O_2$ kinetics. *Medicine & Science in Sports & Exercise* 34: 1351-1359.

Milner-Brown, H.S., Stein, R.B., and Yemin, R. 1973. The orderly recruitment of human motor units during voluntary contractions. *Journal of Physiology* 230: 359-370.

Miranda, H., Fleck, S.J., Simão, R., Barreto, A.C., Dantas, E.H.M., and Novaes, J. 2007. Effect of two different rest period lengths on the number of repetitions performed during resistance training. *Journal of Strength and Conditioning Research* 21: 1032-1036.

Miranda, H., Simão, R., dos Santos Vigário, P., de Salles, B.F., Pacheco, M.T.T., and Willardson, J.M. 2010. Exercise order interacts with different rest interval length during upper-body resistance exercise. *Journal of Strength and Conditioning Research* 24: 1573-1577.

Misner, S.E., Broileau, R.A., Massey, B.H., and Mayhew, J. 1974. Alterations in the body composition of adult men during selected physical training. *Journal of the American Geriatrics Society* 22: 33-38.

Miyamoto, N., Kanehisa, H., Fukunaga, T., and Yasuo, Y. 2011. Effect of post-activation potentiation on the maximal voluntary isokinetic concentric torque in humans. *Journal of Strength and Conditioning Research* 25: 186-192.

Moeckel-Cole, S.A., and Clarkson, P.M. 2009. Rhabdomyolysis in a collegiate football player. *Journal of Strength and Conditioning Research* 23: 1055-1059.

Moffroid, M.T., and Whipple, R.H. 1970. Specificity of speed of exercise. *Physical Therapy* 50: 1693-1699.

Moffroid, M.T., Whipple, R.H., Hofkosh, J., Lowman, E., and Thistle, H. 1969. A study of isokinetic exercise. *Physical Therapy* 49: 735-747.

Mohr, K.J., Pink, N.M., Elsner, C., and Kvitne, R.S. 1998. Electromyographic investigation of stretching: The effect of warm-up. *Clinical Journal of Sports Medicine* 8: 215-220.

Moldoveanu, A.I., Shephard, R.J., and Shek, P.N. 2001. The cytokine response to physical activity and training. *Sports Medicine* 31: 115-144.

Mont, M.A., Cohen, D.B., Campbell, K.R., Gravare, K., and Mathur, S.K. 1994. Isokinetic concentric versus eccentric training of shoulder rotators with functional evaluation of performance enhancement in elite tennis players. *American Journal of Sports Medicine* 22: 513-517.

Monteiro, A.G., Aoki, M.S., Evangelista, A.L., Alveno, D.A., Monteiro, G.A., Picarro, I.D.C., and Ugrinowitsch, C. 2009. Nonlinear periodization maximizes strength gains in split resistance training routines. *Journal of Strength and Conditioning Research* 23: 1321-1326.

Monteiro, W.D., Simao, R., Polito, M.D., Santana, C.A., Chaves, R.B., Bezerra, E. and Fleck, S.J. 2008. Influence of strength training on adult women's flexibility. *Journal of Strength and Conditioning Research* 22: 672-677.

Mookerjee, S., and Ratamess, N.A. 1999. Comparison of strength differences and joint action durations between full and partial range-of-motion bench press exercise. *Journal of Strength Conditioning Research* 13: 76-81.

Moore, C.A., and Fry, A.C. 2007. Nonfunctional overreaching during off-season training for skill position players in collegiate American football. *Journal of Strength and Conditioning Research* 21: 793-800.

Moore, C.A., Weiss, L.W., Schilling, B.K., Fry, A.C., and Li, Y. 2007. Acute effects of augmented eccentric loading on jump squat performance. *Journal of Strength and Conditioning Research* 21: 372-377.

Moore, D.R., Burgomaster, K.A., Schofield, L.M., Gibala, M.J., Sale, D.G., and Phillips, S.M. 2004. Neuromuscular adaptations in human muscle following low intensity resistance training with vascular occlusion. *European Journal of Applied Physiology* 92: 399-406.

Moore, M.A., and Hutton, R.S. 1980. Electromyographic investigation of muscle stretching techniques. *Medicine & Science in Sports & Exercise* 12: 322-329.

Morales, J., and Sobonya, S. 1996. Use of submaximal repetition tests for predicting 1-rm strength in class athletes. *Journal of Strength and Conditioning Research* 10: 186-189.

Moran, K.A., Clarke, M., Reilly, F., Wallace, E.S., Brabazon, D., and Marshall, B. 2009. Does endurance fatigue increase the risk of injury when performing drop jumps? *Journal of Strength and Conditioning Research* 23: 1448-1455.

Moran, K., McNamara, B., and Luo, J. 2007. Effect of vibration training in maximal effort (70% 1 RM) dynamic bicep curls. *Medicine & Science in Sports & Exercise* 39: 526-533.

Morehouse, C. 1967. Development and maintenance of isometric strength of subjects with diverse initial strengths. *Research Quarterly* 38: 449-456.

Morganti, C.M., Nelson, M.E., Fiatarone, M.A., Dallal, G.E., Economos, C.D., Crawford, B.M., and Evans, W.J. 1995. Strength improvements with 1 yr of progressive resistance training in older women. *Medicine & Science in Sports & Exercise* 27: 906-912.

Moritani, T. 1992. Time course of adaptations during strength and power training. In *Strength and power in sport*, edited by P.V. Komi, 226-278. Oxford: Blackwell.

Moritani, T., and DeVries, H.A. 1979. Neural factors versus hypertrophy in the time course of muscle strength gain. *American Journal of Physical Medicine* 82: 521-524.

Moritani, T., and DeVries, H.A. 1980. Potential for gross hypertrophy in older men. *Journal of Gerontology* 35: 672-682.

Morrey, M.A., and Hensrud, D.D. 1999. Risk of medical events in a supervised health and fitness facility. *Medicine & Science in Sports & Exercise* 31: 1233-1236.

Morris, C.J., Tolfroy, K., and Coppack, R.J. 2001. Effects of short-term isokinetic training on standing long-jump performance in untrained men. *Journal of Strength and Conditioning Research* 15: 498-502.

Morrissey, M.C., Harman, E.A., Frykman, P.N., and Han, K.H. 1998. Early phase differential effects of slow and fast barbell squat training. *American Journal of Sports Medicine* 26: 221-230.

Morrison, R.S., Chassin, M.R., and Siu, A.L. 1998. The medical consultant's role in caring for patients with hip fracture. *Annals of Internal Medicine* 128: 1010.

Morton, S.K., Whitehead, J.R., Brinkert, R.H., and Caine, D.J. 2011. Resistance training vs. static stretching: Effects on flexibility and strength. *Journal of Strength and Conditioning Research* 25: 3391-3398.

Mosher, P.E., Underwood, S.A., Ferguson, M.A., and Arnold, R.O. 1994. Effects of 12 weeks of aerobic circuit weight training on anaerobic capacity, muscular strength, and body composition in college-age women. *Journal of Strength and Conditioning Research* 8: 144-148.

Moskwa, C.A., and Nicholas, J.A. 1989. Musculoskeletal risk factors in the young athlete. *Physician and Sportsmedicine* 17: 45-59.

Moss, B.M., Refsnes, P.E., Abildgaard, A., Nicolaysen, K., and Jensen, J. 1997. Effects of maximal effort strength training with different loads on dynamic strength, cross-sectional area, load-power, and load-velocity relationships. *European Journal of Applied Physiology* 75: 193-199.

Mujika, I., and Padilla, S. 2001. Muscular characteristics of detraining in humans. *Medicine & Science in Sports & Exercise* 33: 1297-1303.

Mulligan, S.E., Fleck, S.J., Gordon, S.E., Koziris, L.P., Triplett-McBride, N.T., and Kraemer, W.J. 1996. Influence of resistance exercise volume on serum growth hormone and cortisol concentrations in women. *Journal of Strength and Conditioning Research* 10: 256-262.

Murphy, A.J., Wilson, G.J., Pryor, J.F., and Newton, R.U. 1995. Isometric assessment of muscular function: The effect of joint angle. *Journal of Applied Biomechanics* 11: 205-215.

Murray, M.P., Duthie, E.H., Gambert, S.T., Sepic, S.B., and Mollinger, L.A. 1985. Age-related differences in knee muscle strength in normal women. *Journal of Gerontology* 40: 275-280.

Nader, G.A. 2006. Concurrent strength and endurance training from molecules to man. *Medicine & Science in Sports & Exercise* 38: 1965-1970.

Nakamura, Y., Aizawa, K., Imai, T., Kono, I., and Mesaki, N. 2011. Hormonal responses to resistance exercise during different menstrual cycle states. *Medicine & Science in Sports & Exercise* 43: 967-973.

Nakamaru, Y., and Schwartz, A. 1972. The influence of hydrogen ion concentration on calcium binding and release by skeletal muscle sarcoplasmic reticulum. *Journal of General Physiology* 59: 22-32.

Nakao, M., Inoue, Y., and Murakami, H. 1995. Longitudinal study of the effect of high-intensity weight training on aerobic capacity. *European Journal of Applied Physiology* 70: 20-25.

Narici, M.V., Maffulli, N., and Maganaris, C.M. 2008. Aging of human muscles and tendons. *Disability and Rehabilitation* 30: 1548-1554.

Narici, M.V., Roi, G.S., Landoni, L., Minetti, A.E., and Cerretelli, P. 1989. Changes in force, cross-sectional area and neural activation during strength training and detraining of the human quadriceps. *European Journal of Applied Physiology* 59: 310-319.

Narin, P.D., Bunker, D., Rhea, M.R., and Ayllon, F.N. 2009. Neuromuscular activity during whole-body vibration of different amplitudes and footwear conditions: Implications for prescription of vibratory stimulation. *Journal of Strength and Conditioning Research* 23: 2311-2316.

National Association for Sport and Physical Education. 2008. *Strength training for children and adolescence.* Reston, VA.

National Strength and Conditioning Association. 2009. Youth resistance training: Updated position statement paper from the National Strength and Conditioning Association. *Journal of Strength and Conditioning Research* 23: S60-S79.

Nattiv, A., Agonstini, R., Drinkwater, B., and Yeager, K.K. 1994. The female athlete triad: The inter-relatedness of disorder eating, amenorrhea, and osteoporosis. *Clinics in Sports Medicine* 13: 405-418.

Nattiv, A., Loucks, A.B., Manore, M.M., Sanborn, C.F., Sundgot-Borgen, J., and Warren, M.P. 2007. American College of Sports Medicine position stand. The female athlete triad. *Medicine & Science in Sports & Exercise* 39: 1867-1882.

Naughton, G., Farpour-Lambert, N.J., Carlson, J., Bradney, M., and Van Praagh, E. 2000. Physiological issues surrounding the performance of adolescent athletes. *Sports Medicine* 30: 309-325.

Naylor, L.H., George, K., O'Driscoll, G., and Green, D.J. 2008. The athlete's heart: A contemporary appraisal of the "Morganroth hypothesis." *Sports Medicine* 38: 69-90.

Naylor, N.H., Watts, K., Sharpe, J.A., Jones, T.W., Davis, E.A., Thompson, A., George, K., Ramsay, J.M., O'Driscoll, G., and Green, D.J. 2008. Resistance training and diastolic myocardial tissue velocities in obese children. *Medicine & Science in Sports & Exercise* 40: 2027-2032.

Neder, J.A., Luiz, E.N., Shinzato, G.T., Andrade, M.S., Peres, C., and Silva, A.C. 1999. Reference values for concentric knee isokinetic strength and power in nonathletic men and women from both 20 to 80 years old. *Journal of Orthopedic and Sports Physical Therapy* 29: 116-126.

Neely, K.R., Terry, J.G., and Morris, M.J. 2010. A mechanical comparison of linear and double-looped on a supplemental heavy chain resistance to the back squat: A case study. *Journal of Strength and Conditioning Research* 24: 278-281.

Neils, C.M., Udermann, B.E., Brice, G.A., Winchester, J.B., and McGuigan, M.R. 2005. Influence of contraction velocity in untrained individuals over the initial early phase of resistance training. *Journal of Strength and Conditioning Research* 19: 883-887.

Nelson, A.G., Allen, J.D., Cornwell, C., and Kookonen, J. 2001. Inhibition of maximal voluntary isometric torque production by acute stretching is joint-angle specific. *Research Quarterly for Exercise and Sport* 72: 68-70.

Nelson, A.G., Guillory, I.K., Cornwell, C., and Kookonen, J. 2001. Inhibition of maximal voluntary isokinetic torque production following stretching is velocity specific. *Journal of Strength and Conditioning Research* 15: 241-246.

Nelson, G.A., Arnall, D.A., Loy, S.F., Silvester, L.J., and Conlee, R.K. 1990. Consequences of combining strength and endurance training regimens. *Physical Therapy* 70: 287-294.

Nelson, M.E., Fiatarone, M.A., Morganti, C.M., Trice, I., Greenberg, R.A., and Evans, W.J. 1994. Effects of high-intensity strength training on multiple risk factors for osteoporotic fractures. *Journal of the American Medical Association* 272: 1909-1914.

Nemoto, E.M., Hoff, J.T., and Sereringhaus, W.J. 1974. Lactate uptake and metabolism by brain during hyperlactacidemia and hypoglycemia. *Stroke* 5: 353-359.

Newton, R.U., Häkkinen, K., Kraemer, W.J., McCormick, M., Volek, J., Gordon, S.E., Campbell, W.W., and Evans, W.J. 1995. Resistance training and the development of muscle strength and power in young versus older men. In *XV Congress of the International Society of Biomechanics*, University of Jyväskylä, Finland, pp. 672-673.

Newton, R.U., and Kraemer, W.J. 1994. Developing explosive muscular power: Implications for a mixed methods training strategy. *Journal of Strength and Conditioning Research* 16: 20-31.

Newton, R.U., Kraemer, W.J., and Häkkinen, K. 1999. Effects of ballistic training on preseason preparation of elite volleyball players. *Medicine & Science in Sports & Exercise* 31: 323-330.

Newton, R.U., Kraemer, W.J., Häkkinen, K., Humphries, B.J., and Murphy, A.J. 1996. Kinematics, kinetics, and muscle activation during explosive upper body movements: Implications for power development. *Journal of Applied Biomechanics* 12: 31-43.

Newton, R.U., and Wilson, G.J. 1993a. The kinetics and kinematics of powerful upper body movements: The effects of load. Abstracts of the International Society of Biomechanics XIVth Congress, Paris, 4-8 July, p. 1510.

Newton, R.U., and Wilson, G.J. 1993b. Reducing the risk of injury during plyometric training: The effect of dampeners. *Sports Medicine, Training and Rehabilitation* 4: 1-7.

Nichols, D.L., Sanborn, C.F., Bonnick, S.L., Gench, B., and DiMarco, N. 1995. Relationship of regional body composition to bone mineral density in college females. *Medicine & Science in Sports & Exercise* 27: 178-182.

Nichols, D.L., Sanborn, C.F., and Essery, E.V. 2007. Bone density and young athletic women. An update. *Sports Medicine* 37: 1001-1014.

Nichols, D.L., Sanborn, C.F., and Love, A.M. 2001. Resistance training and bone mineral density in adolescent females. *Journal of Pediatrics* 139: 494-499.

Nichols, J.F., Hitzelberger, L.M., Sherman, J.G., and Patterson, P. 1995. Effects of resistance training on muscular strength and functional abilities of community-dwelling older adults. *Journal of Aging and Physical Activity* 3: 238-250.

Nicol, C., Avela, J., and Komi, P.V. 2006. The stretch-shortening cycle a model for studying naturally occurring neuromuscular fatigue. *Sports Medicine* 36: 977-999.

Nindl, B.C., Alemany, J.A., Tuckow, A.P., Rarick, K.R., Staab, J.S., Kraemer, W.J., Maresh, C.M., Spiering,

B.A., Hatfield, D.L., Flyvbjerg, A., and Frystyk, J. 2010. Circulating bioactive and immunoreactive IGF-I remain stable in women, despite physical fitness improvements after 8 weeks of resistance, aerobic, and combined exercise training. *Journal of Applied Physiology* 109: 112-120.

Nindl, B.C., Harman, E.A., Marx, J.O., Gotshalk, L.A., Frykman, P.N., Lammi, E., Palmer, C., and Kraemer, W.J. 2000. Regional body composition changes in women after 6 months periodized physical training. *Journal of Applied Physiology* 88: 2251-2259.

Nindl, B.C., Hymer, W.C., Deaver, D.R., and Kraemer, W.J. 2001. Growth hormone pulsability profile characteristics following acute heavy resistance exercise. *Journal of Applied Physiology* 91: 163-172.

Nindl, B.C., Kraemer, W.J., Gotshalk, L.A., Marx, J.O., Volek, J.S., Bush, J.A., Häkkinen, K., Newton, R.U., and Fleck, S.J. 2001. Testosterone responses after acute resistance exercise in women: Effects of regional fat distribution. *International Journal of Sports Nutrition and Metabolism* 11: 451-465.

Nindl, B.C., Kraemer, W.J., Marx, J.O., Arciero, P.J., Dohi, K., Kellogg, M.D., and Loomis, G.A. 2001. Overnight responses of the circulating IGF-1 system after acute heavy-resistance exercise. *Journal of Applied Physiology* 90: 1319-1326.

Nindl, B.C., Kraemer, W.J., Marx, J.O., Tuckow, A.P., and Hymer, W.C. 2003. Growth hormone molecular heterogeneity and exercise. *Exercise and Sport Science Reviews* 31: 161-166.

Nindl, B.C., and Pierce, J.R. 2010. Insulin-like growth factor I as a biomarker of health, fitness, and training status. *Medicine & Science in Sports & Exercise* 42: 39-49.

Nordstrom, A., Olsson, T., and Nordstrom, P. 2005. Bone gained from physical activity and lost through detraining: A longitudinal study in young males. *Osteoporosis International* 16: 835-841.

Norris, D.O. 1980. *Vertebrate endocrinology*. Philadelphia: Lea and Febiger.

Norwood, J.T., Anderson, G.S., Gaetz, M.B., and Twist, P.W. 2007. Electromyographic activity of the trunk stabilizers during stable and unstable bench press. *Journal of Strength and Conditioning Research* 21: 343-347.

Nosaka, K., and Clarkson, P.M. 1995. Muscle damage following repeated bouts of high force eccentric exercise. *Medicine & Science in Sports & Exercise* 27: 1263-1269.

Nosaka, K., Clarkson, P.M., McGuiggin, M.E., and Byrne, J.M. 1991. Time course of muscle damage after high force eccentric exercise. *European Journal of Applied Physiology* 63: 70-76.

Nosaka, K., and Newton, M. 2002. Difference in the magnitude of muscle damage between maximal and submaximal eccentric loading. *Journal of Strength and Conditioning Research* 16: 202-208.

Nozaki, D. 2009. Torque interaction among adjacent joints to the action of biarticular muscles. *Medicine & Science in Sports & Exercise* 41: 205-209.

Nunes, J.A., Crewther, B.T., Ugrinowitsch, C., Tricoli, V., Viveiros, L., de Rose, D. Jr., and Aoki, M.S. 2011. Salivary hormone and immune responses to three resistance exercise schemes in elite female athletes. *Journal of Strength and Conditioning Research* 25: 2322-2327.

Nyburgh, K.H., Bachrach, L.K., Lewis, B., Kent, K., and Marcus, R. 1993. Low bone mineral density at axial and appendicular sites in amenorrheic athletes. *Medicine & Science in Sports & Exercise* 25: 1197-1202.

O'Bryant, H.S., Byrd, R., and Stone, M.H. 1988. Cycle ergometer performance and maximum leg and hip strength adaptations to two different methods of weight training. *Journal of Applied Sport Science Research* 2: 27-30.

O'Connor, P.J., Bryant, C.X., Veltri, J.P., and Gebhardt, S.M. 1993. State anxiety and ambulatory blood pressure following resistance exercise in females. *Medicine & Science in Sports & Exercise* 25: 516-521.

O'Hagan, F.T., Sale, D.G., MacDougall, J.D., and Garner, S.H. 1995a. Comparative effectiveness of accommodating and weight resistance training modes. *Medicine & Science in Sports & Exercise* 27: 1210-1219.

O'Hagan, F.T., Sale, D.G., MacDougal, J.D., and Garner, S.H. 1995b. Response to resistance training in young women and men. *International Journal of Sports Medicine* 16: 314-321.

Ohberg, L., Lorentzen, R., and Alfredson, H. 2004. Eccentric training in patients with chronic Achilles tendinosis: Normalized tendon structure and decreased thickness at follow up. *British Journal of Sports Medicine* 38: 8-11.

Ohtsuki, T. 1981. Decrease in grip strength induced by simultaneous bilateral exertion with reference to finger strength. *Ergonomics* 24: 37-48.

Ojanen, T., Rauhala, T., and Häkkinen, K. 2007. Strength and power profiles of the lower and upper extremities in master throwers at different ages. *Journal of Strength and Conditioning Research* 21: 216-222.

Ojastro, T., and Hakkinen, K. 2009. Effects of different accentuated eccentric load levels in eccentric-concentric actions on acute neural muscular, maximal force and power responses. *Journal of Strength and Conditioning Research* 23: 996-1004.

Oliver, G.D., and Di Brezzo, R.D. 2009. Functional balance training in collegiate women athletes. *Journal of Strength and Conditioning Research* 23: 2124-2129.

Orsatti, F.L., Nahas, E.A., Maesta, N., Nahas-Neto, J., and Burini, R.C. 2008. Plasma hormones, muscle mass and strength in resistance-trained postmenopausal women. *Maturitas* 59: 394-404.

Ortego, A.R., Dantzler, D.K., Zaloudek, A., Tanner, J., Khan, T., Panwar, R., Hollander, D.B., and Kraemer, R.R. 2009. Effects of gender on physiological responses to strenuous circuit resistance exercise and recovery. *Journal of Strength and Conditioning Research* 23: 932-938.

O'Shea, K.L., and O'Shea, J.P. 1989. Functional isometric weight training: Its effects on dynamic and static strength. *Journal of Applied Sport Science Research* 3: 30-33.

O'Shea, P. 1966. Effects of selected weight training programs on the development of strength and muscle hypertrophy. *Research Quarterly* 37: 95-102.

Osternig, L.R., Robertson, R.N., Troxel, R.K., and Hansen, P. 1990. Differential responses to proprioceptive neuromuscular facilitation (PNF) stretch techniques. *Medicine & Science in Sports & Exercise* 22: 106-111.

Ostrowski, K., Wilson, G.J., Weatherby, R., Murphy, P.W., and Lyttle, A.D. 1997. The effect of weight training volume on hormonal output and muscular size and function. *Journal of Strength and Conditioning Research* 11: 148-154.

Oteghen, S.L. 1975. Two speeds of isokinetic exercise as related to the vertical jump performance of women. *Research Quarterly* 46: 78-84.

Otto, W.H., Coburn, J.W., Brown, L.E., and Spiering, B.A. 2012. Effects of weightlifting vs. kettlebell training on vertical jump, strength, and body composition. *Journal of Strength and Conditioning Research* 26: 1199-1202.

Ozmun, J.C., Mikesky, A.E., and Surburg, P.R. 1994. Neuromuscular adaptations following prepubescent strength training. *Medicine & Science in Sports & Exercise* 26: 510-514.

Paasuke, M., Ereline, J., Gapeyeva, H., Sirkel, S., and Sander, P. 2000. Age-related differences in twitch contractile properties of plantarflexor muscles in women. *Acta Physiologica Scandinavica* 170: 51-57.

Paasuke, M., Saapar, L., Ereline, J., Gapeyeva, H., Requena, B., and Oopik, V. 2007. Postactivation potentiation of knee extensor muscles in power-and endurance-trained, and untrained women. *European Journal of Applied Physiology* 101: 577-585.

Paavolainen, L., Häkkinen, K., Hamalainen, I., Nummela, A., and Rusko, H. 1999. Explosive-strength training improves 5-km running time by improving running economy and muscle power. *Journal of Applied Physiology* 86: 1527-1533.

Pacak, K., Palkovits, M., Yadid, G., Kvetnansky, R., Kopin, I.J., and Goldstein, D.S. 1998. Heterogeneous neurochemical responses to different stressors: A test of Selye's doctrine of nonspecificity. *American Journal of Physiology* 275: R1247-R1255.

Paddon-Jones, D., and Abernathy, P.J. 2001. Acute adaptation to low-volume eccentric exercise. *Medicine & Science in Sports & Exercise* 33: 1213-1219.

Padua, D.A., DiStefano, L.J., Marshall, S.W., Beutler, A.I., de la Motte, S.J., and DiStefano, M.J. 2012. Retention of movement pattern changes after a lower extremity injury prevention program is affected by program duration. *American Journal of Sports Medicine* 40: 300-306.

Paffenbarger, R.S., Hyde, R.T., Wing, A.L., and Steinmetz, C.H. 1984. A natural history of athleticism and cardiovascular health. *Journal of the American Medical Association* 252: 491-495.

Parkhouse, W.S., Coupland, D.C., Li, C., and Vanderhoek, K.J. 2000. IGF-1 bioavailability is increased by resistance training in older women with low bone mineral density. *Mechanisms of Aging Development* 113: 75-83.

Path, G., Bornstein, S.R., Ehrhart-Bornstein, M., and Scherbaum, W.A. 1997. Interleukin-6 and the interleukin-6 receptor in the human adrenal gland: Expression and effects on steroidogenesis. *Journal of Clinical Endocrinology and Metabolism* 82: 2343-2349.

Patton, J.F., Kraemer, W.J., Knuttgen, H.G., and Harman, E.A. 1990. Factors in maximal power production and in exercise endurance relative to maximal power. *European Journal of Applied Physiology* 60: 222-227.

Paulsen, G., Myklestad, D., and Raastad, T. 2003. The influence of volume of exercise on early adaptations to strength training. *Journal of Strength and Conditioning Research.* 17: 115-120.

Pavlath, G.K., Rich, K., Webster, S.G., and Blau, H.M. 1989. Localization of muscle gene products in nuclear domains. *Nature* 337: 570-573.

Payne, V.G., Morrow, J.R., Jr., Johnson, L., and Dalton, S.N. 1997. Resistance training in children and youth: A meta-analysis. *Research Quarterly for Exercise and Sport* 68: 80-88.

Pearson, A.C., Schiff, M., Mrosek, D., Labovitz, A.J., and Williams, G.A. 1986. Left ventricular diastolic function in weight lifters. *American Journal of Cardiology* 58: 1254-1259.

Pearson, D.R., and Costill, D.L. 1988. The effects of constant external resistance exercise and isokinetic exercise training on work-induced hypertrophy. *Journal of Applied Sport Science Research* 3: 39-41.

Peng, H-E. 2011. Changes in biomechanical properties during drop drops of incremental height. *Journal of Strength and Conditioning Research* 25: 2510-2518.

Perls, T.H., Reisman, N.R., and Olshansky, S.J. 2005. Provision or distribution of growth hormone for "Antiaging." *Journal of the American Medical Association* 294: 2086-2090.

Perrault, H., and Turcotte, R.A. 1994. Exercise-induced cardiac hypertrophy fact or fallacy? *Sports Medicine* 17: 288-308.

Perrone, C.E., Fenwick-Smith, D., and Vandenburgh, H.H. 1995 Collagen and stretch modulate autocrine secretion of insulin-like growth factor-1 and insulin-like growth factor binding proteins from differentiated skeletal muscle cells. *Biological Chemistry* 270: 2099-106.

Pesta, D.H., Hoppel, F., Macek, C., Messner, H., Faulhaber, M., Kobel, C., Parson, W., Burtscher, M., Schocke, M.F., and Gnaiger, E. 2011. Similar qualitative and quantitative changes of mitochondrial respiration following strength and endurance training in normoxia and hypoxia in sedentary humans. *American Journal of Physiology, Regulatory, Integrative and Comparative Physiology* 301: R1078-R1087.

Petersen, S., Wessel, J., Bagnall, K., Wilkens, H., Quinney, A., and Wenger, H. 1990. Influence of concentric resistance training on concentric and eccentric strength. *Archives of Physical Medicine and Rehabilitation* 71: 101-105.

Petersen, S.R., Miller, G.D., Quinney, H.A., and Wenger, H.A. 1987. The effectiveness of a mini-cycle on velocity-specific strength acquisition. *Journal of Orthopaedic and Sports Physical Therapy* 9: 156-159.

Peterson, J.A. 1975. Total conditioning: A case study. *Athletic Journal* 56: 40-55.

Peterson, M.D., Rhea, M.R., and Alvar, B.A. 2004. Maximizing strength development and athletes: A meta-analysis to determine the dose-response relationship. *Journal of Strength and Conditioning Research* 18: 377-382.

Petit, M.A., Prior, J.C., and Barr, S.L. 1999. Running and ovulation positively change cancellous bone in premenopausal women. *Medicine & Science in Sports & Exercise* 31: 780-787.

Petrella, J.K., Kim, J.S., Mayhew, D.L., Cross, J.M., and Bamman, M.M. 2008. Potent myofiber hypertrophy during resistance training in humans is associated with satellite cell-mediated myonuclear addition: A cluster analysis. *Journal of Applied Physiology* 104: 1736-1742.

Petrella, J.K., Kim, J.S., Tuggle, S.C., and Bamman, M.M. 2007. Contributions of force and velocity to improved power with progressive resistance training in young and older adults. *European Journal of Applied Physiology* 99: 343-351.

Pette, D., and Staron, R.S. 1990. Cellular and molecular diversities of mammalian skeletal muscle fibers. *Review of Physiology, Biochemistry and Pharmacology* 116: 2-75.

Pette, D., and Staron, R.S. 1997. Mammalian skeletal muscle fiber type transitions. *International Review of Cytology* 170: 143-223.

Pette, D., and Staron, R.S. 2001. Transitions of muscle fiber phenotypic profiles. *Histochemistry and Cell Biology* 115: 359-372.

Pfeiffer, R., and Francis, R. 1986. Effects of strength training on muscle development in prepubescent, pubescent and postpubescent males. *Physician and Sportsmedicine* 14: 134-143.

Phillips, S.K., Bruce, S.A., Newton, D., and Woledge, R.C. 1992. The weakness of old age is not due to failure of muscle activation. *Journal of Gerontology: Medical Sciences* 47: 45-49.

Phillips, S.M., Tipton, K.D., Aarsland, A., Wolf, S.E., and Wolfe, R.R. 1997. Mixed muscle protein synthesis and breakdown after resistance exercise in humans. *American Journal of Physiology* 273: E99-E107.

Phillips, S.M., Tipton, K.D., Ferrando, A.A., and Wolfe, R.R. 1999. Resistance training reduces the acute exercise-induced increase in muscle protein turnover. *American Journal of Physiology* 276: E118-E124.

Pichon, C.E., Hunter, G.R., Morris, M., Bond, R.L., and Metz, J. 1996. Blood pressure and heart rate response and metabolic cost of circuit versus traditional weight training. *Journal of Strength and Conditioning Research* 10: 153-156.

Pierce, K., Rozenek, R., and Stone, M.H. 1993. Effects of high volume weight training on lactate, heart rate, and perceived exertion. *Journal of Strength and Conditioning Research* 7: 211-215.

Piirainen, J.M., Tanskanen, M., Nissila, J., Kaarela, J., Vaarala, A., Sippola, N., and Linnamo, V. 2011. Effects of a heart rate-based recovery period on hormonal, neuromuscular, and aerobic performance responses during 7 weeks of strength training in men. *Journal of Strength and Conditioning Research* 25: 2265-2273.

Pikosky, M., Faigenbaum, A., Westcott, W., and Rodriguez, N. 2002. Effect of resistance training on protein utilization in healthy children. *Medicine & Science in Sports & Exercise* 34: 820-827.

Pillard, F., Laoudj-Chenivesse, D., Carnac, G., Mercier, J., Rami, J., Riviere, D., and Rolland, Y. 2011. Physical activity and sarcopenia. *Clinics in Geriatric Medicine* 27: 449-470.

Pincivero, D.M., Campy, R.M., and Karunakara, R.G. 2004. The effects of rest interval and resistance training on quadriceps femoris muscle. Part II: EMG and perceived exertion. *Journal of Sports Medicine and Physical Fitness* 44: 224-232.

Pincivero, D.M., Gear, W.S., Sterner, R.L., and Karunakara, R.G. 2000. Gender differences in the relationship between quadriceps work and fatigue during high-intensity exercise. *Journal of Strength and Conditioning Research* 14: 202-206.

Pincivero, D.M., Lephart, S.M., and Karunakara, R.G. 1997. Effects of rest interval on isokinetic strength and functional performance after short term high intensity training. *British Journal of Sports Medicine* 31: 229-234.

Pipes, T.V. 1978. Variable resistance versus constant resistance strength training in adult males. *European Journal of Applied Physiology* 39: 27-35.

Pipes, T.V. 1979. Physiological characteristics of elite body builders. *Physician and Sportsmedicine* 7: 116-126.

Pizzimenti, M.A. 1992. Mechanical analysis of the Nautilus leg curl machine. *Canadian Journal of Sport Science* 17: 41-48.

Ploutz, L.L., Tesch, P.A., Biro, R.L., and Dudley, G.A. 1994. Effect of resistance training on muscle use during exercise. *Journal of Applied Physiology* 76: 1675-1681.

Ploutz-Snyder, L.L., and Giamis, E.L. 2001. Orientation and familiarization to 1 RM strength testing in old and young women. *Journal of Strength and Conditioning Research* 15: 519-523.

Ploutz-Snyder, L.L., Giamis, E.L., and Rosenbaum, A.E. 2001. Resistance training reduces susceptibility to eccentric exercise-induced muscle dysfunction in older women. *Journal of Gerontology: Biological Sciences, Medical Sciences* 56: B384-B390.

Pluim, B.M., Zwinderman, A.H., van der Laarse, A., and van der Wall, E.E. 1999. The athlete's heart: A meta-analysis of cardiac structure and function. *Circulation* 100: 336-344.

Polhemus, R., Burkhart, E., Osina, M., and Patterson, M. 1981. The effects of plyometric training with ankle and vest weights on conventional weight training programs for men and women. *National Strength Coaches Association Journal* 2: 13-15.

Pollock, M.H., Graves, J.E., Bamman, M.M., Leggett, S.H., Carpenter, D.M., Carr, C., Cirulli, J., Makozich, J., and Fulton, M. 1993. Frequency and volume of resistance training: Effect on cervical extension strength. *Archives of Physical Medicine and Rehabilitation* 74: 1080-1086.

Poole, H. 1964. Multi-poundage sets. *Muscle Builder* 14: 20-21.

Pope, R.P., Herbert, R.D., Kirwan, J.D., and Graham, B.J. 2000. A randomized trial of preexercise stretching for prevention of lower-limb injury. *Medicine & Science in Sports & Exercise* 32: 271-277.

Porter, M.M. 2006. Power training for older adults. *Applied Physiology, Nutrition, and Metabolism* 31: 87-94.

Porter, M.M., Vandervoort, A.A., and Lexell, J. 1995. Aging of human muscle: Structure, function and adaptability. *Scandinavian Journal of Medicine & Science in Sports* 5: 129-142.

Poston, B., Holcomb, W.R., Guadagnoli, M.A., and Linn, L.L. 2007. The acute effects of mechanical vibration on power output in the bench press. *Journal of Strength and Conditioning Research* 21: 199-203.

Potteiger, J.A., Lockwood, R.H., Haub, M.D., Dolezal, B.A., Almuzaini, K.S., Schroeder, J.M., and Zebras, C.J. 1999. Muscle power and fiber characteristics following 8 weeks of plyometric training. *Journal of Strength and Conditioning Research* 13: 275-279.

Powers, W.E., Browning, F.M., and Groves, B.R. 1978. The super overload: The new method for improving muscular strength. *Journal of Physical Education* (March/April): 10-12.

Prestes, J., De Lima, C., Frollini, A.B., Donatto, F.F., and Conte, M. 2009. Comparison of linear and reverse linear periodization effects on maximal strength and body composition. *Journal of Strength and Conditioning Research* 23: 266-274.

Prestes, J., Frollini, A.B., De Lima, C., Donatto, F.F., Foschini, D., DeCassia Marqueti, R., Figueira, A., Jr., and Fleck, S.J. 2009. Comparison between linear and daily undulating periodized resistance training to increase strength. *Journal of Strength and Conditioning Research* 23: 2437-2442.

Prestes, J., Shiguemoto, G., Botero, J.P., Frollini, A., Dias, R., Leite, R., Pereira, G., Magosso, R., Baldissera, V., Cavaglieri, C., and Perez, S. 2009. Effects of resistance training on resistin, leptin, cytokines, and muscle force in elderly post-menopausal women. *Journal of Sports Sciences* 27: 1607-1615.

Prior, J.C., Vigna, Y.M., and McKay, D.W. 1992. Reproduction for the athletic female: New understandings of physiology and management. *Sports Medicine* 14: 190-199.

Prokopy, M.P., Ingersoll, C.D., Nordenschild, E., Katch, F.I., Gaesser, G.A., and Weltman, A. 2008. Closed-kinetic chain upper-body training improves throwing performance of NCAA division I softball players. *Journal of Strength and Conditioning Research* 22: 1790-1798.

Pruit, L.A., Jackson, R.D., Bartels, R.L., and Lehnard, H.J. 1992. Weight-training effects on bone mineral density in early post-menopausal women. *Journal of Bone Mineral Research* 7: 179-185.

Pyka, G., Wiswell, R.A., and Marcus, R. 1992. Age-dependent effect of resistance exercise on growth hormone secretion in people. *Journal of Clinical Endocrinology and Metabolism* 75: 404-407.

Quaedackers, M.E., Van Den Brink, C.E., Wissink, S., Schreurs, R.H., Gustafsson, J.K., Van Der, J.A., Saag, P.T., and Van Der Burg, B.B. 2001. 4-hydroxy-tamoxifen trans-represses nuclear factor-kappa B activity in human osteoblastic U2-OS cells through estrogen receptor (ER) alpha, not through ER beta. *Endocrinology* 142: 1156-1166.

Quatman, C.E., Myer, G.D., Khoury. J., Wall, E.J., and Hewett, T.E. 2009. Sex differences in "weightlifting" injuries presenting to United States emergency rooms. *Journal of Strength and Conditioning Research* 23: 2061-2067.

Queiroz, A.C.C., Gagliardi, J.F.L., Forjaz, C.L.M., and Rezk, C.C. 2009. Clinic and ambulatory blood pressure responses after resistance exercise. *Journal of Strength and Conditioning Research* 23: 571-578.

Raastad, T., Bjoro, T., and Hallen, J. 2000. Hormonal responses to high- and moderate-intensity strength exercise. *European Journal of Applied Physiology* 82: 121-128.

Rack, D.M.H., and Westbury, D.R. 1969. The effects of length and stimulus rate on isometric tension in the cat soleus. *Journal of Physiology* 204: 443-460.

Rahimi, R., Qaderi, M., Faraji, H., and Boroujerdi, SS. 2010. Effects of very short rest periods on hormonal responses to resistance exercise in men. *Journal of Strength and Conditioning Research* 24: 1851-1859.

Rains, C.B., Weltman, A.W., Cahil, B.R., Janney, C.A., Tippett, S.R., and Katch, F.I. 1987. Strength training for prepubescent males: Is it safe? *American Journal Sports Medicine* 15: 483-489.

Ramos, E., Frontera, W.R., Llopart, A., and Feliciano, D. 1998. Muscle strength and hormonal levels and adolescents: Gender related differences. *International Journal of Sports Medicine* 19: 526-531.

Ramsay, J.A., Blimkie, C.J.R., Smith, K., Garner, S., MacDougall, J.D., and Sale, D.G. 1990. Strength training effects and prepubescent boys. *Medicine & Science in Sports & Exercise* 22: 605-614.

Rana, S.R., Chleboun, G.S., Gilders, R.M., Hagerman, F.C., Herman, J.R., Hikida, R.S., Kushnick, M.R., Staron, R.S., and Toma, K. 2008. Comparison of early phase adaptations for traditional strength and endurance, and low velocity resistance training programs in college-aged women. *Journal of Strength and Conditioning Research* 22: 119-127.

Rarick, G.L., and Larson, G.L. 1958. Observations on frequency and intensity of isometric muscular effort in developing static muscular strength in post-pubescent males. *Research Quarterly* 29: 333-341.

Rasch, P., and Morehouse, L. 1957. Effect of static and dynamic exercises on muscular strength and hypertrophy. *Journal of Applied Physiology* 11: 29-34.

Rasch, P.J., and Pierson, W.R. 1964. One position versus multiple positions in isometric exercise. *American Journal of Physical Medicine* 43: 10-12.

Rasch, P.J., Preston, W.R., and Logan, G.A. 1961. The effect of isometric exercise upon the strength of antagonistic muscles. *Internationale Zeitschrift für Angewandte Physiologie Einschliesslich Arbeitsphysiologie* 19: 18-22.

Ratamess, N.A., Faigenbaum, A.D., Hoffman, J.R., and Kang, J. 2008. Self-selected resistance training intensity in healthy women: The influence of a personal trainer. *Journal of Strength and Conditioning Research* 22: 103-111.

Ratamess, N.A., Kraemer, W.J., Volek, J.S., Maresh, C.M., Vanheest, J.L., Sharman, M.J., Rubin, M.R., French, D.N., Vescovi, J.D., Silvestre, R., Hatfield, D.L., Fleck, S.J., and Deschenes, M.R. 2005. Androgen receptor content following heavy resistance exercise in men. *Journal of Steroid Biochemistry and Molecular Biology* 93: 35-42.

Rawson, E.S., and Volek, J.S. 2003. Effects of creatine supplementation and resistance training on muscle strength and weightlifting performance. *Journal of Strength and Conditioning Research* 17: 822-831.

Read, M.M., and Cisar, C. 2001. The influence of varied rest interval lengths on depth jump performance. *Journal of Strength and Conditioning Research* 15: 279-283.

Reeves, N.D., Maganaris, C.N., Longo, S., and Narici, M.V. 2009. Differential adaptations to eccentric versus conventional resistance training and older humans. *Experimental Physiology* 94: 825-833.

Reeves, N.D., Maganaris, C.N., and Narici, M.V. 2003. Effect of strength training on human patella tendon mechanical properties of older individuals. *Journal of Physiology* 548: 971-981.

Rehn, B., Lidstrom, J., Skoglund, J., and Lindstrom, B. 2007. Effects on leg muscular performance from whole-body vibration exercise: A systematic review. *Scandinavian Journal of Medicine & Science in Sports* 17: 2-11.

Reis, E., Frick, U., and Schmidbleicher, D. 1995. Frequency variations of strength training sessions triggered by the phases of the menstrual cycle. *International Journal of Sportsmedicine* 16: 545-550.

Reyes, G.F., and Doly, D. 2009. Acute effects of various weighted bat warm-up protocols on bat velocity. *Journal of Strength and Conditioning Research* 23: 2114-2118.

Rhea, M.R., 2004. Synthesizing strength and conditioning research: The meta-analysis. *Journal of Strength and Conditioning Research* 18: 921-923.

Rhea, M.R., and Alderman, B.L. 2004. A meta-analysis of periodized versus nonperiodized strengthen

and power training programs. *Research Quarterly for Exercise and Sport* 75: 413-422.

Rhea, M.R., Alvar, B.A., and Burkett, L.N. 2002. Single versus multiple sets for strength: A meta-analysis to address the controversy. *Research Quarterly for Exercise and Sport* 73: 485-488.

Rhea, M.R., Alvar, B.A., Burkett, L.N., and Ball, S.D. 2003. A meta-analysis to determine the dose response for strength development. *Medicine & Science in Sports & Exercise* 35: 456-464.

Rhea, M.R., Ball, S.D., Phillips, W.T., and Burkett, L.N. 2002. A comparison of linear and daily undulating periodized programs with equated volume and intensity for strength. *Journal of Strength and Conditioning Research* 16: 250-255.

Rhea, M.R., Phillips, W.T., Burkett, L.N., Stone, W.J., Ball, S.D., Alvar, B.A., and Thomas, A.B. 2003. A comparison of linear and daily undulating periodized programs with equated volume and intensity for local muscular endurance. *Journal of Strength and Conditioning Research* 17: 82-87.

Richford, C. 1966. *Principles of successful body building.* Alliance, NE: Iron Man Industries.

Rico, H., Gonzalez-Riola, J., Revilla, L.F., Gomez-Castresana, F., and Escribano, J. 1994. Cortical versus trabecular bone mass: Influence of activity on both bone components. *Calcified Tissue International* 37: 325-330.

Rimmer, E., and Sleivert, G. 2000. Effects of a plyometrics intervention program on sprint performance. *Journal of Strength and Conditioning Research* 14: 295-301.

Rixon, K.P., Lamont, H.S., and Bemben, M.G. 2007. Influence of type of muscle contraction, gender, and lifting experience on postactivation potentiation performance. *Journal of Strength and Conditioning Research* 21: 500-505.

Rizzo, M.R., Mari, D., Barbieri, M., Ragno, E., Grella, R., Provenzano, R., Villa, I., Esposito, K., Giugliano, D., and Paolisso, G. 2005. Resting metabolic rate and respiratory quotient in human longevity. *Journal of Clinical Endocrinology and Metabolism* 90: 409-413.

Robbins, D.W. 2005. Postactivation potentiation and its practical applicability: A brief review. 2005. *Journal of Strength and Conditioning Research* 19: 453-458.

Robbins, D.W., Young, W.B., and Behm, D.G. 2010. The effect of an upper-body agonist-antagonist resistance training protocol on volume load and efficiency. *Journal of Strength and Conditioning Research* 24: 2632-2640.

Robbins, D.W., Young, W.B., Behm, D.G., and Payne, W.R. 2010a. Agonist–antagonist paired set resistance training: A brief review. *Journal of Strength and Conditioning Research.* 24: 2873-2882.

Robbins, D.W., Young, W.B., Behm, D.G., and Payne, W.R. 2010b. The effect of a complex agonist and antagonist training protocol on volume load, power output, electromyographic responses, and efficiency. *Journal of Strength and Conditioning Research* 24: 1782-1789.

Robbins, D.W., Young, W.B., Behm, D.G., Payne, W.R., and Klimstra, M.D. 2010c. Physical performance and electromyographic responses to an acute bout of paired set strength training versus traditional strength training. *Journal of Strength and Conditioning Research* 24: 1237-1245.

Robergs, R.A., Ghiasvand, F., and Parker, D. 2004. Biochemistry of exercise-induced metabolic acidosis. *American Journal of Physiology Regulatory Integrative and Comparative Physiology* 287: R502-R516.

Roberts, J.M., and Wilson, K. 1999. Effect of stretching duration on active and passive range of motion in the lower extremity. *British Journal of Sports Medicine* 33: 259-263.

Robinson, J.M., Stone, M.H., Johnson, R.L., Penland, C.M., Warren, B.J., and Lewis, R.D. 1995. Effects of different weight training exercise/rest intervals on strength, power, and high intensity exercise endurance. *Journal of Strength and Conditioning Research* 9: 216-221.

Roelants, M., Verschuern, S.M.P., Delecluse, C., Levin, O., and Stijnen, V. 2006. Whole-body-vibration-induced increase in leg muscle electricity during different squat exercises. *Journal of Strength and Conditioning Research* 20: 124-129.

Rogers, M.A., and Evans, W.J. 1993. Changes in skeletal muscle with aging: Effects of exercise training. In *Exercise and sport sciences reviews*, vol. 21, edited by J.O. Holloszy. Baltimore: Williams & Wilkins.

Roltsch, M.H., Mendez, T., Wilund, K.R., and Hagberg, J.M. 2001. Acute resistive exercise does not affect ambulatory blood pressure in young men and women. *Medicine & Science in Sports & Exercise* 33: 881- 886.

Ronnestad, B.R., Egeland, W., Kvamme, N.H., Refsnes, P.E., Kadi, F., and Raastad, T. 2007. Dissimilar effects of one-and three-set strength training on strength and muscle mass gains in upper and lower body in untrained subjects. *Journal of Strength and Conditioning Research* 21: 157-163.

Ronnestad, B.R., Hansen, E.A., and Raastad, T. 2012a. Strength training affects tendon cross-sectional area and freely chosen cadence differently in noncyclists and well-trained cyclists. *Journal of Strength and Conditioning Research* 26: 158-166.

Rønnestad, B.R., Hansen, E.A., Raastad, T. 2012b. High volume of endurance training impairs adaptations to 12 weeks of strength training in well-trained endurance athletes. *European Journal of Applied Physiology* 112: 1457-1466.

Rønnestad, B.R., Nygaard, H., and Raastad, T. 2011. Physiological elevation of endogenous hormones results in superior strength training adaptation. *European Journal of Applied Physiology* 111: 2249-2259.

Ronnestad, B.R., Nymark, B.S., and Raastad, T. 2011. Effects of in-season strength maintenance training frequency in professional soccer players. *Journal of Strength and Conditioning Research* 25: 2653-2660.

Rooney, K.J., Herbert, R.D., and Balwave, R.J. 1994. Fatigue contributes to the strength training stimulus. *Medicine & Science in Sports & Exercise* 26: 1160-1164.

Rooyackers, O.E., and Nair, K.S. 1997. Hormonal regulation of human muscle protein metabolism. *Annual Reviews in Nutrition* 17: 457-485.

Roth, D.A., Stanley, W.C., and Brooks, G.A. 1988. Induced lactacidemia does not affect postexercise O_2 consumption. *Journal of Applied Physiology* 65: 1045-1049.

Roth, S.M., Martel, G.F., Ivey, F.M., Lemmer, J.T., Tracy, B.L., Hurlbut, D.E., Metter, E.J., Hurley, B.F., and Rogers, M.A. 1999. Ultrastructural muscle damage in young vs. older men after high-volume, heavy resistance strength training. *Journal of Applied Physiology* 86: 1833-1840.

Roth, S.M., Martel, G.F., Ivey, F.M., Lemmer, J.T., Tracy, B.L., Hurlbut, D.E., Metter, E.J., Hurley, B.F., and Rogers, M.A. 2000. High-volume, heavy-resistance strength training and muscle damage in young and older women. *Journal of Applied Physiology* 86: 1112-1118.

Rothenberg, E.M., Bosaeus, I.G., and Steen, B.C. 2003. Energy expenditure at age 73 and 78—a five year follow-up. *Acta Diabetologica* 40 (Suppl. 1): S134-138.

Roubenoff, R. 2001. Origins and clinical relevance of sarcopenia. *Canadian Journal of Applied Physiology* 26: 78-89.

Roubenoff, R. 2003. Sarcopenis: Effects on body composition and function. *Journal of Gerontology* 58A: 1012-1017.

Roupas, N.D., and Georgopoulos, N.A. 2011. Menstrual function in sports. *Hormones* (Athens) 10: 104-116.

Rowell, L.B., Kranning, K.K., Evans, T.O., Kennedy, J.W., Blackman, J.R., and Kusumi, F. 1966. Splanchnic removal of lactate and pyruvate during prolonged exercise in man. *Journal of Applied Physiology* 21: 1773-1783.

Rowland, T., and Fernhall, B. 2007. Cardiovascular responses to static exercise: A re-appraisal. *International Journal of Sports Medicine* 28: 905-908.

Rowlinson, S.W., Waters, M.J., Lewis, U.J., and Barnard, R. 1996. Human growth hormone fragments 1-43 and 44-191: In vitro somatogenic activity and receptor binding characteristics in human and non-primate systems. *Endocrinology* 137: 90-95.

Roy, B.D., Tarnopolsky, M.A., MacDougall, J.D., Fowles, J., and Yarasheski, K.E. 1997. Effect of glucose supplement timing on protein metabolism after resistance training. *Journal of Applied Physiology* 82: 1882-1888.

Rubin, M.R., Kraemer, W.J., Maresh, C.M., Volek, J.S., Ratamess, N.A., Vanheest, J.L., Silvestre, R., French, D.N., Sharman, M.J., Judelson, D.A., Gómez, A.L., Vescovi, J.D., and Hymer, W.C. 2005. High-affinity growth hormone binding protein and acute heavy resistance exercise. *Medicine & Science in Sports & Exercise* 37: 395-403.

Ruggiero, C., Metter, E.J., Melenovsky, V., Cherublnl, A., Najjer, S.S., Ble, A., Senin, U., Longo, D.L., and Ferrucci, L. 2008. High basal metabolic rate is a risk factor for mortality: The Baltimore Longitudinal Study of Aging. *Journals of Gerontology Series A: Biological Sciences and Medical Sciences* 63: 698-706.

Ruiz, J.R., Moran, M., Arenas, J., and Lucia, A. 2011. Strenuous endurance exercise improves life expectancy: It's in our genes. *British Journal of Sports Medicine* 45: 159-161.

Ruiz, J.R., Sui, X., Lobelo, F., Morrow, J.R., Jackson, A.W., Sjostrom, M. and Blair, S.N. 2008. Association V. muscular strength and mortality in men: Prospective cohort study. *British Medical Journal* 337: 92-95.

Ruiz, R.J., Simão, R., Sacomani, M.G., Casonatto, J., Alexander, J.L., Rhea, M., and Polito, M.D. 2011. Isolated and combined effects of aerobic and strength exercise on post-exercise blood pressure and cardiac vagal reactivation in normotensive men. *Journal of Strength and Conditioning Research* 25: 640-645.

Russell-Jones, D.L., Umpleby, A., Hennessey, T., Bowes, S., Shojaee-Moradies, F., Hopkins, K., Jackson, N., Kelly, J., Jones, R., and Sonksen, P. 1994. Use of leucine clamp to demonstrate that IGF-I actively stimulates protein synthesis in normal humans. *American Journal of Physiology* 267: E591-598.

Ryan, A.S., Ivey, F.M., Hurlbut, D.E., Martel, G.F., Lemmer, J.T., Sorkin, J.D., Metter, E.J., Fleg, J.L., and Hurley, B.F. 2004. Regional bone mineral density after resistive training in young and older men and women. *Scandinavian Journal of Medicine and Science in Sports* 14: 16-23.

Ryan, E.D., Beck, T.W., Herda, T.J., Hull, H.R., Hartman, M.J., Costa, P.B, Defreitas, J.M., Stout, J.R., and Cramer, J.T. 2008. The time course of musculotendinous stiffness responses following different durations of passive stretching. *Journal of Orthopedic and Sports Physical Therapy* 38: 632-639.

Ryushi, T., Häkkinen, K., Kauhanen, H., and Komi, P.V. 1988. Muscle fiber characteristics, muscle cross-sectional area and force production in strength athletes, physically active males and females. *Scandinavian Journal of Sports Science* 10: 7-15.

Sadamoto, T., Bonde-Peterson, F., and Suzuki, Y. 1983. Skeletal muscle tension, flow pressure and EMG during sustained isometric contractions in humans. *European Journal of Applied Physiology* 51: 395-408.

Saeterbakken, A.H., van den Tillaar, R., and Seiler, S. 2011. Effect of core stability training and throwing velocity in female handball players. *Journal of Strength and Conditioning Research* 25: 712-718.

Saez Saez deVillarreal, E., Gonzalez-Badillo, J.J., and Izquierdo, M. 2007. Optimal warm-up stimuli of muscle activation to enhance short and long-term acute jumping performance. *European Journal of Applied Physiology* 100: 393-401.

Saez Saez deVillarreal, E., Gonzalez-Badillo, J.J., and Izquierdo, M. 2008. Low and moderate plyometric training frequency produces greater jumping and spending gains compared with high frequency. *Journal of Strength and Conditioning Research* 22: 715-725.

Saez Saez de Villarreal, E., Kellis, E., Kraemer, W.J., and Izquierdo, M. 2009. Determining variables of plyometric training for improving vertical jump height performance: A meta-analysis. *Journal of Strength and Conditioning Research* 23: 495-506.

Sahlin, K., and Ren, J.M. 1989. Relationship of contraction capacity to metabolic changes during recovery from a fatiguing contraction. *Journal of Applied Physiology* 67: 648-654.

Sailors, M., and Berg, K. 1987. Comparison of responses to weight training in pubescent boys and men. *Journal of Sports Medicine* 27: 30-37.

Sale, D.G. 1992. Neural adaptations to strength training. In *Strength and power in sport,* edited by P.V. Komi, 249-265. Boston: Blackwell Scientific.

Sale, D.G., MacDougall, J.D., Alway, S.E., and Sutton, J.R. 1987. Voluntary strength and muscle characteristics in untrained men and women and male bodybuilders. *Journal of Applied Physiology* 62: 1786-1793.

Sale, D.G., MacDougall, J.D., Jacobs, I., and Garner, S. 1990. Interaction between concurrent strength and endurance training. *Journal of Applied Physiology* 68: 260-270.

Sale, D.G., MacDougall, J.D., Upton, A.R.M., and McComas, A.J. 1983. Effect of strength training upon motoneuron excitability in man. *Medicine & Science in Sports & Exercise* 15: 57-62.

Sale, D.G., Moroz, D.E., McKelvie, R.S., MacDougall, J.D., and McCartney, N. 1993. Comparison of blood pressure response to isokinetic and weight-lifting exercise. *European Journal of Applied Physiology* 67: 115-120.

Sale, D.G., Moroz, D.E., McKelvie, R.S., MacDougall, J.D., and McCartney, N. 1994. Effect of training on the blood pressure response to weight lifting. *Canadian Journal of Applied Physiology* 19: 60-74.

Sallinen, J., Fogelholm, M., Pakarinen, A., Juvonen, T., Volek, J.S., Kraemer, W.J., Alen, M., and Häkkinen, K. 2005. Effects of strength training and nutritional counseling metabolic health indicators and aging women. *Canadian Journal of Applied Physiology* 30: 690-707.

Sallinen, J., Fogelholm, M., Volek, J.S., Kraemer, W.J., Alen, M., and Häkkinen, K. 2007. Effects of strength training and reduced training on functional performance and metabolic health indicators in middle-aged men. *International Journal of Sports Medicine* 28: 815-822.

Sallinen, J., Pakarinen, A., Fogelholm, M., Sillanpaa, E., Alen, M., Volek, J.S., Kraemer, W.J., and Häkkinen, K. 2006. Serum basal hormone concentrations and muscle mass in aging women: Effects of strength training and diet. *International Journal of Sport Nutrition and Exercise Metabolism* 16: 316-331.

Saltin, B., and Astrand, P.O. 1967. Maximal oxygen uptake in athletes. *Journal of Applied Physiology* 23: 353-358.

Sanborn, K., Boros, R., Hruby, J., Schilling, B., O'Bryant, H., Johnson, R., Hoke, T., Stone, M., and Stone, M.H. 2000. Performance effects of weight training with multiple sets not to failure versus a single set to failure in women. *Journal of Strength and Conditioning Research* 14: 328-331.

Sanchez-Medina, L., and Gonzalez-Badillo, J.J. 2011. Velocity loss as an indicator of neuromuscular fatigue during resistance training. *Medicine in Science in Sports and Exercise* 43: 1725-1734.

Sandberg, J.B., Wagner, D.R., Willardson, J.M., and Smith, G.A. 2012. Acute effects of antagonist stretching on jump height, torque, and electromyography of agonist musculature *Journal of Strength and Conditioning Research* 26: 1249-1256.

Sands, W.A., McNeal, J.R., Stone, Haff, G.G., and Kinser, A.M. 2008. Effect of vibration on forward split flexibility and pain perception in young male gymnasts. *International Journal of Physiology and Performance* 3: 469-481.

Sands, W.A., McNeal, J.R., Stone, M.H., Russell, E.M., and Jemni, M. 2006. Flexibility enhancement with vibration: Acute and long-term. *Medicine & Science in Sports & Exercise* 38: 720-725.

Santos, A.P., Marinho, D.A., Costa, A.M., Izquierdo, M., and Marques, M.C. 2012. The effects of concurrent resistance and endurance training follow a detraining period in elementary school students. Musculature. *Journal of Strength and Conditioning Research* 26: 1708-1716.

Santos, E., Rhea, M.R., Simão, R., Dias, I., de Salles, B.F., Novaes, J., Leite, T., Blair, J.C., and Bunker, D.J. 2010. Influence of moderately intense strength training on flexibility in sedentary young women. *Journal of Strength and Conditioning Research* 24: 3144-3149.

Santos, E.J.A.M., and Janeira, M.A.A.S. 2008. Effects of complex training on explosive strength in adolescent male basketball players. *Journal of Strength and Conditioning Research* 22: 903-909.

Santos, E.J.A.M., and Janeira, M.A.A.S. 2009. Effects of reduced training and detraining on upper and lower body explosive strength in adolescent male basketball players. *Journal of Strength and Conditioning Research* 23: 1737-1744.

Santos, E.J.A.M., and Janeira, M.A.A.S. 2011. The effects of plyometric training the effects of plyometric training followed by detraining and reduced training periods explosive in adolescent male basketball players. *Journal of Strength and Conditioning Research* 25: 441-452.

Sapolsky, R.M., Romero, L.M., and Munck, A.U. 2000. How do glucocorticoids influence stress responses? Integrating permissive, suppressive, stimulatory, and preparative actions. *Endocrine Reviews* 21: 55-89.

Sarna S., Sahi T., Koskenvuo M., and Kaprio, J. 1993. Increased life expectancy of world class male athletes. *Medicine & Science in Sports & Exercise* 25: 237-244.

Saxton, J.M., Clarkson, P.M., James, R., Miles, M., Westerfer, M., Clark, S., and Donnelly, A.E. 1995. Neuromuscular dysfunction following eccentric exercise. *Medicine & Science in Sports & Exercise* 27: 1185-1193.

Saxton, J.M., and Donnelly, A.E. 1995. Light concentric exercise during recovery from exercise-induced muscle damage. *International Journal of Sports Medicine* 16: 347-351.

Sayers, S.P., and Clarkson, P.M. 2001. Force recovery after eccentric exercise in males and females. *European Journal of Applied Physiology* 84: 122-126.

Sayers, S.P., Clarkson, P.M., Rouzier, P.A., and Kamen, G. 1999. Adverse events associated with eccentric exercise protocols: Six case studies. *Medicine & Science in Sports & Exercise* 31: 1697-1702.

Sayers, S.P., Guralnik, J.M., Thombs, L.A., and Fielding, R.A. 2005. Impact of leg muscle contraction velocity on functional performance in older men and women. *Journal of the American Geriatric Society* 53: 467-471.

Schantz, P. 1982. Capillary supply in hypertrophied human skeletal muscle. *Acta Physiologica Scandinavica* 114: 635-637.

Schantz, P., Randall-Fox, E., Hutchinson, W., Tyden, A., and Astrand, P.O. 1983. Muscle fibre type distribution, muscle cross-sectional area and maximal voluntary strength in humans. *Acta Physiologica Scandinavica* 117: 219-226.

Schantz, P., Randall-Fox, E., Norgen, P., and Tyden, A. 1981. The relationship between the mean muscle fibre area and the muscle cross-sectional area of the thigh in subjects with large differences in thigh girth. *Physiologica Scandinavica* 113: 537-539.

Scharf, H.-P., Eckhardt, R., Maurus, M., and Puhl, W. 1994. Metabolic and hemodynamic changes during

isokinetic muscle training. *International Journal of Sports Medicine* 15: S56-S59.

Scher, J.M.L., Ferriolli, E., Moriguti, J.C., Scher, R., and Lima, N.K.C. 2011. The effect of different volumes of acute resistance exercise on elderly individuals with treated hypertension. *Journal of Strength and Conditioning Research* 25: 1016-1023.

Schilling, B.K., Falvo, M.J., Karlage, R.E., Weiss, L.W., Lohnes, C.A., and Chiu, L.Z.F. 2009. Effects of unstable surface training on measures of balance in older adults. *Journal of Strength and Conditioning Research* 23: 1211-1216.

Schiotz, M.K., Potteiger, J.A., Huntsinger, P.G., and Denmark, D.C. 1998. The short-term effects of periodized and constant-intensity training on body composition, strength, and performance. *Journal of Strength and Conditioning Research* 12: 173-178.

Schlumberger, A., Stec, J., and Schmidtbleicher, D. 2001. Single- vs. multiple-set strength training in women. *Journal of Strength and Conditioning Research* 15: 284-289.

Schmidtbleicher, D. 1994. Training for power events. In *Strength and power and sport*, edited by P.V. Komi, 381-395. London: Blackwell Scientific.

Schmidtbleicher, D., and Gollhofer, A. 1982. Neuromuskulare Untersuchungen zur Bestimmung individueller Belatungsgrossen für ein Tiefsprungtraining. *Leistungssport* 12: 298-307.

Schmidtbleicher, D., Gollhofer, A., and Frick, U. 1988. Effects of stretch-shortening type training on the performance capability and innervation characteristics of leg extensor muscles. In *Biomechanics XI-A*, edited by G. deGroot, A. Hollander, P. Huijing, and G. van Ingen Schenau, vol. 7-A, 185-189. Amsterdam: Free University Press.

Schneider, V., Arnold, B., Martin, K., Bell, D., and Crocker, P. 1998. Detraining effects in college football players during the competitive season. *Journal of Strength and Conditioning Research* 12: 42-45.

Schnoebelen-Combes, S., Louveau, I., Postel-Vinay, M.C., and Bonneau, M. 1996. Ontogeny of GH receptor and GH-binding protein in the pig. *Journal of Endocrinology* 148: 249-255.

Schoenfeld, B.J. 2010. The mechanisms of muscle hypertrophy and their application to resistance training. *Journal of Strength and Conditioning Research* 24: 2857-2872.

Schott, J., McCully, K., and Rutherford, O.M. 1995. The role of metabolites in strength training II. Short versus long isometric contractions. *European Journal of Applied Physiology* 71: 337-341.

Schroeder, E.T., Hawkins, S.A., and Jaque, S.V. 2004. Musculoskeletal adaptations 16 weeks of eccentric progressive resistance training in young women. *Journal of Strength and Conditioning Research* 18: 227-235.

Schuenke, M.D., Herman, J.R., Gliders, R.M., Hagerman, F.C., Hikida, R.S., Rana, S.R., Ragg, K.E., and Staron, R.S. 2012. Early-phase muscular adaptations in response to slow-speed versus traditional resistance-training regimens. *European Journal of Applied Physiology* 112: 3585-3595.

Schuenke, M.D., Herman, J., and Staron, R.S. 2013. Preponderance of evidence proves "big" weights optimize hypertrophic and strength adaptations. *European Journal of Applied Physiology* 113: 269-271.

Schultz, R.W. 1967. Effect of direct practice and repetitive sprinting and weight training on selected motor performance tasks. *Research Quarterly* 38: 108-118.

Schwab, R., Johnson, G.O., Housh, T.J., Kinder, J.E., and Weir, J.P. 1993. Acute effects of different intensities of weight lifting on serum testosterone. *Medicine & Science in Sports & Exercise* 25: 1381-1385.

Schweizer, A., Schneider, A., and Goehner, K. 2007. Dynamic eccentric-concentric strength training of the finger flexors to improve rock climbing performance. *Isokinetics and Exercise Science* 15: 131-136.

Scofield, D.E., McClung, H.L., McClung, J.P., Kraemer, W.J., Rarick, K.R., Pierce, J.R., Cloutier, G.J., Fielding, R.A., Matheny, R.W., Jr., Young, A.J., and Nindl, B.C. 2011. A novel, noninvasive transdermal fluid sampling methodology: IGF-I measurement following exercise. *American Journal of Physiology Regulatory Integrative and Comparative Physiology* 300: R1326-R1332.

Scoles, G. 1978. Depth jumping! Does it really work? *Athletic Journal* 58: 48-75.

Seaborne, D., and Taylor, A.W. 1984. The effect of speed of isokinetic exercise on training transfer to isometric strength in the quadriceps. *Journal of Sports Medicine* 24: 183-188.

Seals, D.R. 1993. Influence of active muscle size on sympathetic nerve discharge during isometric contractions in humans. *Journal of Applied Physiology* 75: 1426-1431.

Secher, N.H. 1975. Isometric rowing strength of experienced and inexperienced oarsmen. *Medicine & Science in Sports & Exercise* 7: 280-283.

Secher, N.H., Rorsgaard, S., and Secher, O. 1978. Contralateral influence on recruitment of curarized muscle fibers during maximal voluntary extension of the legs. *Acta Physiologica Scandinavica* 130: 455-462.

Sedano Campo, S., Vaeyens, R., Philippaerts, R.M., Redondo, J.C., De Benito, A.M., and Cuadrado, G. 2009. Effects of lower-limb plyometric training on body composition, explosive strength, and kicking speed in female soccer players. *Journal of Strength and Conditioning Research* 23: 1714-1722.

Seger, J.Y., Arvidsson, B., and Thorstensson, A. 1998. Specific effects of eccentric and concentric training on muscle strength and morphology in humans. *European Journal of Applied Physiology* 79: 49-57.

Selye, H. 1936. A syndrome produced by diverse nocuous agents. *Nature* 138: 32.

Serra-Rexach, J.A., Bustamante-Ara, N., Villarán, M.H., Gil, P.G., Sanz Ibáñez, M.J., Blanco Sanz, N., Ortega Santamaría, V., Gutiérrez Sanz, N., Marín Prada, A.B., Gallardo, C., Rodríguez Romo, G., Ruiz, J.R., and Lucia, A. 2011. Short-term, light-moderate intensity exercise training improves leg muscle strength in the oldest old: A randomized controlled trial. *Journal of the American Geriatric Society* 59: 594-602.

Serresse, O., Lortie, G., Bouchard, C., and Boulay, M.R. 1988. Estimation of the contribution of the various energy systems during maximal work of short duration. *International Journal of Sports Medicine* 9: 456-460.

Sewall, L., and Micheli, L. 1986. Strength training for children. *Journal of Pediatric Orthopedics* 6: 143-146.

Sewright, K.A., Hubal, M.J., Kearns, A., Holbrook, M.T., and Clarkson, P.M. 2008. Sex differences in response to maximal eccentric exercise. *Medicine & Science in Sports & Exercise* 40: 242-251.

Sforzo, G.A., and Touey, P.R. 1996. Manipulating exercise order affects muscular performance during a resistance exercise training session. *Journal of Strength and Conditioning Research* 10: 20-24.

Sgro, M., McGuigan, M.R., Pettigrew, S., and Newton, R.U. 2009. The effect of duration of resistance training interventions in children who are overweight or obese. *Medicine & Science in Sports & Exercise* 23: 1263-1270.

Shaharudin, S., Ghosh, A.K., and Ismail, A.A. 2011. Anaerobic capacity of physically active eumenorrheic females at mid-luteal and mid-follicular phases of ovarian cycle. *Journal of Sports Medicine and Physical Fitness* 51: 576-582.

Shaibi, G.Q., Cruz, M.L., Ball, G.D., Weigensberg, M.J., Salem, G.J., Crespo, N.C., and Goran, M.I. 2006. Effects of resistance training on insulin sensitivity in overweight Latino adolescent males. *Medicine & Science in Sports & Exercise* 38: 1208-1215.

Sharman, M.J., Newton, R.U., Triplett-McBride, T., McGuigan, M.R., McBride, J.M., Häkkinen, A., Häkkinen, K., and Kraemer, W.J. 2001. Changes in myosin heavy chain composition with heavy resistance training in 60- to 70-year-old men and women. *European Journal of Applied Physiology* 84 (1-2): 127-132.

Sharp, M.A. 1994. Physical fitness and occupational performance of women in the U.S. Army. *Work* 2: 80-92.

Shaw, B.S., Shaw, I., and Brown, G.A. 2009. Comparison of resistance and concurrent resistance and endurance training regimes in the development of strength. *Journal of Strength and Conditioning Research* 23: 2507-2514.

Shaw, C.E., McCully, K.K., and Posner, J.D. 1995. Injuries during the one repetition maximum assessment in the elderly. *Journal of Cardiopulmonary Rehabilitation* 15: 283-287.

Shellock, F.G., and Prentice, W.E. 1985. Warming-up and stretching for improved physical performance and prevention of sports related injuries. *Sports Medicine* 2: 267-278.

Shephard, R.J. 2000a. Exercise and training in women, part I: Influence of gender on exercise and training responses. *Canadian Journal of Applied Physiology* 25: 19-34.

Shephard, R.J. 2000b. Exercise and training in women, part II: Influence of menstrual cycle and pregnancy on exercise responses. *Canadian Journal of Applied Physiology* 25: 35-54.

Shepstone, T.N., Tang, J.E., Dallaire, S., Schuenke, M.D., Staron, R.S., and Phillips, S.M. 2005. Short-term high- vs low-velocity isokinetic lengthening training results in greater hypertrophy of the elbow in young men. *Journal of Applied Physiology* 98: 1768-1776.

Shimano, T., Kraemer, W.J., Spiering, B.A., Volek, J.S., Hatfield, D.L., Silvestre, R., Vingren, J.L., Fragala, M.S., Maresh, C.M., Fleck, S.J., Newton, R.U., Spreuwenberg, L.P., and Häkkinen, K. 2006. Relationship between the number of repetitions and selected percentages of one repetition maximum in free weight exercises in trained and untrained men. *Journal of Strength and Conditioning Research* 20: 819-823.

Shinohara, M., Kouzaki, M., Yoshihisa, T., and Fukunaga, T. 1998. Efficacy of tourniquet ischemia for strength training with low resistance. *European Journal of Applied Physiology* 77: 189-191.

Shultz, S.J., Schmitz, R.J., Kong, Y., Dudley, W.N., Beynnon, B.D., Nguyen, A-D., Kim, H., and Montgomery, M.M. 2012. Cyclic variations in multiplanar knee laxity influence landing biomechanics. *Medicine & Science in Sports & Exercise* 44: 900-909.

Siegal, J., Camaione, D., and Manfredi, T. 1989. The effects of upper body resistance training in prepubescent children. *Pediatrics Exercise Science* 1: 145-154.

Siewe, J., Rudat, J., Röllinghoff, M., Schlegel, U.J., Eysel, P., and Michael, J.W. 2011. Injuries and overuse syndromes in powerlifting. *International Journal of Sports Medicine.* 32: 703-711.

Sigal, R.J., Kenny, G.P., Boulé, N.G., Wells, G.A., Prud'homme, D., Fortier, M., Reid, R.D., Tulloch, H., Coyle, D., Phillips, P., Jennings, A., and Jaffey, J. 2007. Effects of aerobic training, resistance training, or both on glycemic control in type 2 diabetes: A randomized trial. *Annals of Internal Medicine* 147: 357-369.

Sillanapaa, E., Laaksonen, D.E., Häkkinen, A., Karavirta, L., Jensen, B., Kraemer, W.J., Nyman, K., and Häkkinen, K. 2009. Body composition, fitness, and metabolic health during strength and endurance training and their combination in middle-aged and older women. *European Journal of Applied Physiology* 106: 286-296.

Silva, H.R., Couto, B.P., and Szmuchrowski, L.A. 2008. Effects of mechanical vibration applied in the opposite direction of muscle shortening on maximal isometric strength. *Journal of Strength and Conditioning Research* 22: 1031-1036.

Silva, R.F., Cadore, E.L., Kothe, G., Guedes, M., Alberton, C.L., Pinto, S.S., Pinto, R.S., Trindade, G., and Kruel, L.F. 2012. Concurrent training with different aerobic exercises. *International Journal of Sports Medicine* 33: 627-634.

Silvester, L.J., Stiggins, C., McGown, C., and Bryce, G. 1984. The effect of variable resistance and free-weight training programs on strength and vertical jump. *National Strength and Conditioning Association Journal* 5: 30-33.

Silvestre, R., Kraemer, W.J., West, C., Judelson, D.A., Spiering, B.A., Vingren, J.L., Hatfield, D.L., Anderson, J.M., and Maresh, C.M. 2006. Body composition and physical performance during a national collegiate athletic association division I men's soccer season. *Journal of Strength and Conditioning Research* 20: 962-970.

Simão, R., Farinatti Pde., T., Polito, M.D., Viveiros, L., and Fleck, S.J. 2007. Influence of exercise order on the number of repetitions performed and perceived exertion during resistance exercise in women. *Journal of Strength and Conditioning Research* 21: 23-28.

Simão, R., Fleck, S.J., Polito, M., Monteiro, W., and Farinatti, P.T.V. 2005. Effects of resistance training intensity, volume, and session format on the post exercise hypotensive response. *Journal of Strength and Conditioning Research* 19: 853- 858.

Simão, R., Spineti, J., Freitas de Salles, B., Matta, T., Fernandes, L.,Fleck, S.J., Rhea, M.R., and Strom-Olsen, H.E. 2012. Comparison between inear and nonlinear periodized resistance training: Strength and muscle thickness effects. *Journal of Strength and Conditioning Research* 26: 1389-1395.

Simenz, C.J., Dugan, C.A., and Ebben, W.P. 2005. Strength and conditioning practices of National Basketball Association strength and conditioning coaches. *Journal of Strength and Conditioning Research* 19: 1495-1504.

Singh, M.A., Ding, W., Manfredi, T.J., Solares, G.S., O'Neill, E.F., Clements, K.M., Ryan, N.D., Kehayias, J.J., Fielding, R.A., and Evans, W.J. 1999. Insulin-like growth factor I in skeletal muscle after weight-lifting exercise in frail elders. *American Journal of Physiology* 277: E135-E143.

Sinnett, A.M., Berg, K., Latin, R.W., and Noble, J.M. 2001. The relationship between field tests of anaerobic power and 10-km run performance. *Journal of Strength and Conditioning Research* 15: 405-412.

Sinning, W.E. 1974. Body composition assessment of college wrestlers. *Medicine and Science in Sports* 6: 139-145.

Skinner, J.S., Jaskólski, A., Jaskólska, A., Krasnoff, J., Gagnon, J., Leon, A.S., Rao, D.C., Wilmore, J.H., and Bouchard, C. 2001. Age, sex, race, initial fitness, and response to training: The HERITAGE Family Study. *Journal of Applied Physiology* 90: 1770-1776.

Skutek, M., van Griensven, M., Zeichen, J., Brawer, N., and Bosch, U. 2001. Cyclic mechanical stretching modulates secretion pattern of growth factors in human tendon fibroblasts. *European Journal of Applied Physiology* 86: 48-52.

Smith, E.L., Smith, P.E., Ensign, C.J., and Shea, M.M. 1984. Bone involution decrease in exercising middle-aged women. *Calcified Tissue International* 36 (Suppl.): S129-S138.

Smith, J.C., and Fry, A.C. 2007. Effects of a ten-second maximum voluntary contraction on regulatory myosin light-chain phosphorylation and dynamic performance measures. *Journal of Strength and Conditioning Research* 21: 73-76.

Smith, K., Winegard, K., Hicks, A.L., and McCartney, N. 2003. Two years of resistance training in older men and women: The effects of three years of detraining on the retention of dynamic strength. *Canadian Journal of Applied Physiology* 28: 462-474.

Smith, L.L. 2000. Cytokine hypothesis of overtraining: A physiological adaptation to excessive stress? *Medicine & Science in Sports & Exercise* 32: 317-331.

Smith, M.J., and Melton, P. 1981. Isokinetic versus isotonic variable resistance training. *American Journal of Sports Medicine* 9: 275-279.

Smith, M.L., and Raven, B.P. 1986. Cardiovascular responses to lower body negative pressure in endurance and static exercise trained men. *Medicine & Science in Sports & Exercise* 18: 545-550.

Smith, R.C., and Rutherford, O.M. 1995. The role of metabolites in strength training I. A comparison of eccentric and concentric contractions. *European Journal of Applied Physiology* 71: 332-336.

Snoecky, L.H.E.H., Abeling, H.F.M., Lambrets, J.A.C., Schmitz, J.J.F., Verstappen, F.T.J., and Reneman, R.S. 1982. Echocardiographic dimensions in athletes in relation to their training programs. *Medicine & Science in Sports & Exercise* 14: 42-54.

Snow, C.M., Rosen, C.J., and Robinson, T.L. 2000. Serum IGF-I is higher in gymnasts than runners and predicts bone and lean mass. *Medicine & Science in Sports & Exercise* 32: 1902-1907.

Snow, C.M., Williams, D.P., LaRiviere, J., Fuchs, R.K., and Robinson, T.L. 2001. Bone gains and losses follow seasonal training and detraining in gymnasts. *Calcified Tissue International* 60: 7-12.

Sorichter, S., Mair, J., Koller, A., Secnik, P., Parrak, V., Haid, C., Muller, E., and Puschendorf, B. 1997. Muscular adaptation and strength during the early phase of eccentric training: Influence of the training frequency. *Medicine & Science in Sports & Exercise* 29: 1646-1652.

Sparti, A., DeLany, J.P., de la Bretonne, J.A., Sander, G.E, and Bray, G.A. 1997. Relationship between resting metabolic rate and the composition of the fat-free mass. *Metabolism* 46: 1225-1230.

Spataro, A., Pellicca, A., Proschan, M.A., Granata, M., Spataro, A., Bellone, P., Caselli, G., Biffi, A., Vecchio, C., and Maron, B.J. 1994. Morphology of the "athlete's heart" assessed by echocardiography in 947 elite athletes representing 27 sports. *American Journal of Cardiology* 74: 802-806.

Spence, A.L., Carter, H.H., Murray, C.P., Oxborough, D., Naylor, L.H., George, K.P., and Green, D.J. 2013. Magnetic resonance imaging-derived right ventricular adaptations to endurance versus resistance training. *Medicine and Science in Sports and Exercise* 45: 534-541.

Spencer, M., Bishop, D., Dawson, B., and Goodman, C. 2005. Physiological and metabolic responses of repeated-sprint activities specific to field-based team sports. *Sports Medicine* 35: 1025-1044.

Speroff, L., and Redwine, D.B. 1980. Exercise and menstrual function. *Physician and Sportsmedicine* 8: 42-48.

Spiering, B.A., Kraemer W.J., Anderson, J.M., Armstrong, L.E., Nindl, B.C., Volek, J.S., Judelson, D.A., Joseph, M., Vingren, J.L., Hatfield, D.L., Fragala, M.S., Ho, J.Y., and Maresh, C.M. 2008a. Effects of elevated circulating hormones on resistance exercise-induced Akt signaling. *Medicine & Science in Sports & Exercise* 40: 1039-1048.

Spiering, B.A., Kraemer, W.J., Anderson, J.M., Armstrong, L.E., Nindl, B.C., Volek, J.S., and Maresh, C.M. 2008b. Resistance exercise biology: Manipulation of resistance exercise programme variables determines the responses of cellular and molecular signaling pathways. *Sports Medicine* 38: 527-540.

Spiering, B.A., Kraemer, W.J., Vingren, J.L., Ratamess, N.A., Anderson, J.M., Armstrong, L.E., Nindl, B.C., Volek, J.S., Häkkinen, K., and Maresh, C.M. 2009. Elevated endogenous testosterone concentrations potentiate muscle androgen receptor responses to resistance exercise. *Journal of Steroid Biochemistry and Molecular Biology* 114: 195-199.

Spitzer, J.J. 1974. Effect of lactate infusion on canine myocardial free fatty acid metabolism in vivo. *American Journal of Physiology* 22: 213-217.

Spreuwenberg, L.P.B., Kraemer, W.J., Spiering, B.A., Volek, J.S., Hatfield, D.L., Silvestre, R., Vingren, J.L., Fragala, M.S., Häkkinen, K., Newton, R.U., Maresh, C.M., and Fleck, S.J. 2006. Influence of exercise order in a resistance-training exercise session. *Journal of Strength and Conditioning Research* 20: 141-144.

Sprynarova, S., and Parizkova, J. 1971. Functional capacity and body composition in top weight lifters, swimmers, runners, and skiers. *Internationale Zeitschrift für Angewandte Physiologie* 29: 184-194.

Spurrs, R.W., Murphy, A.J., and Watsford, M.L. 2003. The effect of plyometric training on distance running performance. *European Journal of Applied Physiology* 89: 1-7.

Staff, P.H. 1982. The effect of physical activity on joints, cartilage, tendons and ligaments. *Scandinavian Journal of Social Medicine* 290 (Suppl.): 59-63.

Stanforth, P.R., Painter, T.L., and Wilmore, J.H. 1992. Alteration in concentric strength consequent to powercise and universal gym circuit training. *Journal of Applied Sport Science Research* 6: 152-157.

Stanley, W.C. 1991. Myocardial lactate metabolism during exercise. *Medicine & Science in Sports & Exercise* 23: 920-924.

Stanton, R., Reaburn, P.R., and Humphries, B. 2004. The effect of short-term Swiss ball training on core stability and running economy. *Journal of Strength and Conditioning Research* 18: 522-528.

Starkey, D.B., Pollock, M.L., Ishida, Y., Welsch, M.A., Brechue, W.F., Graves, J.E., and Feigenbaum, M.S. 1996. Effect of resistance training volume on strength and muscle thickness. *Medicine & Science in Sports & Exercise* 28: 1311-1320.

Staron, R.S., Hagerman, F.C., and Hikida, R.S. 1981. The effects of detraining on an elite power lifter. *Journal of Neurological Sciences* 51: 247-257.

Staron, R.S., Hagerman, F.C., Hikida, R.S., Murray, T.F., Hostler, D.P., Crill, M.T., Ragg, K.E., and Toma, K. 2000. Fiber type composition of the vastus lateralis muscle of young men and women. *Journal of Histochemistry and Cytochemistry* 48: 623-629.

Staron, R.S., and Hikida, R.S. 2001. Muscular responses to exercise and training. In *Exercise and Sport Science*, edited by W.E. Garrett Jr. and D.T. Kirkendall. Philadelphia: Lippincott Williams & Wilkins.

Staron, R.S., Hikida, R.S., and Hagerman, F.C. 1983. Reevaluation of human muscle fast-twitch subtypes: Evidence for a continuum. *Histochemistry* 78: 33-39.

Staron, R.S., and Johnson, P. 1993. Myosin polymorphism and differential expression in adult human skeletal muscle. *Comparative Biochemical Physiology* 106B: 463-475.

Staron, R.S., Karapondo, D.L., Kraemer, W.J., Fry, A.C., Gordon, S.E., Falkel, J.E., Hagerman, F.C., and Hikida, R.S. 1994. Skeletal muscle adaptations during the early phase of heavy-resistance training in men and women. *Journal of Applied Physiology* 76: 1247-1255.

Staron, R.S., Leonardi, M.J., Karapondo, D.L., Malicky, E.S., Falkel, J.E., Hagerman, F.C., and Hikida, R.S. 1991. Strength and skeletal muscle adaptations in heavy-resistance-trained women after detraining and retraining. *Journal of Applied Physiology* 70: 631-640.

Staron, R.S., Malicky, E.S., Leonardi, M.J., Falkel, J.E., Hagerman, F.C., and Dudley, G.A. 1989. Muscle hypertrophy and fast fiber type conversions in heavy resistance-trained women. *European Journal of Applied Physiology* 60: 71-79.

Stauber, W.T., Clarkson, P.M., Fritz, V.K., and Evans, W.J. 1990. Extracellular matrix disruption and pain after eccentric muscle action. *Journal of Applied Physiology* 69: 868-874.

Steben, R.E., and Steben, A.H. 1981. The validity of the stretch-shortening cycle in selected jumping events. *Journal of Sports Medicine* 21: 28-37.

Steinhaus, A.H. 1954. Some selected facts from physiology and the physiology of exercise applicable to physical rehabilitation. Paper presented to the study group on body mechanics, Washington, DC.

Stoessel, L., Stone, M.H., Keith, R., Marple, D., and Johnson, R. 1991. Selected physiological, psychological and performance characteristics of national-caliber United States women weightlifters. *Journal of Strength and Conditioning Research* 5: 87-95.

Stojanovic, M.D., and Ostojic, S.M. 2011. Stretching and injury prevention in football: Current perspectives. *Research in Sports Medicine* 19: 73-91.

Stone, M.H. 1992. Connective tissue and bone response to strength training. In *Strength and power training in sport*, edited by P.V. Komi, 279-290. Oxford: Blackwell Scientific.

Stone, M.H., Fleck, S.J., Triplett, N.R., and Kraemer, W.J. 1991. Physiological adaptations to resistance training exercise. *Sports Medicine* 11: 210-231.

Stone, M.H., Johnson, R.C., and Carter, D.R. 1979. A short term comparison of two different methods of resistance training on leg strength and power. *Athletic Training* 14: 158-160.

Stone, M.H., Nelson, J.K., Nader, S., and Carter, D. 1983. Short-term weight training effects on resting and recovery heart rates. *Athletic Training*, Spring: 69-71.

Stone, M.H., O'Bryant, H., and Garhammer, J.G. 1981. A hypothetical model for strength training. *Journal of Sports Medicine and Physical Fitness* 21: 342-351.

Stone, M.H., Plisk, S.S., Stone, M.E., Schilling, B.K., O'Bryant, H.S., and Pierce, K.C. 1998. Athletic performance development: Volume load—1 set vs. multiple sets, training velocity and training variation. *Strength and Conditioning* 20: 22-31.

Stone, M.H., Potteiger, J.A., Pierce, K.C., Proulx, C.M., O'Bryant, H.S., Johnson, R.L., and Stone, M.E. 2000. Comparison of the effects of three different weight-training programs on the one repetition maximum squat. *Journal of Strength and Conditioning Research* 14: 332-337.

Stone, M.H., Sands, W.A., Pierce, K.C., Ramsey,. M.W., and Haff, G.G. 2008. Power and power potentiation among strength-power athletes: Preliminary study. *International Journal of Sports Physiology and Performance* 3: 55-67.

Stone, M.H., Wilson, G.D., Blessing, D., and Rozenek, R. 1983. Cardiovascular responses to short-term Olympic style weight-training in young men. *Canadian Journal of Applied Sport Science* 8: 134-139.

Stone, W.J., and Coulter, S.P. 1994. Strength/endurance effects from three resistance training protocols with women. *Journal of Strength and Conditioning Research* 8: 231-234.

St-Onge, M-P., and Gallagher, D. 2010. Body composition changes with aging: The cause or the result of alterations in metabolic rate and macronutrient oxidation? *Nutrition* 26: 152-155.

Stowers, T., McMillian, J., Scala, D., Davis, V., Wilson, D., and Stone, M. 1983. The short-term effects of three different strength-power training methods. *National Strength and Conditioning Association Journal* 5: 24-27.

Strasburger, C.J., Wu, Z., Pfaulm, C., and Dressendorfer, R.A. 1996. Immunofunctional assay of human growth hormone (hGH) in serum: A possible consensus of quantitative hGH measurement. *Journal of Clinical Endocrinology and Metabolism* 81: 2613-2620.

Strasser, B., Keinrad, M., Haber, P., and Schobersberger, W. 2009. Efficacy of systematic endurance and resistance training on muscle strength and endurance performance in elderly adults—a randomized controlled trial. *Wiener Klinische Wochenschrift* 121: 757-764.

Strasser, B. and Schobersberger, W. 2011. Evidence for resistance training as a treatment therapy in obesity. *Journal of Obesity* pii: 482564.

Sugiura, T., Matoba, H., Miyata, H., Kawai, Y., and Murakami, N. 1992. Myosin heavy chain isoform transition in aging fast and slow muscles of the rat. *Acta Physiological Scandinavica* 144: 419-423.

Sullivan, M.K., Dejulia, J.J., and Worrell, T.W. 1992. Effect of pelvic position and stretching method on hamstring muscle flexibility. *Medicine & Science in Sports & Exercise* 24: 1383-1389.

Sumide, T., Sakuraba, K., Sawaki, K., Ohmura, H., and Tamura, Y. 2009. Effect of resistance exercise training combined with relatively low vascular occlusion. *Journal of Science and Medicine in Sport* 12: 107-112.

Swanson, S.C., and Caldwell, G.E. 2000. An integrated biomechanical analysis of high speed incline and level treadmill running. *Medicine & Science in Sports & Exercise* 32: 1146-1155.

Swinton, P.A., Lloyd, R., Agouris, I., and Stewart, A. 2009. Contemporary training practices in elite British powerlifters: Survey results from an international competition. *Journal of Strength and Conditioning Research* 23: 380-384.

Swinton, P.A., Stewart, A.D., Keogh, J.W.L., and Agouris, I. 2011. Kinematic and kinetic analysis of maximal velocity deadlifts performed with and without the inclusion of chain resistance. *Journal of Strength and Conditioning Research* 25: 3163-3174.

Syrovy, I., and Gutmann, E. 1970. Changes in speed of contraction and ATPase activity in striated muscle during old age. *Experimental Gerontology* 5: 31-35.

Szanberg, E., Jefferson, L.S., Lundholm, K., and Kimball, S.R. 1997. Postprandial stimulation of muscle protein synthesis is independent of changes in insulin. *American Journal of Physiology* 272: E841-847.

Szczypaczewska, M., Nazar, K., and Kaciuba-Uscilko, H. 1989. Glucose tolerance and insulin response to glucose load in body builders. *International Journal of Sports Medicine* 10: 34-37.

Szymanski, D.J., Beiser, E.J., Bassett, K.E., Till, M.E., Medlin, G.L., Beam, J.R., and DeRenne, C. 2011. Effect of warm-up devices on bat velocity of intercollegiate baseball players. *Journal of Strength and Conditioning Research* 25: 287-292.

Szymanski, D.J., DeRenne, C., and Spaniol, F.J. 2009. Contributing factors for increased bat swing velocity. *Journal of Strength and Conditioning Research* 23: 1338-1352.

Szymanski, D.J., Szymanski, J.M., Bradford, T.J., Schade, R.L., and Pascoe, D.D. 2007. Effect of twelve weeks of medicine ball training on high school baseball players. *Journal of Strength and Conditioning Research* 21: 894-901.

Szymanski, D.J., Szymanski, J.M., Molloy, J.M., and Pascoe, D.D. 2004. Effects of 12-weeks of wrist and forearm training on high school baseball players. *Journal of Strength and Conditioning Research* 18: 432-440.

Taaffe, D.R., Henwood, T.R., Nalls, M.A., Walker, D.G., Lang, T.F., and Harris, T.B. 2009. Alterations in muscle attenuation following detraining and retraining in resistance-trained older adults. *Gerontology* 55: 217-223.

Taaffe, D.R., and Marcus, R. 1997. Dynamic muscle strength alterations to detraining and retraining in elderly men. *Clinical Physiology* 17: 311-324.

Takarada, Y., and Ishii, N. 2002. Effects of low-intensity resistance exercise with short interset rest period on muscular function in middle-aged women. *Journal of Strength and Conditioning Research* 16: 123-128.

Takarada, Y., Nakamura, Y., Aruga, S., Onda, T., Miyazaki, S., and Ishi, N. 2000. Rapid increase in plasma growth hormone after low-intensity resistance exercise with vascular reclusion. *Journal of Applied Physiology* 88: 61-65.

Takarada, Y., Sato, Y., and Ishii, N. 2002. Effects of resistance exercise combined with vascular occlusion on muscle function and athletes. *European Journal of Applied Physiology* 86: 308-314.

Takarada, Y., Takazawa, H., Sato, Y., Takebayashi, S., Tanaka, Y., and Ishii, Y. 2000. Effects of resistance exercise combined with moderate vascular occlusion on muscular function in humans. *Journal of Applied Physiology* 88: 2097-2106.

Talag, T.S. 1973. Residual muscular soreness as influenced concentric, eccentric, and static contractions. *Research Quarterly* 44: 458-461.

Tanasescu, M., Leitzmann, M.F., Rimm, E.B., Willett, M.C., Stampfer, M.J., and Hu, F.B. 2002. Exercise type and intensity in relation to coronary heart disease in men. *Journal of the American Medical Association* 288: 1994-2000.

Tanner, J.M. 1964. *The physique of the Olympic athlete.* London: Allen and Unwin.

Tarnopolsky, M.A., Atkinson, S.A., MacDougall, J.D., Senor, B.B., Lemon, P.W., and Schwarcz, H. 1991. Whole body leucine metabolism during and after resistance exercise in fed humans. *Medicine & Science in Sports & Exercise* 23: 326-333.

Tarnopolsky, M.A., MacDougall, J.D., and Atkinson, S.A. 1988. Influence of protein intake and training status on nitrogen balance and lean body mass. *Journal of Applied Physiology* 64: 187-193.

Tatro, D.L., Dudley, G.A., and Convertino, V.A. 1992. Carotid cardiac baroreflex response and LBNP tolerance following resistance training. *Medicine & Science in Sports & Exercise* 24: 789-796.

Taube, W., Kullmann, N., Leukel, C., Kurz, O., Amtage, F., and Gollhofer, A. 2007. Differential reflex adaptations following sensorimotor and strengths training in young elite athletes. *International Journal of Sports Medicine* 28: 999-1005.

Taylor, A.C., McCartney, N., Kamath, M.V., and Wiley, R.L. 2003. Isometric training lowers resting blood pressure and modulates autonomic control. *Medicine & Science in Sports & Exercise* 35: 251-256.

Taylor, J.M., Thompson, H.S., Clarkson, P.M., Miles, M.P., and DeSouza, M.J. 2000. Growth hormone response to an acute bout of resistance exercise in weight-trained and non-weight-trained women. *Journal of Strength and Conditioning Research* 14: 220-227.

Terzis, G., Stratkos, G., Manta, P., and Georgiadis, G. 2008. Throwing performance after resistance training and detraining. *Journal of Strength and Conditioning Research* 22: 1198-1204.

Tesch, P.A. 1987. Acute and long-term metabolic changes consequent to heavy-resistance exercise. *Medicine & Science in Sports & Exercise* 26: 67-89.

Tesch, P.A. 1992. Short- and long-term histochemical and biochemical adaptations in muscle. In *Strength and power in sport*, edited by P.V. Komi, 239-248. Oxford: Blackwell Scientific.

Tesch, P.A., and Dudley, G.A. 1994. *Muscle meets magnet*. Published by P.A. Tesch, Stockholm, Sweden. Distributed by BookMaster, Inc., Mansfield, OH.

Tesch, P.A., Dudley, G.A., Duvoisin, M.R., Hather, B.M., and Harris, R.T. 1990. Force and EMG signal patterns during repeated bouts of concentric or eccentric muscle actions. *Acta Physiologica Scandinavica* 138: 263-271.

Tesch, P.A., Hjort, H., and Balldin, U.I. 1983. Effects of strength training on G tolerance. *Aviation, Space, and Environmental Medicine* 54: 691-695.

Tesch, P.A., Komi, P.V., and Häkkinen, K. 1987. Enzymatic adaptations consequent to long-term strength training. *International Journal of Sports Medicine* 8 (Suppl.): 66-69.

Tesch, P.A., and Larsson, L. 1982. Muscle hypertrophy in bodybuilders. *European Journal of Applied Physiology* 49: 301-306.

Tesch, P.A., Thorsson, A., and Colliander, E.B. 1990. Effects of eccentric and concentric resistance training on skeletal muscle substrates, enzyme activities and capillary supply. *Acta Physiologica Scandinavica* 140: 575-580.

Tesch, P.A., Thorsson, A., and Essen-Gustavsson, B. 1989. Enzyme activities of FT and ST muscle fibers in heavy-resistance trained athletes. *Journal of Applied Physiology* 67: 83-87.

Tesch, P.A., Thorsson, A., and Kaiser, P. 1984. Muscle capillary supply and fiber type characteristics in weight and power lifters. *Journal of Applied Physiology* 56: 35-38.

Tesch, P.A., Wright, J.E., Vogel, J.A., Daniels, W.L., Sharp, D.S., and Sjodin, B. 1985. The influence of muscle metabolic characteristics on physical performance. *European Journal of Applied Physiology* 54: 237-243.

Thacker, S.B., Gilchrist, J., Stroup, D.F., and Kimsey, C.D. Jr. 2004. The impact of stretching on sports injury risk: A systematic review of the literature. *Medicine & Science in Sports & Exercise* 36: 371-378.

Tharion, W.J., Rausch, T.M., Harman, E.A., and Kraemer, W.J. 1991. Effects of different resistance exercise protocols on mood states. *Journal of Applied Sport Science Research* 5: 60-65.

Thepaut-Mathieu, C., Van Hoecke, J., and Martin, B. 1988. Myoelectrical and mechanical changes linked to length specificity during isometric training. *Journal of Applied Physiology* 64: 1500-1505.

Thissen, J.P., Ketelslegers, J.M., and Underwood, L.E. 1994. Nutritional regulation of the insulin-like growth factors. *Endocrine Reviews* 15: 80-101.

Thistle, H.G., Hislop, H.J., Moffroid, M., and Lowman, E.W. 1967. Isokinetic contraction: A new concept in resistive exercise. *Archives of Physical Medicine and Rehabilitation* 48: 279-282.

Thomas, G.A., Kraemer, W.J., Kennett, M.J., Comstock, B.A., Maresh, C.M., Denegar, C.R., Volek, J.S., and Hymer, W.C. 2011. Immunoreactive and bioactive growth hormone responses to resistance exercise in men who are lean or obese. *Journal of Applied Physiology* 111: 465-472.

Thomas, G.A., Kraemer, W.J., Spiering, B.A., Volek, J.S., Anderson, J.M., and Maresh, C.M. 2007. Maximal power at different percentages of one repetition maximum: Influence of resistance and gender. *Journal of Strength and Conditioning Research* 21: 336-342.

Thompson, C.W., and Martin, E.T. 1965. Weight training and baseball throwing speed. *Journal of the Association of Physical and Mental Rehabilitation* 19: 194-196.

Thompson, D.B., and Chapman, A.E. 1988. The mechanical response of active human muscle during and after stretch. *European Journal of Applied Physiology* 57: 691-697.

Thorner, M.O. 2009. Statement by the Growth Hormone Research Society on the GH/IGF-I axis in extending health span. *Journals of Gerontology Series A: Biological Sciences and Medical Sciences* 64A: 1039-1044.

Thorstensson, A. 1977. Observations on strength training and detraining. *Acta Physiologica Scandinavica* 100: 491-493.

Thorstensson, A., Hulten, B., von Dolben, W., and Karlsson, J. 1976. Effect of strength training on enzyme activities and fibre characteristics in human skeletal muscles. *Acta Physiologica Scandinavica* 96: 392-398.

Thorstensson, A., Karlsson, J., Viitasalo, J., Luhtanen, P., and Komi, P. 1976. Effect of strength training on EMG of human skeletal muscle. *Acta Physiologica Scandinavica* 98: 232-236.

Thrash, K., and Kelly, B. 1987. Flexibility and strength training. *Journal of Applied Sports Science Research* 1: 74-75.

Tikkanen, H.O., Naverl, H., and Harkonen, M. 1996. Skeletal muscle fiber distribution influences serum high-density lipoprotein cholesterol level. *Atherosclerosis* 120: 1-5.

Tillin, N.A., and Bishop, D. 2009. Factors modulating post-activation potentiation and its effect on performance of subsequent explosive activities. *Sports Medicine* 39: 147-166.

Timiras, P.S., ed. 2003. *Physiological basis of aging and geriatrics*, 3rd ed. Boca Raton, FL: CRC Press.

Timmons, J.A. 2011. Variability in training-induced skeletal muscle adaptation. *Journal of Applied Physiology* 110: 846-853.

Timonen, S., and Procope, B.J. 1971. Premenstrual syndrome and physical exercise. *Acta Obstetrica et Gynaecologica Scandinavica* 50: 331-337.

Timson, B.F., Bowlin, B.K., Dudenhoeffer, G.A., and George, J.B. 1985. Fiber number, area, and composition of mouse soleus muscle following enlargement.

Journal of Applied Physiology: Respiratory, Environmental and Exercise Physiology 58: 619-624.

Tipton, C.M., Matthes, R.D., Maynard, J.A., and Carey, R.A. 1975. The influence of physical activity on ligaments and tendons. *Medicine and Science in Sports* 7: 34-41.

Tipton, K.D., Rasmussen, B.B., Miller, S.L., Wolf, S.E., Owens-Stovall, S.K., Petrini, B.E., and Wolfe, R.R. 2001. Timing of amino acid-carbohydrate ingestion alters anabolic response of muscle to resistance exercise. *American Journal of Physiology* 281: E197-206.

Tipton, K.D., and Wolfe, R.R. 1998. Exercise-induced changes in protein metabolism. *Acta Physiologica Scandinavica* 162: 377-387.

Todd, T. 1985. The myth of the muscle-bound lifter. *National Strength and Conditioning Association Journal* 7: 37-41.

Toji, H., and Kaneko, M. 2004. Effect of the multiple-load training on the force-velocity relationship. *Journal of Strength and Conditioning Research* 18: 792-795.

Tomberline, J.P., Basford, J.R., Schwen, E.E., Orte, P.A., Scott, S.C., Laughman, R.K., and Ilstrud, D.M. 1991. Comparative study of isokinetic eccentric and concentric quadriceps training. *Journal of Orthopaedic and Sports Physical Therapy* 14: 31-36.

Tomlin, D.L., and Wenger, H.A. 2001. The relationship between aerobic fitness and recovery from high intensity intermittent exercise. *Sports Medicine* 31: 1-11.

Tomten, S.E., Falch, J.A., Birkenland, K.I., Hemmersbach, P., and Hostmark, A.T. 1998. Bone mineral density and menstrual irregularities. A comparative study on cortical and trabecular bone structures in runners with alleged normal eating behavior. *International Journal of Sportsmedicine* 19: 92-97.

Too, D., Wakatama, E.J., Locati, L.L., and Landwer, G.E. 1998. Effect of precompetition bodybuilding diet and training regime on body composition and blood chemistry. *Journal of Sports Medicine and Physical Fitness* 238: 45-52.

Torres, E.M., Kraemer, W.J., Vingren, J.L., Volek, J.S., Hatfield, D.L., Spiering, B.A., Ho, J.Y., Fragala, M.S., Thomas, G.A., Anderson, J.M., Häkkinen, K., and Maresh, C.M. 2008. Effects of stretching on upper-body muscular performance. *Journal of Strength and Conditioning Research* 22: 1279-1285.

Trebs, A.A., Brandenburg, J.P., and Pitney, W.A. 2010. An electromyography analysis of 3 muscles surrounding the shoulder joint during the performance of a chest press exercise at several angles. *Journal of Strength and Conditioning Research* 24: 1925-1930.

Trivedi, B., and Dansforth, W.H. 1966. Effect of pH on the kinetics of frog muscle phosphofructokinase. *Journal of Biology Chemistry* 241: 4110-4112.

Tsolakis, C., Messinis, D., Stergiolas, A., and Dessypris, A. 2000. Hormonal responses after strength training and detraining in prepubertal and pubertal boys. *Journal of Strength and Conditioning Research* 14: 399-404.

Tsolakis, C.K., Vagenas, G.K., and Dessypris, A.G. 2004. Strength adaptations and hormonal responses to resistance training and detraining in preadolescent males. *Journal of Strength and Conditioning Research* 18: 65-69.

Tsuzuku, S., Ikegami, Y., and Yabe, K. 1998. Effects of high-intensity resistance training on bone mineral density in young male powerlifters. *Calcification Tissue International* 63: 283-286.

Tsuzuku, S., Shimokata, H., Ikegami, Y., Yabe, K., and Wasnich, R.D. 2001. Effects of high versus low-intensity resistance training on bone mineral density in young males. *Calcification Tissue International* 68: 342-347.

Tucci, J.T., Carpenter, D.M., Pollock, M.L., Graves, J.E., and Leggett, S.H. 1992. Effect of reduced frequency of training and detraining on lumbar extension strength. *Spine* 17: 1497-1501.

Turner, A.P., Sanderson, M.F., and Attwood, L.A. 2011. The acute effect of different frequencies of whole-body vibration comfort performance. *Journal of Strength and Conditioning Research* 25: 1592-1597.

Turto, H., Lindy, S., and Halme, J. 1974. Protocollagen proline hydroxylase activity in work-induced hypertrophy of rat muscle. *American Journal of Physiology* 226: 63-65.

Twisk, J.W.R. 2001. Physical activity guidelines for children and adolescents: A critical review. *Sports Medicine* 31: 617-627.

Twisk, J.W.R., Kemper, H.C.G., and van Mechelen, W. 2000. Tracking of activity and fitness and the relationship with cardiovascular disease risk factors. *Medicine & Science in Sports & Exercise* 32: 1455-1461.

Ugarkovic, D., Matavuji, D., Kukoji, M., and Jaric, S. 2002. Standard anthropometric, body composition, and strength variables as predictors of jumping performance in elite junior athletes. *Journal of Strength and Conditioning Ressearch* 16: 227-230.

Ullrich, B., Kleinoder, H., and Bruggemann, P. 2010. Influence of length-restricted strength training on

athlete's power-load curves of knee extensors and flexors. *Journal of Strength and Conditioning Research* 24: 668-678.

Urhausen, A., and Kindermann, W. 1992. Echocardiographic findings in strength- and endurance-trained athletes. *Sports Medicine* 13: 270-284.

Van Der Heijden, G., Wang, Z.J., Chu, Z., Toffolo, G., Manesso, E., Sauer, P.J.J., and Sunehag, A.L. 2010. Strength exercise improves strength exercise improves muscle mass insulin sensitivity in obese youth. *Medicine & Science in Sports & Exercise* 42: 1973-1980.

Van der Ploeg, G.E., Brooks, A.G., Withers, R.T., Dollman, J., Leaney, F., and Chatterton, B.E. 2001. Body composition changes in female bodybuilders during preparation for competition. *European Journal of Clinical Nutrition* 55: 268-277.

Vandervoort, A.A. 2009. Potential benefits of warm-up for neuromuscular performance of older athletes. *Exercise and Sport Sciences Reviews* 37: 60-65.

Vandervoot, A.A., Sale, D.G., and Moroz, J. 1984. Comparison of motor unit activation during unilateral and bilateral leg extensions. *Journal of Applied Physiology: Respiratory, Environmental and Exercise Physiology* 56: 46-51.

Vandervoot, A.A., and Symons, T.B. 2001. Functional and metabolic consequences of sarcopenia. *Canadian Journal of Applied Physiology* 26: 90-101.

Vanhelder, W.P., Radomski, M.W., and Goode, R.C. 1984. Growth hormone responses during intermittent weight lifting exercise in men. *European Journal of Applied Physiology and Occupational Physiology* 53: 31-34.

Vardar, S.A., Tezel, S., Ozturk, L., and Kaya, O. 2007. The relationship between body composition and anaerobic performance of elite young wrestlers. *Journal of Sport Science and Medicine* 6: 34-38.

Verhoshanski, V. 1967. Are depth jumps useful? *Track and Field* 12: 9.

Vermeulen, A., Rubens, R., and Verdonck, L. 1972. Testosterone secretion and metabolism in male senescence. *Journal of Clinical Endocrinology* 34: 730-735.

Vikne, H., Refsnes, P.E., Ekmark, M., Medbo, J.I., Gundersen, V., and Gundersen, K. 2006. Muscular performance after concentric and eccentric exercise in trained men. *Medicine & Science in Sports & Exercise* 38: 1770-1781.

Vincent, H.K., Bourguignon, C., and Vincent, K.R. 2006. Resistance training lowers exercise-induced oxidative stress and homocysteine levels in overweight and obese older adults. *Obesity (Silver Spring)* 14: 1921-1930.

Vincent, K.R., and Braith, R.W. 2002. Resistance exercise and bone turnover in elderly men and women. *Medicine & Science in Sports & Exercise* 34: 17-23.

Vingren, J.L., Kraemer, W.J., Hatfield, D.L., Volek, J.S., Ratamess, N.A., Anderson, J.M., Häkkinen, K., Ahtiainen, J., Fragala, M.S., Thomas, G.A., Ho, J.Y., and Maresh, C.M. 2009. Effect of resistance exercise on muscle steroid receptor protein content in strength-trained men and women. *Steroids* 74: 1033-1039.

Vingren, J.L., Kraemer, W.J., Ratamess, N.A., Anderson, J.M., Volek, J.S., and Maresh, C.M. 2010. Testosterone physiology in resistance exercise and training: The up-stream regulatory elements. *Sports Medicine* 40: 1037-1053.

Vitcenda, M., Hanson, P., Folts, J., and Besozzi, M. 1990. Impairment of left ventricular function during maximal isometric dead lifting. *Journal of Applied Physiology* 691: 2062-2066.

Volek, J.S. 2004. Influence of nutrition on responses to resistance training. *Medicine & Science in Sports & Exercise* 36: 689-696.

Volek, J.S., Duncan, N.D., Mazzetti, S.A., Staron, R.S., Putukian, M.P., Gomez, A.L., Pearson, D.R., Fink, W.J., and Kraemer, W.J. 1999. Performance and muscle fiber adaptations to creatine supplementation and heavy resistance training. *Medicine & Science in Sports & Exercise* 31: 1147-1156.

Volek, J.S., and Kraemer, W.J. 1996. Creatine supplementation: Its effect on human muscular performance and body composition. *Journal of Strength and Conditioning Research* 10: 200-210.

Volek, J.S., Kraemer, W.J., Bush, J.A., Incledon, T., and Boetes, M. 1997. Testosterone and cortisol in relationship to dietary nutrients and resistance exercise. *Journal of Applied Physiology* 82: 49-54.

Vorobyev, A.N. 1988. Part 12: Musculo-skeletal and circulatory effects of weightlifting. *Soviet Sports Review* 23: 144-148.

Vossen, J.E., Kramer, J.E., Burke, D.G., and Vossen, D.P. 2000. Comparison of dynamic push-up training and plyometric push-up training on upper-body power and strength. *Journal of Strength and Conditioning Research* 14: 248-253.

Vrijens, J. 1978. Muscle strength development in the pre- and post-pubescent age. *Medicine and Sports* (Basel) 11: 152-158.

Wagner, D.R., and Kocak, M.S. 1997. A multivariate approach to assessing anaerobic power following a plyometric training program. *Journal of Strength and Conditioning Research* 11: 251-255.

Wahl, M.J., and Behm, D.G. 2008. Not all instability training devices enhance muscle activation in highly resistance-trained individuals. *Journal of Strength and Conditioning Research* 22: 1360-1370.

Walberg, J.L., and Johnston, C.S. 1991. Menstrual function and eating behavior in female recreational weight lifters and competitive body builders. *Medicine & Science in Sports & Exercise* 23: 30-36.

Walberg-Rankin, J., Edmonds, C.E., and Gwazdauskas, F.C. 1993. Diet and weight changes of female bodybuilders before and after competition. *International Journal of Sports Medicine* 3: 87-102.

Walberg-Rankin, J., Franke, W.D., and Gwazdauskas, F.C. 1992. Response of beta-endorphin and estradiol to resistance exercise in females during energy balance and energy restriction. *International Journal of Sports Medicine* 13: 542-547.

Waldman, R., and Stull, G. 1969. Effects of various periods of inactivity on retention of newly acquired levels of muscular endurance. *Research Quarterly* 40: 393-401.

Walker, D.K., Dickinson, J.M., Timmerman, K.L., Drummond, M.J., Reidy, P.T., Fry, C.S., Gundermann, D.M., and Rasmussen, B.B. 2011. Exercise, amino acids, and aging in the control of human muscle protein synthesis. *Medicine & Science in Sports & Exercise* 43: 2249-2258.

Walker, P.M., Brunotte, F., Rouhier-Marcer, I., Cottin, Y., Casillas, J.M., Gras, P., and Didier, J.P. 1998. Nuclear magnetic resonance evidence of different muscular adaptations after resistance training. *Archives of Physical Medicine and Rehabilitation* 79: 1391-1398.

Wall, C., Byrnes, W., Starek, J., and Fleck, S.J. 2004. Prediction of performance in female rock climbers. *Journal of Strength and Conditioning Research* 18: 77-83.

Wallace, B.J., Kernozek, T.W., White, J.M., Kline, D.E., Wright, G.A., Peng, H-T, and Huang, C-F. 2010. Quantification of vertical ground reaction forces of popular bilateral plyometric exercise. *Journal of Strength and Conditioning Research* 24: 207-212.

Wallace, J.D., Cuneo, R.C., Bidlingmaier, M., Lundberg, P.A., Carlsson, L., Luiz, C., Boguszewski, C.L., Hay, J., Healy, M.L., Napoli, R., Dall, R., Rosén, T., and Strasburger, C.J. 2001. The response of molecular isoforms of growth hormone to acute exercise in trained adult males. *Journal of Clinical Endocrinology and Metabolism* 86: 200-206.

Wallace, M.B., Moffatt, R.J., Haymes, E.M., and Green, N.R. 1991. Acute effects of resistance exercise on parameters of lipoprotein metabolism. *Medicine & Science in Sports & Exercise* 23: 199-204.

Walters, P.H., Jezequel, J.J., and Grove, M.B. 2012. Case study: Bone mineral density of two elite senior female powerlifters. *Journal of Strength and Conditioning Research* 26: 867-972.

Wang, N., Hikida, R.S., Staron, R.S., and Simoneau, J.-A. 1993. Muscle fiber types of women after resistance training-quantitative ultrastructure and enzyme activity. *Pflugers Archives* 424: 494-502.

Warburton, D.E.R., and Bredin, S.S.D. 2006. Health benefits of physical activity: The evidence. *Canadian Medical Association Journal* 174: 801-809.

Ward, J., and Fisk, G.H. 1964. The difference in response of the quadriceps and biceps brachii muscles to isometric and isotonic exercise. *Archives of Physical Medicine and Rehabilitation* 45: 612-620.

Ware, J.S., Clemens, C.T., Mayhew, J.L., and Johnston, T.J. 1995. Muscular endurance repetitions to predict bench press and squat strength in college football players. *Journal of Strength and Conditioning Research* 9: 99-103.

Warren, B.J., Stone, M.H., Kearney, J.T., Fleck, S.J., Johnson, R.L., Wilson, G.D., and Kraemer, W.J. 1992. Performance measures, blood lactate and plasma ammonia as indicators of overwork in elite junior weightlifters. *International Journal of Sports Medicine* 13: 372-376.

Warren, G.L., Hermann, K.M., Ingallis, C.P., Masselli, M.A., and Armstrong, R.B. 2000. Decreased EMG median frequency during a second bout of eccentric contractions. *Medicine & Science in Sports & Exercise* 32: 820-829.

Wasserman, D.H., Connely, C.C., and Pagliassotti, M.J. 1991. Regulation of hepatic lactate balance during exercise. *Medicine & Science in Sports & Exercise* 23: 912-919.

Weaver, C.M., Teegarden, D., Lyle, R.M., McCabe, G.P., McCabe, L.D., Proullx, W., Kern, M., Sedlock, D., Anderson, D.D., Hillberry, B.M., Peacock, M., and Johnston, C.C. 2001. Impact of exercise on bone health and contraindication of oral contraceptive use in young women. *Medicine & Science in Sports & Exercise* 33: 873-880.

Weber, K.R., Brown, L.E., Coburn, J.W., and Zinder, S.M. 2008. Acute effects of heavy-load squats on consecutive squat jump performance. *Journal of Strength and Conditioning Research* 22: 726-730.

Weider, J. 1954. Cheating exercises build the biggest muscles. *Muscle Builder* 3: 60-61.

Weir, J.P., Housh, D.J., Housh, T.J., and Weir, L.L. 1997. The effect of unilateral concentric weight training and detraining on joint angle specificity, cross-training, and the bilateral deficit. *Journal of Orthopedic Sports Physical Therapy* 25: 264-270.

Weir, J.P., Housh, T.J., and Weir, L.L. 1994. Electromyographic evaluation of joint angle specificity and cross-training after isometric training. *Journal of Applied Physiology* 77: 197-201.

Weir, J.P., Housh, T.J., Weir, L.L., and Johnson, G.O. 1995. Effects of unilateral isometric strength training and joint angle specificity and cross training. *European Journal of Applied Physiology* 70: 337-343.

Weiss, L.W., Coney, H.D., and Clark, F.C. 1999. Differential functional adaptations to short-term low-, moderate-, and high-repetition weight training. *Journal of Strength and Conditioning Research* 13: 236-241.

Weiss, L.W., Cureton, K.J., and Thompson, F.N. 1983. Comparison of serum testosterone and androstenedione responses to weight lifting in men and women. *European Journal of Applied Physiology* 50: 413-419.

Wells, J.B., Jokl, E., and Bohanen, J. 1973. The effects of intense physical training upon body composition of adolescent girls. *Journal of the Association for Physical and Mental Rehabilitation* 17: 63-72.

Wernbom, M., Augustsson, J., and Thomee, R. 2007. The influence of frequency, intensity, volume and mode of strength training on whole muscle cross-sectional area in humans. *Sports Medicine* 37: 225-264.

West, D.J., Cunningham, D.J., Bracken, R.M., Bevan, H.R., Crewther, B.T., Cook, C.J., and Kilduff, L.P. 2013. Effects of resisted sprint training on acceleration in professional rugby union players. *Journal of Strength and Conditioning Research* 27: 1014-1018.

Westcott, W. 1994. High-intensity training. *Nautilus* 4: 5-8.

Westcott, W. 1995. High intensity strength training. *IDEA Personal Trainer* 6: 9.

Westcott, W.L., Winett, R.A., Anderson, E.S., Wojcik, J.R., Loud, R.L.R., Cleggett, E., and Glover, S. 2001. Effects of regular and slow speed resistance training on muscle strength. *Journal of Sports Medicine and Physical Fitness* 41: 154-158.

Whipple, T.J., Le, B.H., Demers, L.H., Chinchilli, V.M., Petit, M.A., Sharkey, N., and Williams, N.I.

2004. Acute effects of moderate intensity resistance exercise on bone cell activity. *International Journal of Sports Medicine* 25: 496-501.

Wickiewicz, T.L., Roy, R.R., Powell, P.L., Perrine, J.J., and Edgerton, B.R. 1984. Muscle architecture and force-velocity relationships in humans. *Journal of Applied Physiology: Respiratory, Environmental and Exercise Physiology* 57: 435-443.

Wickwire, P.J., McLester, J.R., Green, J.M., and Crews, T.R. 2009. Acute heart rate, blood pressure, and RPE responses during super slow versus traditional machine resistance training protocols using small muscle group exercises. *Journal of Strength and Conditioning Research* 23: 72-79.

Widholm, O. 1979. Dysmenorrhea during adolescence. *Acta Obstetricia et Gynecologica Scandinavica* 87: 61-66.

Wiemann, K., and Hahn, K. 1997. Influences of strength, stretching, and circulatory exercises on flexibility parameters of the human hamstrings. *International Journal of Sports Medicine* 18: 340-346.

Wieser, M., and Haber, P. 2007. The effects of systematic resistance training in the elderly. *International Journal of Sports Medicine* 28: 59-65.

Wilkinson, S.B., Phillips, S.M., Atherton, P.J., Patel, R., Yarasheski, K.E., Tarnapolsky, M.A., and Rennie, M.J. 2008. Differential effects of resistance and endurance exercise in the fed state on signaling molecule phosphorylation and protein synthesis in human muscle. *Journal of Physiology* 586: 3701-3717.

Willardson, J.M. 2006. A brief review: Factors affecting the length of the rest interval between resistance exercise sets. *Journal of Strength and Conditioning Research* 20: 978-984.

Willardson, J.M. 2007a. The application of training to failure in periodized multi-set resistance exercise programs. *Journal of Strength and Conditioning Research* 21: 628-631.

Willardson, J.M. 2007b. Core stability training: Applications to sports conditioning programs. *Journal of Strength and Conditioning Research* 21: 979-985.

Willardson, J.M., and Burkett, L.N. 2005. A comparison of three different rest intervals on the exercise volume completed during a workout. *Journal of Strength and Conditioning Research* 19: 23-26.

Willardson, J.M., and Burkett, L.N. 2006. The effect of rest interval length on the sustainability of squat and bench press repetitions. *Journal of Strength and Conditioning Research* 20: 396-399.

Willardson, J.M., Emmett, J., Oliver, J.A., and Bressel, E. 2008. Effect of short-term failure versus non-failure training lower body muscular endurance. *International Journal of Sports Physiology and Performance* 3: 279-293.

Willardson, J.M., Kattenbraker, M.S., Khairallah, M., and Fontana, F.E. 2010. Research note: Effect of load reductions over consecutive sets on repetition performance. *Journal of Strength and Conditioning Research* 24: 879-884.

Willett, G.M., Hyde, J.E., Uhrlaub, M.B., Wendl, C.L., and Karst, G.M. 2001. Relative activity of abdominal muscles during commonly prescribed strengthening exercises. *Journal of Strength and Conditioning Research* 15: 480-485.

Williams, A.G., Ismail, A.N., Sharma, A., and Jones, D.A. 2002. Effects of resistance exercise volume and nutritional supplementation on anabolic and catabolic hormones. *European Journal of Applied Physiology* 86 (4): 315-321.

Williams, C.A., Oliver, J.L., and Faulkner, J. 2010. Seasonal monitoring of strength and jump performance in a soccer youth academy. *International Journal of Sports Physiology and Performance* 6: 264-275.

Williams, M.A., Haskell, W.L., Ades, P.A. Amsterdam, E.A., Bittner, V., Franklin, B.A., Gulanick, M., Laing, S.T., and Stewart, K.J. 2007. Resistance exercise in individuals with and without cardiovascular disease: 2007 update: A scientific statement from the American Heart Association Council on Clinical Cardiology and Council on Nutrition, Physical Activity, and Metabolism. *Circulation* 116: 572-584.

Williams, M., and Stutzman, L. 1959. Strength variation throughout the range of joint motion. *Physical Therapy Review* 39: 145-152.

Williams, N.I., Young, J.C., McArthur, J.W., Bullen, B., Skrinar, G.S., and Turnbull, B. 1995. Strenuous exercise with caloric restriction: Effect on luteinizing hormone secretion. *Medicine & Science in Sports & Exercise* 27: 1390-1398.

Williams, P.T., Stefanick, M.L., Vranizan, K.M., and Wood, P.D. 1994. The effects of weight loss of exercise or by dieting on plasma high-density lipoprotein (HDL) levels in man with low, intermediate, and normal-to-high HDL at baseline. *Metabolism* 43: 917-924.

Willoughby, D.S. 1992. A comparison of three selected weight training programs on the upper and lower body strength of trained males. *Annual Journal Applied Research in Coaching Athletics* March: 124-146.

Willoughby, D.S. 1993. The effects of meso-cycle-length weight training programs involving periodization and partially equated volumes on upper and lower body strength. *Journal of Strength and Conditioning Research* 7: 2-8.

Willy, R.M., Kyle, B.A., Moore, S.A., and Chileboun, G.S. 2001. Effect of cessation and resumption of static hamstring muscle stretching on joint range of motion. *Journal of Orthopedic Sports Physical Therapy* 31: 138-144.

Wilmore, J.H. 1974. Alterations in strength, body composition, and anthropometric measurements consequent to a 10-week weight training program. *Medicine and Science in Sports* 6: 133-138.

Wilmore, J.H., Parr, R.B., Girandola, R.N., Ward, P., Vodak, P.A., Barstow, T.J., Pipes, T.V., Romero, G.T., and Leslie, P. 1978. Physiological alterations consequent to circuit weight training. *Medicine and Science in Sports* 10: 79-84.

Wilson, G.J. 1994. Strength and power in sport. In *Applied anatomy and biomechanics in sport*, edited by J. Bloomfield, T.R. Aukland, and B.C. Elliott, 110-208. Boston: Blackwell Scientific.

Wilson, G.J., and Murphy, A.J. 1996. The use of isometric tests of muscular function in athletic assessment. *Sports Medicine* 22: 19-37.

Wilson, G.J., Murphy, A.J., and Walshe, A.D. 1997. Performance benefits from weight and plyometric training: Effects of initial strength level. *Coaching and Sport Science Journal* 2 (1): 3-8.

Wilson, G.J., Newton, R.U., Murphy, A.J., and Humphries, B.J. 1993. The optimal training load for the development of dynamic athletic performance. *Medicine & Science in Sports & Exercise* 25: 1279-1286.

Wilson, J.M., Marin, P.J., Rhea, M.R., Wilson, S.M., Loenneke, J.P., and Anderson, J.C. 2012. Concurrent training: A meta-analysis examining interference of aerobic and resistance exercise. *Journal of Strength and Conditioning Research* 26: 2293-2307.

Winchester, J.B., Nelson, A.G., Landin, D., Young, M.A., and Schexnayder, I.C. 2008. Static stretching impairs sprint performance in collegiate track and field athletes. *Journal of Strength and Conditioning Research* 22: 13-19.

Winters, K.M., and Snow, C.M. 2000. Detraining reverses positive effects of exercise on the musculoskeletal system in premenopausal women. *Journal of Bone and Mineral Research* 15: 2495-2503.

Winters-Stone, K.M., and Snow, C.M. 2006. Site-specific response of bone to exercise in premenopausal women. *Bone* 39: 1203-1209.

Winwood, P.W., Keogh, J.W.L., and Harris, N.K. 2011. The strength and conditioning practices of strongmen competitors. *Journal of Strength and Conditioning Research* 25: 3118-3128.

Wiswell, R.A., Hawkins, S.A., Jaque, S.V., Hyslop, D., Constantino, N., Tarpenning, K., Marcell, T., and Schroeder, E.T. 2001. Relationship between physiological loss, performance decrement, and age in master athletes. *Journal of Gerontology: Biological Sciences, Medical Sciences* 56: M618-M626.

Withers, R.T. 1970. Effect of varied weight-training loads on the strength of university freshmen. *Research Quarterly* 41: 110-114.

Withers, R.T., Noell, C.J., Whittingham, N.O., Chatterton, B.E., Schultz, C.G., and Keeves, J.P. 1997. Body composition changes in elite male bodybuilders during preparation for competition. *Australian Journal of Science and Medicine in Sport* 29: 11-16.

Witzke, K.A., and Snow, C.M. 1999. Lean body mass and leg power best predict bone mineral density in adolescent girls. *Medicine & Science in Sports & Exercise* 31: 1558-1563.

Wolfe, L.A., Cunningham, D.A., and Boughner, D.R. 1986. Physical conditioning effects on cardiac dimensions: A review of echocardiographic studies. *Canadian Journal of Applied Sport Science* 11: 66-79.

Wolfe, B.L., LeMura, L.M., and Cole, P.J. 2004. Quantitative analysis of single- vs. multiple-set programs in resistance training. *Journal of Strength and Conditioning Research* 18: 35-47.

Wolfe, R.R. 2000. Effects of insulin on muscle tissue. *Current Opinion in Clinical Nutrition and Metabolic Care* 3: 67-71.

Wolfe, R.R., Miller, S.L., and Miller, K.B. 2008. Optimal protein intake in the elderly. *Clinical Nutrition* 27: 675-684.

Wolinsky, F.D., and Fitzgerald, J.F. 1994. Subsequent hip fracture among older adults. *American Journal of Public Health* 84: 1316-1318.

Wolinsky, F.D., Fitzgerald, J.F., and Stump, T.E. 1997. The effect of hip fracture on mortality, hospitalization, and functional status: A prospective study. *American Journal of Public Health* 87: 398-403.

Wong, P-L., Chamari, K., and Wisloff, U. 2010. Effects of 12 week on-field combined strength and power training on physical performance among U-14 young soccer players. *Journal of Strength and Conditioning Research* 24: 644-652.

Wood, R.H., Reyes, R., Welsch, M.A., Favarolo-Sabatier, J., Sabatier, M., Lee, C.M., Johnson, L.G., and Hooper, P.F. 2001. Concurrent cardiovascular and resistance training in healthy older adults. *Medicine & Science in Sports & Exercise* 33: 1751-1758.

Woolf, K., Reese, C.E., Mason, M.P., Beaird, L.C., Tudor-Locke, C., and Vaughan, L.A. 2008. Physical activity is associated with risk factors for chronic disease across adult women's life cycle. *Journal of the American Dietetic Association* 108: 948-959.

Wright, J.E. 1980. Anabolic steroids and athletics. In *Exercise and sport sciences reviews,* edited by R.S. Hutton and D.I. Miller, 149-202. The Franklin Institute: Philadelphia, PA.

Wright, J.R., McCloskey, D.I., and Fitzpatrick, R.C. 2000. Effects of systemic arterial blood pressure on the contractile force of a human hand muscle. *Journal of Applied Physiology* 88: 1390-1396.

Yao, W., Fuglevand, R.J., and Enoka, R.M. 2000. Motor-unit synchronization increases EMG amplitude and decreases force steadiness of simulated contractions. *Journal of Neurophysiology* 83: 441-452.

Yarasheski, K.E., Zachwieja, J.J., and Bier, D.M. 1993. Acute effects of resistance exercise on muscle protein synthesis rate in young and elderly men and women. *American Journal of Applied Physiology* 265: 210-214.

Yarrow, J.F., Borsa, P.A., Borst, S.E., Sitren, H.S., Stevens, B.R., and White, L.J. 2008. Early-phase neurendocrine responses and strength adaptations following eccentric-enhanced resistance training. *Journal of Strength and Conditioning Research* 22: 1205-1214.

Yasuda, T., Fujita, S., Ogasawara, R., Sato, Y., and Abe, T. 2010. Effects of low-intensity bench press training with restricted arm muscle blood flow on chest muscle hypertrophy: A pilot study. *Clinical Physiology and Functional Imaging* 30: 338-343.

Yates, J.W., and Kamon, E. 1983. A comparison of peak and constant angle torque-velocity curves in fast and slow twitch populations. *European Journal of Applied Physiology* 51: 67-74.

Yoshioka, S., Nagano, A., Hay, D.C., and Fukashiro, S. 2010. The effect of bilateral asymmetry of muscle strength on jumping height of the countermovement jump: A computer simulation study. *Journal of Sports Sciences* 28: 209-218.

Yoshioka, S., Nagano, A., Hay, D.C., and Fukashiro, S. 2011. The effect of bilateral asymmetry of muscle strength on the height of a squat jump: A computer simulation study. *Journal of Sports Sciences* 29: 867-877.

Young, A., and Skelton, D.A. 1994. Applied physiology of strength and power in old age. *International Journal of Sports Medicine* 15: 149-151.

Young, A., Stokes, M., and Crowe, M. 1984. Size and strength of the quadriceps muscles of old and young women. *European Journal of Clinical Investigation* 14: 282-287.

Young, M.A., Cook, J.L., Purdam, C.R., Kiss, Z.S., and Alfredson, H. 2005. Eccentric decline squat protocol offers superior results at 12 months compared with traditional eccentric protocol for patellar tendinopathy in volleyball players. *British Journal of Sports Medicine* 39: 102-105.

Young, N., Formica, C., Szmukler, G., and Seeman, E. 1994. Bone density at weight-bearing and non-weight-bearing sites in ballet dancers: The effects of exercise, hypogonadism, and body weight. *Journal of Endocrinology Metabolism* 78: 449-454.

Young W., and Elliott, S. 2001. Acute effects of static stretching, proprioceptive neuromuscular facilitation stretching, and maximum voluntary contractions on explosive force production and jumping performance. *Research Quarterly Exercise and Sport* 72: 273-279.

Young, W.B., and Bilby, G.E. 1993. The effect of voluntary effort to influence speed of contraction on strength, muscular power, and hypertrophy development. *Journal of Strength and Conditioning Research* 7: 172-178.

Young W.B., McDowell, M.H., and Scarlett, B.J. 2001. Specificity of sprint and agility training methods. *Journal of Strength and Conditioning Research* 15: 315-319.

Young, W.B., and Rath, D.A. 2011. Enhancing foot velocity in soccer kicking: The role of strength training. *Journal of Strength and Conditioning Research* 25: 561-566.

Yudkin, J., and Cohen, R.D. 1974. The contribution of the kidney to the removal of a lactic acid load under normal and acidotic conditions in the conscious rat. *Clinical Science and Molecular Medicine* 46: 9.

Zapf, J. 1997. Total and free IGF serum levels. *European Journal of Endocrinology* 136: 146-147.

Zatsiorsky, V. 1995. *Science and practice of strength training.* Champaign, IL: Human Kinetics.

Zemper, E.D. 1990. Four year study of weight room injuries in national sample of college football teams. *National Strength and Conditioning Association Journal* 12: 32-34.

Zernicke, R.F., and Loitz, B.J. 1992. Exercise related adaptations in connective tissue. In *Strength and power in sport,* edited by P.V. Komi, 77-95. Oxford: Blackwell Scientific.

Ziliak, J.P., Gundersen, C., and Haist, M.P. 2008. The causes, consequences, and future of senior hunger in America. Meals on Wheels Association of America Foundation Technical Report.

Zinovieff, A. 1951. Heavy resistance exercise: The Oxford technique. *British Journal of Physical Medicine* 14: 129-132.

Zrubak, A. 1972. Body composition and muscle strength of body builders. *Acta Facultatis Rerum Naturalium Universitatis Comenianae Anthropologia* 11: 135-144.

Zupan, M.F., Arata, A.W., Dawson, L.H., Wile, A.L., Payn, T.L., and Hannon, M.E. 2009. Wingate anaerobic test peak power and anaerobic capacity classifications for men and women intercollegiate athletes. *Journal of Strength and Conditioning Research* 23: 2598-2604.

INDEX

Page numbers followed by an *f* or a *t* indicate a figure or table, respectively.

ABOUT THE AUTHORS

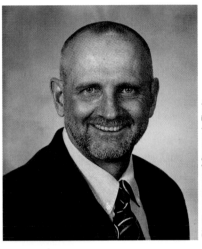

Photo courtesy of Steven J. Fleck.

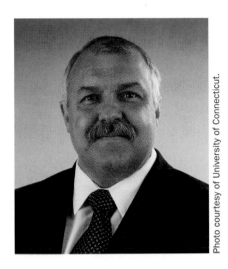

Photo courtesy of University of Connecticut.

Steven J. Fleck, PhD, is an associate professor in health, exercise science, and sport management at the University of Wisconsin-Parkside. He earned a PhD in exercise physiology from Ohio State University in 1978. He has headed the physical conditioning program of the U.S. Olympic Committee; served as strength coach for the German Volleyball Association; and coached high school track, basketball, and football. Fleck is a former vice president of basic and applied research and the current president of the National Strength and Conditioning Association (NSCA). He is a fellow of the American College of Sports Medicine (ACSM) and the NSCA. He was honored in 1991 as the NSCA Sport Scientist of the Year and received that organization's Lifetime Achievement Award in 2005.

William J. Kraemer, PhD, is a professor in the department of kinesiology in the Neag School of Education at the University of Connecticut. He holds joint appointments as a professor in the department of physiology and neurobiology and as a professor of medicine at the UConn Health School of Medicine Center on Aging.

He earned a PhD in physiology from the University of Wyoming in 1984. Kraemer held the John and Janice Fisher Endowed Chair in Exercise Physiology and was director of the Human Performance Laboratory and a professor at Ball State University from 1998 until June of 2001. He also was a professor at the Indiana School of Medicine. At Pennsylvania State University, he was professor of applied physiology, director of research in the Center for Sports Medicine, associate director of the Center for Cell Research, and faculty member in the kinesiology department and the Noll Physiological Research Center. He is a fellow of the ACSM and past president of the NSCA. Kraemer has been honored by the NSCA with both their Outstanding Sport Scientist Award and Lifetime Achievement Award. In 2006, the NSCA's Outstanding Sport Scientist Award was named in his honor. He is editor in chief of the *Journal of Strength and Conditioning Research*.

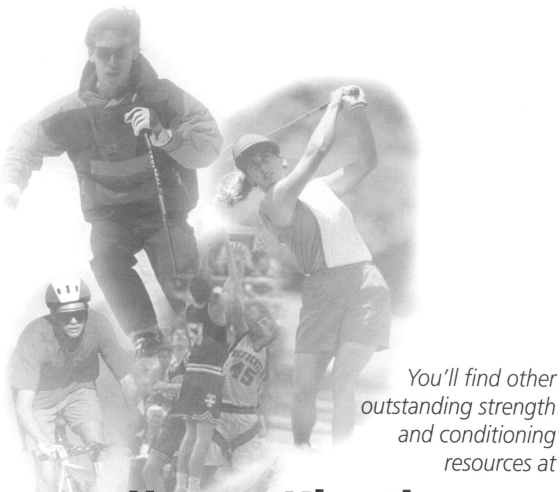